TIME WILL TELL

TIME WILL TELL

A Theory of Dynamic Attending

MARI RIESS JONES

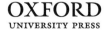
OXFORD
UNIVERSITY PRESS

OXFORD
UNIVERSITY PRESS

Oxford University Press is a department of the University of Oxford. It furthers the University's objective of excellence in research, scholarship, and education by publishing worldwide. Oxford is a registered trade mark of Oxford University Press in the UK and certain other countries.

Published in the United States of America by Oxford University Press
198 Madison Avenue, New York, NY 10016, United States of America.

Library of Congress Cataloging-in-Publication Data
Names: Jones, Mari Riess, author.
Title: Time will tell : a theory of dynamic attending / Mari Riess Jones.
Description: New York, NY : Oxford University Press, [2019]
Identifiers: LCCN 2018006108 |
ISBN 978–0–19–061821–6
Subjects: LCSH: Attention. | Synchronization. | Rhythm.
Classification: LCC BF321.J57 2018 | DDC 153.7/33—dc23
LC record available at https://lccn.loc.gov/2018006108

1 3 5 7 9 8 6 4 2

Printed by Sheridan Books, Inc., United States of America

This book is dedicated to the memory of Ellen Kimberly Riess.

O body swayed to music, O brightening glance,
How can we know the dancer from the dance?

—"Among School Children," WILLIAM BUTLER YEATS

CONTENTS

PREFACE

It was a long time ago when I began to doubt my interpretations of my own psychological experiments designed to study serial pattern learning. It seemed to me that explanations of my findings in terms of codes, storage, and retrieval were missing something important about how people were responding in time to a succession of items. Over the years, these doubts grew as I recurrently confronted powerful effects of timing and its regularity in my research. Eventually, I simply took a different path, one that is traced out in this book.

Along this path, there were many turning points sparked by the great researchers of the day. Among those most influential in my early thinking were Al Bregman, Wendel Garner, J. J. Gibson, Roger Shepard, and Paul Fraisse. All offered different, provocative perspectives from which to view my studies. As I continued on this path, I was also influenced by the work of James Martin and Robert Port, among other trail blazers. Closer to home, I found, in the lively interdisciplinary academia of Ohio State Studies, that I could learn from musical scholars such as David Butler and David Huron and from thoughtful linguists such as Ilse Lehiste and Mary Beckman. And I am also indebted to my colleagues in psychology, Caroline Palmer, Richard Jagacinski, and Trish Van Zandt. In addition, in the past few years, I have spent much time reading widely from scholarship in a range of different fields (e.g., neuroscience, music cognition, and psycholinguistics) with the aim of finding integrating themes. This endeavor humbled me. I was impressed and inspired by the vigor and dedication of many scholars working across these fields. The ones discussed in this book are those I found most admirable.

Finally, in this journey, the people who have had the most influence on the development of these ideas are my graduate students and post-doctoral fellows. They brought not only enthusiasm and skill to the development of ideas about attending and timing, but also keen insights and critical thinking. There are too many of these good people to name here. However, their contributions are priceless and hopefully evident in the pages of this book.

Last, not to be overlooked are the invaluable colleagues who assisted in the production of this book. I am especially grateful for the insightful and very helpful comments of Laura Dilley, Robert Port, and W. Jay Dowling who read a semi-final copy of the whole book. I am also indebted to Susan Holleran and June Skelly for their critical reading of various chapters. Finally, I am very thankful to Richard Jones who reviewed all book chapters.

—Mari Riess Jones
The Ohio State University
The University of California, Santa Barbara

1

Time Will Tell

An Overview of Dynamic Attending

This is a book about time and synchrony. The time in question is not the time of an alarm clock, nor is it the time consumed while processing something. Instead, it is the time of rhythms that we live by. Among other things, our biological rhythms influence how we interact with our surroundings. And with this, synchrony enters the story. Our interactions with events in the world depend on synchrony, on being able to engage with an event *as it happens* . . . in the moment. Of course, what we mean by "event" will matter, and we need to be more specific about terms like "engagement." These and related terms take shape over the first few chapters on this book. But, for the moment, imagine an event as a happening that unfolds with structure over time. It can be a spoken phrase, a song, a fleeting vision of a running child, and so on. The basic idea is that events are things in our environment to which we commonly attend, either on command or willingly. In this book, our interactions with these events are viewed through the lens of the psychological phenomenon of attending. And attending is conceived as a synchronous interaction between a perceiver and an engaging event.

SYNCHRONOUS INTERACTIONS

Attending is portrayed as a dynamic activity that involves the interaction of an attender's internal rhythms with the external rhythms that make up an event in the world around us. It is an activity so natural to us that we are hardly aware of its roots in synchrony. It may be obvious to claim that "paying attention" to something requires that one's attention activity occurs "at the right moment" in order for attending to promote perception. Perhaps because this is so obvious, the qualifying requirement of synchrony between an attender and a to-be-attended event is overlooked in most approaches to attention. It is an unacknowledged "given." Nevertheless, the primacy of synchrony is present in our conversational exchanges, in our ability to follow a sporting event, in listening to a synchrony, in driving a car, and even in our mesmerizing response to the purring of a pet cat. Inherent in such varied interactions is the common property of synchrony between the internal rhythms of an individual attender and the rhythms supplied by some external event. To fully understand such interactions, we need to reexamine how we think about attenders, external events, and the way these entities interact.

Dynamic Attending Theory (DAT), as described in this book, begins this reexamination. It places a major emphasis on the time structure of biological rhythms inherent to an individual attender as well as on the rhythmic patterning of an external (to-be-attended) event, an event we must perceive and even learn about. In this, I try to illustrate how such an event can be conceived as a structure in time, offering one or several external rhythms that essentially function in synchronous interactions with the internal, cortical rhythms of an attender.

Dynamic Interactions

The interactive activity that defines attending in its simplest form can be described as *synchrony* between an individual's internal (cortical) rhythms with an event's external stimulus rhythm (or rhythms). Consider a familiar example that involves a conversation between two people. Most of us would agree that some level of attending by participants must support this exchange. A speaker creates a phrase (an acoustic event), while the other person, a listening attender, simultaneously tracks this speech signal in real time, albeit with greater internal energy occurring at some moments in the phrase than others. The idea is that in both the acoustic event and in the listener's brain are rhythms, and this sets the stage for a discussion about synchrony between these rhythms. This interactive setting involves attending.

Elements of such a setting are found in the popular attention paradigm, the Cocktail Party, where several different talkers simultaneously plague a single listener who must focus attending energy onto one speaker while simultaneously "tuning out" others.[1,2] Various versions of this paradigm have decorated the research on this topic over the years. Oddly enough, most research along these lines does not interpret a given speaker's utterance as a dynamically changing event nor does it portray a listener's attending as a neural synchronization with the event. In fact, research on attention in conversational exchanges usually does not treat the speaker–listener setting as source of interactions in which listeners rely on temporal biases that govern their natural ability to "keep pace" with a talker's utterance. In short, we know relatively little about how people coordinate their attending *in time* with unfolding events during speaker–listener exchanges.

Kernels of the dynamic view of attending were sown long ago.[3] However, its broader implications fed very slowly into mainstream thinking about attending. Reasons for this are understandable. We are used to thinking about time as a vacuous continuum within which processing of some sort transpires; in fact, often a time interval is seen as an empty void that we fill with encoded information about objects that draw *real* attention. Once filled with processing, time now serves as a measure of an individual's processing efficiency. Such approaches view time very differently from that suggested by DAT. Among other things, they typically preclude questions about relative time structure, which requires considering the context in which some time interval appears. Overlooked is the possibility that a time interval, which is normally deemed a void or a silence, is actually serving a function within some larger temporal context. That is, in this larger context, time intervals become part of rhythms that may offer ways for an attender to interact in the moment with that context. Instead, it is common to view the brain activity of an attender in terms of receptive responses to discrete time intervals, not as synchronized activity that interacts with an external pattern of time intervals. But exciting new neuroscience research offers cause for rethinking both these patterns of thought.[4]

Broadly speaking, tenets of synchronous interactions, as described in DAT, may not have reached a wide audience because they conflict with the contemporary *zeitgeist* embodied in information theory, where, given sufficient processing time, encoded chunks of information are economically stored in a lexicon or an analogous brain region. Accordingly, this book is an attempt to offer an alternative picture. It provides a few examples of the explanatory potential of a dynamic approach to attending for a range of psychologists and cognitive scientists who are unfamiliar with this theory.

Attending in Real Time

Attending can be viewed as an activity that relies on the in-the-moment activities of an attender to unfolding event relationships. This book focuses mainly on communicative acoustic events where there is a long history of documenting event time structures. However, the principles involved are not modality specific. In general, an event is presumed to offer a series of time spans marked by tones, phonemes, or the like that form some sort of rhythm. One premise of DAT is that the event's time structure, specifically its rate and its semi-regularity, affords a basis for both capturing and guiding a listener's attending. More formally, the time structure of an event is assumed to provide one or several rhythms that drive a listener's attending in time; hence, they are termed *driving rhythms*.

The story of driving rhythms and their capacity to engage attending continues as we consider the inner workings of a listener's brain in response to such a driving rhythm. A second premise of DAT holds that listeners are equipped with cortical oscillations capable of synchronizing with an external (event) periodicity. This internal periodicity is termed a *driven rhythm*. A driven rhythm is awakened, via resonance, by a related driving rhythm, forming a basic theoretical unit, the *driving/driven dyad*. In most listening situations, the state of dyadic synchrony between a driving and driven rhythm has a strong appeal, so strong that certain states of synchrony are termed *attractors*. Simply put, we are wired to draw toward synchrony as a moth is drawn to light. The future "click" of synchrony between two rhythms serves as an automatic pull on attending; more precisely, the goal of synchrony is attractive. In its simplest form, we feel this draw as we nod our head or tap our foot to the regular *tap, tap, tap* of a marching drum. There is something special, even reinforcing, about this alignment. Synchrony is a guiding force in the interactions between an attender's driven rhythm and externally produced driving rhythm (in music or speech).

Varieties of Synchronous Interactions

Synchrony refers to specially timed interactions between a driving and driven rhythm. The mechanisms that describe the workings of synchrony together fall under the topic of *entrainment*. Most simply, entrainment refers to the activity of becoming synchronized. Indeed, the most elementary theoretical unit is a *driving-driven dyad*. The dyad refers to the interaction of two rhythms, where typically the driven rhythm changes its phase relationship to the driving rhythm to realize a fixed (stable) coupling of the two rhythms. However, synchrony comes in many forms or *modes*. The simplest mode is one where driving and driven rhythms have similar *periods* (e.g., peak amplitudes in both recur with a period of 1 second). Entrainment is the process that ensures that those amplitude peaks come into a fixed relationship: that is, they are either aligned or one consistently precedes the other by fixed amount (e.g., half a second). This represents the simplest mode of synchrony. This typically involves acquired synchrony between one periodic driving rhythm and a different driven periodicity, where n cycles of a driving rhythm's period equals m cycles of the driven rhythm's period: n:m = 1:1. But there are many other, more complex modes of synchrony that support entrainment and figure into our real-time interactions with various, e.g., acoustic events. Different *modes of synchrony* offer a range of ways of explaining attending in real time as people tune *into* the world around them.

Attending and Selectivity

A key feature of attending is its selectivity. This refers to an individual's ability to focus on one event and ignore another. Conventional explanatory attending mechanisms call on filters, spotlights, limited resources and the like to explain how we succeed in focusing on one event to the exclusion of others. Thus, for example, in the Cocktail Party paradigm, we might have only enough attending resources to focus on one of three simultaneous talkers.

A different approach to selectivity of focal attending is offered by DAT. It depends on two factors. One is synchrony. In a speaker–listener interaction, a listener must be able to ensure that his driving–driven dyad for a given talker enables synchronous tracking of that particular speaker's driving rhythms. In other words, attending must be synchronized so that a listener can allocate focal energy to a speaker's dialogue

"at the right time." This brings us to the second factor, which involves the momentary amplitude of a driven rhythm in a dyad and its regulation. Peak amplitudes of the driven rhythm must be sufficiently strong relative to surrounding neural activities. Higher amplitudes of a driven rhythm are correlated with stronger focal attending. Both factors are the subject of discussion throughout later chapters.

Themes

The main themes of this book center on the roles of time and synchrony in explaining momentary attending. To advance these themes, principles of resonance and entrainment are introduced as enablers of attending dynamics. I attempt to show how these principles lead to hypotheses about attending and attending energy carried by an attender's neural oscillations. *Resonance* involves the amplitude heightening of an oscillation by frequency matching with the frequency of its driving rhythm; resonance can add a "boost" of neural energy at the right time. *Entrainment* refers to phase and frequency adjustments of a driven oscillation in response to properties of a driving rhythm. In short, a recurring idea is that attending is a process of one individual "tuning" into a signal created by another individual.

Another theme surrounds special mode-locking relationships, termed *attractors*. Attractors are compelling states of synchrony that are assumed to be innate. Thus, as explanatory constructs, they weave in and out of themes surrounding innate versus acquired skills. Some dyads reflect simple attractors, others involve complex ones. Nevertheless, all reflect states of synchrony, whether simple or complex, that carry some degree of "attractor pull."

Two broad DAT hypotheses set the stage for other recurring themes. One is the *general attending hypothesis,* which concerns entrainment constraints on a dyad's driving rhythm; the other is the *aging hypothesis*, which addresses age-specific resonance constraints on a dyad's driven rhythm properties, along with life span changes in entrainment.

Another theme springs from basic principles of resonance and entrainment. Because these are universal principles, the concepts developed in this book are not domain-specific. As the next section on book organization reveals, dynamic attending is adaptable to the driving rhythm of speech as well as music. Applications differ in certain domain-specific ways, but overarching themes of both innateness and universality of these concepts weave in and out of the chapters in Part II.

Finally, an overriding theme in this book involves "keeping in time" with world events. This involves paying attention, at some level, to the sounds around us. *Keeping time* refers to one's implicit aim to achieve a compatible synchronous relationship between an attender's current internal state and that of a preferred (i.e., attractor) state. Throughout the following chapters, a goal is to illustrate how various events in different situations translate into driving rhythms that allow people to effortlessly synchronize a driven rhythm with an ongoing event.

Admittedly, this theory represents a significant departure from currently popular psychological views about attending. For this reason, the discussions of these and related ideas in this book assume that the reader has little knowledge of entrainment and its applications to attending. With respect to terminology, it is new; the next section lightly sketches out some of the novel terms and concepts to be encountered in various chapters. In this, it will strike some readers as odd that many familiar terms and concepts are missing. For instance, information processing terms such as *coding*, *processing time*, or *retrieval* are absent. This is because their explanatory job has been replaced by other constructs.

ALTERNATIVE VIEWS OF ATTENDING

The preceding overview outlines a perspective of attention that will be new to many readers. Its grounding in time, entrainment, and resonance brings new terminology and unfamiliar concepts such as *oscillator clusters*. Especially psychologists familiar with contemporary approaches to attention will find this dynamic approach puzzling. For this reason, a brief rationale for this theoretical departure is warranted.

Generally, psychologists have conceived of attention as a selective cognitive process that eliminates distracting information. For instance, Broadbent's[5] early theory of attention and communication attributed attentional selectivity to the operation of a passive internal filter located early in a specific processing channel. In dichotic listening tasks, listeners had to focus on one of two sounds (dichotically presented); each ear, then, opened a processing channel that could be blocked by the filter, a means of suppressing distracting sounds. Debates about selectivity centered on the location of the filter: Is the filter (or bottleneck) located early or late in processing?[6]

Following a persuasive critique of filter theory by Kahneman,[7] thinking shifted to embrace a new concept of attention based on limited resources that could be flexibility allocated to certain stimulus items (and not others). Around this time, a new paradigm also entered the scene, one that employed visual stimuli instead of auditory ones. *Visual search tasks* required a new approach to attention in which selective suppression applied to distracting visual items in a search for a target item was defined by a conjunction of two features (e.g., yellow color plus circular shape). Although selectivity here may be affected by limited resources, other search-based concepts have also been enlisted to describe allocation of attention resources to specific stationary items in a visual display.

In this era, Triesman's *Feature Integration Theory* introduced a different metaphor to explain attention that moves over a static visible array. Visual search paradigms are more likely to describe our trip through the Metropolitan Museum, where we shift focus from one spatial location of a visual item (e.g., a portrait) to the next. Presumably, a spotlight of focal attention is guided to focus on one item while suppressing attention to distracting items in a visual array.[8] Pre-attention automatically registered (in parallel) individual features of all items, such as color or shape. However, if told to search for a particular portrait or, in a laboratory setting, to find a target that combines two features (yellow-plus-circle), serial search allows for feature integration (or "gluing") of designated target features. In this view, selectivity of attention depends on serial search to points in space and coincidental feature integration. Wolfe further modeled key processes of guided spatial searches to precisely explain selectivity of visual attending.[9,10] More recently, different mechanisms have been proposed as the source of attention selectivity. For instance, Lavie proposed limits on attention due to an individual's perceptual load. [11,12] (For an overview, see Nobre and Kastner.[13])

Admittedly, this is a most truncated trip through many of the consequential concepts that have come to dominate thinking about attending. Nevertheless, it is sufficient to establish an important point: namely, a majority of approaches to attention minimize the role of timing in both the tasks employed and with the concepts proposed. The search paradigm, for instance, features a kind of attending that motivates us when searching for a lost item ("*Where* did I leave my keys?"). The emphasis is on selective attention in space, not time. Certainly, with tasks involving stationary visual displays, positing a role for the external event rate and rhythm of to-be-attended items seems problematic. Nevertheless, in search theories it remains unclear "what" attention is and how it is oriented in time to coincide with a target.[14,15,16] Recently, more dynamic approaches to visual search tasks have begun to struggle with such issues.[17,18]

A striking feature of research on attention is the predominant concentration with attention to static visual objects or scenes, as described earlier. Although there are notable exceptions (e.g., Broadbent's channel theory), in general, relatively few theories have addressed attention to dynamic objects whether visual or auditory. Yet, much of our lives is devoted to conversing with others, listening to music, and even watching movies and TV. In part, this predisposition to study static visual scenes is responsible for the limited role assigned to time in describing attending.

Contrasting Views of Attention

This brief overview of mainstream approaches suggests significant differences between current thinking on attention and a dynamic approach to this topic. Although these differences may become clearer in forthcoming chapters, it is instructive to underscore a few fundamental differences of these contrasting views.

- *Spatial versus temporal arrays.* Many attention theories are designed to explain "spatial" attention. Typically, these approaches depict an initial involuntary (pre-attention processing) reaction to a visual-spatial scene followed by voluntarily (task-specific) guided attention directed toward a "where" in the space of a static target.
  Alternatively, DAT is designed to explain involuntary and voluntary attending to temporally unfolding events (auditory or visual) that serve as driving rhythms. This emphasizes the "when" of forthcoming targets.
- *Neural correlates of attention.* Current attention models typically confine neural correlates to heightened reactive (e.g., event-related potential [ERP]) activity located in certain spatial brain regions (e.g., the parietal cortex).
  Alternatively, DAT assumes that correlates of attending depend on driving–driven dyads in which neural correlates (i.e., driven rhythms) are limit-cycle (adaptive) oscillations that carry attending energy

and may be specific to several related brain regions.
- *Selective attention.* Internal origins of selectivity in contemporary attention models have graduated from filters to guided search/spotlight activity, among other things.
  Alternatively, in DAT, attending is tied to momentary amplitudes of one or several entraining (driven) rhythms. Two mechanisms contribute to selectivity. One is synchrony: some event driving rhythms lead to preferred modes of synchrony that favor entrainment of a driven rhythm (of a specific amplitude) with one driving rhythm rather than a different driving rhythm. The other determinant of selectivity involves a listener's voluntary heightening of the amplitude of a particular driven rhythm during its entrainment.

BOOK ORGANIZATION

This book is organized into two parts. Part I introduces the major concepts and themes of DAT. These include basic assumptions about resonance and entrainment and various forms of synchronous dyads and attractors that realize different interactions between a speaker/musician and a listener. Part II applies these theoretical concepts to psychological phenomena involving a listener's responses to communicative acoustic events drawn from two important domains: music and speech. Although there is no question that events in these domains differ, thereby justifying some segregation, a case can be made that people accommodate domain differences by applying dynamic attending principles to both musical and speech patterns in somewhat different ways. This implies a fundamental commonality in how people react to distinctive time structures of events in the two domains.

Part I: Theoretical Framework

Part I includes a preliminary background chapter (Chapter 2) on popular experimental paradigms and hypotheses used to study how people respond to and use time. It sets the stage for the six following chapters (Chapters 3–8).

A fundamental assumption of dynamic attending theory holds that attending involves a synchronous interaction of a driven with a driving rhythm (i.e., of a dyad). Chapter 3 supplies evidence for the existence and entraining capacity of driven rhythms as neural brain oscillations.

A tunable brain depends on adaptable neural oscillations, meaning that one oscillation may briefly change its phase and period to synchronize either with an external rhythm, exogenous entrainment, or with another neural oscillation, namely endogenous entrainment. Hence, the introduction of entrainment and of *limit cycle oscillations* begins in this chapter. Limit cycle oscillations specify, for instance, how one cortical oscillation adjusts to follow (i.e., track) another oscillation. Many endogenous entrainments follow a common entrainment recipe for coupling of two rhythms: the *traditional mode-locking protocol*. The governing goal of traditional mode locking is maximum stability, which is expressed by a special relative time state of synchrony termed an *attractor state*. Finally, this chapter also introduces certain configurations of nested cortical oscillations, based on traditional mode-locking, termed *oscillator clusters*. Other configurations are also described as *oscillator rings* and *oscillator networks*. In these ways, brains follow the maxim: "Tune thyself."

The following two chapters introduce two major hypotheses. The *general attending hypothesis* (Chapter 4) outlines dyadic entrainment constraints based on driving rhythm properties. The next chapter, on temporal niches (Chapter 5), outlines aging constraints on the driven rhythm, summarized in an *aging hypothesis*. These constraints lead to predictions of age-related slowing of attending.

Subsequent chapters extend the generality of an entrainment framework to events that some argue defy entrainment: namely, fast events and non-isochronous events. Chapter 6 tackles exogenous and endogenous entrainments involving fast events, defined by micro-driving rhythms. This takes us into predictions involving oscillator clusters that apply to pitch perception phenomena. By contrast, in the following chapter (Chapter 7), the tricky issues for entrainments to slow events (macro-driving rhythms) involve seeming unevenness, specifically, irregularity in driving rhythms. Hence, unpacked here is a new entrainment protocol termed the *transient mode-locking protocol*. And, instead of oscillator clusters, a new entrainment construct of *attractor profile* is developed.

Chapter 8 ends Part I by scrutinizing how people produce entrainable rhythms. Following a brief review of *zietgebers* as time markers of driving rhythms, this chapter focuses on parallelisms between produced and perceived rhythms (using musical examples). *Motor productions* of a (musical) performer are shown to create events (i.e.,

driving rhythms) that express parallelism of *temporal expectancies* carried by listeners' driven rhythms.

In sum, Part I introduces basic theoretical principles and constructs. All return in Part II in various forms that cross the barriers of domains of music and speech.

Part II: Theoretical Applications

The chapters of Part II illustrate applications of the dynamic attending concepts introduced in Part I. Part II is divided into two subparts. Chapters 9–11 are devoted to describing DAT applications to musical events, whereas as Chapters 12–14 concentrate on attending to speech events. Each chapter in Part II focuses on a typically familiar topic, whether the topic involves musical meter or tonality or concerns well-known speech phenomena involving percepts of phonemes or words. All topics deal with communicative time patterns that grab and/or sustain a listener's attending. Each chapter in Part II begins with a brief overview of background thinking about this topic, while the body of the chapter applies major entrainment hypotheses (general attending, aging hypotheses) to specific situations in order to illustrate the breadth of entrainment mechanisms (e.g., adaptive, tracking, oscillator clusters, and/or attractor profiles).

The Music Domain

Chapter 9 continues with a focus on slow (macro-rhythmic) events from Chapter 8. It tackles the canonical crafted hierarchical timing of musical meter and its differences from rhythmic structure. Translated into DAT terminology, metric hierarchies create simultaneously unfolding, nested, driving rhythms. Concepts such as oscillator clusters are applied to explain meter perception using *metric oscillator clusters*. Meter perception is juxtaposed with rhythm perception, which is shown to depend on a *rhythm attractor profile*.

Musical skill, especially in meter perception, is addressed in Chapter 10. A new concept is introduced to address explain learning. This chapter argues that learning, while distinct from entrainment, also depends on stable synchronies delivered by entrainment that binds entraining oscillation in a metric oscillator cluster. In this, a familiar Hebbian learning adage is translated for metric binding (learning) as "*oscillations that frequently fire in phase bind in phase.*"

Musical melodies in Chapter 11 revive the micro-driving rhythms of fast events described in

Part I (Chapter 6). Melodies are tone sequences wherein tones are conceived as micro-driving rhythms. This allows an entrainment explanation of attending to both tonality and melodic contour, following Jay Dowling's[19] classic distinctions. Again, oscillator clusters and attractor profiles return to explain familiar findings about various tonal melodies.

The Speech Domain

Speech timing is a topic famous for long-standing debates over isochrony and timing in general. Chapter 12 reviews this background from early isochrony theories to current prosody theories (e.g., *Prosodic Bootstrapping Theory*). Also, DAT is contrasted with contemporary theories. Both oscillator clusters and attractor profiles are enlisted to illustrate both metrical and rhythmic properties in speech timing.

Speech melodies, in Chapter 13, invite an explanation of intonation contour that parallels the explanation of musical contours. In particular, to follow the ups and downs of a speaker's vocal pitch, listeners engage in frequency-following activities (i.e., *pitch tracking entrainment*). As with music, speech melodies afford other entrainment mechanisms, namely *oscillator clusters* and *attractor profiles*.

The final chapter, Chapter 14, is a substantive one which pulls together many preceding constructs to address the challenge of skill acquisition. Here, instead of explaining the mastery of metric categories (Chapter 10), the task is to explain speech learning (e.g., of categories of phonemes, syllables, and words). Both infant learning of real phoneme categories and adult learning of nonsense words are explained using oscillator clusters and attractor profiles. Various entrainment mechanisms, together with binding/learning concepts, are contrasted with other skill acquisition theories (e.g., Magnet Theory, Statistical Learning Theory).

Concluding Speculations

Chapter 15 speculates on the implications of a dynamic view of attending for understanding the changing soundscapes of our contemporary environment, raising concerns about the rates and rhythms of the current Information Age on attending. A rapidly changing technological world presents us with new and challenging mechanical driving rhythms that are increasingly likely to grab and entrain the attending of young children who are preferentially oriented to fast events.

This chapter also speculates on generalizing DAT to other species, given the universality of resonance and entrainment principles. It raises questions about the inherent commonality of communicative activities of species in which vocalizations register many different potential driving rhythms that reveal species-specific differences in rate and relative timing.

HOW TO READ THIS BOOK

The organization of this book allows for different reading strategies depending on the goals of a reader. The book is aimed at readers who are cognitive scientists in fields of music, speech, psycholinguistics, and attending/perception in general. It also assumes that readers will have little or no knowledge of DAT. For this reason I tried to avoid special jargon, complex mathematical descriptions, and exotic terminology. That is, because unifying research of diverse specialty areas is one goal of this book, subject matter throughout is explained with a minimum of domain-specific jargon. Nevertheless, the organization also allows readers of different fields to concentrate on some chapters and not others depending on their background and immediate interests. The basic ideas and concepts presented in Part I are developed in somewhat different guises across chapters, meaning that there is unescapable redundancy. This redundancy derives from the fact that one important message is that entrainment, in its various forms, is universal and hence evident in different forms and applicable to different domains.

In short, various options for speed reading and/or selective reading are offered for busy scholars. Part I lays out most of the basic theoretical concepts, and Part II applies these to music and speech in related subsections.

NOTES

1. E. Colin Cherry, "Some Experiments on the Recognition of Speech, with One and with Two Ears," *The Journal of the Acoustical Society of America* 25, no. 5 (1953): 975, doi:10.1121/1.1907229.

2. D. E. Broadbent, *Perception and Communication* (Elmsford, NY: Pergamon Press, 1958), http://content.apa.org/books/10037-000.

3. Mari R. Jones, "Time, Our Lost Dimension: Toward a New Theory of Perception, Attention, and Memory," *Psychological Review* 83, no. 5 (1976): 323.

4. P. Lakatos et al., "Entrainment of Neuronal Oscillations as a Mechanism of Attentional Selection," *Science* 320, no. 5872 (April 4, 2008): 110–13, doi:10.1126/science.1154735.

5. Broadbent, *Perception and Communication.*

6. J. A. Deutsch and D. Deutsch, "Attention: Some Theoretical Considerations," *Psychological Review* 70, no. 1 (1963): 80–90, doi:10.1037/h0039515.

7. Daniel Kahneman, *Attention and Effort* (Citeseer, 1973), http://citeseerx.ist.psu.edu/viewdoc/download?doi=10.1.1.398.5285&rep=rep1&type=pdf.

8. Anne M. Treisman and Garry Gelade, "A Feature-Integration Theory of Attention," *Cognitive Psychology* 12, no. 1 (January 1980): 97–136, doi:10.1016/0010-0285(80)90005-5.

9. Jeremy M. Wolfe, Kyle R. Cave, and Susan L. Franzel, "Guided Search: An Alternative to the Feature Integration Model for Visual Search," *Journal of Experimental Psychology: Human Perception and Performance* 15, no. 3 (1989): 419–33, doi:10.1037/0096-1523.15.3.419.

10. Jeremy M. Wolfe, "Guided Search 2.0: A Revised Model of Visual Search," *Psychonomic Bulletin & Review* 1, no. 2 (June 1994): 202–38, doi:10.3758/BF03200774.

11. Nilli Lavie, "Perceptual Load as a Necessary Condition for Selective Attention," *Journal of Experimental Psychology: Human Perception and Performance* 21, no. 3 (1995): 451.

12. Nilli Lavie, "Attention, Distraction, and Cognitive Control Under Load," *Current Directions in Psychological Science* 19, no. 3 (June 1, 2010): 143–48, doi:10.1177/0963721410370295.

13. *The Oxford Handbook of Attention*, accessed January 27, 2016, https://books-google-com.proxy.library.ucsb.edu:9443/books/about/The_Oxford_Handbook_of_Attention.html?id=_sjRAgAAQBAJ.

14. C. Miniussi et al., "Orienting Attention in Time," *Brain* 122, no. 8 (August 1, 1999): 1507–18, doi:10.1093/brain/122.8.1507.

15. Jennifer T. Coull and Anna C. Nobre, "Where and When to Pay Attention: The Neural Systems for Directing Attention to Spatial Locations and to Time Intervals as Revealed by Both PET and fMRI," *The Journal of Neuroscience* 18, no. 18 (September 15, 1998): 7426–35.

16. Kia Nobre and Jennifer Theresa Coull, *Attention and Time* (New York: Oxford University Press, 2010).

17. Robert Desimone and John Duncan, "Neural Mechanisms of Selective Visual Attention," *Annual Review of Neuroscience* 18, no. 1 (1995): 193–222.

18. Mark Stokes and John Duncan, "Dynamic Brain States for Preparatory Attention and Working Memory," In *Oxford's Handbook of Attention* (New York: Oxford University Press, 2013), Edited by Anna C. Nobre and Sabine Kastner, 152–82.

19. W. Jay Dowling, "Scale and Contour: Two Components of a Theory of Memory for Melodies.," *Psychological Review* 85, no. 4 (1978): 341–54, doi:10.1037/0033-295X.85.4.341.

PART I

Theoretical Framework

2

Time . . . and How We Study It

J. J. Gibson[1] famously claimed that we "don't perceive time, we perceive events." This is hard to dispute if we think of how often we "lose track of time" when absorbed in some project. We certainly do not fill elapsed time with counting as we experience some compelling event. In important ways, Gibson's position on this matter is captured in this book, which emphasizes how people "use" time in attending to nontemporal features. Nevertheless, the view advanced here departs from Gibson's behavioristic position because it assumes that perceivers, as animate creatures, rely on distinctive internal rhythmic structures to guide attending.

The concept of time and theories about it pose unresolved puzzles for contemporary psychology. Some psychologists continue to embrace Gibson's skepticism about event time perception. Others reject Gibson's argument to demonstrate that people really *do perceive time*. However, often this becomes a battle of different tasks, which are numerous. Not surprisingly, we are left with many different task-specific outcomes that shed little light on time perception and its link to attending. This has led some to question the relevance of studying time and time perception for understanding basic psychological concepts such perception and attending. For instance, a common cry from these psychologists is that time estimation/perception has little to do with attention. That is, it is . . . well, after all . . . "*only time estimation.*" Yet, despite such travails and critiques, the field of time perception remains a respected area of study. Furthermore, time perception theories actually may offer links to basic concepts such as attention.

Nevertheless, an argument can be made that laboratory tasks designed to study time perception are remote from the role of timing in daily life. Consider the two basic laboratory paradigms for studying time: prospective and retrospective paradigms. *Prospective paradigms* instruct people in advance that they must judge two forthcoming time intervals. *Retrospective paradigms*, on the other hand, present certain to-be-judged time intervals in a disguised format and later test

a listener's percept of these intervals. A case can be made that neither task captures how we deal with time as it happens in everyday activities. For instance, how often do we tell someone with whom we are talking, "I am going to ask you to judge whether or not the time spans of my last two words are the same or different." That just doesn't happen. Nor do we typically encounter prospective situations that require us to merely judge two forthcoming time spans in isolation.

The generality of findings from a retrospective paradigm is also questionable. That is, if we are suddenly asked to estimate the duration of one word, relative to the duration of a neighboring word within a preceding utterance, it is likely we would fail miserably. In normal situations, people don't explicitly attend to individual time intervals. So, this paradigm also fails to capture how people respond to timing in ordinary settings. Yet, if someone waved a wand that suddenly changed the phrased timing of words and syllables in such an utterance even slightly, this change would likely evoke a keen response in a listener. Indeed, a listener's quick response suggests that, at some level, s/he implicitly operates with an attending mechanism that tracks stimulus timing. Yet popular laboratory timing tasks do not readily apply to the way people use timing in everyday life. Such tasks are predicated on a tacit—and false—assumption that we have evolved to judge isolated time intervals.

It is more likely that we have evolved a capacity to *use* the timing relationships of dynamic events that fill our world in order to connect with that world, *not* to estimate individual time intervals as such. In this, it is useful to distinguish between those tasks in which people implicitly (involuntarily) *use* event time structure to guide attending and other tasks which require explicit (voluntary) *attending* to certain features of events. Specifically, many time perception tasks require explicit attending to event timing, whereas general perception of certain events features invites implicit attending to event timing.

Most daily activities fall into the latter category of general perception. As such, these activities involve tacitly "using" event timing to track events in real time. Such default activities grant priority to attending about what is going on in our immediate environment. This means the time perception that psychologists typically study is rarely found in everyday activities. We are too busy involuntarily using time to guide anticipatory attending to forthcoming happenings, than to "pay attention" to time, qua time, as discrete intervals. In tacit acknowledgment of this, societies over millennia developed clocks and wristwatches to precisely correct for this common human deficiency involving time perception.

Finally, the internal timing mechanisms we use to track events do not mirror mechanical clocks, for good reasons. Our biological clocks are ongoing neural oscillations that fluctuate spontaneously, hence they are less precise than mechanical clocks in certain respects. However, they compensate for their imprecision in capturing discrete time intervals with a potential for adapting to variable timing, enabling them to track changing events and to even adjust to unexpected timings. This adaptive facility of biological, i.e., neural, rhythms makes them capable of synchronizing to dynamically changing time patterns of real-world events. Had we inherited internal clocks that operate like wristwatches or hourglasses instead of adaptive oscillators, we would perform better in traditional time perception tasks but much worse in everyday tasks that require flexible attending to dynamically changing contexts in our environment

CHAPTER GOALS

For psychologists, a common answer to "how" we study time is obvious: we march into our laboratories to design tasks that manipulate discrete time intervals in order to measure people's response to this manipulation. This chapter describes the most common of these tasks. One goal is to compare time perception/judgment tasks with general perception tasks that tap into how people "use" time (versus perceive it).

A brief background section distinguishes explicit attending *to* time, as in time judgment tasks, from tasks designed to study general perception, which encourage *using* time to attend elsewhere. Next, the two following sections flesh out these distinctions with a focus on the role of temporal contexts in both kinds of tasks. Traditionally, the topic of context is ignored. These sections make a case for the relevance of dynamic contexts in studying time perception.

A second goal is to introduce aspects of Dynamic Attending Theory (DAT). DAT constructs such as anticipatory attending, entrainment, and driving–driven dyads, among others, are developed. These constructs are shown to figure into various attention/perception tasks, such as the well-known foreperiod (FP) task and others familiar to most psychologists.

A third goal aims to lay a foundation for linking DAT concepts to brain activities. Thus, a final section provides a sample of emerging research relevant to DAT concepts of driven rhythms and their capacity for entrainment.

BACKGROUND: ATTENDING "TO" TIME VERSUS ATTENDING THAT "USES" TIME

The time dimension is necessarily acknowledged in studies of time perception, where people are told to "pay attention" to time. However, it is noteworthy that a potential role for the time dimension is not acknowledged in many general perception tasks where people are simply told to "pay attention" to e.g., red dots or high-pitched sounds, for instance.

The theoretical divide between research on time perception and that on attention is wide. Whereas approaches to attention/general perception rarely acknowledge the impact of time structure on attending, time perception theories often relegate attention to a minor role (e.g., as an on–off attention switch). This is despite the fact that certain attentional phenomena, such as attentional capture, for example, have an important temporal component.

TIME PERCEPTION: STUDIES ON ATTENDING *TO* TIME

There is a long history of research on time perception, Gibson's position not withstanding.[2,3,4] (For reviews[5,6,7,8]). The favored tasks stipulate time as the relevant property: people are explicitly told to attend to certain time intervals and judge their elapsed time intervals.

Theoretical Perspectives

Against this backdrop, two approaches to time perception are of theoretical interest. Both address how people judge time in a conventional laboratory task where they must "pay attention" to a standard time interval followed by a comparison time interval. The task is simple: people judge whether a comparison is *shorter,* the *same,* or *longer* than a preceding standard. Experimental interest typically focuses on people's ability to compare only two isolated time intervals. Less interest is directed to the fact that such judgments happen in laboratory tasks wherein a series of trials (a session) provides a larger, potentially salient temporal context.

One prominent time perception approach emphasizes coding of *time intervals.* People are assumed to independently encode standard and comparison time intervals, regardless of the temporal context established by prior trials in a session. An alternative approach emphasizes *temporal expectancies* presumably based on contextual time relationships.

Time Interval Encoding Models

Interval time models of time perception feature encoding by an internalized clock that typically functions as an hourglass or interval coding device.[9,10,11,12,13,14] Most influential is *Scalar Expectancy Theory* (SET), shown schematically in Figure 2.1.[15,16] Central to this school of thought is a neural pacemaker that generates stochastic ticks that "fill" a time interval. Attention is included as an agent of control via an "on–off" switch that regulates tick flow to a counter/accumulator. Finally, the sums of ticks accumulated, respectively for standard and comparison intervals, are stored in memory (reference versus working memories, respectively). Next, remembered counts are compared, allowing a perceiver to report that a comparison interval is either the "same," "longer," or "shorter" than a preceding standard. Finally, see Matthews & Meck (2016) for a masterful review of various SET models.[17]

Temporal Expectancy Models

Models of temporal expectancies, based on DAT, provide a contrasting approach which features a role for temporal contexts. These models differ from SET models in that they are fundamentally attending models.[18,19,20,21] DAT rests on the assumption that people's judgments of standard and comparison intervals are inevitably influenced by a prevailing context (local and/session). A local context (i.e., a single trial) entails inter–onset-time intervals (IOIs), shown in Figure 2.2, that form a regular or irregular rhythmic context. In this figure, the regular rhythm putatively paces one's attending rhythm, leading to anticipatory attending about "when" future onsets will occur. This is because as a stimulus driving rhythm (black), this external periodicity *exogenously* entrains an individual's internal oscillator (gray) via synchrony. Entrainment depends on the capacity of a driven (oscillator) rhythm to adapt to a driving rhythm (recurring IOIs) of this stimulus context as well as to timings of standard and comparison intervals. Oscillations forming the driven rhythm adapt by changing their phase (and period), thereby correcting momentary temporal expectancies. The resulting (corrected) expectancy, then, delivers more attending energy at expected future times. For this reason, unexpected standards should lead to distorted time judgments.[22,23,24]

Theoretically, two distinctions between DAT and SET models are important. First, SET assumes that people *independently* encode all successive time intervals, including standards and comparisons, as discrete intervals. By contrast, DAT assumes that momentary responses to all these time intervals are *dependent* on people's reliance on the period of a common driven rhythm. Second, theoretical timing mechanisms differ. SET expresses the internal timing mechanism as a pacemaker-plus-counter, whereas DAT relies on adaptive properties of driven (neural) oscillations. Reflecting on contexts featured in Figure 2.2, Devin McAuley considered whether the brain's time-keeper for short time intervals operates like an hourglass, which can be started and stopped at arbitrary points in time, or perhaps resembles a self-sustaining oscillator with rhythmic characteristics. These options lead to respectively different predictions.

Evidence from Time Judgment Studies

Contrasting predictions about the influence of isochronous temporal contexts on time judgments were

Scalar expectancy theory (SET) and *the perceptual clock*

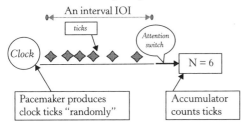

The N value for a standard interval in this task is stored in memory for later comparisons.

FIGURE 2.1 Outline of a hypothesized time-keeper of the Scalar Expectancy Theory (SET).

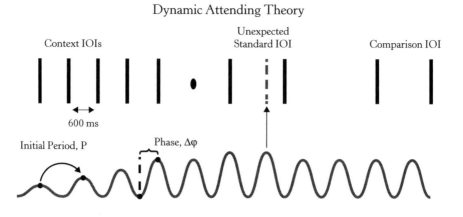

Dynamic Attending Theory

DAT prediction:
If a standard ends unexpectedly
partial phase correction, yields poor time judgements

FIGURE 2.2 Outline of driving-driven entrainment activity hypothesized by DAT. Driving rhythm is outlined by time-markers (black bars); entraining driven rhythm shows periodic expectancy pulses adjusting phase of pulse peaks for a time judgment task.

Modified from J. Devin McAuley and Mari Riess Jones, "Modeling Effects of Rhythmic Context on Perceived Duration: A Comparison of Interval and Entrainment Approaches to Short-Interval Timing," *Journal of Experimental Psychology: Human Perception and Performance* 29, no. 6 (2003): 1102–25, doi:10.1037/0096-1523.29.6.1102.

addressed in experiments designed by McAuley.[25] Using contexts of Figure 2.2, SET predicts no influence of context rhythm, whereas DAT does.

Specifically, these contexts exhibited a fixed 600 ms period followed by a standard/comparison pair. Over trials, equally often a standard, S, ended on-time (S = 600 ms), early (S = 540 ms), or late (660 ms); the comparison, C, was yoked to S (C = S + Δt ms); that is, C could differ from the preceding standard. People were explicitly told to "ignore the context" and "attend to standard/comparison intervals." They simply had to report if a comparison was the "same," "shorter," or "longer" than its standard.

According to DAT, this context will automatically govern an individual's attending, thereby shaping subsequent perception of standard intervals. In particular, phase-sensitive rhythmic expectancies will facilitate judgments of an expected standard while degrading judgments of unexpected standards. DAT predicts a partial phase correction for unexpected standards, thus guaranteeing distorted percepts. In short, regardless of instructions to ignore context, involuntary attending guarantees best performance with expected ("on-time") standards.

Alternatively, SET predicts uniformly good performance for all standards, expected and unexpected. This is because pacemaker models operate like mechanical, not biological, clocks. Accordingly, accumulated counts correctly reflect standard and comparison time intervals *regardless of a prior context*.

Results supported DAT predictions: people were best with on-time standards. McAuley sleuthed out reasons for SET failures. These stemmed from the fact that a canonical SET model mimics *complete* correction of the code for an unexpected standard. In fact, SET versions that mimicked partial phase correction were shown to perform better than the canonical model. Interestingly, only SET versions that mimicked partial phase corrections of adaptive oscillations worked. In short, people don't correctly perceive unexpected standards. Similar problems for interval encoding theories are documented in related studies.[26,27,28] In sum, time perception involves fallible rhythmic expectancies.

Evidence from Time Discrimination Studies
Other evidence about time perception comes from research on temporal acuity. In these tasks, people must discriminate intervals that differ by much smaller time changes, Δt. In practice, psychometric functions used to assess acuity focus

primarily on the magnitude of a change, but rarely do these paradigms consider the impact of a surrounding context on temporal acuity. Nevertheless, a surrounding temporal context, comprising various time spans, T, may help or hurt temporary acuity as confirmed by emerging evidence.[29,30,31,32]

A common finding is that acuity, expressed by threshold Weber fraction ($\Delta t/T$), is around 5% in time discrimination tasks. But these estimates can drop to 2%, given a highly regular temporal context, or exceed 10% in irregular contexts.[33,34] Furthermore, detection of a near-threshold time change embedded in a longer sequence depends on both near and remote temporal regularities in a session context.[35,36] This body of research is enlightening for another reason. It demonstrates that a simple statistical description of temporal contexts (e.g., variance in T values) does not explain time discrimination. That is, different context rhythms with the same statistical variance lead to acuity differences. Furthermore, both local and global (session) contexts matter. Clearly, temporal acuity depends temporal context.

Summary of Approaches to Time Perception

Time perception is a relative affair. It depends on how the duration of a to-be-judged stimulus "fits" into a contextually induced expected time frame set. This describes a contextually oriented approach which challenges an alternative view that people independently encode successive time intervals. In fact, it appears that hypotheses based on independence of successive T values incorrectly predict performance that is "too good." Instead, time perception is more malleable and flawed. It is biased by a temporal expectancy that is induced by temporal contexts which people are told to ignore. The strong impact of surrounding stimulation on people's percepts of time intervals suggests that dynamic contexts levy an involuntary, stimulus-driven draw on attending.

The main points in this section are:

- People's time perception in realistic settings is influenced by relative timing (rate, rhythm) of a local and/or global context even when people try to ignore this context.
- Consistent with DAT, temporal expectancies based on an internal oscillator activity selectively influence judgments of expected and unexpected time intervals.
- An alternative appropriate is expressed by interval encoding models, consistent

with SET. These models fail to predict time judgments; they incorrectly predict equally accurate judgments of both expected and unexpected time intervals.

ATTENDING "IN" TIME: USING TIME IN GENERAL PERCEPTION

Let's next consider the impact of dynamic attending on general perception. For instance, how do we perceive the shape of brief visual target or the pitch of a designated sound? In these tasks, technically, time is defined as a task-irrelevant feature because people are explicitly told to focus only on a nontemporal property. A second goal centers on aspects of DAT that are not confined to time perception; rather they speak to perception in general.

Let's begin with an observation about how we study perception. A passing observation is warranted regarding an inherent contradiction between our methods of studying perception and laboratory treatments of time. On one hand, psychological methodology reflects great care in designing timing in these experiments: trial timing and other temporal factors surrounding presentations of to-be-judged (non-temporal) targets are typically carefully controlled. On the other hand, theoretical implications of these methodological constraints are rarely acknowledged as qualifiers of observed results. For instance, many perception/attention studies rely on default timing of stimuli and trials that are roughly isochronous over the course of an experimental session. That is, "deep down," we all know that temporal regularly is helpful, and, if we screw up timing, then the experimental results we seek might be jeopardized. Scrambling the relative timing of stimuli and trials is an option most experimenters would balk at. Why? In part, such a reaction suggests an intuitive knowledge of the importance of time, yet this is formally denied.

So, instead, let us acknowledge the importance of timing in our methodology. It is difficult to imagine encounters with events that are devoid of some temporal context. Time is ever present; it is one of those things that can never be totally eliminated. Most events we encounter have some time signature, whether the event happens in a laboratory study, as a series of to-be-judged pictures, or outside the laboratory in the fast-paced chatter of a friend. A single item in each stimulus setting (e.g., a picture or a word) happens within a larger, unfolding temporal context. Yet, we often fail to acknowledge the temporal context in such settings. Perhaps this is because people, including experimenters, rarely "pay attention" to durations of stimulus items such as pictures, syllables, words. Nevertheless, it can be argued that participants in our experiments do involuntarily *use* sequential timing to effortlessly guide their attending in such settings. That is, people serving in laboratory studies may nonetheless implicitly take advantage of crafted time constraints on putatively irrelevant information, such as onsets of successive stimuli or trials, to orient their attending to the "when" of forthcoming target information. That is, methodology that regularizes the timing of seemingly "irrelevant" aspects of a laboratory paradigm can surreptitiously shape both time perception and perception more generally.

This section challenges the unspoken assumption that the time structure of a context is inevitably irrelevant to general perception. One aim is to highlight the role of temporal contexts and related rhythmic expectancies in four common laboratory perception tasks: foreperiod (FP) tasks, discrete cueing tasks, sequential targeting and selective attending tasks. A second aim is to illustrate that people who serve in these diverse tasks unwittingly "use" event time structure to direct attending to targets of interest.

Foreperiod Tasks and Temporal Expectancies

The FP paradigm, dating from Woodrow's[37] seminal studies, provides a classic example of how we study time. This is an elegantly simple laboratory task renowned for its assessment of temporal expectancies. On each trial, an individual is presented with a single warning signal, which is followed after a specific period of time—termed the *foreperiod*—by a target stimulus to which a rapid response is required. Typically, neither the warning signal nor the target stimulus change over trials. A governing idea is that people will react more quickly (i.e., yield a faster reaction time [RT]) for expected than unexpected targets. The main independent variable is the FP time interval (e.g., FPs may range from 200 ms to longer than 3 seconds).

This paradigm is a crucible for studying the impact of temporal context on people's tacit temporal expectancies about "when" a target might occur. In fact, temporal context enters the picture as a critical variable because it is reflected in the time schedule of FPs over trials. Typically, two different types of sessions have, respectively, variable and constant FP values over trials and these sessions are typically summarized by FP probability distributions.

However, it should be noted that there is an often overlooked catch: inevitably, the variable condition not only has a higher statistical variance of FPs than the constant condition, but it also has a more irregular temporal context (over trials in a session) due to different, randomly occurring FP time intervals. By contrast, the constant condition, with a very low statistical variance, consists of a repeating FP over all trials in a session, thereby creating a highly regular temporal context.

Both FP and session context affect people's reaction times to a target. In fact, they interact to yield different profiles of reaction time to FPs for variable and constant conditions: the variable condition shows falling (speeding) RTs as the FP lengthens, whereas the constant condition shows rising (slowing) RTs as the FP lengthens.

Popular explanations of this interaction appeal to different probabilistic uncertainties created, respectively, by stochastic properties of session contexts (cf. Niemi and Näätänen[38]; Nobre, Correa, and Coull[39]; Los[40]; Wagener and Hoffman[41] for reviews). The variable condition has many different FPs that lead to high target uncertainty on each trial, particularly with a uniform FP probability distribution (i.e., equi-probable FPs in a session). Accordingly, probabilistic predictions (e.g., by a hazard or aging function) that specify the decreasing likelihood of short FP on a given trial create decreasing temporal uncertainty. These statistical expectancies, due to reduced uncertainty, then explain faster responding to longer FPs in variable conditions. By contrast, because the constant condition lacks session uncertainty (due to FP repetitions), RT should (and does) mirror expected FP durations, meaning slower RTs to longer FPs.

These replicable FP findings are diagnostic of strong session context effects. Most explanations assume that FP statistical uncertainties lead people to compute likelihoods of target times (e.g., hazard functions). Generally, psychological concepts such as certainty and temporal expectancy are framed probabilistically. This practice converges with a debatable, but popular, tradition of equating expectancy with statistical probability. Such a practice, however, ignores the impact of certain quasi-deterministic context properties, such as the sequential constraints in variable FP schedules (cf. Steinborn[42]). For instance, Sander Los has incisively shown that people's reaction time on one FP trial is strongly affected by the FP of the immediately preceding trial.[43] According to Los, sequential effects challenge explanations based on probabilistic session contexts. This sparks a rethinking of session contexts: Is a temporal context most fruitfully expressed as a probability distribution of time intervals (e.g., FPs), or might the critical factor be a correlated regularity (constant) versus irregularity (variable) of the two conditions?

This is not a radical idea. It has long been known that run structures in sequences capture attention, evident in the gamblers' fallacy phenomena.[44] For instance, Sanabria and colleagues showed rate effects (fast, slow) associated with session contexts in FP designs.[45,46] Others find pronounced rhythmic influences in FP contexts.[47,48] The gist of the latter can be illustrated in a simplistic example of two different variable sequences with the same long (L) and short (S) FP intervals distributed over nine trials as: S,S,L, S,S,L, S,S, **L** or as S, L, S,S,S, L, S,S, **L**. Although statistically both variable conditions are identical, intuitively it seems that expectancies about the final **L** FP interval will differ in these conditions.

Recent research pursues this issue. For example, Rob Ellis[49] conducted an FP study in which many session contexts fell into one of two different, but statistically identical, variable FP conditions. Specifically, sequences in one FP condition were rhythmically coherent (regular), but in the other FP condition, all sequences were incoherent (irregular). Sessions in both conditions conveyed the *same probability distribution of time intervals*. If probabilistic session properties are determinants of falling RT profiles of variable FP conditions, then both conditions should yield identical shortening RTs as FP intervals lengthened. But, they did not. Neither group showed a typical variable RT profile. Instead, mean RT was slow and flat over FPs in the incoherent temporal context; by contrast, the mean RT was overall faster for the coherent condition, slowing as FPs lengthened. These and related findings suggest that attending and temporal expectancies reflect rhythmic, not probabilistic, certainty.[50,51] (Cravo et al.[52] also report endogenous brain oscillations reacting to session contexts.)

In sum, the FP design occupies an honored seat in the pantheon of paradigms developed to study time and temporal expectancies. It poses the simplest of goals: "react quickly to a target." There is general agreement that temporal expectancies speed this response. There is also agreement that these expectancies depend on a temporal context developed over trials (i.e., a session context). However, there is less agreement on how temporal context operates. For some scholars, temporal context creates temporal expectancies based on acquired probabilities. For others, the origin of temporal expectancies resides in people's default sensitivity to sequential invariants of session. Finally, a view compatible with DAT is that a "tacit," possibly involuntary, "use" of sequential time patterns in a given session invites temporal expectancies in FP designs.

Cueing Tasks and Temporal Expectancies

Temporal expectancies are also found in certain cueing tasks that resemble FP paradigms. Instead of a warning stimulus, on each trial, people are presented with a distinctive cue that may predict "when" a future target will occur. These tasks combine aspects of an FP paradigm with features of Posner's classic spatial cueing task,[53] in which a valid visual cue (e.g., an arrow) reliably orients a viewer's attention to a particular spatial locus. Similarly, temporal cuing presents valid stimulus cues that successfully orient one's attention to a locus in time.[54] Two important FP features remain in cueing tasks: first, RTs remain the dependent variable of choice for assessing temporal expectancies. Second, session context is again probabilistically manipulated. What is new is cue validity. *Cue validity* reflects the relative frequency of cue–target time intervals in a probabilistic session context.

In 1998, Coull and Nobre developed a temporal cue validity to elegantly illustrate that probabilistically valid symbolic cues orient attending in time. Resulting temporal expectancies paralleled spatial expectancies discovered by Posner et al. To appreciate this approach, imagine a laboratory task with a goal of target identification (e.g., targets are + or −). Although the target is variably timed, a valid static cue to its timing precedes each target, allowing one to reliably predict "when" a future target may occur. For instance, a valid cue may be a large visual circle that frequently precedes a long pre-target time interval (800 ms), whereas a smaller circle is frequently paired with a shorter pre-target interval (400 ms). In such contexts, people respond faster to temporally expected than to unexpected targets, especially for shorter pre-target target times.[55,56] According to Coull and Nobre, valid cueing stimuli function internally as *endogenous cues that voluntarily orient attending to moments in time*.[57]

Much evidence favors this approach (cf. reviews of Nobre and Coull[58,59]. For instance, using functional magnetic resonance imaging (fMRI) and also positron emission tomography (PET) recordings, they stablished that spatial and temporal cueing tasks elicit brain activity in right and left parietal brain regions, respectively. Selective enhancements to anticipated target times appear to be mediated by a left hemisphere–dominant parietal system that partially overlaps with spatial orienting networks (for task generality, see Miniussi et al.[60]; Nobre et al.[61]).

In sum, cueing tasks illustrate how people use the "what" of one stimulus to anticipate the "when" of another stimulus. It reflects one way we have learned to guide attending in time within our daily lives. Attentional orienting in time is viewed as goal-directed, endogenous, and under voluntary control.[62,63] A mundane example of this resides in citizens' ability to operate safely in traffic. In many cultures, a yellow traffic light signals that a red light (stop) will appear soon. Our driving behaviors testify that, while conscious of the yellow light, we have also internalized the meaning of both stimuli—the cue (yellow) and target (red)—as well as their temporal separation. It illustrates that, with clear task goals, people readily learn to associate a discrete stimulus with a specific time span. Without such skills, at the least, we may find more traffic accidents. We know a good deal more about this kind of temporally oriented attending than we did a few decades ago.

Sequential Targeting Tasks and Temporal Expectancies

Another paradigm for studying time involves a sequential targeting task. This task embeds a to-be-identified target stimulus in a sequence of nontarget stimuli, where the surrounding sequence provides a temporal context. Unlike cueing tasks, which engage voluntary, goal-oriented attending to probabilistic cues, these tasks are designed to study stimulus-driven attending that is not necessarily under voluntary control. Importantly, this temporal context may not even be relevant to task goals.

A dynamic attending view of such paradigms holds that sequences in these tasks provide external rhythms that entrain attending of neural correlates, more or less effectively. As such, they induce temporal expectancies. However, unlike the probabilistic expectancies featured in FP and cueing tasks, these are dynamic expectancies which are fundamentally sensitive to contextual time and rhythm, *where the latter may be irrelevant to task goals.*

Ideas surrounding dynamic expectancies date back to the debut of temporally oriented attending in 1976, when entrained attending was "off the radar" for psychologists.[64] Moreover, understanding of the stimulus-driven nature of dynamic attending and related concepts such as entrainment has developed slowly. Nevertheless, a consistent prediction of DAT has been that temporal context can influence percepts of future targets even if context timing is deemed "irrelevant" to task goals. Targeted attending in time should facilitate general feature perception of various (nontemporal) targets (e.g., pitch, intensity, color, etc.) because it facilitates a synchronicity between temporally allocated attending energy and a target item.

Originally, DAT predictions were pursued in ecologically valid experiments using general perception tasks involving music-like stimuli with meaningful manipulations of melody and rhythm. It addressed listeners' tacit "use" of stimulus timing to perceive nontemporal (e.g., melodic) targets; also, conventional accuracy measures (e.g., proportion correct, PC, as well as signal detection metrics, e.g. d') are stressed over the RT measures popular in FP and cueing tasks. For example, Marilyn Boltz [65]showed that people listening to folk tunes generate temporal expectancies based on the accompanying rhythm which, in turn, enhanced the accuracy of detecting pitch changes in future, temporally expected, tones. Finally, in such tasks, temporal context refers not simply to stimuli preceding a target on a single trial, but it also speaks to a larger context, namely session context over trials.[66,67,68,69]

A number of studies converge to highlight the unrecognized relevance of putatively "irrelevant" rhythmic contexts in enhancing general perception of nontemporal targets.[70,71,72] Thus, Figure 2.3b shows that pitch judgments of target tones embedded in different isochronous melodies are better (higher accuracy, d') for temporally expected than for unexpected (early, late) targets.[73] Rhythmic contexts also facilitate detection of intensity changes[74] Finally, Geiser and colleagues[75] directly manipulated task relevance to show that temporal perturbations in an otherwise coherent rhythmic context produced event-related potentials (ERPs) in both a time-relevant task (time-change detection) and, more importantly, in a time-irrelevant task (pitch change detection). Related results from other studies converge with this.[76,77,78] In sum, consistent with DAT predictions, in auditory sequences, perception of target sounds is influenced by surrounding temporal contexts that are 'technically' task irrelevant.

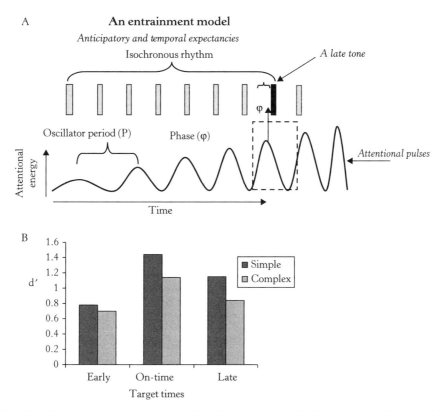

FIGURE 2.3 Outline of entrainment for a tone identification task. Panel **A** shows driving–driven dyad for a target tone (pitch; black bar) identification task which could appear with early, on-time, or late phase (late is shown) relative to temporal context of an isochronous driving rhythm. Entraining oscillations show increasing energy of attentional pulses. Panel **B** shows target detection performance (d′) as function of target phase and melodic complexity of context.

Modified from figure 3 in Mari Riess Jones, Heather Moynihan Johnston, and Jennifer Puente, "Effects of Auditory Pattern Structure on Anticipatory and Reactive Attending," *Cognitive Psychology* 53: 59–96, doi:10.1016/j.cogpsych.2006.01.003.

Time Is Amodal

The inherent amodality of time implies that temporal context should be important to perception of visual as well as auditory sequences. Indeed, Olsen and Chun[79] showed that temporally structured visual sequences successfully guided attending to "when" a visual target might occur. Others also find that regular visual rhythms (vs irregular ones) improve detection of embedded targets as well as boost perceptual acuity.[80,81,82,83] Finally, commonalities among auditory and visual modes find ecological validation in dynamics of natural visual scenes, as Marilyn Boltz has demonstrated.[84]

Cross-modal effects transcend modality. Thus, a rhythmic sequence presented to an individual through one modality affects this person's responses to a sequence of another modality. For instance, background music synchronized with on-beat visual stimulus facilitates perception of

visual targets[85,86,87,88] Interestingly, cross-modal effects may reflect unidirectional effects where auditory rhythms prime tracking visual events but not the reverse.[89]

In sum, regardless of modality, when people respond to target stimuli embedded within a larger sequence, the timing of a prevailing sequential context affects target perception. This is true whether or not the context is deemed task-relevant; stimulus-driven attending involuntarily governs performance. Furthermore, relative to incoherent contexts, rhythmically coherent contexts enhance performance. These findings are consistent with long-standing predictions of DAT regarding anticipatory attending. Alternatively, they pose problems for traditional attention theories, past and present, which provide no rationale for including putatively irrelevant contextual timing as a basis for guiding attending.

Selective Attending Tasks

Selective orienting is a diagnostic of attention, as described in Chapter 1. It refers to the ability to focus on one aspect of a complex scene (auditory or visual) while simultaneously "tuning out" (i.e., suppressing) other co-occurring features. Typically, selective attending tasks aim to discover how people voluntarily comply with instructions to attend to certain stimuli and ignore others.

The classic Cocktail Party scenario suggests that people can selectively attend to one talker among many others.[90,91,92] Recently, Zion-Golumbic and colleagues pursued a neural entrainment approach to selective attending using a version of the Cocktail Party phenomenon that featured a role for temporal context.[93,94] Both voluntary and involuntary attending appear to be involved. In this study, task instructions affected listeners' voluntary control of attention, whereas speech stimuli, which carried a temporal context, appeared to govern stimulus-driven attending. Thus, both voluntary and involuntary attending contribute to selective attending to events that unfold in time. However, questions remain surrounding the interaction of voluntary and involuntary attending.

Rokenhokl et al.[95] tackled some of these questions. Using visual stimuli, they presented people with a bouncing ball as a temporal context. Viewers had to "pay attention" either to the ball's color (ignore its rhythm) or its rhythmic rate (ignore its color) as a "cue" to the time of forthcoming target stimulus. People readily complied with instructions to ignore color, but they failed to comply with instructions to ignore rhythm. Furthermore, the effect of instructions did not interact with variations in stimulus properties, leading the authors to conclude that these factors are dissociable. In short, voluntary attending, linked to instructions, operates independently of involuntary attending which is linked to a stimulus rhythm.

But this story may not be so simple. Selective attending tasks are often complex, so that general claims of dissociable mechanisms are premature. This is suggested in a sequential target task of Klein and Jones[96] using auditory stimuli. They varied instructions to listeners who had to either selectively attend to one of two pitch streams (high [H] or low [L] pitch) in a complex rhythm or to divide their attention between the two pitch streams. Also rhythmic structure was varied by manipulating the timing of low pitch tones (simple, moderate, complex). Listeners had to detect a timbre change of a tone that occurred randomly within the isochronous stream of high-pitched tones.

Unlike Rokenhol et al., this study revealed a significant interaction of instructions with rhythmic structure. People who followed instructions to divide attending to both H and L tones performed best when the overall rhythmic context was simple. Surprisingly, people told to selectively attend only to the high-pitch stream performed best in complex temporal context! Logically, such an outcome should reflect voluntarily heightened attending to high tones in both rhythms. In retrospect, this intriguing result prefigures contemporary hypotheses about the voluntary control of entrainment via inhibitory oscillations.[97,98] Perhaps instructions to selectively attend facilitates a "tuning out" of distractor tones in complex rhythms due to heightened entrainment of well-timed neural inhibitory pulses. In short, this interaction suggests interdependencies among voluntary and involuntary attending of people listening to ecologically valid sequences in music and speech.

In sum, selective attending is influenced both by instructions about "what" to attend to and by rhythmic complexity that affects anticipations about "when" a target might happen. Although these factors may respectively control voluntary and involuntary attending activities, they do not necessarily operate independently.

Summary of Attending

People either explicitly or implicitly use information in temporal contexts to orient attending in time via temporal expectancies. However, both context and expectancies are interpreted differently across the four paradigms discussed in this section. In FP and cueing designs, temporal context is often defined probabilistically, whereas in sequential targeting tasks, including selective attending ones, temporal context is conceived in a quasi-deterministic fashion as external rhythms. These different portrayals invite respectively different views about internal mechanisms underlying temporal expectancies. Probabilistic descriptions of context spawn hypotheses that temporal expectancies depend on statistical computations such as hazard functions. Alternatively, descriptions of rhythmic contexts lead to hypotheses about entrained attending and temporal expectancies based on anticipatory attending.

Finally, the main points of this section are:

- Temporal expectancies may arise from temporal contexts in various tasks, including both time perception and general attention/perception tasks.

- Theoretically, temporal context can be described either stochastically (i.e., as a probability distribution of time intervals) or, alternatively as a quasi-deterministic time pattern.
- Hypotheses about temporal expectancies may feature either probability computations or anticipatory attending due to entrainment.
- Two DAT predictions find support in sequential targeting tasks: (1) a "task-irrelevant" temporal context can influence attention/perception of targets, and (2) regardless of modality, coherent driving rhythms lead to better target detection/identification than do incoherent ones.

TUNING IN: NEURAL TIMING MECHANISMS

This chapter opened with portraits of two different internal timing mechanisms. One depicts a prominent time perception theory (SET) based on an internal pacemaker mechanism that encodes discrete time spans. This is a widely endorsed view that recurs in future chapters. For instance, it supports certain theories of pitch perception and speech prosody in a shared assumption that pitch and speech stimuli represent strings of independent time intervals.

An alternative portrait appeals to internal mechanisms involving temporal dependencies expressed by biological oscillations and entrainment principles. DAT presumes that people rely on neural oscillations that adapt to successive time intervals during real-time tracking of stimulus rhythms. More precisely, an external rhythm comprising stimulus IOIs functions as a driving rhythm, which enforces synchrony of an internal rhythm—a neural oscillation—that functions as a driven rhythm. The hypothesized oscillation, then, has a capacity for entrainment; in this case it is *exogenous entrainment* because the driving rhythm is an external rhythm. The internal, driven rhythm is powered by self-sustaining energy and postulated to expend work and energy in tasks ranging from time perception to general attention/perception. Yet the word "hypothesized" is telling. The research reviewed to this point is largely behavioral in nature, whereas the explanatory mechanisms of DAT involve neural oscillations.

Accordingly, it is fair to ask of DAT: "What evidence exists for exogenous entrainment of neural oscillations?"

The remainder of this chapter (and the next) addresses this question. This final section presents four illustrative "cross-over" studies. Each addresses a different question about biological oscillations and their putative entrainment power. But, first, it is useful to review some oscillator terminology.

Elementary Oscillation Terminology

The term "rhythm" can be unpacked in several ways. In both speech and music, stimulus-driving rhythms are associated with pitch contours and/or certain recurring time patterns (e.g., long-short-short). They live in the sound patterns we produce during communications. Internal rhythms, on the other hand, are brain rhythms that listeners use as *driven rhythms* during attending. It is useful to review a few basics of brain oscillations in preparation for the next chapter on the "tunable brain." This chapter, then outlines some fundamental oscillator properties of frequency, amplitude, and phase. Although these properties hold for linear and nonlinear oscillations, linear oscillations generate very simple (i.e., perfectly sinusoidal) waveforms, whereas this is not the case for nonlinear oscillations.

It is well-known that individual neurons produce spikes with firing rates that vary with stimulus intensity. Although rates are rarely considered rhythmical, the emergence of whole ensembles of neurons firing synchronously offers clear collective evidence of a neural (i.e., endogenous) rhythm. Jointly, assemblies of active neurons create waves of alternating excitatory and inhibitory activity that form rhythmic fluctuations of Local Field Potentials (LFPs; in micro-volts [μV]). This multi-unit activity (MUA) embeds multiple frequencies that vary in amplitude/energy and phase; nevertheless, together, they contribute to a raw signal, as shown in Figure 2.4 (from Hanslmayr et al., 2011[99]). This figure offers a clear illustration of brain oscillations recorded by electroencephalograms (EEGs) that indirectly reflect LFP rhythms. When appropriately filtered, oscillator frequencies representative of common rhythmic categories can be isolated (e.g., frequencies of 4, 10, 40 Hz, etc.). Box 2.1 details relevant features and notations for three critical properties of a neural oscillation: frequency, amplitude and phase. This terminology facilitates understanding the studies described next.

BOX 2.1
OSCILLATOR TERMINOLOGY

Frequency components extracted from complex brain signals are conventionally categorized by rate (Hz). Oscillator frequencies range from very high frequencies (>15 kHz) to very low ones (<.01 Hz), where the latter include circadian rhythms (periods of ~24 hours). Figure 2.4B shows three different (common) frequency components: a theta frequency (~4 Hz), a faster alpha frequency (10 Hz), and a high-frequency gamma component (e.g., 40 Hz). Standard frequency categories (from EEG bands) are useful in part because grouped frequencies may serve different functions. For instance, theta and gamma frequencies tend to show increasing amplitudes in response to external stimulation, whereas alpha and beta often decrease in response to this stimulation.

Generally, frequency, f, reflects cycles per seconds in units of Hertz of internal oscillations (F specifies stimulus frequencies based on external periodicities). In discussing an oscillator's period, p (p = 1/f) milliseconds are often used for fast rhythms; when considering momentary frequency (or angular velocity), the formula $\omega = 2\pi f (= 2\pi/t)$ in radians is used.

Amplitude of an oscillation varies with the number of active, synchronized, neural units. It also changes momentarily throughout an oscillation's cycle. In a vibrating signal, amplitude reflects signal strength given by displacements of matter. Importantly, instantaneous amplitude of an oscillation is correlated with its momentary energy. *Energy*, an abstract concept, is the ability to work (i.e., to force a displacement in matter away from an equilibrium). Moreover, energy (or work) takes place over time, leading to a related term, *power*, which reflects the rate of work per unit time. Over the time of a cycle, if average amplitude, measured in several ways (e.g., peak-to-peak, root-mean square amplitude), is identical for two different oscillations, one with a period of 100 ms, the other with p = 200 ms, then the power of the former is greater than that of the lower frequency oscillation because the higher frequency oscillation is working at a faster rate. Particularly in autonomous neural oscillations, energy is intrinsic; that is, it is internal to the system and not imposed by an external force. The LFP neural rhythms can be thought of as preserving an equilibrium between an internal energy supply and its dissipation over time. A *stable oscillation* is one in which just enough internal energy is created on each cycle to compensate for the energy dissipated in work on that cycle.

Instantaneous amplitude changes reflect LPF fluctuations within a cycle. From a dynamic attending perspective, these feed into fleeting changes in attending energy. A resulting pattern of amplitude changes is usually referred to as a potential. However, to avoid confusions, the terms amplitude and changing amplitudes are retained throughout this book. So, Figure 2.4C shows amplitude changes at two time scales, one involving instantaneous changes within the period of an alpha cycle and the other reflecting envelop changes that rise and fall over longer time spans. Overall these energy levels are created by joint activities of multiple oscillations in which energy levels change over time. This flexibility makes oscillatory energy an important factor in understanding attending because it instantiates the idea that internal energies of driven rhythms determine momentary attending.

Phase φ, of an oscillation is illustrated Figure 2.4D (for an alpha oscillation). Typically, phase refers to a point in time, t, within a cycle; in radians, it corresponds to an angle within a 2π closed oscillator path for an oscillator with period, p. Phase at time t is $\varphi(t) = \Delta t/p$, whereas in an oscillation Δt is a time difference between a reference point, t_0, for $\varphi(0)$ in a cycle. Thus, phase is a time change normalized by an oscillator's period, assuming $t - t_0 = \Delta t$. For example, if $\Delta t = 25$ ms with an oscillator with p = 100 ms (10 Hz), then, using the general formula: $\varphi(t) = \varphi(0) + 2\pi(t - t_0)/p$, the $\varphi(t) = 1.57$ radians (i.e., an angle of 90 degrees). In practice, the referent phase point, $\varphi(0)$, can be strategically defined according to task, theory, or the like. For instance, it may reflect a theoretically defined peak expectancy time point in a periodic cycle. Once stipulated, all subsequent time points separated by 2π from the referent are identical (i.e., = 0 radians; mod 2π).

Phase is important in several respects. First, it can specify optimal phase points within a cycle, such as peak energy points and/or phase regions in a cycle of greater sensitivity. Such points then many function as reference phase points, φ (0). Second, phase is useful in describing relationships between driving and driven oscillations. Given specified phase points within each of two oscillations, (O_i, O_j), if their relative phase, $\Delta\varphi$ ($\Delta\varphi = \varphi_i - \varphi_j$) is constant, this reflects a *stable time relationship* between a pair of oscillators. In other words, interactions between two oscillations can be gauged by the variability of the relative phase, $\Delta\varphi$, such that if a measure of its variability, Var ($\Delta\varphi$), is low over cycles, then these oscillations are likely interacting. Low variability is a symptom of phase-locking, also termed *phase coupling*, discussed in the next chapter.

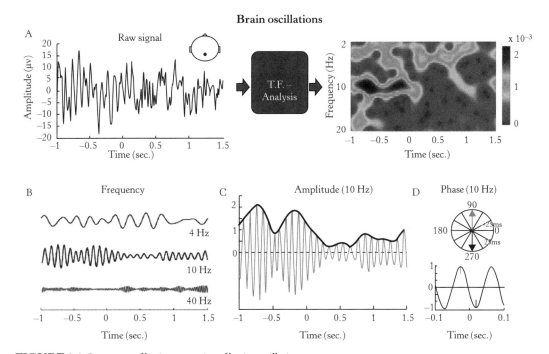

FIGURE 2.4 Summary of basic properties of brain oscillation.

Reprinted from figure 1 in Simon Hanslmayr et al., "The Role of Alpha Oscillations in Temporal Attention," *Brain Research Reviews* 67, no. 1–2 (June 24, 2011): 331–43, doi:10.1

EVIDENCE FOR NEURAL ATTENDING RHYTHMS: SOME REPRESENTATIVE STUDIES

Early in the past century, psychologists knew of only one type of neural oscillation, aptly termed the *alpha rhythm*.[100] For decades, alpha rhythms remained a poorly understood curiosity. Even with discoveries of other brain oscillations (e.g.,

theta, delta), some skepticism remained regarding these curious findings. Indeed, not so long ago, neural oscillations were considered epiphenomena or mere by-products of the "real work" of the brain. However, in recent decades, advanced EEG and magnetoencephalography (MEG) technologies have motivated some psychologists to take a second look at brain oscillations. This has led to promising findings that forecast a greater theoretical role for neural oscillations in psychology.

Discoveries of brain oscillations reinforce dynamic attending theory. They validate the idea of external driving rhythms that activate internal tunable rhythms which function as driven rhythms. In turn, this paves the way for exploring the explanatory potential of principles of entrainment. Each of the four studies described in the next section tackles a different piece of the puzzle surrounding driving and driven (oscillator) rhythms and entrainment.

Driven Oscillator Rhythms: Do They Figure in Anticipatory Attending?

One concern about neural oscillations involves their entrainment capacity. Do neural oscillations really function as rate-specific, tunable, driven rhythms? If so, they can support anticipatory attending.

Anticipatory attending reflects a sustaining neural oscillatory activity that precedes a future stimulus. Theoretically, attending is initially induced by an external (context) rhythm with a rate close to its ongoing oscillation's intrinsic rate. Thus, contextually activated oscillations can facilitate attending to future targets at the "right" (i.e., expected) time, as implied in Figure 2.3. To test this hypothesis, Rohenkohl and Nobre[101] used the clever bouncing-ball paradigm (described previously). The ball trajectory initially supplied either a regular or irregular temporal context, at fast or slow rates. Each trial terminated with a short or long occlusion period (i.e., lacking stimulation)

prior to appearance of a future target. A time-frequency EEG analysis of cortical activity during this occlusion period confirmed that only the regular rhythms, not irregular ones, induced recurrent desynchronizations of inhibitory alpha-band amplitudes at phases *preceding* expected targets. This activity correlated with attending that culminated in better performance due to anticipatory attending (in the occlusion period) that ensured synchrony with the expected target (cf. Cravo et al.[102]).

In sum, it appears that neural oscillations realize anticipatory attending due to their sustained periodicities following entrainment to a preceding, external driving rhythm.

Oscillations as Driven Rhythms: How Do They Work?

If neural oscillations entrain to an external stimulus, how does this work? One possibility is that some induced rhythms "clean up the neural stage" for entry of an expected stimulus. This implicates a role for inhibitory properties of neural oscillations.

Alpha rhythms have inhibitory properties that can "tune out" interfering stimulation.[103,104,105] Mathewson and colleagues pursued this aspect of alpha rhythms.[106,107,108] They argued that entrained alpha oscillations produce phase-specific *pulses of inhibition* such that peaks of alpha power "tune-out" percepts of ill-timed stimuli (i.e., early or late stimuli). Moreover, both ERP and EEG recordings suggest that phases immediately preceding on-time targets correspond to an oscillatory trough

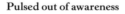

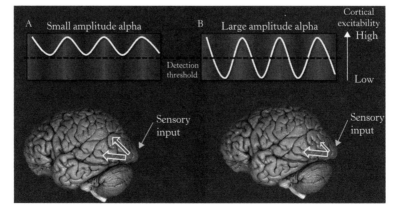

FIGURE 2.5 Effects of alpha band cortical inhibition proposed by Mathewson and colleagues.

Reprinted from figure 4 in Kyle E. Mathewson et al., "Pulsed Out of Awareness: EEG Alpha Oscillations Represent a Pulsed-Inhibition of Ongoing Cortical Processing," *Frontiers in Psychology* 2 (May 19, 2011), doi:10.3389/fpsyg.2011.00099.

(i.e., lowered alpha inhibition), suggesting that they pinpoint times of released energy that improves target detections (cf. Strauß et. al.[109]).

Inhibitory alpha-band oscillations, championed by Mathewson and his colleagues, reflect one-way oscillations operate during entrainment. These researchers hypothesized phase-specific predictions in which alpha-band power produces both a general decrease in performance due to greater cortical inhibition and phase-specific effects wherein inhibitory alpha pulses boost performance at particular phase points vis-a-vis a stimulus, as suggested in Figure 2.5.

Is Neural Entrainment by External Driving Rhythms a "Real" Phenomenon?

A question popular since biologists first discovered entrainment (i.e., of circadian rhythms) concerns its determinants. Skeptics commonly ask if external driving rhythms are *really* capable of eliciting neural correlates in animate creatures. In the simplest case, an external driving rhythm is an approximately isochronous time pattern; it may be a continuous waveform or consist of a regular series of discrete stimuli, termed *time-markers*. For instance, auditory time-markers, such as tone onsets, can deliver temporally regular local physical changes such as frequency modulation (FM) or amplitude modulation (AM) which function as a driving rhythm.

Skepticism surrounding entrainment has led some to claim that responses to rhythmic time-markers do not reflect *real* entrainment; rather, they reflect *faux entrainments*. Echoing early naysayers of circadian entrainment, contemporary critics note that discrete physical changes in amplitude simply evoke *reactive pulses* that are mistaken for rhythmically induced *expectancy pulses* of an entraining neural oscillation.

So how "real"—indeed, how general—is the phenomenon of neural entrainment? An answer is found in a compelling study of Henry and Obleser.[110] They used continuously undulating complex sounds as driving rhythms with a modulation frequency (FM with a delta period of 333 ms; Figure 2.6A). Listeners had to detect brief silences (i.e., short time gaps) staggered evenly throughout each delta cycle. If entrainment is real, then detection should be best when a listener relies on his or her own optimal phase of an entraining neural oscillation. Despite individual differences, EEGs revealed neural entrainment at the appropriate delta periodicity. Moreover, each listener operated with his or her optimal phase for target detection, given the entraining oscillation. In other words, detection behavior (in hit rates, ERPs) was mediated by a neural oscillation entrained by continuous external frequency modulations. This research not only establishes the reality of neural entrainment, but it also suggests a generality of driving rhythms.

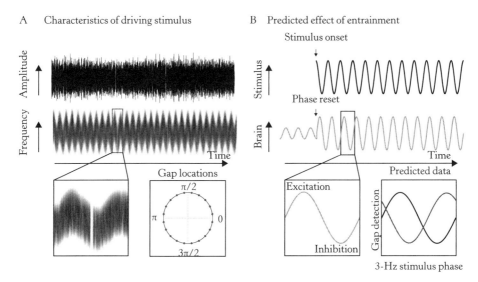

FIGURE 2.6 Driving rhythms and predicted entrainment effects in gap detection task. Frequency modulated stimuli.

Reproduced from Molly J. Henry and Jonas Obleser, "Dissociable Neural Response Signatures for Slow Amplitude and Frequency Modulation in Human Auditory Cortex," *PLoS ONE* 8, no. 10 (October 29, 2013): e78758, doi:10.1371/journal.pone.0078758.

Generalizing Driving Rhythms: Can Nonisochronous Rhythms Drive Attending?

Another criticism of entrainment theory rests on the claim that isochronous driving rhythms are unrealistically limiting. They rightly note that most natural signals (visual, auditory) are either quasi-isochronous or downright non-isochronous. So if neural entrainment is limited to isochronous driving rhythms, how general can it be?

But neural entrainments in fact are not limited to isochronous events. Not only can an entraining oscillation directly adapt to certain forms of non-isochrony, it is also the case that many non-isochronous external rhythms embed (e.g., hide) temporal regularities that a sensitive neural oscillation can find. To illustrate, consider two kinds of non-isochronous candidates for driving rhythms: rhythmically coherent, but non-isochronous time patterns that embed ('hide') a *regular beat* versus incoherent sequences that lack any hidden beat.[111,112] Grahn and colleagues exposed listeners to both kinds of non-isochronous rhythms.[113,114,115] Using fMRI recordings they found enhanced neural activity to rhythms with "hidden" temporal regularities over a broad neural timing network (including the cerebellum, basal ganglia, parietal cortex, and motor areas such as the premotor cortex [PMC], supplementary motor area [SMA], and auditory cortices). Especially interesting was the selective response of the putamen (in basal ganglia) to coherent (non-isochronous) time patterns with strongest reactions to very regular (but hidden!) beats. Intriguingly, once a strong internalized beat response is established, this beat persists even in the absence of stimulation. This is intriguing for it suggests that putamen activity not only reacts to certain non-isochronous rhythms, but it also supports anticipatory attending and persisting temporal expectancies.[116] By contrast, other basal ganglia regions (caudate nucleus, ventral striatum) only became active when beat-induced expectancies were violated (i.e., by early or late stimuli relative to an expected beat).

In short, one way that non-isochronous stimulus rhythms participate in entrainment is through putamen activity. It is fair to conclude that such rhythms are effective external driving rhythms if they embed some temporal regularity. Finally, together with other findings, a broad neural timing network exists that includes motor areas.[117]

This research supports the idea that various non-isochronous time patterns in our environment ignite in an attender's brain coherent neural responses—responses that in turn carry an oscillatory beat evident even in motor regions of the brain. This lends credence to the intuition that some compelling rhythmic patterns can spur one to "get up and dance!"

In summary, the following points are highlighted in these examples.

- Driven neural oscillations are rate-specific in their response to certain driving rhythms.
- Some entrainable rhythms are inhibitory (e.g., alpha rhythms); they carry phased inhibitory pulses that can "tune-out" certain stimuli even in fast sequential contexts.
- Driving rhythms based on frequency modulations (time-markers) induce phase-specific neural entrainments in the range of delta frequency oscillations.
- Non-isochronous, as well as isochronous, sequences can function as driving rhythms if they embed a temporal regularity, such as a recurring beat.

Interpreting Attention and Temporal Expectancies

This final section turns a corner to focus on implications of oscillatory entrainments for understanding dynamic attending and temporal expectancies that will figure in future chapters. The checkered history of attention theories suggests that attempts to define attention should be justly viewed with caution. Yet it is also true that prior, now abandoned approaches to attention have added to our understanding of this topic by stimulating new avenues of exploration. In this spirit, DAT offers a new interpretation of attending that links the energy of entraining oscillations to momentary states of attending.

Other formalizations of attention rest on contrasting assumptions. As mentioned in Chapter 1, many approaches to attention rest on metaphors of filters or spotlights, while others emphasize perceptual loads or even agency, seen as turning an on–off switch (e.g., SET). More recently Summerfield and Egner,[118] proposed even greater attentional agency, wherein attention is equated with a process of "prioritizing" information according to task relevance. All these approaches contrast with a dynamic approach to attending that is rooted in biological activity governed by universal physical principles. Specifically, DAT differs in that it proposes what attention *is*, not what it *is like* or what it *does*.

Admittedly, DAT promises a challenging adventure into neural activities. That is, attending is a natural activity that involves the momentary, aggregated power of multiple fluctuating, entraining neural oscillations. Within an entrainment narrative, its simplest manifestation resides in the synchrony between one internal (driven) oscillation and another external (driving) oscillation, which together form an *exogenous driving–driven dyad*. In this view, it takes at least two to "tango."

Attending Energy Fluctuates

According to DAT, multiple dyads are involved in attending. Each dyad is putatively based on an external driving rhythm that is coupled with an internal (i.e., neural) driven rhythm. At any moment such a dyad defines a fleeting entrainment state associated with internal, renewable oscillator energy. In theory, allocations of attending energy are targeted toward a future occurrence of an external stimulus change; they are automatically assigned by involuntary (task-irrelevant) factors with associated energy levels then modulated by voluntary (task-relevant) factors.

One implication of this framework is that attending can express a range of energy levels from low levels of activity due to involuntary forces to higher energy levels arising from voluntary modulations.[119] This configuration then allows for vanishingly low energy levels in the absence of voluntary factors. And, lacking involuntary reactions to external stimulations as well as voluntary forces, neural oscillatory activity is "on its own": oscillations of various rates fluctuate spontaneously. Neural oscillations of all frequencies bubble along at resting energy levels. Given this portrait, one implication is that a driving rhythm that captures a related driven rhythm may result in the involuntary entrainment of a dyad with very low energy levels. Such routine entrainments tether us to our environment in subtle ways, quite outside our awareness; yet attending in some measure is nonetheless involved. Conversely, high neural energy levels may accompany entrainment due to many (yet unknown) factors, including driving rhythm force and task relevance. Finally, attending energy is core to this puzzling construct termed "attention." Therefore, it is implausible that attention is an all-or-none phenomenon. Rather, attending is an activity that rides on graded levels of internal energy.

Are Attending and Temporal Expectancies Independent Activities?

The answer is "No." Temporal expectancies depend on attending. These two activities are related, but separable. This is evident in Figure 2.7. *Attending* refers to momentary interactions of a driven with an external driving rhythm. It happens in the presence of a stimulus. By contrast, anticipatory attending, which carries temporal expectancies, can happen in the absence of a stimulus.

Figure 2.7 summarizes this distinction. This figure also highlights the complexity implied by DAT. It illustrates entrainment activities of four different (nested) oscillations responding respectively to different external driving rhythms. These nested neural oscillations operate simultaneously in a coordinated fashion to govern attending. Such a configuration of several co-occuring oscillations can function as an *oscillator cluster*.

- One neural oscillation is induced by a slow driving rhythm with an external period, T (sounds are light gray). This *low frequency oscillation* paces expectancy pulses (dark gray triangles) with a period, p (p ~T).
- A second oscillation is a high-frequency, e.g., a beta oscillation, defining *expectancy pulses* (e.g., beta pulses). These pulses, in turn, are carried by the slower (low) frequency oscillation allowing beta pulses to precede future sound onsets.
- Third, a different high-frequency *reactive pulse* (open triangles) is not anticipatory. Instead it is evoked by each time a stimulus marker generates a sound.
- A fourth oscillation is an *alpha rhythm* (vertical black bars). Peaks of this rhythm also reflect entrainment via localized inhibition of responses to distractions prior to a sound onset.

Finally, a comment is in order concerning the higher frequency pulses evoked by individual stimulus items. These are included in this set of oscillators merely for completeness. That is, high-frequency (beta, gamma) oscillations define pulses that have not been discussed in this chapter. However, later chapters do elaborate on beta and gamma pulses, hence this previews those discussions.

Figure 2.7 also captures the idea that repetition of the same time span (T, between sound onsets) reflects the "when" of stimulus occurrences. This stimulus periodicity then "grows" internal localized beta pulses (these expectancy pulses appear as dark gray triangles) which recur with period, p (p ~T). Note that expectancy (beta) pulses precede sound onsets, shown (above) as

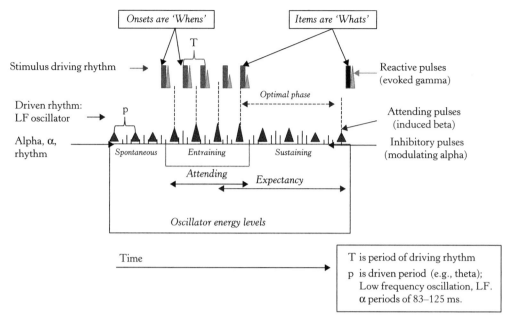

FIGURE 2.7 Distinguishing driving from driven rhythms and attending from expectancy. Stimulus driving rhythm (bars), with period, T, and driven oscillations with period, p, with attention/expectancy pulses (dark gray triangles) during entrainment (p ~ T). Attending energy is higher in the presence of driving rhythm (i.e., attending) and persists in the absences of the driving rhythm (i.e., expectancy), both following low frequency (LF) timing. Two high-frequency internal oscillation are also shown: reactive pulses (gamma) and attending pulse (beta); also shown are moderate rate inhibiting pulses (alpha).

light gray bars. In this way, the period, p, of recurring beta pulses becomes *phase-locked* with the external T rhythm. (cf. Large and Snyder[120]). In contrast, this figure also shows that evoked gamma pulses (empty outlined triangles) react to driving rhythm sounds *only after* they occur (i.e., as time-locked gamma pulses). Finally, this figure also implicates *repetition suppression* such that over time a repeating stimulus item weakens gamma pulses.

In sum, this overview of attending and temporal expectancies distinguishes three stages of oscillator activity: spontaneous, entrained attending, and sustained (anticipatory) expectancies. Initially, oscillations engage in low-level spontaneous activity prior to arrival of an external driving rhythm. Once present, however, a stimulus driving rhythm sparks involuntary attending based on entrainment; this entails a phase/frequency locking with an ongoing oscillation, hence producing a driving–driven dyad. Entrainment consists of momentary states of attending involving driving/driven synchronies (*see black arrow in Figure 2.7*). And, if the driving rhythm is removed from its partner, the driven

rhythm (an oscillation) persists for a time, as sustaining temporal expectancy (*see gray arrow in this figure*). This last stage also suggests how a sustaining oscillation supports a temporal expectancy or anticipatory attending. This implies that although attending and expectancy (i.e., anticipatory attending) differ, they are closely related.

The main points of these section are:

- Attending depends on an interaction of a driven (neural) rhythm with an external driving rhythm.
- This interaction is expressed by phase-locking (entrainment) of a driven with an external driving rhythm, which has been observed in behaviors of neural oscillations.
- Multiple entraining oscillations exist, including ones bearing timed inhibitory actions.

CHAPTER SUMMARY

This chapter about how we study time casts a wide net. It includes tasks centered on how we *judge* time (time perception tasks) as well tasks that explore how we *use* time (attention tasks).

One goal was to provide background on the limited research and theory addressing the role of temporal context in shaping performance in such tasks. It turns out that even in tasks where time structure is deemed irrelevant, timing continues to noticeably affect people's performance. This presents a problem for conventional approaches to attention that deny a role for time structure.

A second goal was to introduce pertinent DAT concepts such as driving and driven rhythms, as well as entrainment. These aid in explaining the effects of anticipatory attending and its relationship to temporal expectancies. In this narrative, driving–driven dyads describe an individual's real-time response to a temporal context, which is shown to convey driving rhythms to which spontaneous neural oscillations (driven rhythms) may entrain. Throughout this chapter, these constructs were applied in order to explain a range of findings in familiar behavioral tasks.

A third goal aimed to lay a foundation for describing driven rhythms as neural oscillations. Accordingly, the final section of this chapter presents examples of emerging neuroscience research that document (e.g., EEG measures) activities of various neural oscillations that function as driven rhythms that respond to a variety of driving rhythms.

NOTES

1. J. J. Gibson, "Events Are Perceivable But Time Is Not," in *The Study of Time II*, ed. J. T. Fraser and N. Lawrence (Berlin, Heidelberg: Springer, 1975), 295–301, http://link.springer.com.proxy.library.ucsb.edu:2048/chapter/10.1007/978-3-642-50121-0_22.

2. Paul Fraisse, *The Psychology of Time* (Oxford: Harper & Row, 1963).

3. William James, *The Principles of Psychology* (vol. 1) (New York: Holt, 1890).

4. Herbert Woodrow, "Time Perception," in *Handbook of Experimental Psychology* edited by S.S. Stevens (Oxford: Wiley, 1951), 1224–36.

5. Lorraine G. Allan, "The Perception of Time," *Perception & Psychophysics* 26, no. 5 (September 1979): 340–54, doi:10.3758/BF03204158.

6. Simon Grondin, "Timing and Time Perception: A Review of Recent Behavioral and Neuroscience Findings and Theoretical Directions," *Attention, Perception, & Psychophysics* 72, no. 3 (April 2010): 561–82, doi:10.3758/APP.72.3.561.

7. *The Oxford Handbook of Attention*, accessed January 27, 2016, https://books-google-com.proxy.library.ucsb.edu:9443/books/about/The_Oxford_Handbook_of_Attention.html?id=_sjRAgAAQBAJ.

8. J. Devin McAuley, "Tempo and Rhythm," in *Music Perception* edited by Mari Riess Jones (Springer, 2010), 165–199, http://link.springer.com.proxy.library.ucsb.edu:2048/chapter/10.1007/978-1-4419-6114-3_6.

9. Richard B. Ivry and R. Eliot Hazeltine, "Perception and Production of Temporal Intervals Across a Range of Durations: Evidence for a Common Timing Mechanism," *Journal of Experimental Psychology: Human Perception and Performance* 21, no. 1 (1995): 3.

10. Steven W. Keele et al., "Mechanisms of Perceptual Timing: Beat-Based or Interval-Based Judgements?," *Psychological Research* 50, no. 4 (April 1989): 251–56, doi:10.1007/BF00309261.

11. Dan Zakay and Richard A. Block, "Temporal Cognition," *Current Directions in Psychological Science* 6, no. 1 (1997): 12–16.

12. Russell M. Church and Hilary A. Broadbent, "Special Issue Animal Cognition: Alternative Representations of Time, Number, and Rate," *Cognition* 37, no. 1 (November 1, 1990): 55–81, doi:10.1016/0010-0277(90)90018-F.

13. Matell, Mathew S., Meck, Warren H. and Nicolelis, Miguel A. L, "Interval Timing and the Encoding of Signal Duration by Ensembles of Cortical and Striatal Neurons," *Behavioral Neuroscience* 117, no. 4 (2003): 760–73, doi:10.1037/0735-7044.117.4.760.

14. Sundeep Teki, "A Citation-Based Analysis and Review of Significant Papers on Timing and Time Perception," *Frontiers in Neuroscience* 10 (July 15, 2016), doi:10.3389/fnins.2016.00330.

15. Russell M. Church, Warren H. Meck, and John Gibbon, "Application of Scalar Timing Theory to Individual Trials," *Journal of Experimental Psychology: Animal Behavior Processes* 20, no. 2 (1994): 135–55, doi:10.1037/0097-7403.20.2.135.

16. Michel Treisman, "Temporal Discrimination and the Indifference Interval: Implications for a Model of the 'Internal Clock,'" *Psychological Monographs: General and Applied* 77, no. 13 (1963): 1–31, doi:10.1037/h0093864.

17. William J. Matthews and Warren H. Meck, "Temporal Cognition: Connecting Subjective Time to Perception, Attention, and Memory," *Psychological Bulletin* 142, no. 8 (2016): 865–907

18. J. Devin McAuley, "Perception of Time as Phase: Toward an Adaptive-Oscillator Model of Rhythmic Pattern Processing," 1995, ftp://html.soic.indiana.edu/pub/techreports/TR438.pdf.

19. Nathaniel S. Miller and J. Devin McAuley, "Tempo Sensitivity in Isochronous Tone Sequences: The Multiple-Look Model Revisited," *Perception & Psychophysics* 67, no. 7 (October 2005): 1150–60, doi:10.3758/BF03193548.

20. J. Devin McAuley and Mari Riess Jones, "Modeling Effects of Rhythmic Context on Perceived Duration: A Comparison of Interval and Entrainment Approaches to Short-Interval Timing," *Journal of Experimental Psychology: Human Perception and Performance* 29, no. 6 (2003): 1102–25, doi:10.1037/0096-1523.29.6.1102.

21. Edward W. Large and Mari Riess Jones, "The Dynamics of Attending: How People Track Time-Varying Events," *Psychological Review* 106, no. 1 (1999): 119–59, doi:10.1037/0033-295X.106.1.119.

22. Mari R. Jones and Marilyn Boltz, "Dynamic Attending and Responses to Time," *Psychological Review* 96, no. 3 (1989): 459–91, doi:10.1037/0033-295X.96.3.459.

23. Arilyn Boltz, "Time Judgments of Musical Endings: Effects of Expectancies on the 'filled Interval Effect,'" *Perception & Psychophysics* 46, no. 5 (1989): 409–418.

24. Mari Riess Jones, Marilyn G. Boltz, and James M. Klein, "Expected Endings and Judged Duration," *Memory & Cognition* 21, no. 5 (1993): 646–665.t

25. McAuley and Riess Jones, "Modeling Effects of Rhythmic Context on Perceived Duration."

26. Ralph Barnes and Mari Riess Jones, "Expectancy, Attention, and Time," *Cognitive Psychology* 41, no. 3 (November 2000): 254–311, doi:10.1006/cogp.2000.0738.

27. J. Devin McAuley and Gary R. Kidd, "Temporally Directed Attending in the Discrimination of Tempo: Further Support for an Entrainment Model," *The Journal of the Acoustical Society of America* 97, no. 5 (May 1, 1995): 3278, doi:10.1121/1.411574.

28. J. Devin McAuley and Gary R. Kidd, "Effect of Deviations from Temporal Expectations on Tempo Discrimination of Isochronous Tone Sequences," *Journal of Experimental Psychology: Human Perception and Performance* 24, no. 6 (1998): 1786.

29. Gary R. Kidd, Charles S. Watson, and Brian Gygi, "Individual Differences in Auditory Abilities," *The Journal of the Acoustical Society of America* 122, no. 1 (July 1, 2007): 418–35, doi:10.1121/1.2743154.

30. Caroline B. Monahan and Ira J. Hirsh, "Studies in Auditory Timing: 2. Rhythm Patterns," *Perception & Psychophysics* 47, no. 3 (May 1990): 227–42, doi:10.3758/BF03204998.

31. Carolyn Drake and Marie-Claire Botte, "Tempo Sensitivity in Auditory Sequences: Evidence for a Multiple-Look Model," *Perception & Psychophysics* 54, no. 3 (May 1993): 277–86, doi:10.3758/BF03205262.

32. Andrea R. Halpern and Christopher J. Darwin, "Duration Discrimination in a Series of Rhythmic Events," *Perception & Psychophysics* 31, no. 1 (January 1982): 86–89, doi:10.3758/BF03206204.

33. Large and Riess Jones, "The Dynamics of Attending."

34. William Yee, Susan Holleran, and Mari Riess Jones, "Sensitivity to Event Timing in Regular and Irregular Sequences: Influences of Musical Skill," *Perception & Psychophysics* 56, no. 4 (July 1994): 461–71, doi:10.3758/BF03206737.

35. Mari Riess Jones and William Yee, "Sensitivity to Time Change: The Role of Context and Skill," *Journal of Experimental Psychology: Human Perception and Performance* 23, no. 3 (1997): 693.

36. Yee, Holleran, and Riess Jones, "Sensitivity to Event Timing in Regular and Irregular Sequences."

37. Herbert Woodrow, "The Measurement of Attention," *The Psychological Monographs* 17, no. 5 (1914): i-158, doi:10.1037/h0093087.

38. Pekka Niemi and Risto Näätänen, "Foreperiod and Simple Reaction Time," *Psychological Bulletin* 89, no. 1 (1981): 133.

39. "ScienceDirect Snapshot," accessed January 30, 2016, http://www.sciencedirect.com.proxy.library.ucsb.edu:2048/science/article/pii/S095943880700089X.

40. Sander A. Los, "Foreperiod and the Sequential Effect: Theory and Data," *Attention and Time*, 2010, 289–302.

41. Annika Wagener and Joachim Hoffmann, "Behavioural Adaptations to Redundant Frequency Distributions in Time," *Attention and Time*, 2010, 217–26.

42. Michael B. Steinborn et al., "Sequential Effects Within a Short Foreperiod Context: Evidence for the Conditioning Account of Temporal Preparation," *Acta Psychologica* 129, no. 2 (October 2008): 297–307, doi:10.1016/j.actpsy.2008.08.005.

43. Los, "Foreperiod and the Sequential Effect."

44. Blase Gambino and Jerome L. Myers, "Role of Event Runs in Probability Learning," *Psychological Review* 74, no. 5 (1967): 410.

45. Daniel Sanabria, Mariagrazia Capizzi, and Ángel Correa, "Rhythms That Speed You Up," *Journal of Experimental Psychology: Human Perception and Performance* 37, no. 1 (2011): 236.

46. Daniel Sanabria and Ángel Correa, "Electrophysiological Evidence of Temporal Preparation Driven by Rhythms in Audition," *Biological Psychology* 92, no. 2 (February 2013): 98–105, doi:10.1016/j.biopsycho.2012.11.012.

47. Tim Martin et al., "Chronometric Evidence for Entrained Attention," *Perception & Psychophysics* 67, no. 1 (January 2005): 168–84, doi:10.3758/BF03195020.

48. Mariagrazia Capizzi et al., "Foreperiod Priming in Temporal Preparation: Testing Current Models of Sequential Effects," *Cognition* 134 (January 2015): 39–49, doi:10.1016/j.cognition.2014.09.002.

49. Robert J. Ellis and Mari Riess Jones, "Rhythmic Context Modulates Foreperiod Effects," *Attention, Perception, & Psychophysics* 72, no. 8 (November 2010): 2274–88, doi:10.3758/BF03196701.

50. María Dolores de la Rosa et al., "Temporal Preparation Driven by Rhythms Is Resistant to Working Memory Interference," *Frontiers in Psychology* 3 (August 28, 2012), doi:10.3389/fpsyg.2012.00308.

51. Deirdre Bolger, Wiebke Trost, and Daniele Schön, "Rhythm Implicitly Affects Temporal Orienting of Attention Across Modalities," *Acta Psychologica* 142, no. 2 (February 2013): 238–44, doi:10.1016/j.actpsy.2012.11.012.

52. Andre M. Cravo et al., "Endogenous Modulation of Low Frequency Oscillations by

Temporal Expectations," *Journal of Neurophysiology* 106, no. 6 (December 1, 2011): 2964–72, doi:10.1152/jn.00157.2011.

53. Michael I. Posner, Charles R. Snyder, and Brian J. Davidson, "Attention and the Detection of Signals," *Journal of Experimental Psychology: General* 109, no. 2 (1980): 160.

54. Jennifer T. Coull and Anna C. Nobre, "Where and When to Pay Attention: The Neural Systems for Directing Attention to Spatial Locations and to Time Intervals as Revealed by Both PET and fMRI," *The Journal of Neuroscience* 18, no. 18 (September 15, 1998): 7426–35.

55. Coull and Nobre, "Where and When to Pay Attention."

56. Joanna R. Doherty et al., "Synergistic Effect of Combined Temporal and Spatial Expectations on Visual Attention," *The Journal of Neuroscience* 25, no. 36 (September 7, 2005): 8259–66, doi:10.1523/JNEUROSCI.1821-05.2005.

57. J. T. Coull and A. C. Nobre, "Dissociating Explicit Timing from Temporal Expectation with fMRI," *Current Opinion in Neurobiology, Cognitive Neuroscience*, 18, no. 2 (April 2008): 137–44, doi:10.1016/j.conb.2008.07.011.

58. Kia Nobre and Jennifer Theresa Coull, *Attention and Time* (Oxford: Oxford University Press, 2010).

59. A. C. Nobre, A. Correa, and J. T. Coull, "The Hazards of Time," *Current Opinion in Neurobiology, Sensory Systems*, 17, no. 4 (August 2007): 465–70, doi:10.1016/j.conb.2007.07.006.

60. C. Miniussi et al., "Orienting Attention in Time," *Brain* 122, no. 8 (August 1, 1999): 1507–18, doi:10.1093/brain/122.8.1507.

61. Nobre, Correa, and Coull, "The Hazards of Time."

62. Coull and Nobre, "Dissociating Explicit Timing from Temporal Expectation with fMRI."

63. Gustavo Rohenkohl and Anna C. Nobre, "Alpha Oscillations Related to Anticipatory Attention Follow Temporal Expectations," *The Journal of Neuroscience* 31, no. 40 (October 5, 2011): 14076–84, doi:10.1523/JNEUROSCI.3387-11.2011.

64. Mari R. Jones, "Time, Our Lost Dimension: Toward a New Theory of Perception, Attention, and Memory," *Psychological Review* 83, no. 5 (1976): 323.

65. Marilyn G. Boltz, "The Generation of Temporal and Melodic Expectancies during Musical Listening," *Perception & Psychophysics* 53, no. 6 (November 1993): 585–600, https://doi.org/10.3758/BF03211736.

66. Gary Kidd, Marilyn Boltz, and Mari Riess Jones, "Some Effects of Rhythmic Context on Melody Recognition," *The American Journal of Psychology* 97, no. 2 (1984): 153–73, doi:10.2307/1422592.

67. Mari R. Jones, Gary Kidd, and Robin Wetzel, "Evidence for Rhythmic Attention," *Journal of Experimental Psychology: Human Perception and Performance* 7, no. 5 (1981): 1059.

68. Large and Riess Jones, "The Dynamics of Attending," 119.

69. Orsolya Szalárdy et al., "The Effects of Rhythm and Melody on Auditory Stream Segregation," *The Journal of the Acoustical Society of America* 135, no. 3 (March 1, 2014): 1392–405, doi:10.1121/1.4865196.

70. Marilyn Boltz, "Perceiving the End: Effects of Tonal Relationships on Melodic Completion," *Journal of Experimental Psychology: Human Perception and Performance* 15, no. 4 (1989): 749–61, doi:10.1037/0096-1523.15.4.749.

71. Mari Riess Jones et al., "Temporal Aspects of Stimulus-Driven Attending in Dynamic Arrays," *Psychological Science* 13, no. 4 (2002): 313–9.

72. Mari Riess Jones, Marilyn Boltz, and Gary Kidd, "Controlled Attending as a Function of Melodic and Temporal Context," *Perception & Psychophysics* 32, no. 3 (1982): 211–8.

73. Mari Riess Jones, Heather Moynihan Johnston, and Jennifer Puente, "Effects of Auditory Pattern Structure on Anticipatory and Reactive Attending," *Cognitive Psychology* 53, no. 1 (August 2006): 59–96, doi:10.1016/j.cogpsych.2006.01.003.

74. Eveline Geiser, Michael Notter, and John D. E. Gabrieli, "A Corticostriatal Neural System Enhances Auditory Perception through Temporal Context Processing," *The Journal of Neuroscience* 32, no. 18 (May 2, 2012): 6177–82, doi:10.1523/JNEUROSCI.5153-11.2012.

75. Marijtje L. A. Jongsma et al., "Expectancy Effects on Omission Evoked Potentials in Musicians and Non-Musicians," *Psychophysiology* 42, no. 2 (March 1, 2005): 191–201, doi:10.1111/j.1469-8986.2005.00269.x.

76. Jongsma et al., "Expectancy Effects on Omission Evoked Potentials in Musicians and Non-Musicians."

77. Peter Vuust et al., "To Musicians, the Message Is in the Meter: Pre-Attentive Neuronal Responses to Incongruent Rhythm Are Left-Lateralized in Musicians," *NeuroImage* 24, no. 2 (January 15, 2005): 560–64, doi:10.1016/j.neuroimage.2004.08.039.

78. Jessica A. Grahn and James B. Rowe, "Feeling the Beat: Premotor and Striatal Interactions in Musicians and Nonmusicians During Beat Perception," *The Journal of Neuroscience* 29, no. 23 (June 10, 2009): 7540–48, doi:10.1523/JNEUROSCI.2018-08.2009.

79. Bolger, Trost, and Schön, "Rhythm Implicitly Affects Temporal Orienting of Attention Across Modalities."

80. Mari R. Jones and June J. Skelly, "The Role of Event Time in Attending," *Time & Society* 2, no. 1 (January 1, 1993): 107–28, doi:10.1177/0961463X93002001008.

81. Jennifer L. Marchant and Jon Driver, "Visual and Audiovisual Effects of Isochronous Timing on

Visual Perception and Brain Activity," *Cerebral Cortex*, April 16, 2012, bhs095, doi:10.1093/cercor/bhs095.

82. Rohenkohl et al., "Temporal Expectation Improves the Quality of Sensory Information."

83. Doherty et al., "Synergistic Effect of Combined Temporal and Spatial Expectations on Visual Attention."

84. Marilyn Boltz, "Temporal Accent Structure and the Remembering of Filmed Narratives," *Journal of Experimental Psychology: Human Perception and Performance* 18, no. 1 (1992): 90–105, doi:10.1037/0096-1523.18.1.90.

85. Sanne ten Oever, Charles E. Schroeder, David Poeppel, Nienke van Atteveldt, Elana Zion-Golumbic., "Rhythmicity and Cross-Modal Temporal Cues Facilitate Detection," *Neuropsychologia* 63 (October 2014): 43–50, https://doi.org/10.1016/j.neuropsychologia.2014.08.008.

86. Bolger, Trost, and Schön, "Rhythm Implicitly Affects Temporal Orienting of Attention Across Modalities."

87. Bolger, Trost, and Schön, "Rhythm Implicitly Affects Temporal Orienting of Attention Across Modalities."

88. J. Devin McAuley and Molly J. Henry, "Modality Effects in Rhythm Processing: Auditory Encoding of Visual Rhythms Is Neither Obligatory nor Automatic," *Attention, Perception, & Psychophysics* 72, no. 5 (July 2010): 1377–89, doi:10.3758/APP.72.5.1377.

89. Jessica A. Grahn, Molly J. Henry, and J. Devin McAuley, "FMRI Investigation of Cross-Modal Interactions in Beat Perception: Audition Primes Vision, but Not Vice Versa," *NeuroImage* 54, no. 2 (January 15, 2011): 1231–43, doi:10.1016/j.neuroimage.2010.09.033.

90. *Auditory Scene Analysis*, accessed January 30, 2016, https://books-google-com.proxy.library.ucsb.edu:9443/books/about/Auditory_Scene_Analysis.html?id=jI8muSpAC5AC.

91. E. Colin Cherry, "Some Experiments on the Recognition of Speech, with One and with Two Ears," *The Journal of the Acoustical Society of America* 25, no. 5 (September 1, 1953): 975–79, doi:10.1121/1.1907229.

92. Rhodri Cusack et al., "Effects of Location, Frequency Region, and Time Course of Selective Attention on Auditory Scene Analysis," *Journal of Experimental Psychology: Human Perception and Performance* 30, no. 4 (2004): 643–56, doi:10.1037/0096-1523.30.4.643.

93. Elana M. Zion Golumbic et al., "Mechanisms Underlying Selective Neuronal Tracking of Attended Speech at a 'Cocktail Party,'" *Neuron* 77, no. 5 (March 2013): 980–91, doi:10.1016/j.neuron.2012.12.037.

94. E. Zion Golumbic et al., "Visual Input Enhances Selective Speech Envelope Tracking in Auditory Cortex at a 'Cocktail Party,'" *Journal of Neuroscience* 33, no. 4 (January 23, 2013): 1417–26, doi:10.1523/JNEUROSCI.3675-12.2013.

95. Gustavo Rohenkohl, Jennifer T. Coull, and Anna C. Nobre, "Behavioural Dissociation between

Exogenous and Endogenous Temporal Orienting of Attention," *PLoS One* 6, no. 1 (2011): e14620–e14620.

96. Mari Riess Jones, Heather Moynihan Johnston, and Jennifer Puente, "Effects of Auditory Pattern Structure on Anticipatory and Reactive Attending," *Cognitive Psychology* 53, no. 1 (August 2006): 59–96, doi:10.1016/j.cogpsych.2006.01.003.

97. Kyle E. Mathewson et al., "Pulsed Out of Awareness: EEG Alpha Oscillations Represent a Pulsed-Inhibition of Ongoing Cortical Processing," *Frontiers in Psychology* 2 (May 19, 2011), doi:10.3389/fpsyg.2011.00099.

98. N. Ding and J. Z. Simon, "Neural Coding of Continuous Speech in Auditory Cortex during Monaural and Dichotic Listening," *Journal of Neurophysiology* 107, no. 1 (January 1, 2012): 78–89, doi:10.1152/jn.00297.2011.

99. Simon Hanslmayr et al., "The Role of Alpha Oscillations in Temporal Attention," *Brain Research Reviews* 67, no. 1–2 (June 24, 2011): 331–43, doi:10.1016/j.brainresrev.2011.04.002.

100. Hans Berger, "Über das Elektrenkephalogramm des Menschen," *Archiv für Psychiatrie und Nervenkrankheiten* 87, no. 1 (December 1929): 527–70, doi:10.1007/BF01797193.

101. Rohenkohl and Nobre, "Alpha Oscillations Related to Anticipatory Attention Follow Temporal Expectations."

102. Gustavo Rohenkohl et al., "Temporal Expectation Improves the Quality of Sensory Information," *The Journal of Neuroscience* 32, no. 24 (2012): 8424–8.

103. Ali Mazaheri et al., "Region-Specific Modulations in Oscillatory Alpha Activity Serve to Facilitate Processing in the Visual and Auditory Modalities," *NeuroImage* 87 (February 15, 2014): 356–62, doi:10.1016/j.neuroimage.2013.10.052.

104. Wolfgang Klimesch, "EEG Alpha and Theta Oscillations Reflect Cognitive and Memory Performance: A Review and Analysis," *Brain Research Reviews* 29, no. 2–3 (April 1999): 169–95, doi:10.1016/S0165-0173(98)00056-3.

105. Wolfgang Klimesch, Paul Sauseng, and Simon Hanslmayr, "EEG Alpha Oscillations: The Inhibition–Timing Hypothesis," *Brain Research Reviews* 53, no. 1 (January 2007): 63–88, doi:10.1016/j.brainresrev.2006.06.003.

106. Kyle E. Mathewson et al., "To See or Not to See: Prestimulus α Phase Predicts Visual Awareness," *The Journal of Neuroscience* 29, no. 9 (March 4, 2009): 2725–32, doi:10.1523/JNEUROSCI.3963-08.2009.

107. Kyle E. Mathewson et al., "Rescuing Stimuli from Invisibility: Inducing a Momentary Release from Visual Masking with Pre-Target Entrainment," *Cognition* 115, no. 1 (April 2010): 186–91, doi:10.1016/j.cognition.2009.11.010.

108. Mathewson et al., "Pulsed Out of Awareness."

109. Antje Strauß et al., "Alpha Phase Determines Successful Lexical Decision in Noise," *The Journal of*

Neuroscience 35, no. 7 (February 18, 2015): 3256–62, doi:10.1523/JNEUROSCI.3357-14.2015.

110. Molly J. Henry and Jonas Obleser, "Dissociable Neural Response Signatures for Slow Amplitude and Frequency Modulation in Human Auditory Cortex," *PLoS One* 8, no. 10 (October 29, 2013): e78758, doi:10.1371/journal.pone.0078758.

111. Dirk-Jan Povel and Peter Essens, "Perception of Temporal Patterns," *Music Perception: An Interdisciplinary Journal* 2, no. 4 (1985): 411–40.

112. Ellis and Jones, "Rhythmic Context Modulates Foreperiod Effects."

113. Grahn and Rowe, "Feeling the Beat."

114. Grahn, Henry, and McAuley, "FMRI Investigation of Cross-Modal Interactions in Beat Perception."

115. Jessica A. Grahn and J. Devin McAuley, "Neural Bases of Individual Differences in Beat Perception," *NeuroImage* 47, no. 4 (October 1, 2009): 1894–1903, doi:10.1016/j.neuroimage.2009.04.039.

116. Jessica A. Grahn and James B. Rowe, "Finding and Feeling the Musical Beat: Striatal Dissociations Between Detection and Prediction of Regularity," *Cerebral Cortex*, April 11, 2012, bhs083, doi:10.1093/cercor/bhs083.

117. Coull and Nobre, "Dissociating Explicit Timing from Temporal Expectation with fMRI."

118. Christopher Summerfield and Tobias Egner, "Expectation (and Attention) in Visual Cognition," *Trends in Cognitive Sciences* 13, no. 9 (September 2009): 403–09, doi:10.1016/j.tics.2009.06.003.

119. Jones, Mari Riess, and Boltz, Marilyn. Dynamic Attending and responses to time. Psychological Review, vol 96 (3) 1989: 459–491.

120. Edward W. Large and Joel S. Snyder, "Pulse and Meter as Neural Resonance," *Annals of the New York Academy of Sciences* 1169, no. 1 (July 2009): 46–57, doi:10.1111/j.1749-6632.2009.04550.x.

3

The Tunable Brain

Ideally, a book about psychological time must not only speak to the time of observable events but also to people's unobservable responses to such events. What happens inside our heads as we experience dynamic changes in our environment? Does our brain actually follow happenings in real time? Only recently has science acquired techniques that address these questions. Previously, neuroscience concentrated on spatial mappings of brain regions, identifying modules specialized for certain skills. Nowadays, a revolution is under way that probes neurodynamic brain activities. With this, new discoveries of endogenous rhythms and their interactions, even among spatially remote brain regions, raise questions about the role of timing relationships among spatially disparate brain modules. More intriguing is surfacing evidence of a *tunable*—that is, an entrainable—brain. This research promises to reveal interesting secrets of the inner workings about how a brain "tunes itself."

This chapter offers glimpses of emerging research on brain tuning. It selectively focuses on synchrony and its many forms in brain activity. In this regard, this chapter lays a foundation for all following chapters that tackle fundamental psychological phenomena such as attention and perception from the perspective of synchronous tuning of brain rhythms. Nevertheless, this overview remains a snapshot in time of this fast-breaking area of study, which is in its infancy:

"The fundamental and so far unresolved problem for neuroscience remains to understand how oscillatory activity in the brain codes information for cognition."[1][p.1]

CHAPTER GOALS

This chapter outlines a journey into the inner world of a tunable brain. It begins with a single workhorse oscillation, then travels through interactions between pairs of neural oscillations (as dyads) to consider whole groups of interacting oscillations. In snapshots, it attempts to convey ways in which multiple neural dyads within a tunable brain may participate in larger oscillatory groups/configurations, using principles of resonance, and entrainment.

In this journey, a primary goal is to illustrate how current neuroscience converges with long-standing ideas of dynamic attending theory. The preceding chapter provides supporting behavioral evidence for Dynamic Attending Theory (DAT) hypotheses that postulate a major role for internal (i.e., endogenous) neural oscillations, nevertheless what do we actually *know* about these hypothetical oscillations? This chapter offers a partial answer. It extends a path opened by Molly Henry and Björn Herrmann[2] who document relationships between fast-breaking neuroscience research on tunable brain oscillations and DAT.

A secondary goal involves acquainting readers unfamiliar with entrainment and brain rhythms with elementary constructs relevant to studying psychological phenomena. A path is outlined that begins with defining a single limit cycle oscillation and ends with some speculative postulations regarding formations of larger oscillator configurations. Along this path, topics such as endogenous dyads (simple vs. complex) and oscillator gradients, as well as concepts involving multi-oscillator configurations, are considered. A recurring theme holds that basic properties of *limit cycle oscillations*, such as frequency, phase, and amplitude, enable the formation of brain synchronies that unite multiple endogenous dyads within larger collections of oscillations. Along the way, relevant trends in neuroscience pertinent to various modes of endogenous synchrony are reviewed. All this is aimed at preparing the reader for understanding a key psychological construct, *attending,* addressed in the following chapter.

Finally, this chapter has a tutorial flavor. It is aimed at readers unfamiliar with what may seem exotic topics. For this reason, presentations of limit cycle oscillations, phase adaptation, and entrainment dyads, as well as oscillator interactions, are highly simplified to convey their gist and relevance to familiar psychological phenomena such as attending. Despite this tutorial goal, some sections necessarily become detailed; in these cases, boxes, notes, and section summaries aim to distill the main points.

BACKGROUND: WHAT ARE NEURAL OSCILLATIONS?

Neural oscillations were first discovered by Berger in 1929.[3] He employed electroencephalograms (EEGs) to record a pervasive cortical periodicity now known as the *alpha rhythm*. However, the full explanatory potential of such oscillations went unrecognized for a long time. In fact, only in recent decades, with a multiplication of EEG oscillations, has the status/function of neural oscillations been questioned.

So what exactly *is* a cortical oscillation? This section tackles this question by selectively outlining a few properties of a special oscillation relevant to the entrainment story. In particular, these properties enable an oscillation to synchronize with other internal (brain) oscillations. This chapter concentrates on this self-tuning aspect of cortical oscillations. Specifically, it addresses *endogenous synchronizing connections among two or more cortical oscillations*.

A Neural Oscillation as a Tunable Brain Rhythm

Let's begin with a single, independent endogenous brain rhythm, one unencumbered by an external (driving) stimulus rhythm. This oscillation is said to be *spontaneous* when its activity persists over time without any obvious force. Such brain activity is created by cycles of a local field potential (LFP). Recall from the preceding chapter that the LFP refers to neuroelectrical changes collectively created from synchronous activities among the spiking frequencies of many neurons comprising a larger neuronal population. Aggregated spiking patterns lead to a single, emergent LFP periodicity with alternating spells of positive (i.e., excitatory [depolarization]) and negative (i.e., inhibitory [hyper-polarization]) activities that reflect postsynaptic chemoelectrical currents flowing through dendrites. In other words, an oscillation, tied to LFP neurodynamics, emerges from the coordinated actions of many individual nerve cells (i.e., neurons). And, over time an LFP traces out aggregated amplitude changes that are evident as the oscillatory ups and downs of an endogenous rhythmic waveform.

Neural Oscillations

Abstractly, the behaviors of an oscillation, O_i, can be formalized using the concept of a *phase space*. A *phase space* reflects all possible phase states an oscillation may inhabit given the polar coordinate dimensions of amplitude and phase.

Amplitude and Phase in a limit cycle oscillation

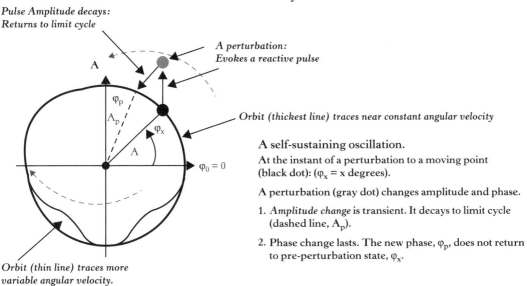

Pulse Amplitude decays: Returns to limit cycle

A perturbation: Evokes a reactive pulse

Orbit (thickest line) traces near constant angular velocity

A self-sustaining oscillation.

At the instant of a perturbation to a moving point (black dot): (φ_x = x degrees).

A perturbation (gray dot) changes amplitude and phase.

1. *Amplitude change* is transient. It decays to limit cycle (dashed line, A_p).

2. Phase change lasts. The new phase, φ_p, does not return to pre-perturbation state, φ_x.

Orbit (thin line) traces more variable angular velocity.

Limit cycle of sustaining oscillation with coordinates phase angle, amplitude.

FIGURE 3.1 A schematic of trajectory paths of a limit cycle, sustaining oscillation with coordinates phase angle and amplitude. Phase portraits of two attractors: a point attractor (smaller black dot) and a periodic attractor (thick black circle) in a phase space of all possible phase points.

Figure 3.1 shows two subsets of special states (a thick black orbit and a thin black orbit). Let us focus upon the subset of special states for the thicker lines that outline an almost *circular orbit* for oscillator O_i within a larger phase space. Such a path is a *phase portrait*. Here, the states of both orbits express closed paths of a phase portrait, but the thinly outlined phase portrait expresses greater variability. Let states along these paths reflect momentary values of an oscillation's amplitude and phase at different time points within an orbit.[4] A momentary measure of amplitude is expressed as a radius,[5] and phase is given by the corresponding polar angle. In short, this path traces instantaneous amplitude levels for all phases of an orbit. A perfectly circular orbit is one with a constant angular velocity throughout. Neither of these orbits in Figure 3.1 express this, but one is closer to perfect (heavier black lines) than the other.

The intrinsic frequency of any oscillation, O_i is $\omega_{oi} = 2\pi f$. Because frequency is inversely related to oscillator period, angular velocity of any oscillation is $\omega_i = 2\pi/p_i$ (p_i is oscillator period). Generally, points along a phase portrait's path express momentary amplitudes, a (t), over all phases given by φ (t) $= \omega_i\, t + \varphi_0$ (φ_0 connotes a starting phase).

The interesting feature of phase portraits involving orbits is that recurring trips around a given orbit generates a distinctive waveform. A perfectly circular orbit path leads to the common sinusoidal waveform; that is, x (t) $\approx$ A sin $(\omega_i t + \varphi_0)$]. The amplitude (A) indexes an oscillator's overall strength, while this formula specifies a timed series of instantaneous amplitudes.[6] Yet, we rarely encounter sinusoidal perfection; more often we encounter *almost sine waves*. Although the two portraits of Figure 3.1 specify imperfect sine waves, other phase portraints, generated by patterns of fast/slow angular velocities along an orbit's path, implicate different waveforms. For instance, saw-toothed waveforms, distorted square waves or still other rhythms (as with Van der Pol oscillations) arise from respectively different phase portraits.

Finally, the main point is that the different phase portraits, mentioned above, all describe oscillations. Hence, by definition they all yield some type of rhythmic periodicity. This is because a fixed phase portrait dictates periodic constancy due to repetitions of the same profile of angular velocities within a cycle. Finally, three basic properties of any neural oscillation contribute to these formulations: frequency, phase, and amplitude. These and other pertinent properties are defined in Box 3.1.

Tunable Neural Rhythms: Limit Cycle Oscillations

In the dynamical systems of interest here, the focus will be upon rhythms emerging from the simplest kinds of phase portraits, those which deliver almost regular rhythms. The underlying oscillations are limit cycle oscillations. As such, they yield a limiting periodicity that exerts a *attractive pull* of trajectories (dashed convergent lines) surrounding their limiting path in phase space (e.g., thicker orbit in Figure 3.1). More generally, the pull of a limiting path theoretically captures the idea of "tuning in" to an underlying relationship. In other words, even rather remote deviant points in phase space may survive in this account if they can gravitate toward a nearby powerful orbit. Informally, we might say that they jump onto one of these dashed trajectories to catch a ride toward the nearest stable ('attracting') orbit.

Attracting orbits of many limit cycle oscillations are not as simple that shown in Figure 3.1. For instance, a common biological oscillation is a relaxation oscillation that has a more complex orbit and delivers a jagged waveform with momentary amplitude peaks at regular time points. Indeed, some rightly argue that relaxation oscillations are especially suited for phase-coupling because amplitude peaks precisely identify narrow, but highly sensitive, phase regions of peak energy within an orbit.[7] Nevertheless, to convey entrainment concepts in this book, simplicity wins out. Consequently, the "almost sine wave" version of limit cycle oscillations is the tutorial vehicle of choice. Despite limitations, approximately circular phase portraits permit teachable explanations of the roles of three critical limit cycle oscillator properties discussed in this book: *self-sustaining, adaptive,* and *stability* properties.

The Self-Sustaining Property

A *self-sustaining oscillation* persists over time without "outside" help. As a spontaneous oscillation, it simply bubbles along with a favored (i.e., intrinsic) period; its amplitude is likely to be low, i.e., resting level. On reflection, this self-sustaining activity conveys a rather magical aspect of living things. With life comes ongoing vibrating energies. Unlike mechanical pace-maker/counter clocks (Chapter 2), these are biological clocks that exhibit natural rhythms which afford self-restoring internal energy. That is, their energy continues to ebb and flow even in the absence of outside forces. Energy flow within a cycle alternates between a positive energy flow (depolarized neural membranes) and a negative ebb (i.e., dissipative

BOX 3.1
DEFINITIONS OF OSCILLATOR CONSTRUCTS

Construct	Notation	Metrics	Description
Oscillator *i*	Oi	None	Periodic activity of a neuron or neuron population
Local field potential	*LFP*	μVolt	Aggregated electrical synaptic currents of local neurons
Oscillator frequency	*f*	Hertz, Hz	Periods (cycles) per second of an oscillation
Intrinsic oscillator frequency	$\omega_i = 2\pi f$	Radians	Characteristic angular velocity of oscillation
Intrinsic oscillator period	p_i	ms (milliseconds)	Characteristic neural period; recurrent wavelength, λ
Manifest oscillator frequency	Ω_i	Radians	Temporary, observable form of ω_i
Manifest oscillator period	p_i'	ms	Temporary, observable form of p_i
Oscillator phase: referent	$\varphi_0 = 0$	Degrees	Starting or referent phase (often = 0^0); also notated as φ_0
Phase angle	$\varphi_x - \varphi_0$	Degrees	Angle of point *x* at time t; polar coordinates
Relative phase	$\Delta\varphi_{(t)} = \varphi_1 - \varphi_2$	Degrees	Phase difference (two oscillations) same time, t
Oscillator amplitude	A	Pascal, Pa	Radial displacement, as pressure
Instantaneous amplitude	a_t	Pa	Pressure/force of displacement at time t
Pressure/Force	F	Volts	Electrical brain currents (microvolts, uV)
Oscillator energy	E	Erg	Capacity for work; depends on duration of power
Power	*P*	Watts	Rate of work; i. e., energy, E
Stimulus time span	T	Ms	External cycle duration (continuous or discrete)
Inter-onset-time interval	IOI =T	Ms	External onset-to-onset time (discrete rhythm)
Pi	π	Degrees/Radians	For a circle, π = 180 degrees and 3.14159. . . radians
Phi	φ	Golden ratio	Fibonacci sequence: 1, 2, 3, 5, 13 . . . ($\varphi = F_{n+1}/F_n = 1.6180327\ldots$ F_1, F_2, F_n, F_{n+1})

energy, hyperpolarized membranes). These ebbs and flows elegantly balance out within each recurring cycle. Self-restoration ensures that an oscillation with a given frequency persists at or near threshold levels. As dynamical systems, living things effortlessly sustain many biological rhythms that undulate continuously at very low resting levels. Importantly, this self-sustaining property of limit cycle oscillations means that they operate *spontaneously*; namely, without external forces. Just as infants are born with moving arms and legs, they also arrive in this world equipped with spontaneously modulating brain oscillations.

Finally, although admittedly simplified, this conceptual framework opens new ways to conceive of psychological activities. For instance, we can imagine situations in which spontaneous oscillations, active at low resting levels, may suddenly ramp up to higher, suprathreshold energy levels for some purpose. Perhaps this purpose reflects a person's need to explicitly attend to some relevant event. The sustaining property of limit cycle oscillations invites new hypotheses surrounding their takeover by certain voluntary forces to boost energy levels.[8] Generally, self-sustaining brain activity includes spontaneous rhythms that lie "in wait," ready to be of service when needed. Brains are continuously "busy"; they never really sleep.[9] Sleep merely reflects activities of another set of oscillations.

The Adaptive Property

Adaptivity refers to an oscillation's potential for adjusting to change. This is the core of a brain oscillation's tunability. Adaptive changes in the phase, frequency, and/or amplitude of a limit cycle oscillation happen if one oscillation is perturbed, perhaps by another. Or, an oscillation can be perturbed by an external event. In either case, the resulting perturbation automatically elicits changes in a resting limit cycle oscillation. That's what limit cycles oscillations are born to do.

Imagine traveling along an oscillation's orbit (e.g., as the large black dot in Figure 3.1). Suddenly an "unexpected" loud sound happens as this perturbation "hits" this orbit at phase, φ_p (gray dot). This unexpected stimulation disrupts an otherwise smooth "trip" of the black dot along this orbit in two ways: the oscillation adaptively shifts phase and increases its amplitude.

Phase adaptive behavior automatically arises from the "push" of this external, perturbing, stimulus at φ_p. It entails a shift from the original oscillator phase, φ_x, toward a new phase, that of the perturbation, φ_p. This is *phase-resetting*. The original phase instantly resets (i.e., corrects) to a new phase. Here, this new phase accurately "marks" stimulus time. Notice, however, that the new phase does not vanish (i.e., return to φ_x) after the perturbing stimulus is removed. Rather, a *phase change persists*.

Amplitude changes of a perturbed oscillation also happen. But, unlike phase changes, these changes are temporary. Following a single 'push' of the perturbing stimulus, a limit cycle oscillation automatically emits an instantaneous amplitude change (Ap) that is a burst of added energy which then decays rapidly. This fleeting response constitutes a time-locked heightening of reactive energy. As Figure 3.1 shows, this entails a rapid rise and fall of energy (*arrows*); it suggests a sort of "surprise" neural response to a sudden stimulus. The neural signature of such an *evoked* response in EEG recordings is an *event-related potential* (ERP).

Not shown in Figure 3.1 is another important oscillation modification. An oscillator's local amplitude may also change gradually if such a perturbing force is repeated regularly in time. This effectively transforms the psychological task into one wherein a repeated sound generates an external driving rhythm. As such, over longer stretches of time, regular driving rhythms begin to *induce* phased bursts of amplitude increases that *anticipate* stimulus onsets.

Capture Versus Expectancy

The preceding discussion warrants additional comments about *evoked* versus *induced* amplitude changes, here conceived as pulses in localized orbit regions. Although a single perturbing stimulus *evokes* an after-the-fact *reactive pulse* in amplitude, driving rhythm regularities can elicit a different kind of amplitude pulse, namely the anticipatory *expectancy pulse*. This distinction is familiar to psychologists as it echoes differences between *attentional capture* and *expectancy*. Evoked reactive responses refer to capture scenarios because they involve rapid involuntary reactions to a surprising stimulus.[10,11,12,13] By contrast, induced anticipatory responses are hypothesized to arise in contextually driven expectancy scenarios (not shown in this figure). This important distinction is revived in future chapters.

Stability

A third limit cycle feature is stability. Stability refers to oscillator tendencies to *resist* permanent change. Limit cycles have "bounce-back" capacity. When perturbed, they react fast, but just as quickly they then "pull" back to a favored state, suggested by the dashed lines of trajectories in Figure 3.1. So, imagine a gentle poke to a full balloon; its stability is evident in its quick return to its former, unperturbed state.

Stability of oscillations is important because it supports long-term predictability conferred by an *attractor*. Formally, an attractor implicates a region in a phase space to which other states gravitate. One such region surrounds the circular orbit path of certain phase states in Figure 3.1. The thin-lined orbit in this figure, for example, falls under the attractor potential of this limit cycle. Also victims of the pull of the thicker cycle are more remote points in phase space which are shown along the path of other trajectories (dashed converging lines) in this figure.

Finally, an attractor "pull" opposes a "perturbing push" from an single discrete external perturbation as shown in this figure shown in Figure 3.1. These pulls occur in a phase space region near an attractor. This region is termed an *entrainment region* or a *basin of attraction*. For instance, if the larger black dot is mildly pushed off its path, it will land in an entrainment region where attractor stability "pulls" it back to the path. This is a *periodic attractor*, one that, in this case, happens to be defined by phase states with constant angular velocities. An attractor can also be a single phase state, namely a *point attractor* (e.g., the small central black dot in Figure 3.1). In more complex systems, attractors refer to special patterns of angular velocities, or they may exhibit *strange* configurations of phase states (e.g., chaos).

This framework also sets the stage for an interesting type of tension. Whereas a perturbation functions to "push" a system off track, i.e., away from an attractor, the attractor relationship operates in the opposite direction, "pulling" the system back to its path. This amounts to push–pull tension between a perturbing stimulus and its potential attractor state, where the "pull" of stable attractors is expressed as implied velocity trajectories that "point to" attractor states, indicating a goal state. In short, attractors ensure regions of stability within a dynamical system.

Stability is a general feature of attractors. Figure 3.2 shows additional examples of oscillator stability using more complex—but "toy"—biological oscillations. Two stable phase portraits (*top row*) and two unstable ones (*bottom row*) are shown. Implied velocity trajectories (*dashed lines*)

of a single perturbing event (large black dot) are shown "pointing to" their simple (*top left*) or complex (*top right*) periodic attractors (resembling a Van der Pol oscillation). In these examples, converging trajectories connote pulls toward stable limit cycles, whereas diverging trajectories push away (i.e., repel) connoting unstable limit cycles. These distinctions are critical to understanding categorization in later chapters.

An example. Assume that a periodic attractor has several trajectories converging to its orbit. And let the attractor orbit represent a category prototype. For instance, a prototype might be an isochronous rhythm with a 1 second period, meaning it has a circular attractor path in phase space. Trajectories of slightly deviant (i.e., quasi-isochronous) rhythms represent category tokens (e.g., thin black orbit in Figure 3.1). Within the attractor's entrainment region these trajectories converge to the signature, limiting, orbit. Consequently, perceivers judge such quasi-isochronous rhythms to be members (tokens) of the category of isochronous rhythms.[14]

Limit Cycles and Bifurcations

Stability is a very nice property. Yet, even stable limit cycle oscillations can lose stability! In fact, instabilities are interesting because they can spark reorganizations within a phase space and/

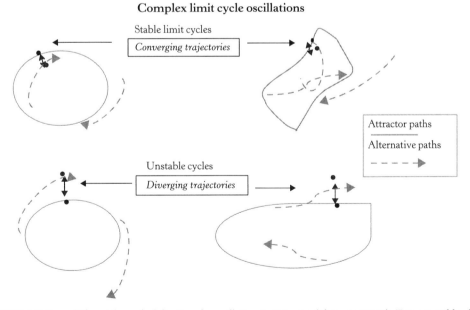

FIGURE 3.2 Four different (complex) limit cycle oscillation trajectories (phase portraits). Two are stable: dashed lines of other (nearby) converging trajectories are pulled toward these (solid line) paths. Two are unstable: diverging (dashed) trajectories. Dots reflect individual moments along a trajectory.

or motivate transitions to new attractor states. As suggested above, some states that are "off-path," but close to an attractor path, are taken to "belong" to the attractor's category. Alternatively, states in phase space remote from a particular attractor cannot "feel its pull." These footloose states are often unstable, eventually following another crowd of trajectories converging to a different attractor. In other words, in the grand playground of a phase space, several attractors with related entrainment regions stake claim to different phase space regions, regions with different sets of converging trajectories.

Entrainment regions of attractors are delineated by *bifurcations* in phase space. Bifurcations are analogous to category boundaries. For instance, the two attractors in Figure 3.1 (period and point attractors) should attract different converging trajectories. Somewhere between these two sets of trajectories an imagery bifurcation line (i.e., not shown) separates these attractor regions. Close to a bifurcation line is an unstable region where states "go either way." To preview later chapters on speech categories, if a bifurcation separates two different phoneme categories, then the psychologist's job is to discover (1) What modulates the pull of a phoneme attractor levied on tokens in this phoneme category (e.g., find a prototype)? And (2) What affects phoneme category boundaries (e.g., identify category bifurcations)?

Bifurcations: Limits of Categories

Bifurcations assume different forms (with catchy names, e.g., Saddle nodes, Andronov-Hopf bifurcations, etc.) with different properties. For instance, saddle node bifurcations may prolong transient instability between two stable (attractor) states, whereas Andronov-Hopf bifurcations are more courteous, often offering transition paths facilitating a flow from one attractor state (a resting state) to another (an oscillator spiking state).

Figure 3.3 shows an Andronov-Hopf bifurcation transition.[15][p.117] Here, a brain oscillation begins in a resting state as a point attractor. Next, it is exposed to external stimulation in the form of a control parameter that moves states as a function of the intensity of an external rhythm (**I,** an injected current, on abscissa). A dependent variable registers momentary system states as excitation levels of a neuron's membrane (in microvolts). As forced changes to the underlying state of this oscillation reach a critical point (e.g., for **I** = 12), a bifurcation is recorded: the resting level of this oscillation suddenly awakens into periodic spiking, indicating arrival of a new, and periodic, attractor.[16] Others supply details.[17,18,19,20]

Summary of Limit Cycle Oscillations

Limit cycle oscillations are the workhorses of a tunable brain. They have periodic attractor orbits with self-sustaining, closed trajectories. A single

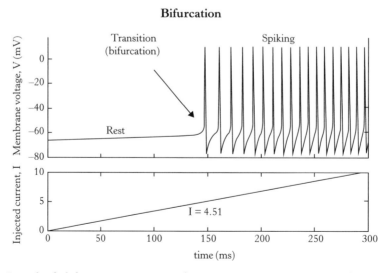

Bifurcation

FIGURE 3.3 Example of a bifurcation as a transition from a resting state to a repetitive spiking state (upper graph) as a function of injected ramp current I (lower graph). Note that the initial spike frequency is slow but becomes faster as the injected current increases.

Reprinted from Eugene M. Izhikevich, *Dynamical Systems in Neuroscience: The Geometry of Excitability and Bursting* (Cambridge, MA: MIT Press, 2006; figure 4.33). By permission of the MIT Press.

perturbation of such an oscillation by an external force (e.g., a sudden auditory or visual stimulus) evokes both a reactive phase adaptation and a fleeting amplitude increase of the oscillation. By contrast, regularly repeated perturbations create a driving rhythm and induced expectancies. Generally, limit cycle oscillations have stability, conferred by attractors, that portends new interpretations of categories and their boundaries.

Major points of this section are:

- *Neural oscillations* are defined by frequency, amplitude, and phase, formally expressed in a two-dimensional phase space as a phase portrait.
- *Limit cycle oscillations* are characterized by phase-adaptive, self-sustaining, and stable behaviors associated with periodic attractors.
- *Amplitude of a limit cycle oscillation* is briefly responsive to a single perturbation (i.e., an evoked response), a rapid reactive energy burst that returns to a limit cycle attractor.
- *Amplitude of a limit cycle oscillation* in other contexts can increase gradually in response to stimulus regularities.
- *Stability of limit cycle oscillations* depends on an attractor that "pulls" trajectories in phase space toward a delimited region in phase space.
- *Bifurcations* divide a phase space into different attractor regions.

DANCING DYADS

The brain is awash with rhythms. These are related to neural waveforms of different limit cycle oscillations. Moreover, those rhythmic interactions that involve two limit cycle oscillations form a fundamental entrainment unit: the *driving–driven dyad*. The adaptive properties of such oscillations, which involve adjustments of phase, period, and sometimes amplitude, glue together two oscillations into a synchronized *endogenous dyad*. In other words, endogenous dyads showcase the brain's self-tuning activity. The brain is an inherently self-tuning organ based on oscillator synchronies.

This section describes the emergence of synchronies in many and varied endogenous dyads. To understand the pertinent dynamical contexts, we must face the fact that the relevant phase space for dyads is more complex than that of a single limit cycle (e.g., Figure 3.1). It has more than two dimensions.[21] Hence, the relevant phase portrait for a dyad must also change. A dyad expresses oscillator interactions. Often the changing phase

relations between two such intersecting circular paths are traced out along a donut configuration where the faster oscillation winds about the slower one within an enlarged three dimensional phase space. Figure 3.4 shows a phase-portrait of such a configuration where the two limit cycle oscillations observe an attractor relationship based upon their time relations; thus, one period ($n = 1$) of the slow oscillation covers four periods of the faster one ($m = 4$). Unfortunately, often donut (and more complex) configurations provoke painful head-scratching in many readers. It is also possible to convey the gist of such dyadic interactions more simply—as a dance[22].

Attractors and Oscillator Synchrony

When two cortical oscillations interact, they create synchronies that resemble the timing of a *pas-de-deux* performed by two dancers. For instance, when a leading dancer produces a particular tempo (i.e., a recurring period), the other dancer may follow by exactly matching this tempo while gradually adjusting the phase of each step to coincide, over time, with steps of the leading dancer. Eventually, the two dancing periods synchronize, as gauged by a minimum of calibrated phase differences. This may happen, for instance, when the number of cycles of leading dancer, n, exactly equals the number of cycles, m, of the following dancer (i.e., $n{:}m = 1{:}1$). Similarly, if a leading dancer steps twice as fast as his partner but retains a small fixed-phase difference, then this dancing dyad preserves a rational periodic relationship of $n{:}m = 2{:}1$. Specifically, n is the number of cycles of a driving rhythm and m the number of driven

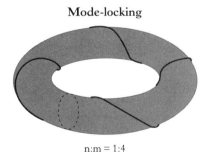

Mode-locking

n:m = 1:4

FIGURE 3.4 Phase space of a two coupled oscillators. Two limit cycle oscillations endogenously couple to form a doughnut manifold. A driving neural oscillation is the slower oscillation which mode-locks with a faster, driven oscillation, that supplies a pattern of phase-locking within the slower rhythm. This results in a phase space formulated as product of two circles expressing a n:m attractor relationship of 1:4.

rhythm cycles. When n and m are commensurate integers, opportunities for synchrony are high, especially for simple $n:m$ ratios (i.e., low variance of phase differences, $\Delta\varphi$). And returning to the donut configuration of Figure 3.4, the dyadic relationship here follows an attractor based upon an $n:m = 1:4$ driving: driven relationship.

A dyadic attractor then is often simply expressed as a ratio of oscillator periods (i.e., $n:m$). Specifically, an $n:m$ ratio is an attractor whenever n cycles of a driving rhythm equal m cycles of a driven period. More formally, any qualifying $n:m$ ratio defines a synchronous *attractor mode* which may be more or less complex. Nevertheless, these relationships define a goal state of synchrony to which a dynamic system moves.

Entrainment is all about the many modes of synchrony. Thus, the goal of a dancing dyad is synchrony. To achieve this goal, oscillator dyads must gravitate to a synchronous state. Two limit cycle oscillations that do not initially exhibit a commensurate $n:m$ will eventually gravitate to their nearest rational $n:m$ ratio by adapting their phases and/or periods. In a dance scenario, for instance, each dancer's stepping period and phase shift is pulled toward synchronizing these motions with his or her partner. Such a goal may involve quite simple attractors, such as $n:m = 1:1$ or $2:1$, or more complex ones, such as $n:m = 1:10$ or $5:8$. Synchronous modes vary in complexity along a continuum from *low-order synchronies*, with simplest ratios (e.g., $n:m = 1:1, 1:2, 1:3, 1:4 \dots$), to complex *high-order synchronies* (e.g., $n:m = 3:4, 2:5, 5:8 \dots$).

The synchronizing quality of attractors is recognized in *mode-locking* of neural oscillations. That is, mode-locking brain relationships are no longer mathematical abstractions; contemporary neuroscience has provided real glimpses into these tunable brain activities. Box 3.2 shows familiar EEG/magnetoencephalography (MEG) categories of neural oscillations registered as electrical brain activity in scalp electrodes. More invasive electrodes involve subdural electrode brain implacements (electrocorticography [ECoG]); these electrodes are applied to different cortical levels (i.e., laminal analyses) in human patients, monkeys, and even rats.

Simple Endogenous Entrainment Depends on Simple Attractors

Let's begin with simple dyads involving oscillations with different, but similar, frequencies. For instance, in the *pas de deux*, let the leader have a stepping frequency of 2 Hz (a 500 ms period). Imagine that his partner, after watching and nodding to this tempo, follows suit at almost the same rate but slightly out-of-phase. Nevertheless, the powerful "pull" of a simple attractor (i.e., $n:m$ is 1:1) quickens the partner's phase corrections, leading to dyadic synchrony where the two periods match, and the phase differences ($\Delta\varphi$) of the steps are minimized.

Oscillator Frequencies, Simple Attractors, and Attractor Categories

Next, replace this observable *pas de deux* of humans with an unobservable neural analog: two dancing brain oscillations (labeled O_1, O_2) with different, but similar, intrinsic frequencies ($\omega_{o1} \sim \omega_{o2}$). Each frequency/velocity leads to a limit cycle oscillation with a near sinusoidal waveform (cf. Figure 3.1). Specifically, the periods of these two oscillations entrain, creating *loosely coupled oscillations,* where both oscillations have moderate amplitudes. Finally, assume that one oscillation, here O_2, functions as a driving rhythm.[23] Of primary interest is the way frequencies of loosely coupled oscillations achieve the binding goal of synchrony.

Figure 3.5 shows how this happens when oscillations have related, but different, intrinsic frequencies. The goal of dyadic synchrony is attained with period adjustments of the driven oscillation, O_1.[24] This oscillation has an intrinsic period of 9 ms (110 Hz), which comes to match the 10 ms period (100 Hz) of the O_2 driving rhythm. The initial *detuning difference* between oscillations vanishes as the manifest period of O_1, denoted by p', automatically comes to match the latent period of O_2 (10 ms). This leads to frequency-locking in which the n cycles of O_2 equals the m manifest cycles of O_1. Thus, the synchronous goal of $n:m = 1:1$ is achieved.

There is a beguiling aspect to the adaptivity shown in Figure 3.5. A driven oscillation changes its *manifest frequency* (dashed line) to match the frequency of O_2. However, the intrinsic (*latent*) frequencies of both oscillations remain unchanged. This aspect of limit cycle adaptations is important because it is the fleeting manifest versions of adaptive oscillations that we usually observe. Here, notations alert us to these differences. Thus, an oscillation's manifest frequency is denoted as Ω whereas its latent value is ω_o.[25] And a manifest period becomes p' (vs. the latent period, p). Typically, electrical recordings of neural oscillations reflect manifest frequencies/periods (i.e., Ω) at resting levels, $\Omega = \omega_o$.

In addition to showcasing devilishly interesting manifest frequencies, this example also illustrates effects of an attractor pull. Whenever

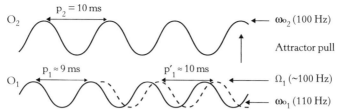

FIGURE 3.5 Two (hypothetical sinewave) cortical oscillations (Oi) are shown with instant latent frequencies of 100 Hz (for ω_{o1}) and ~110 Hz (for ω_{o2}). The faster, weaker oscillation (O_1) *adapts* its manifest frequency (Ω) over time to approximate the slower driving oscillation (ω_{o1}). This manifest frequency (dashed line) is pulled to temporally expand the manifest period, p' of the latent oscillation (9 ms) to a period closer to the period, p_2 = 10 ms of the endogenous driving rhythm, O_2. Note that latent frequency of O_1 remains unchanged.

two oscillations deviate slightly from a nearby attractor, as is the case here, the adaptive pull toward this attractor (here *n:m* = 1:1) motivates emergence of manifest frequencies that yield synchrony in the form of frequency-locking.

Oscillator Amplitudes

An oscillator's amplitude reflects its overall strength. However, amplitude also plays a coordinating role in interactions of cortical oscillations. Although two independent oscillations spontaneously wander as the strength of one increases relative to that of another, a potential for dependency via phase coupling arises, particularly if oscillations have related frequencies. With loosely coupled oscillations, dyadic entrainment is influenced by driving rhythm amplitude: *as driving rhythm strength (amplitude) increases so does entrainment of the driven rhythm to the driving rhythm.*

Figure 3.6 shows three ways in which a driving rhythm's amplitude might figure in dyadic interactions among oscillations (labeled as O_1, O_2) that differ only slightly in intrinsic frequencies (ω_{oi} values). Panel a shows both oscillations adjusting their frequencies (equal manifest shifts in Ω_i) because their amplitudes are identical. Panel b hypothesizes an asymmetrical relationships where the O_2 oscillation, with greater amplitude, pulls more on the manifest frequency (Ω_1) of O_1. Panel c, shows that a strong oscillation may force a complete (but temporary) change in the manifest frequency of O_1 to match that of O_2 which is its intrinsic frequency (ω_{o2}).

These hypothetical pairs involve the role of the amplitude of an endogenous driving rhythm on frequency locking. However, they also raise a related question regarding amplitude. Does driving rhythm amplitude also affect the amplitude of the driven rhythm? Surprisingly, for driving

oscillations of modest amplitudes, a standard answer has been "No." Entrainment principles appear to deny such dependency.[26] *Entrainment of weakly coupled oscillations derives from increased amplitude (strength) of a driving rhythm that enhances phase coupling of its driven rhythm, but this coupling* does not *affect the amplitude of the driven oscillation.*

Cross-Frequency Couplings: Complex Attractors

Dyadic entrainment dances of the preceding section were limited to attractors based on simple frequency relationships (e.g., modes of *n:m* = 1:1, 1:2 etc.). Such "look-alike" oscillations hook up fairly effortlessly. However, recent discoveries show that tunable brains are filled with cortical oscillations that boast more complex relationships. Of special interest are dyads featuring wide frequency differences, termed *cross-frequency couplings* (CFCs).

From an entrainment perspective, CFC dyads engage complex attractors. Consider, for instance, a CFC dyad with a fast neural rhythm, termed a *gamma oscillation* (e.g., 52 Hz), that couples with a much slower theta (e.g., 5 Hz) oscillation. The nearest attractor is complex, as *n:m* = 1:10. As the frequency difference between two oscillations increases, so does the complexity of the nearest attractor. And, synchronous mode-locking also becomes more complex with CFC dyads.[27] And, adding complexity to complexity, recordings of spontaneous brain activities suggest that, with CFC dyads, amplitudes of coupled oscillations may correlate. In other words, CFC dyads do not qualify as *loosely coupled oscillations*. Although the prevalence of such dyads complicates the entrainment story, it commands theoretical generality.

Endogenous Dyads:
Two interacting oscillations

Two intrinsic frequencies: Small (detuning) differences

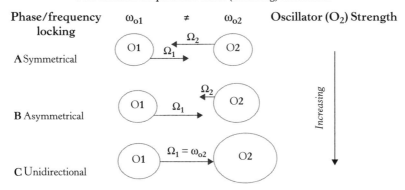

FIGURE 3.6 A schematic of three pairs of oscillations in which intrinsic frequencies (ω_{oi}) reflect small differences, (detuning) differences between oscillations within each pair (rows a,b,c). Amplitudes of the two oscillations in each pair differ, however. With identical amplitudes (symmetrical), adaptive changes in manifest frequencies (Ωi) of each oscillation in a pair are symmetrical. But, as amplitudes within an endogenous dyad differ, greater changes in frequency are hypothesized for the weaker oscillation of a pair, thus leading to unidirectional changes of the manifest frequency of O_1 with its manifest frequency temporally pulled toward the stronger O_2 oscillation.

A succinct review of CFC research by Colgin and Jensen outlines a range of possible neural couplings.[28] Figure 3.7 indicates several different CFC dyads, all involving a slow theta oscillation and a fast gamma oscillation that "link up" via correlations between participating oscillations that involve frequency, phase, and amplitude/power. To illustrate, the following sections focus on two CFC correlations shown in Figure 3.7: one entails phase relationships, the other illustrates phase and amplitude relationships.

Oscillator Phase Relationships in CFC Dyads

A CFC dyad, by definition, combines a slow oscillation with a much faster one. From an entrainment perspective, such dyads are governed by pulls from a nearby complex attractor. Although CFC oscillations follow a more complex dance than do simpler attractors, these complex attractors continue to do what all good attractors do: they afford a goal of synchrony. In theory, these couplings reflect synchronous mode-locking: $n\omega_{oi} = m\omega_{oj}$. In practice, their synchrony is manifest as $n\Omega i \approx m\Omega j$.

Importantly, mode-locking of two very different frequencies follows a generalized phase formulation: $\Delta\varphi_{n,m} = n\varphi_1 - m\varphi_2$. Effectively, mode-locking synchronies enable stable phase relationships between oscillations. The result is

the *phase-to-phase coupling* of Figure 3.7 (panels A and C). Thus, in panel A, a slow-frequency (8 Hz, theta range) couples with a faster oscillation (32 Hz, gamma range) in panel C. This is classic phase coupling based on an *n:m* attractor mode of 1:4 (.25). The dancing dyad of this *pas de deux* neatly fits four short steps of a fast oscillation within each long step of the slower oscillation.

Other support for complex mode-locking couplings involving frequency relations derives from MEG datacollected by Palva et al. They found CFC couplings (*n:m* = 1:2, 1:3, 1:4) in alpha, beta, and gamma ranges (2–80 Hz).[29] Similarly, Holz et al.[30] reported complex mode-locking between a slow theta oscillation (6 Hz) and a fast gamma oscillation (60 Hz; *n:m* = 1:10) recorded as EEGs in parietal-occipital brain regions (cf. Womerlsdorf et al.[31,32]).

In sum, tantalizing evidence confirms the reality of higher order synchronies in dyads comprising neural oscillations with very different CFC frequencies. The role of complex attractors that instill mode-locked synchronies is often overlooked in describing phase-locking. Yet, there are two good reasons to entertain this interpretation. First, from an entrainment perspective, two originally independent limit cycle oscillations, when simultaneously active, *do naturally gravitate* (in frequency) to nearby attractors. Second, even oscillations with very

Cross Frequency Coupling (CFC) types

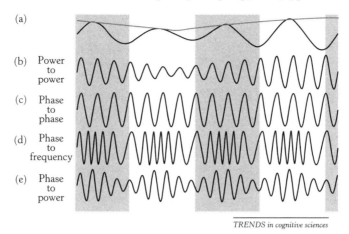

FIGURE 3.7 Five examples of cross-frequency coupling (CFC) entrainments among neural oscillations. Reprint of figure 1 (p. 208) in an article by Ole Jensen and Laura L. Colgin, "Cross-Frequency Coupling Between Neuronal Oscillations," *Trends in Cognitive Sciences* 2007.05.003.

different frequencies (complex attractors) adjust manifest frequencies and phase when pulled by an attractor. [33,34]

Oscillator Amplitudes in CFC Dyads

Complex CFC dyads not only comprise vastly different oscillator frequencies, the two oscillations of a CFC dyad also usually differ in amplitudes (power). Figure 3.7 illustrates one complex CFC dyad that expresses a *phase-to-power correlation* between the theta oscillation's phase (panel A) and the gamma oscillation's amplitude (panel E). Also shown are power-to-power correlations; that is, driving–driven amplitude correlations happen between interacting oscillations (panels A, B).

Evidence for these correlations in the human brain has been reported by Canolty and colleagues.[35,36] Specifically, they used ECoG recordings[37] to tap into CFC interactions of a slow theta (4–8 Hz) rhythm aligning with fast gamma (80–150 Hz) oscillations in the brains of human epileptics. Results appear in Figure 3.8 Panel A shows positions of grid for registering of (MRI) and ECOG in frontal and temporal lobes. A time-frequency plot (panel B) reveals a robust correlation of gamma amplitudes (*top*) with theta phase (*bottom*) suggesting *phase-to-amplitude* coupling in which higher gamma amplitudes happen at theta phases with low amplitudes (μV in panel B, *bottom*). This dovetails with the phase-to-power configuration of Figure 3.7 (panels A, E).

Another important finding of Canolty and Knight confirms power-to-power relationships

of CFC dyads (panels A, B; Figure 3.8). They discovered that the *amplitude of a slow theta driving rhythm is correlated with amplitudes of the fast driven gamma rhythm!* Others report similar findings.[38] Such discoveries strengthen claims that entraining CFC oscillations do not behave as loosely coupled dyads that forbid such correlations.

Finally, Canolty and Knight hypothesized that oscillator correlations result from people's repeated exposure to gamma-plus-theta oscillations. However, this explanation overlooks people's mode-locking tendencies involving oscillator frequencies. That is, CFC paradigms often hide ratios of complex attractors that implicate higher order synchronies.[39] Others also call for closer examinations of frequency/phase variables in these paradigms. For instance, Roopun and colleagues[40[p.148]] describe EEG records in various CFC tasks where "it is possible to discern stable phase relationships between different frequencies" (see also Schyns, Thut, and Gross[41]).

Theoretical Approaches to Complex Endogenous Dyads

Theoretically, what functions are served by CFC couplings? These provocative dyads spark several not mutually exclusive answers. Some explanations are confined to physiological causations. For instance, Colgin and Jenson suggest that CFCs derive from modulated cell excitability (amplitudes) of gamma oscillations by slower theta oscillations. Others appeal to communicative functions between

Cross Frequency Coupling.
Experimental Details and Results

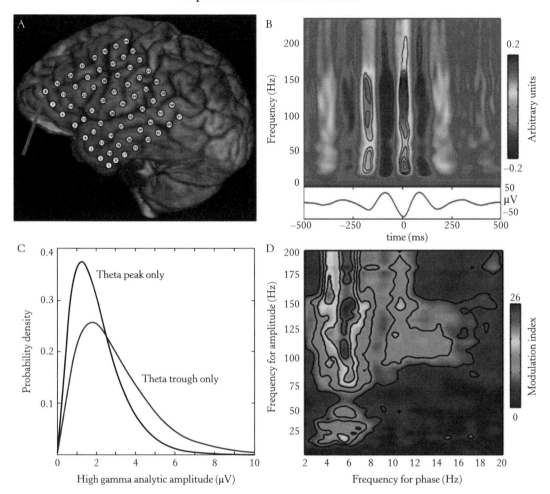

FIGURE 3.8 Details of procedure and results of experiment of Canolty, Knight, and colleagues (2006). High-gamma (80–150 Hz) power is modulated by theta (4–8 Hz) phase. (**A**) Structural magnetic resonance imaging (MRI) showing position of 64-channel (see arrow) electroencephalogram (ECoG) grid over frontal and temporal lobes. (**B**) Example of phase-locked modulation of power in ECoG signal from anterior portion of the middle frontal gyrus (arrow in Fig. 1A). (*Top*) Time–frequency plot of mean power modulation time-locked to the theta trough. Outermost contour indicates statistical significance ($P < 0.001$, corrected). Normalization permits comparison across frequencies; ligher and darker (see right index) regions reflect, respectively, increments and decrements in power relative to the mean power. (*Bottom*) Theta trough-locked average of raw ECoG signal. (**C**) Best-fit gamma distributions for the high-gamma analytic amplitude values of peak (darker; 0 radians) or the trough (lighter, π radians) of the theta waveform as in **B**. (**D**) The modulation index (25) as a function of analytic amplitude (5–200 Hz) and analytic phase (2–20 Hz) for the same electrode as in **B**. Outermost contour indicates statistical significance ($P < 0.001$, corrected). Larger values indicate stronger cross-frequency coupling.

1Reprint of figure 1 from R. T. Canolty et al., "High Gamma Power Is Phase-Locked to Theta Oscillations in Human Neocortex," *Science* 313, no. 5793 (September 15, 2006): 1626–28, doi:10.1126/science.1128115.

remote brain regions because the low-frequency CFC oscillations cover longer distances.[42] Communication here refers to one brain region "talking" to another spatially segregated region. "Talking" may be statistically formalized, as suggested by Canolty and Knight. Thus, a phase/amplitude CFC becomes "a statistical dependence between the phase of a low frequency brain rhythm and the amplitude (or power) of the high frequency component of electrical brain activity."[43][p.507] However, such explanations ignore relational timing constraints, instead granting causality to the mere co-occurrence of any phase with any amplitude.

Pascal Fries[44] offers a different view in his influential *communication through coherence hypothesis*.[45,46] Following pioneering work of Wolf Singer on synchronous feature binding, Fries features a major communicative role for phase relationships, including phase-locking patterns that "telegraph" coherent rhythmic messages between brain regions. Finally, entrainment theories go a step farther along this theoretical path in specifying communications based on synchronies among oscillations, even oscillations in widely separated brain regions. Admittedly, CFC entrainment models become complicated, but so do observed brain rhythms.[47,48,49,50]

Summary of Dancing Dyads

This section illustrates how pairs of oscillations—namely, endogenous driving–driven dyads—function as basic entrainment units. It explores various dependencies between limit cycle oscillations that create dyads. In particular, simple and complex dyads are distinguished largely by frequency dependencies related to attractors. Yet both types of dyads enlist entrainment principles to achieve synchronous modes of coupling driving with driven oscillations.

Application of entrainment principles is most straightforward in simple dyads involving similar frequencies, hence simple attractors. In such dyads, loosely coupled oscillations connect through frequency and phase-locking. By contrast, dyads with complex attractors exhibit CFC arising from interactions of quite different frequencies that implicate complex attractors. Also oscillator amplitudes play respectively different roles in simple versus complex dyads. The main points of this section are:

- *Dyads with similar frequencies* and simple attractors (e.g., *n:m* = 1.1) form loosely coupled oscillations with moderate amplitude levels. Frequency- and phase-locking occur, but driving rhythm amplitudes do not affect the amplitude of a driven rhythm.
- *Dyads with very different frequencies* (CFC dyads) invite complex attractors (e.g., *n:m* ≠ 1:1) which allow for complex synchronization. Yet with high-amplitude levels these dyadic entrainments are not characteristic of entrainments of loosely coupled oscillations.

MULTIPLE OSCILLATIONS: RANDOM OR STRUCTURED DYNAMICS?

"The human system in general, and the perceptual system in particular depend upon the properties of endogenous rhythmic processes in the nervous system. These rhythms differ in frequency and may increase or decrease in amplitude within a given frequency." [51][p.328]

So, how does this work? We are only beginning to probe the mysteries of multiple unit activities in a tunable brain. This section examines the origins and nature of such configurations. If these units are vibrating things (i.e., rhythms), then we must imagine how the dyadic couplings of previous sections operate within larger configurations of many endogenous brain rhythms. As a whole, such brain activity may seem random due to much, seemingly mysterious, spontaneous oscillator activity. But, just as the turbulence of boiling water only *seems* random, it is also the case that the seeming chaos of spontaneous brain oscillations, on closer inspection, hides structured clusters of oscillatory units as dynamically choreographed dances involving three, five, or hundreds of limit cycle brain oscillations. This envisions larger configurations of synchronizing oscillations. A motivating idea in this section holds that these oscillator groups are intrinsically configured not only by topological proximities within brain regions, but also by special time relationships. Here, we peek into an inner world of self-tuning cortical oscillations with timing relationships in mind. And, in addition, this also assumes that external the driving rhythms of environmental events play a minor role. As Buzsaki,[52,53] among others,[54] suggests, the brain's inner timing consists of spontaneous neural activity that variously shapes our intrinsic biases.[55,56,57]

Clearly, extended neural configurations must arise from selective operations (i.e., constraints) that govern both the inclusion of some neural units and the exclusion of other neural units in the formation of multiunit configurations. Three broad categories of selective constraints are *primitive brain topology, neuron physiology*, and *entrainment/resonance principles*.[58]

Primitive Structures and Spontaneous Oscillator Configurations

If, as some argue, the brain at birth is not a blank slate, then what is it?[59] How do newborns, seemingly effortlessly, begin to "tune in" to their booming, buzzing, new world? Instead of randomness or blank slates, let us image that some sort of innate bootstrapping mechanism has evolved that prepares infants to automatically orient to novel, species-relevant sights and sounds. Along these lines, perhaps during gestation, an infant's groups of spontaneous brain oscillations cluster into certain primitive structures. These oscillations begin to selectively engage in self-tuning adaptive activities involving the interactions of multiple oscillations. Instead of a blank slate, let us entertain a more interesting assumption: namely, that *primitive neural configurations* form at, or likely before, birth.

Brain configurations involve groups of vibrating neural units fleshed out as limit cycle oscillations.[60] Broadly speaking, such configurations arise from at least three kinds of constraints. One involves physiological/topological constraints on neural units that shape *frequency gradients*. Other candidates for constraints entail synaptic connection properties found in *conventional connective networks*. A third type of constraint appeals to frequency relationships among neural oscillations that can lead to *synchronized oscillator groupings of various sorts*. Finally, although learning due to exposure frequency undeniably contributes to shaping extended neural configurations, by definition it does not qualify as an innate constraint. Hence, learning is discussed in later chapters.

Frequency Gradients: Architectural and Growth Curve Constraints

A frequency gradient is an important primitive oscillator configuration. Such a gradient corresponds to the topology within a brain region containing multiple neural units spatially distributed along one, two, or three dimensions. Typically, spatial adjacencies between neighboring units

offer strongest gradient connections. Biologically, the emergence of a primitive gradient topology can be attributed to the remarkable rapidity of spontaneous cell divisions in a fetus at conception, which determine the corresponding narrow spacing of units—spacing that widens as growth rate slows.

Spiral Gradients

Although linear spatial gradients are the simplest gradients, curvilinear gradients cannot be ruled out. The latter include two-dimensional rings or three-dimension helixes. Watts and Strogatz[61] proposed rings of neural nodes, later transforming these into the rings/hubs of limit cycle oscillations.[62] As a primitive topological structure, rings exploit spatial proximities between units based on path length between loci.

Spiral gradients also emerge from growth curves. For instance, applying a slowing growth rate to a three-dimensional helix (i.e., including neural brain layers) creates rotating (angular) velocities with dilating oscillator periods, thus leading to a logarithmic spiral or *spira mirabilis*.[63] As growth patterns, logarithmic spirals are ubiquitous in nature (e.g., the nautilus seashell of Figure 3.9). This spiral is famous for its expression of a recursive succession of oscillator frequencies, namely the *Fibonacci sequence*, regulated by the "golden mean" ratio ($\varphi = 1.61803\ldots.$).

Hypotheses about primitive gradients remain to be fleshed out. However, it is interesting that even macaque monkeys exhibit spontaneous tonotopic neural gradients (in their auditor cortex) when responding to different pure tones.[64] Perhaps more telling are related findings that these gradients were curvilinear.

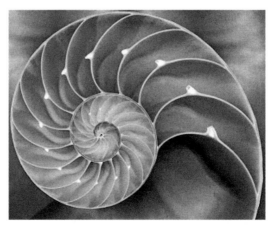

FIGURE 3.9 Depiction of nautilus shell resulting from a logarithmic spiral growth curve.

Connective Networks: Synaptic Constraints
Prominent psychological theories often feature
broad networks of connected neural units, termed
nodes. Typically, selection of the *N* nodes included in a network depends on relative strengths
of internode connections conferred by synaptic
constraints and reinforcements (e.g., exposure
frequency). Such networks are highly popular
for their success in depicting local and global
interactions among nodes in various brain regions.[65] Importantly, network nodes are typically
not conceived as limit cycle oscillations; hence,
node connections do not afford synchrony. These
networks are referred to as *strict* connectionist
networks.

Strict connectionist models typically attribute
connective selectivity among groups of nodes to
two properties: synaptic connection strength
and connective mappings of units. Connection
strength depends on the neurochemistry between a pre-synaptic spiking neuron and a
post-synaptic neuron capable of spiking (e.g.,
gamma-aminobutyric acid [$GABA_A$]; see
Whittington et al. 2000[66]). Specific connective
mapping simply limits *N*, the number of network
nodes.[67,68,69,70,71]

Dynamically Structured Oscillator Groups: Resonance and Entrainment

Dynamic attending models feature groupings
based on synchrony. Unlike strict connection
models, they view nodes as limit cycle oscillations
that can synchronize with other oscillations to
form larger oscillator groups. In fact, synchrony
based on phase-locking is possible across widely
scattered spatial units, as demonstrated by Goel
and Ermentrout,[72] and others.[73,74,75,76,77]

From a DAT perspective, primitive oscillator
configurations arise from *resonance* and *entrainment* constraints. Resulting group members "belong" together by virtue of their synchronizing
potentials. Synchrony depends on entrainment,
which, in turn, relies on resonance supplied by oscillator activities.

Resonance turns out to be essential to the
success of strict connectionist networks (although
this is rarely recognized). Izhikevich and colleagues
demonstrated this using a special (burst) oscillation as a pre-synaptic neuron (i.e., node).[78] They
discovered that a spike burst from this neuron,
designed to stimulate a post-synaptic neuron, selectively activates *only post-synaptic neurons that
resonate to the spiking rate of the pre-synaptic
neuron, regardless of other synaptic properties.* This
is important. It demonstrates the broad power of

resonance in boosting the amplitude of a driven
oscillation.

Entrainment principles are also important. Minimally, they specify phase-locking
among active oscillations as a source of connectivity. Selective entrainment of different pairs of
oscillating units depends on whether or not their
frequency ratios all "point to" the same nearby attractor ratio. As with resonance, the entrainment
concept of an attractor pull, as applied to frequency
relationships between pre- and post-synaptic network units, also influences unit connectivity.

To assess this, Hoppensteadt and Izhikevich[79]
modeled physiological links among neural units
scattered over the thalamo-cortical brain region. Frequency relationships among these units
were cleverly manipulated. And, the results were
stunning. Modeling revealed that two neural units
only interact if their frequency ratios approximate
a rational (i.e., attractor) value. They conclude: "In
a sense, weakly connected cortical oscillators employ an FM radio principle: Frequency encodes
the channel of communication, while phase
modulations encode the information to be
transmitted by the channel."[80][p.92] In other words,
we "tune in" to a particular "beat period" (frequency), then listen for different time patterns
(phase changes) within successive periods.

Emphasis on resonance and entrainment does
not deny the relevance of synapse physiology
in determining connection strength. Rather, it
suggests that physiology *alone* fails to support
neural grouping. Indeed, the chemistry of synaptic physiology contributes to energy levels of
neuronal oscillations. This is evident, for instance,
in parameters of the honored Hodgkin-Huxley
model, which preserves a neuron's status as an
entrainable oscillation while incorporating biological constraints on membrane potential and synaptic chemistry.[81] In brief, network models succeed
when they recognize *both* the right synaptic chemistry and resonant-plus-entraining properties of
oscillatory neurons. Conversely, network models
fail if either property is excluded.

Finally, acknowledging that the primitive
structure of oscillator collections is governed
by resonance and entrainment constraints has
advantages. First, connections among oscillations
are specifically conceived in terms of phase- and
frequency-locking that can operate automatically. Second, coupling among several oscillations
is governed by innate species-specific attractors.
Third, attractors differ in complexity, leading to
testable hypothesis about the role of attractors in
formation of groups as categories.

BOX 3.2
EEG CATEGORIES OF OSCILLATIONS

Category		Category Predictions $f(d_n)$			
Frequency category	Hz	Period (ms)		Bandwidth (center) a	
Very high frequencies	>150 Hz	<6.67 ms			
High frequencies	12–150 Hz	Period (ms)	B_L	Bandwidth (Hz)	B_U
Gamma high	50–110	20–9.09	64.7	(80)	98.9
Beta	12–50	83.3–20	16.18	(25)	32.4
Low frequencies	1–12 Hz				
Alpha 8–12	125–83.3	8.09	(10)	12.4	
Theta	4–8	250–125	4.05	(5)	6.18
Delta	1–4	1,000–250	1.21	(2.5)	3.09
Very low frequencies	<.01Hz	> 100 seconds		$f(d_n) = S \times 2^n$ ($s = 1.25$ Hz)	

aB_L, B_U depend, respectively, on phi: $f(d_n) +/- [1.62 \times = f(d_n)]$

From Klimesch (2013).[104]

Oscillator Categories

Psychology has long recognized certain groups of oscillatory frequencies. These groups have familiar names, like alpha and beta rhythms, and the like. The conventional categories of neural frequencies, as summarized in Box 3.2, represent groups of recorded EEG frequencies. Often these categories are assigned a function (rightly or wrongly).[82] For instance, the category of high gamma frequencies might be linked to sensory responses associated with fine-grained (spectral) stimulation,[83] whereas beta frequencies may serve a motor function.[84,85] Delta rhythms long languished under the label of "sleep rhythms" until they awakened to a new life entraining to slow external time patterns. Similarly, strong alpha rhythms with a widespread cortical EEG resting signal traditionally served a "cortical idling," function, whereas their recent function is seen as an inhibitory force in entrainment tasks.[86,87]

Although functional descriptions can be helpful, they tend to obscure an arguably more important function concerning the role of entrainments in the formation of endogenous brain configurations. A central function of oscillator frequencies is to promote connections between various oscillations; this means connecting one oscillation to another and/or forming larger configurations involving many oscillations united by some selective mechanism.

One approach to connecting neural oscillations into larger configurations builds on the idea of oscillatory hierarchies. Compelling examples of this are found in the research of David Poeppel and his colleagues. For instance, Giraud and Poeppel argue for a principle relationship between neural oscillations in speech. The selective mechanism here involves the embedding (nesting) of bands of faster oscillations, such as low gamma (25–35 Hz) in the range of phonemes, which become nested within slower oscillations of theta (4–8 Hz) and delta (1–3 Hz) in the ranges of words and phrases. Giraud and Poeppel propose that "speech onsets trigger cycles of neuronal encoding at embedded syllabic and phonemic scales."[88]

With respect to embeddings of neural oscillations, we might go further to consider that these connections are strengthened by various attractor relationships among nested oscillations. As special ($n{:}m$) states of synchrony, attractors can unite pairs of similar oscillations to form a category signified by the frequency relationships of oscillator pairs that approximate an n:m attractor. For an analogous hierarchical example, in music, it is easy to hear attractors as harmonic relationships based on special frequency ratios among a several frequencies (e.g., 200, 400, 600, 800 Hz, etc.). In speech, more complex relationships across different frequencies are likely to emerge. The basic idea is that each member of a pair of sounds elicits a resonating neural oscillation in a listener. In this musical example, most pairs will sound rather pleasant if their neural counterparts are simply related (e.g., by an n:m of 1:1 for a unison and 1:2 of an octave).

However, even a slightly mistuned octave (e.g., a ratio of 1:2.2) is recognized as belonging to the octave category. It may sound "off" or mistuned, but an inner "pull" allows inclusion in the octave group. Pairs of oscillations that *just approximate* a compelling attractor ratio nonetheless are perceived as belonging to that attractor category. Following previous distinctions surrounding limit cycle oscillations, various *n:m* pairs of oscillations may all belong to a group/category in the entrainment region of the same attractor. The attractors which spell out these categories realize different rational ratios (e.g., 1:3, 1:4). Attractors, simple or complex, function as selective mechanisms for including neural units in larger brain configurations.

In terms of still larger configurations, whole sets of frequencies belong to EEG categories, as envisioned by Klimesch et al.[89,90,91] Furthermore, Klimesch proposes an elegant algorithm for creating nested categories (i.e., categories within categories) forming larger oscillator configurations. The latter emerges from relationships among the *center frequencies*, f (dn), of many smaller categorical groups of brain oscillations. This is shown in Box 3.2. Frequencies are cast as members of different harmonic configurations in:

$$f(\text{dn}) = s \times 2^n \left(\text{for } n = 0, 1, 2, 3 \ldots \right) \qquad 3.1$$

Each category's center frequency depends on a crafted multiple of a scaling value, **s**.[92] Equation 3.1 spells out constraints for inclusion in a larger configuration of oscillations comprising all related center frequencies (e.g., Hz: 2.5, 5, 10 Hz, etc.) for categories known, respectively, as delta, theta, and so forth (n = 1, 2, 4, etc.). Together, the harmonies specified in the larger configuration form an *oscillatory hierarchy*.

Inclusive Selectivity: Rational Ratios

The group inclusion rule for the larger, hierarchical configuration is seen in Equation 3.1, a constraint not found in conventional networks. From a DAT perspective, this rule implies that oscillations, as neural units, endogenously entrain with other oscillations thereby connecting on the basis of oscillatory frequencies, specifically frequency ratios.[93,94] And the rational frequency ratios that support such endogenous entrainments function as attractors that guarantee (often pleasing) synchronies.

Exclusive Selectivity: A Dash of Irrationality

The central frequency ratios of these categories function as attractors because the inclusion rule of

Equation 3.1 grants synchrony. Logically, then, this rule implies that limits, as category boundaries, should deny synchrony by excluding oscillations that fail to synchronize with other category members. Indeed, category boundaries are defined by very irrational frequency ratios. Basically, these boundaries reflect bifurcations that repel (i.e., exclude) oscillator pairs. As *irrational frequency ratios*, they deny synchrony. Metaphorically, a tunable brain will "sing" harmonically with rational frequency ratios that deliver prized synchronicity, but not with irrational frequency ratios that threaten desynchronization.

These are new and intriguing ideas. Klimesch and colleagues[95,96] propose that category boundaries reflect the most irrational frequency ratio, which corresponds to the golden mean ratio, *phi* (φ). As shown in Box 3.2, lower, B_L, and upper, B_U, EEG category boundaries derive from the infinitely irrational golden mean ratio: φ = 1.681 . . . Famously, this ratio functions as a repellor, denying synchrony of periodicities.[97] Confirming this, Pletzer et al.[98] showed that two simultaneously active oscillations with frequency ratios near φ simply *do not synchronize*. Other fascinating findings from Whittington and colleagues[99] suggest that the repelling aspect of phi plays a role in regulating time patterns of perceivable rhythms.

Ideas surrounding the golden mean are captivating in elegance and explanatory potential. This exclusion mechanism contrasts with more conventional ones such as inhibitory neurons, weakened connections, limits on unit proximities or numbers (e.g., nodes), and so on. Instead, the golden mean delivers a delightful surprise in its simple denial of synchrony. Such discoveries also place this issue within a sweeping historic framework. The golden mean is famous for its role in growth patterns in nature (Figure 3.7) and in art, architecture, and music.[100,101,102] Phi is a ratio that has long fascinated biologists, artists, and scholars. Now it must engage psychologists. In curious ways, this compelling irrationality figures into a grand puzzle of oscillator configurations that we seek to solve.

The Function of Spontaneous Oscillator Configurations

This is a core chapter because it considers ways in which a tunable brain might work. It asserts that the dynamics of spontaneous brain oscillations are not random. Various sorts of gradients, categories, and hierarchies of oscillatory frequencies testify to this. Moreover, given the dynamical heritage of these configurations, rooted in limit cycle oscillations, such groups can spontaneously reorganize, jumping over category boundaries from one endogenous configuration to another.

The psychological functions of brain oscillations discussed in this chapter are relatively new. Not long ago, mainstream thinking concluded that *neural oscillations serve no function.* Many researchers viewed oscillations skeptically; they were dismissed as epiphenomena by scientists who searched in vain for spatial brain loci of modules containing stored memory codes. However, as the exciting news from neuroscience reminds us, this era is waning.

Oscillatory activities, glimpsed in this chapter, signify a revolution in theorizing. They offer novel ways to explain human behaviors associated with attention, perception, and remembering. The tunable brain controls how people dynamically interact with their environment. Momentary inner workings of a self-tuning brain reflect either the inward or outward awareness of an individual. Inward awareness entails a reflective orientation, such as remembering. Outward awareness entails direct orientation to events, as in attending. Because remembering can be seen as a recapitulation of the act of attending,[103] the remainder of this book is devoted to understanding attending.

Attending Dynamics

Attending involves an individual's outward engagement with external events. Unlike remembering, attending entails immediate awareness of current and future events. As noted in the preceding chapter, an event may induce in a perceiver an endogenous rhythm that persists as an *inner temporal context,* preparing this individual (rightly or wrongly) for "what" and "when" happens next. In theory, this persistence depends on self-sustaining oscillator properties. In a tunable brain, limit cycle oscillations create a dynamic internal context that persists to carry an individual's expectancies of forthcoming events.

Of course, expectancies are notoriously fallible. The future has a way of thwarting expectancies. Expectancies based on persisting oscillations cannot guarantee valid percepts of future events; they merely guarantee that people have "built-in" inner contexts that tacitly prepare them (rightly or wrongly) for the "when" of some future happening.

To conclude this chapter Box 3.3 presents a fictional, but real world, example of some of the concepts introduced here and their application in everyday life. The fictional protagonist in this story is Bill, who returns occasionally in later chapters to ground some of the ideas and procedures introduced throughout this book.

The real world example, highlighted in Box 3.3, previews one function of oscillatory brain configurations which concerns endogenous (inner) rhythms. However, it also previews topics in later chapters where other important functions are served by endogenous oscillations as they begin to interact with external world events. Attending dynamics, then, become a central interest. The internal ongoing oscillator configurations described in this chapter pave the way for people to attend to external events. In contrast to the endogenous entrainments featured in this chapter, attending calls forth various kinds of driving/driven dyads connected through exogenous entrainments.

Ideally, the laboratory tasks that psychologists use to isolate attending dynamics capture enough of real-world experiences to illuminate the role of oscillations and their entraining potential in daily events. This chapter lays the groundwork for exploring these roles.

Summary of Multiple Oscillations: Random or Structured Dynamics?

The panoply of multiple oscillator configurations suggested in this chapter implicates activities of many different limit cycle oscillations. The nature of these configurations challenges assumptions that default neural activity is random. To the contrary, cortical oscillations spontaneously interact in various ways, forming various nonrandom multioscillator configurations. Even oscillator configurations that seem random cannot escape the synchronous pull of attractors nor the repelling/desynchronizing push of phi. Also, nonrandom groupings of oscillations derive from structured configurations in which selective inclusion is influenced by growth curves and synaptic constraints, as well as by principles of resonance and entrainment. Nevertheless, an abiding thread relating phenomena explored in this section is the goal of synchrony or, conversely, the loss of this goal.

The main points of this section are:

- Configurations of multiple neural oscillations assume various forms based on inclusive and exclusive constraints on their interactions.

BOX 3.3
A REAL-WORLD EXAMPLE: BILL'S BRAIN

Bill, needing money, volunteered to serve in a psychological experiment. Unfortunately, he arrives late, distracted by ruminations over a recent argument with his girlfriend. His distraction reflects an inward-oriented awareness. It is a state of mind associated with clusters of previously activated cortical oscillations that fill Bill's tunable brain with lingering recapitulations of a preceding argument. Consequently, he brings to the laboratory an inappropriate inner temporal context comprising many ongoing and energetic spontaneous oscillations irrelevant to the task at hand. This task aims to assess people's ability to selectively attend to a music-like tone sequence, a far cry from Bill's preoccupation with romantic difficulties.

Nevertheless, Bill is told to "pay attention only to high tones in presented tone sequences and ignore low pitched tones." Only as the experiment proceeds does Bill begin to comply with instructions. Eventually, he settles in and orients outward, toward tone sequences. Indeed, he becomes involuntarily caught up by the slow rhythm of a succession of tones. During this process, ongoing endogenous oscillations in Bill's brain reorganize as they "bump" up against the external rhythm created by alternating high- and low-pitched tones, each marking a different delta rhythm (500 and 1,000 ms periods, respectively). To follow instructions to "attend only to higher pitched tones," Bill voluntarily heightens the amplitude of a cortical oscillation that has automatically attached itself to the 1,000 ms period of these tones (and/or suppresses amplitudes of other oscillations). Although Bill is hardly aware of this timing, he makes an explicit effort to voluntarily "tune in" to the task-relevant (higher pitched) rhythm.

This example previews one function of oscillatory brain configurations as these endogenous (inner) rhythms begin to interact with external world events. Internal ongoing oscillator configurations pave the way for people to attend to external events using exogenous entrainment (as discussed in the next chapter). Ideally, the tasks that psychologists use to isolate attending dynamics capture enough of real-world experiences to illuminate the role of oscillations and their entraining potential in daily events. This chapter lays the groundwork for exploring these roles.

- Inborn constraints on formations of oscillations configurations are topological, but they also involve sensitivity to resonance and entrainment principles, leading to nonrandom configurations of networks, groups, and oscillator hierarchies.
- Strict connectionist models ignore group formation based on frequencies of neural units (conceived as oscillations), whereas dynamic attending approaches feature inclusive constraints on group formation based on synchrony (rational frequency ratios as attractors) and exclusive constraints based on loss of synchrony (golden mean, phi).

CHAPTER SUMMARY

This chapter introduces readers to the dynamics of cortical oscillations in a tunable brain inspired by recent neuroscience developments. These dynamics lay the necessary groundwork for later chapters on real-time attending which depend on synchronous brain rhythms.

This chapter describes the inner world of a tunable brain in a journey that begins with workhorse oscillation: the limit cycle oscillation. This oscillation, although stable, is also adaptable. These features express the inherent flexibility required for the partnering of two limit cycle oscillations as they form an endogenous dyad. This journey then pursues details of such this partnering as it is governed by special frequency relations (i.e., attractors). Resulting dyads, whether simple or complex, depend on governing attractors. Next, multiple dancing dyads join to form larger groupings of limit cycle oscillations united by various forms of synchrony. Some formations (primitive) happen prior to birth or early in life. Generally, larger groups of adaptive oscillations form, following principles of resonance and entrainment that, together, highlight a uniting role for synchrony in group formations.

The journey ends as oscillations join together in large oscillator configurations. These configurations continue to rely on universal principles of resonance and entrainment to explain synchronous communications among many oscillations. Active brain rhythms relate to one another to form dyads and groups connected synchronously by similar or coherently related periodicities. In turn, such groups can support an individual's development of categories. Together with an opposing phi ratio, an attractor unites spontaneous oscillators within a category cluster in synchrony while the golden mean differentiates categories through a loss of synchrony.

Finally, this journey within a tunable brain features only endogenous rhythms. Once we introduce external events into this narrative (as in Box 3.3), the scenario changes: we then confront external driving rhythms! An individual now has an outward awareness of world events. This begets attending, which is the topic of the next chapter.

NOTES

1. Philippe G. Schyns, Gregor Thut, and Joachim Gross, "Cracking the Code of Oscillatory Activity," *PLoS Biol* 9, no. 5 (May 17, 2011): e1001064, doi:10.1371/journal.pbio.1001064.

2. Molly J. Henry and Björn Herrmann, "Low-Frequency Neural Oscillations Support Dynamic Attending in Temporal Context," *Timing & Time Perception* 2, no. 1 (January 1, 2014): 62–86, doi:10.1163/22134468-00002011.

3. Hans Berger, "Über das Elektrenkephalogramm des Menschen," *Archiv für Psychiatrie und Nervenkrankheiten* 87, no. 1 (December 1929): 527–70, doi:10.1007/BF01797193.

4. The black circle of Figure 3.1 is very close to its attractor (i.e., a perfect circle); a few points on red trajectories render it an almost circular orbit.

5. For instance, amplitude may be measured as electrical current intensity.

6. For our purposes the x dimension is amplitude, hence x(t) is momentary amplitude; that is, a(t).

7. György Buzsáki and Andreas Draguhn, "Neuronal Oscillations in Cortical Networks," *Science* 304, no. 5679 (2004): 1926–29.

8. This previews hypotheses about attentional capture developed in later chapters.

9. "Rhythms of the Brain - György Buzsáki – Oxford University Press, Inc, New York, 2006. accessed February 4, 2016, https://books-google.com.proxy.library.ucsb.edu:9443/books?hl=en&lr=&id=ldz58irprjYC&oi=fnd&pg=PA4&dq=Buzsaki,+2006 &ots=Q1X836eGAS&sig=pvOzjx2ylzrNmQwOmG-Ed1XIPbQ#v=onepage&q=Buzsaki%2C%20 2006&f=false.

10. John Jonides and Steven Yantis, "Uniqueness of Abrupt Visual Onset in Capturing Attention," *Perception & Psychophysics* 43, no. 4 (July 1988): 346–54, doi:10.3758/BF03208805.

11. Steven Yantis and John Jonides, "Abrupt Visual Onsets and Selective Attention: Voluntary versus Automatic Allocation," *Journal of Experimental Psychology: Human Perception and Performance* 16, no. 1 (1990): 121–34, doi:10.1037/0096-1523.16.1.121.

12. Mari Riess Jones et al., "Temporal Aspects of Stimulus-Driven Attending in Dynamic Arrays," *Psychological Science* 13, no. 4 (2002): 313–9.

13. Charles L. Folk, Andrew B. Leber, and Howard E. Egeth, "Made You Blink! Contingent Attentional Capture Produces a Spatial Blink," *Perception & Psychophysics* 64, no. 5 (July 2002): 741–53, doi:10.3758/BF03194741.

14. Phase portraits may not be expressed as two-dimensional rings or trapezoidal orbits, but as three (or more) dimensional forms. Also, individual biological oscillations are more complicated than quasi-linear ones similar to sine-waves. For instance, *burst oscillators* naturally produce spontaneous spikes only within a particular phase region of an oscillator's orbit.

15. Eugene M. Izhikevich -"Dynamical Systems in Neuroscience: The Geometry of Excitability and Bursting." The MIT Press, Cambridge, Massachusetts, 2007. accessed February 6, 2016, https://books-google-com.proxy.library.ucsb.edu:9443/books?hl=en&lr=&id=kVjM6DFk-twC&oi=fnd&pg=PR15&dq=Izhikevich,+2007++book+&ots=KTBxoXg9we&sig=qBGDdXdKlTQKBSD-gNEeknOT0K U#v=onepage&q=Izhikevich%2C%202007%20%20 book&f=false.

16. This is a supercritical Andronov-Hopf bifurcation; a subcritical Andronov-Hopf bifurcation also exists; this section draws from Izhikevich, 2007; see reference 12).

17. Steven H. Strogatz, *Nonlinear Dynamics and Chaos: With Applications to Physics, Biology, Chemistry, and Engineering* (Westview Press, 2014).

18. Diane Kaplan and Leon Glass, *Understanding Nonlinear Dynamics*, accessed February 4, 2016, https://books-google-com.proxy.library.ucsb.edu:9443/books/about/Understanding_Nonlinear_Dynamics.html?id=gh_vBwAAQBAJ.

19. Arkady Pikovsky, Michael Rosenblum, Jurgen Kruths, *Synchronization: A Universal Concept in Nonlinear Science*. Cambridge University Press. Publication date is 2001.

20. Izhikevich, *Dynamical Systems in Neuroscience*, accessed February 4, 2016, Same entry as # 15 https://books-google-com.proxy.library.ucsb.edu:9443/

books/about/Dynamical_Systems_in_Neuroscience.html?id=kVjM6DFk-twC.

21. "Dimension" in dynamical systems is an emergent construct not to be confused with physical dimensions of time and space; it is subject to interpretations too complex for this book.

22. Of course this omits a profile instantaneous phase patterns within the period of the slower oscillation.

23. Typically, oscillator strength is based on amplitude level.

24. This is the simplest case; it is also possible that both oscillations adjust periods.

25. Similarly, the inverse of manifest frequency is a manifest period, denoted by p′.

26. Note, however, this does not preclude increments in amplitude during entrainment due to growing resonance among active oscillations.

27. Later chapters show that the width of a entrainment region decreases with attractor complexity along a continuum termed the *devil's staircase*.

28. Ole Jensen and Laura L. Colgin, "Cross-Frequency Coupling between Neuronal Oscillations," *Trends in Cognitive Sciences* 11, no. 7 (July 2007): 267–69, doi:10.1016/j.tics.2007.05.003.

29. J. Matias Palva, Satu Palva, and Kai Kaila, "Phase Synchrony among Neuronal Oscillations in the Human Cortex," *The Journal of Neuroscience* 25, no. 15 (April 13, 2005): 3962–72, doi:10.1523/JNEUROSCI.4250-04.2005.

30. Elisa Mira Holz et al., "Theta–Gamma Phase Synchronization during Memory Matching in Visual Working Memory," *NeuroImage* 52, no. 1 (August 1, 2010): 326–35, doi:10.1016/j.neuroimage.2010.04.003.

31. Thilo Womelsdorf and Pascal Fries, "The Role of Neuronal Synchronization in Selective Attention," *Current Opinion in Neurobiology*, Cognitive neuroscience, 17, no. 2 (April 2007): 154–60, doi:10.1016/j.conb.2007.02.002.

32. Thilo Womelsdorf et al., "Modulation of Neuronal Interactions Through Neuronal Synchronization," *Science* 316, no. 5831 (June 15, 2007): 1609–12, doi:10.1126/science.1139597.

33. Pikovsky et al. provide a general formula for phase changes in mode-locking: $\Delta\varphi n,m = n\varphi_1(t) - m\varphi_2(t)$ (p.160).

34. This complex continuum is termed the devil's staircase. Although fascinating, details are not helpful in this discussion.

35. R. T. Canolty et al., "High Gamma Power Is Phase-Locked to Theta Oscillations in Human Neocortex," *Science* 313, no. 5793 (September 15, 2006): 1626–28, doi:10.1126/science.1128115.

36. Ryan T. Canolty and Robert T. Knight, "The Functional Role of Cross-Frequency Coupling," *Trends in Cognitive Sciences* 14, no. 11 (November 2010): 506–15, doi:10.1016/j.tics.2010.09.001.

37. ECoG records reflect subdural electrical brain activity (in microvolts, μV).

38. Prasad R. Shirvalkar, Peter R. Rapp, and Matthew L. Shapiro, "Bidirectional Changes to Hippocampal Theta–gamma Comodulation Predict Memory for Recent Spatial Episodes," *Proceedings of the National Academy of Sciences* 107, no. 15 (April 13, 2010): 7054–59, doi:10.1073/pnas.0911184107.

39. Arkady Pikovsky and Michael Rosenblum, "Synchronization," *Scholarpedia* 2, no. 12 (2007): 1459, doi:10.4249/scholarpedia.1459.

40. Anita K. Roopun et al., "Temporal Interactions Between Cortical Rhythms," *Frontiers in Neuroscience* 2, no. 2 (December 15, 2008): 145–54, doi:10.3389/neuro.01.034.2008.

41. Schyns, Thut, and Gross, "Cracking the Code of Oscillatory Activity."

42. Ryan T. Canolty and Robert T. Knight, "The Functional Role of Cross-Frequency Coupling," *Trends in Cognitive Sciences* 14, no. 11 (November 2010): 506–15, doi:10.1016/j.tics.2010.09.001.

43. Canolty and Knight, "The Functional Role of Cross-Frequency Coupling": "[A] statistical dependence between the phase of a low frequency brain rhythm and the amplitude (or power) of the high frequency component of electrical brain activity" (p.507).

44. Pascal Fries, "Neuronal Gamma-Band Synchronization as a Fundamental Process in Cortical Computation," *Annual Review of Neuroscience* 32, no. 1 (2009): 209–24, doi:10.1146/annurev.neuro.051508.135603.

45. Pascal Fries, "A Mechanism for Cognitive Dynamics: Neuronal Communication through Neuronal Coherence," *Trends in Cognitive Sciences* 9, no. 10 (October 2005): 474–80, doi:10.1016/j.tics.2005.08.011.

46. Womelsdorf and Fries, "The Role of Neuronal Synchronization in Selective Attention."

47. Pikovsky and Rosenblum, "Synchronization."

48. Izhikevich, *Dynamical Systems in Neuroscience.*

49. Frank Hoppensteadt and Eugene Izhikevich, "Canonical Neural Models1," 2001, http://www.izhikevich.org/publications/arbib.pdf.

50. Edward W. Large and Felix V. Almonte, "Neurodynamics, Tonality, and the Auditory Brainstem Response," *Annals of the New York Academy of Sciences* 1252, no. 1 (April 1, 2012): E1–7, doi:10.1111/j.1749-6632.2012.06594.x.

51. M. R. Jones, "Time, Our Lost Dimension: Toward a New Theory of Perception, Attention, and Memory," *Psychological Review* 83, no. 5 (September 1976): 323–55.

52. Buzsáki, *Rhythms of the Brain*, accessed February 5, 2016, https://books-google-com.proxy.library.ucsb.edu:9443/books/about/Rhythms_of_the_Brain.html?id=ldz58irprjYC.

53. György Buzsáki and James J. Chrobak, "Temporal Structure in Spatially Organized Neuronal Ensembles: A Role for Interneuronal Networks," *Current Opinion in Neurobiology* 5, no. 4 (August 1995): 504–10, doi:10.1016/0959-4388(95)80012-3.

54. Marcus E. Raichle, "Two Views of Brain Function," *Trends in Cognitive Sciences* 14, no. 4 (April 2010): 180–90, doi:10.1016/j.tics.2010.01.008.

55. Charles E. Schroeder and Peter Lakatos, "Low-Frequency Neuronal Oscillations as Instruments of Sensory Selection," *Trends in Neurosciences* 32, no. 1 (January 2009): 9–18, doi:10.1016/j.tins.2008.09.012.

56. Peter Lakatos et al., "Entrainment of Neuronal Oscillations as a Mechanism of Attentional Selection," *Science* 320, no. 5872 (April 4, 2008): 110–13, doi:10.1126/science.1154735.

57. Womelsdorf and Fries, "The Role of Neuronal Synchronization in Selective Attention."

58. Nancy J. Kopell et al., "Beyond the Connectome: The Dynome," *Neuron* 83, no. 6 (September 17, 2014): 1319–28, doi:10.1016/j.neuron.2014.08.016.

59. Steven Pinker, *The Blank Slate: The Modern Denial of Human Nature* (Penguin, 2003), https://books-google-com.proxy.library.ucsb.edu:9443/books?hl=en&lr=&id=ePNi4ZqYdVQC&oi=fnd&pg=PR7&dq=Pinker,+P.++The+blank+slate++&ots=kKx0CpRmM4&sig=HfDUXqG3sd968Qu56fR8A3vQIVM.

60. It will become clear that units are conceived differently in other approaches, where they are termed *nodes*.

61. Duncan J. Watts and Steven H. Strogatz, "Collective Dynamics of 'Small-World' Networks," *Nature* 393, no. 6684 (June 4, 1998): 440–42, doi:10.1038/30918.

62. Steven H. Strogatz, "Exploring Complex Networks," *Nature* 410, no. 6825 (March 8, 2001): 268–76, doi:10.1038/35065725.

63. T. A. Cook, *The Curves of Life* (Constable and Co., London, 1914).

64. Makoto Fukushima et al., "Spontaneous High-Gamma Band Activity Reflects Functional Organization of Auditory Cortex in the Awake Macaque," *Neuron* 74, no. 5 (June 7, 2012): 899–910, doi:10.1016/j.neuron.2012.04.014.

65. A. C. Nobre and M. M. Mesulam, "Large-Scale Networks for Attentional Biases," *The Oxford Handbook of Attention*, 2014, 105–51.

66. M. A. Whittington et al., "Inhibition-Based Rhythms: Experimental and Mathematical Observations on Network Dynamics," *International Journal of Psychophysiology* 38, no. 3 (December 2000): 315–36, doi:10.1016/S0167-8760(00)00173-2.

67. Where relevant, in some models, it applies to relative numbers of excitatory and inhibitory units.

68. An important exception is the pyramidal interneuronal network gamma (PING) model.

69. Roopun et al., "Temporal Interactions between Cortical Rhythms."

70. Christoph Börgers, Steven Epstein, and Nancy J. Kopell, "Gamma Oscillations Mediate Stimulus Competition and Attentional Selection in a Cortical Network Model," *Proceedings of the National Academy of Sciences* 105, no. 46 (November 18, 2008): 18023–28, doi:10.1073/pnas.0809511105.

71. Christoph Börgers, Steven Epstein, and Nancy J. Kopell, "Background Gamma Rhythmicity and Attention in Cortical Local Circuits: A Computational Study," *Proceedings of the National Academy of Sciences of the United States of America* 102, no. 19 (May 10, 2005): 7002–07, doi:10.1073/pnas.0502366102.

72. Pranay Goel and Bard Ermentrout, "Synchrony, Stability, and Firing Patterns in Pulse-Coupled Oscillators," *Physica D: Nonlinear Phenomena* 163, no. 3–4 (March 15, 2002): 191–216, doi:10.1016/S0167-2789(01)00374-8.

73. Whittington et al., "Inhibition-Based Rhythms."

74. Mette S. Olufsen et al., "New Roles for the Gamma Rhythm: Population Tuning and Preprocessing for the Beta Rhythm," *Journal of Computational Neuroscience* 14, no. 1 (January 2003): 33–54, doi:10.1023/A:1021124317706.

75. Edward W. Large, "Neurodynamics of Music," in *Music Perception*, eds. Mari Riess Jones, Richard R. Fay, and Arthur N. Popper, Springer Handbook of Auditory Research 36 (Springer, New York, 2010), 201–31, doi:10.1007/978-1-4419-6114-3_7.

76. Large and Almonte, "Neurodynamics, Tonality, and the Auditory Brainstem Response."

77. Edward W. Large and John F. Kolen, "Resonance and the Perception of Musical Meter," *Connection Science* 6, no. 2–3 (1994): 177–208.

78. Eugene M. Izhikevich et al., "Bursts as a Unit of Neural Information: Selective Communication via Resonance," *Trends in Neurosciences* 26, no. 3 (March 2003): 161–67, doi:10.1016/S0166-2236(03)00034-1.

79. Frank C. Hoppensteadt and Eugene M. Izhikevich, "Thalamo-Cortical Interactions Modeled by Weakly Connected Oscillators: Could the Brain Use FM Radio Principles?," *Biosystems* 48, no. 1–3 (November 1, 1998): 85–94, doi:10.1016/S0303-2647(98)00053-7.

80. Hoppensteadt and Izhikevich, "Thalamo-Cortical Interactions Modeled by Weakly Connected Oscillators."

81. For instance, variables such as sodium, potassium, and calcium.

82. Paola Malerba et al., "Are Different Rhythms Good for Different Functions?," 2010, http://dcommon.bu.edu:8080/handle/2144/2799.

83. Christoph S. Herrmann, Ingo Fründ, and Daniel Lenz, "Human Gamma-Band Activity: A Review on Cognitive and Behavioral Correlates and Network Models," *Neuroscience & Biobehavioral Reviews*, Binding Processes: Neurodynamics and Functional Role in Memory and Action, 34, no. 7 (June 2010): 981–92, doi:10.1016/j.neubiorev.2009.09.001.

84. Paul Sauseng and Wolfgang Klimesch, "What Does Phase Information of Oscillatory Brain Activity Tell Us about Cognitive Processes?," *Neuroscience & Biobehavioral Reviews* 32, no. 5 (July 2008): 1001–13, doi:10.1016/j.neubiorev.2008.03.014.

85. Malerba et al., "Are Different Rhythms Good for Different Functions?"

86. G. Pfurtscheller, A. Stancák Jr., and Ch. Neuper, "Event-Related Synchronization (ERS) in the Alpha Band—an Electrophysiological Correlate of Cortical Idling: A Review," *International Journal of Psychophysiology*, New Advances in EEG and cognition, 24, no. 1–2 (November 1996): 39–46, doi:10.1016/S0167-8760(96)00066-9.

87. Ole Jensen and Ali Mazaheri, "Shaping Functional Architecture by Oscillatory Alpha Activity: Gating by Inhibition," *Frontiers in Human Neuroscience* 4 (2010): 186.

88. Anne-Lise Giraud and David Poeppel, "Cortical Oscillations and Speech Processing: Emerging Computational Principles and Operations," *Nature Neuroscience* 15, no. 4 (2012): 511–7.

89. Wolfgang Klimesch, "Alpha-Band Oscillations, Attention, and Controlled Access to Stored Information," *Trends in Cognitive Sciences* 16, no. 12 (December 2012): 606–17, doi:10.1016/j.tics.2012.10.007.

90. Wolfgang Klimesch, "An Algorithm for the EEG Frequency Architecture of Consciousness and Brain Body Coupling," *Frontiers in Human Neuroscience* 7 (November 12, 2013), doi:10.3389/fnhum.2013.00766.

91. Belinda Pletzer, Hubert Kerschbaum, and Wolfgang Klimesch, "When Frequencies Never Synchronize: The Golden Mean and the Resting EEG," *Brain Research* 1335 (June 4, 2010): 91–102, doi:10.1016/j.brainres.2010.03.074.

92. In this equation, s = 1.25 Hz (i.e., half a delta frequency of 2.5 Hz).

93. Equation 2 (p. 33 in Jones, 1976; see note 92) is identical to Equation 3.1 here, but it is cast in ratios of oscillator periods.

94. Mari R. Jones, "Time, Our Lost Dimension: Toward a New Theory of Perception, Attention, and Memory," *Psychological Review* 83, no. 5 (1976): 323–55, doi:10.1037/0033-295X.83.5.323.

95. Klimesch, "An Algorithm for the EEG Frequency Architecture of Consciousness and Brain Body Coupling."

96. Pletzer, Kerschbaum, and Klimesch, "When Frequencies Never Synchronize."

97. Roopun et al., "Temporal Interactions Between Cortical Rhythms."

98. Pletzer, Kerschbaum, and Klimesch, "When Frequencies Never Synchronize."

99. Roopun et al., "Temporal Interactions Between Cortical Rhythms."

100. Cook, *The Curves of Life.*

101. Hermann Weyl, *Symmetry* (1952) (Princeton University Press, 1989).

102. Ibid.

103. Marilyn Boltz and Mari Riess Jones, "Does Rule Recursion Make Melodies Easier to Reproduce? If Not, What Does?," *Cognitive Psychology* 18, no. 4 (October 1, 1986): 389–431, doi:10.1016/0010-0285(86)90005-8.

104. Klimesch, "An Algorithm for the EEG Frequency Architecture of Consciousness and Brain Body Coupling."

4

Tuning in to World Events

A General Attending Hypothesis

A tunable brain is a busy brain, continuously alive day and night with spontaneous cortical activities. In fact, even circadian periods of dawn and dusk join in this activity. The preceding chapter traced a path of brain activity from a single limit cycle oscillation to endogenous dyads, then to whole groups of dyads, ultimately leading to configurations of multiple cortical oscillations. Such configurations lay the groundwork for understanding attending. However, they do not represent real attending because a signature component of attending is missing: the to-be-attended event. Attending happens when a tunable brain confronts events in the environment.

Attention is a central construct in the field of psychology, and it is of particular importance in this book. Historically, attention has been variously defined, with a common thread describing it as a process that is focused outward toward the environment. In this view, we selectively orient to happenings (i.e., *events*) in the world: a bird taking flight, the sound of a plane overhead, or a tune hummed by friend. Intuitively, attending represents our momentary engagement with these happenings. These moments of engagement reflect the impact of an external stimulation as an event "bumps into" the ongoing neural activities of an individual's tunable brain: external events force ongoing, spontaneous neural mechanisms to "take notice" of the outside world. In this view, attending is not the stationary construct implied by the label "attention." Instead, it is a real-time activity directed outward to interact with an unfolding event.

Yet, what is this activity termed "attending" that is "directed outward?" And can we be clearer about what constitutes an "event?" These and related constructs are clarified in this chapter.

Attending activity and energy. Unquestionably, to pin down attending is a challenging job. This chapter refrains from comparisons with other attention theories. Instead, it sketches a perspective that is a patently distinguishable theory from earlier approaches with regard to its yoking of attending with entrainment. This chapter makes the case that an entrainment framework can explain attending in terms of amplitude levels of an entraining neural oscillation. In short, *attending begins as an involuntary activity that is correlated with timed amplitudes of an event-driven (entraining) oscillation which may then be shaped by voluntary factors.*

A complete description of attending requires clarifying terms such as "involuntary activity" and "event-driven oscillations." Typically, psychologists distinguish between an activity termed "involuntary attending" from that of "voluntary attending." The latter is considered a selective, even consciously focused, activity whereas involuntary attending is deemed automatic, typically stimulus-driven. We have little control over involuntary attending, but it is there when we need it. On the other hand, voluntary attending, also termed "selective attending," refers to an individual's intentional focus directed toward a particular event.

An event has time structure. As such, it carries one or more external driving rhythms that can support attending. Specifically, a single driving rhythm entrains a corresponding stimulus-driven brain rhythm, creating an exogenous dyad via entrainment. And it is the amplitude of this driven rhythm that carries attending energy. A driven rhythm's amplitude changes to reflect the intensity of attending to an event, whether involuntary or voluntary.

First and foremost, the attended event is a happening in the environment. Events can be common visual happenings, as when a child gestures toward her mother, a kitten leaps on a moving toy mouse, or a friend strides up the stairs, or events may be acoustic patterns conveyed by mechanical or animated sound sources. For instance, the low hum of a washing machine is an acoustic event, as is the sound of a plane overhead.

Animate sources of events are also commonplace. They might assume the form of forceful hammerings or the sounds of a crying infant, a screeching owl. And, of course, there are speech utterances and phrases that deliver sound signals vital to human communication. Such events are ubiquitous; they have beginnings, middles, and ends. Moreover, all embed noticeable regularities as well as distinctive time patterns.

At some level of awareness (i.e., of attending), we register such events, although certain features naturally receive more "attention" than others. That is, at its roots, attending is automatic, requiring little effort/energy. It is because of this involuntary aspect of attending that we can operate effortlessly, with only slight awareness of background events such as the sounds of a washing machine.

But attending also has a voluntary component. This is manifest when attending energy is intentionally focused on a concurrent event, such as an infant's cry. Although infant cries will automatically capture our attending, as these cries persist their relevance commands more concentrated attending than do other less relevant ongoing sounds, such as those of a washing machine. We consciously "pay more attention" to a baby's cry by elevating our attending level directed toward these sounds while simultaneously "tuning out" other, involuntarily registered sounds emitted by a washing machine or an airplane.

It is important to understand how we accomplish these attending activities because together involuntary and voluntary attending enable us to function in our environment. We succeed in the many tasks we effortlessly perform on a daily basis because we have evolved to "use" event time structures, consciously or not, to operate within our environmental niche. Events surrounding us have time structures that afford real-time attending. As preceding examples suggest, attending often is involuntary, as when we automatically react to an event's time pattern. However, as any event unfolds, it reveals its characteristic time structure. For instance, the sound of an airplane is a steady mix of multiple low-frequency continuous micro- and macro-waveforms, whereas a baby's cries will project a series of discrete, complex bursts of high-frequency sound waves. Nevertheless, each of the several waveforms comprising such events can function as an external driving rhythm that elicits a neural oscillation as its driven rhythm. In other words, an event can be a complex thing which leads to the creation of a distinctive combination of exogenous dyads, where exogenous refers to the environmental properties of some event.

Exogenous dyads. Exogenous dyads result from exogenous entrainment, meaning that the driving rhythm of these dyads is an external (stimulus) rhythm; in other words, the driven rhythm is a neural oscillation. Nevertheless, in endogenous as well as exogenous rhythm pairs, entrainment is possible due to the adaptive behaviors of the driven oscillation.[1] To a large degree, the preceding chapter described endogenous entrainments of brain oscillations which yield exogenous dyads (e.g., Figures 3.4 and 3.5). In these cases, both driving and driven rhythms are spontaneous, continuous rhythms, with regularly undulating neural waveforms. Exogenous dyads, by contrast, result from an external driving rhythm which entrains a driven brain oscillation. Furthermore, event-based rhythms may involve more unruly driving rhythms than cortical driving rhythms. That is, world events are not necessarily continuous, nor are they always highly regular. Often external driving rhythms contain unanticipated deviations in time and intensity. In other words, these driving rhythms typically depart from simple isochrony, as in *quasi-isochrony*, and/or they may even project quite complex rhythmic patterns. Nevertheless, when a real-world event "bumps into" the ongoing spontaneous oscillations of an individual's tunable brain, that event demands accommodation from the driven oscillation(s). The result may entail a neural reorganization wherein the end product involves several different dancing exogenous dyads.

This chapter considers interactions of neural rhythms with the time patterns of external events. It concentrates on events with very simple time patterns, such as those of Figure 4.1 (isochronous, quasi-isochronous). To be clear, the events we ordinarily encounter are not as simple as these. In fact, many are downright irregular in time. Eventually, the full story of event engagements must address complex as well as simple event time structures.

In sum, events have time structures (simple or complex) that provide external driving rhythms. In this narrative, events play a central role because they acquire dyadic partners as driven oscillations. In turn, driven rhythms are important because they supply energy for attending outward to the event. Therefore, instead of concentrating on endogenous entrainment, this chapter focuses on *exogenous entrainment*, which describes how external events serve as driving rhythms for neural oscillations. It considers how events around us—ones we often take for granted—subtly shape our attending, often without our awareness. However, the basic principles used to explain endogenous

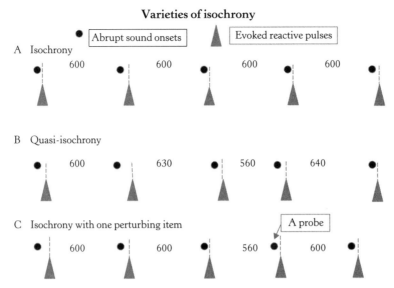

FIGURE 4.1 Three types of isochrony: (**A**) Dots with fixed inter-onset time intervals (T = 600 ms) to which isochronous reactive pulses occur, (**B**) dots with variable inter-onset time intervals forming a quasi- isochrony driving rhythm, (**C**) Isochrony with a single deviant probe item used in perturbation paradigms.

entrainments of brain oscillations remain universal ones of resonance and entrainment.

Attending as a participatory activity. Attending is always an activity that goes on in a listener's head, but it is directed outward by virtue of "when" attending energy is heightened during exogenous entrainment. It resembles a unidirectional dyadic dance that begins with the automatic entrainment of a resonant driven rhythm. This process becomes a dance in which the leading dancer is now an external driving rhythm that partners with an "agreeable" (i.e., adaptable) cortical rhythm. So, there is an undeniable participatory quality to entrainment activities which reflects momentary interactions of an internal oscillation with an external event. As described for endogenous entrainments in the preceding chapter, this driving–driven dyad is always governed by attractors that enable a driven rhythm to adapt to a fluctuating event's driving rhythm. Each moment reflects a new entrainment state (i.e., in a hypothetical phase state). The time course of exogenous entrainments over many moments is indispensable to meaningful engagements with our surroundings. Entrainments allow us to literally partake of an external event. In this way, attending is participatory. An attender's endogenous oscillation literally becomes briefly "glued" (i.e., coupled) to an external event.

Participatory attending emphasizes the dyadic nature of attending. In this regard, it does not equate attending with a decision-making moment prior to the appearance of a relevant (i.e., a to-be-attended) event. A decision-making moment, for example, comes with task instructions when an individual is told to "pay attention to this," where "this" is described as a future "target" item (e.g., "dog faces") among irrelevant items (cats, birds, etc.) in stimulus pictures, or when a motor action is stipulated ("push this button only when you see a dog's face"). These instructions and/or a participant's related intentions are important for their goal-setting prowess vis-à-vis voluntary attending. But these factors cannot substitute for the act of attending. Nor does attending have agency; it does not prioritize stimulus relevance.

In the present view, attending is an engagement activity involving universal biological (neural) mechanisms aroused by an event's time structure. The essence of attending is reflected by dynamically changing states of exogenous dyads, a process possibly set in motion by instructions, but carried out in real time by exogenous entrainments to experimental stimuli. This chapter leads to the conclusion that both involuntary and voluntary attending depend, in different ways, on exogenous entrainments. Involuntary attending ensures automatic entrainments with events at low attending energy levels, whereas voluntary attending builds flexibly on such exogenous entrainments to boost attending energy to targets at the "right" time.

CHAPTER GOALS

An overriding aim of this chapter involves unpacking attending dynamics. Attending is associated with momentary changes in the amplitude (energy) levels of an entraining neural oscillation. This concept is developed over the course of four sections of this chapter. The first section describes events as driving rhythms.

The next two sections detail participatory entrainment activities: the second section aims to place entrainment in an historical context, outlining the classic phase response curves of biological entrainment models, and the third section builds on phase response curves to develop attending energy profiles that propose how phase entrainment fosters temporal targeting of attending energy to expected and unexpected times. Together, these two sections clarify the respective roles of phase and amplitude of the driven oscillation on attending.

A final section pulls together preceding sections to introduce a broad new hypothesis about attending and its dynamic determinants. Here, the *general attending hypothesis* is outlined along with correlated hypotheses and evidence from exciting new neuroscience research on this topic.

EVENTS: WHAT MAKES AN EFFECTIVE DRIVING RHYTHM?

Events with simple time structures make very effective driving rhythms. So, let us begin with the simplest of external driving rhythms: the isochronous time pattern. Why has isochrony been so appealing over the years and yet so often paradoxically dismissed? Isochrony, not surprisingly, turns out to be a powerful driving time structure leading readily to a tacit goal of dyadic synchrony. This is evident in a listener's spontaneous tapping of toes or hands to music that capitalizes on one's need to participate in highly regular events by tapping or moving to their regular "beats." Furthermore, numerous motor tapping studies reveal that people of all ages have a natural (spontaneous) tendency to tap periodically in synchrony with isochronous events and even to continue this tapping after the event ceases.[2,3,4] Audiences at popular music concerts, as well as participants in lab studies, all confirm the power that musical isochrony holds for stimulating observable synchronized motor activities from simple foot-tapping and clapping to heavy metal head-banging behaviors. And—if concerts are reliable examples—then we can infer that participatory engagement increases with the salience of the external sounds (i.e., time markers) of an isochronous rhythm.

Nevertheless, the role of true isochrony remains controversial and elusive. In speech rhythms, for instance, its role is questioned because speech signals are notoriously variable, as discussed in later chapters. Indeed, despite the fact that isochrony supports simple entrainments in certain (e.g., musical) contexts, its function in explaining how we deal with more complex timing relationships (e.g., in music or speech) is less obvious. Yet, it is clear that isochrony describes very effective driving rhythms. As such, it provides an instructive starting point for a story that becomes more complex, one involving non-isochronous rhythmic patterns with fuzzy timing.

An isochronous event appears in the top row of Figure 4.1, where it is shown as a sequence of discrete items (dots). Onsets of successive items (e.g., sounds, lights) are termed *time markers*. In panel a, time markers (dots) outline constant time intervals; thus, let T refer to the time span of a stimulus (event) in this row (e.g., a slow rate has a $T > 200$ ms; i.e., a frequency under 5 Hz). Simple time patterns not only evoke observable motor responses; they also invite neural responses that are not observable, detectable only by electroencephalograms (EEGs) or event-related potentials (ERPs) (i.e., absent motor responses). This figure shows evoked neural responses as pulses (triangles); namely, peak energies of an entraining oscillation. Pulses are phase localized as brief, high-frequency bursts of neural activity (e.g., beta/gamma range of 30–100 Hz). Here, each pulse follows a time marker by a fixed delay, creating a series of *reactive pulses* (termed ERP).[5] Although not shown, reactive pulse amplitudes may also decline as items repeat (i.e., *repetition suppression*). Reactive pulses are automatic bursts of attending energy that follow an item's occurrence. In short, they support local or *reactive attending*.[6,7] (Hermann[8] details various roles/forms of gamma oscillations as induced or evoked pulses.)

Reactive pulses were first observed by Tallon-Baudry as EEG gamma bursts (~40 Hz).[9,10] Eventually, they were distinguished from expectancy pulses (not shown in Figure 4.1). In theory, expectancy pulses are induced by the properties of a preceding temporal context. As noted in preceding chapters, expectancy pulses express *anticipatory attending*.

Compelling evidence for distinctions between expectancy and reactive pulses comes from Fujioka et al.[11,12] who recorded magnetoencephalogram (MEG) oscillations in auditory cortices as people passively listened to either isochronous or non-isochronous sequences of brief sounds at different rates. Results showed that, over time, beta activity increases during moments of synchronized activity (see time–frequency decomposition for 20–22 Hz; Figure 4.2,A–D). Moreover, at each rate, beta power increased *prior to* sound onsets. This suggests the presence of rate-based expectancy pulses (Figure 4.2F; arrows). Relatedly, beta desynchronizations appeared 200 ms after each sound. Importantly, *irregular rhythms only displayed reactive pulses, not expectancy pulses.* Together, these finding suggest that expectancy pulses involve beta oscillations, whereas reactive pulses are gamma oscillations.

In sum, the idea that isochrony of external events invites entrained attending seems plausible. A highly regular event evokes not only reactive pulses; it also induces expectancy pulses. The latter are anticipatory and manifest as high-frequency energy bursts at phase points preceding the onset of an anticipated time marker. Such discoveries reinforce the use of isochronous events as valuable tools for exploring the exogenous entrainment capacities of a tunable brain.

Isochrony: A Special Case

Theoretically, isochronous events are not irrelevant, for several reasons. First, isochrony realizes an important special case of driving–driven dyads with simple attractors. Exogenous entrainment with isochronous events depends on the simplest of attractors: n:m = 1:1, a good starting point for studying this activity.

Second, isochronous events stimulate both expectancy and reactive pulses, as shown in Figure 4.3. Both pulses deliver timed bursts of energy directed outward toward this driving rhythm. By

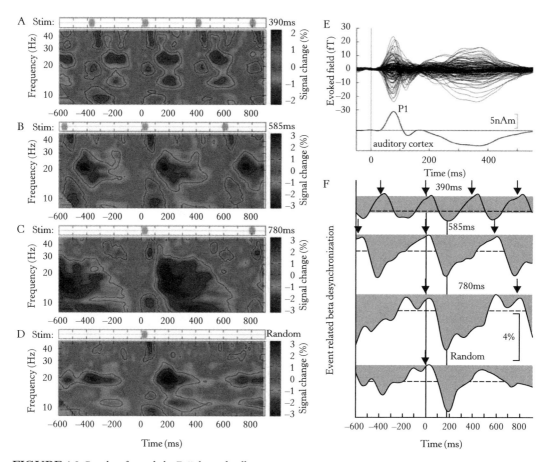

FIGURE 4.2 Results of a study by Fujioka and colleagues.

Reprinted from T. Fujioka et al., "Internalized Timing of Isochronous Sounds Is Represented in Neuromagnetic Beta Oscillations," *Journal of Neuroscience* 32, no. 5 (February 1, 2012): 1791–802, doi:10.1523/JNEUROSCI.4107-11.2012.

contrast, often highly irregular events fail to induce expectancy pulses, evoking only reactive pulses.

Third, isochrony highlights two different kinds of event-related attending. *Anticipatory attending* rides on expectancy pulses set in motion by a regular driving rhythm. *Reactive attending* signals the points of phase correction. Both pulses reflect brief, high-frequency bursts of internal energy instantiating subjective salience.

Admittedly, everyday events are rarely isochronous. But often their timing is "good enough" to support attending. If they display temporal jitter, as in quasi-isochrony, often these happenings fall within an attractor region implicating an isochronous waveform. In other words, such variability automatically forces people to continuously update dyadic phase relationships. Typically, we are unaware of updating because adaptive neural responses are largely automatic. Nevertheless, the effectiveness of minor phase adjustments keeps us effortlessly "in touch" with our surroundings. For these reasons, discussions of exogenous entrainments begin with this simplest of all event rhythms.

Exogenous Entrainments

Exogenous entrainment depicts the journey of a driven oscillator from an *out-of-sync* state to a completely *in-sync* state as this oscillator locks onto an isochronous event. Factors responsible for such entrainments involve an event's driving rhythm properties. Generalizing from internal rhythms described in the preceding chapter, important external driving rhythm properties are frequency, phase, and amplitude/force. In the special case of "near isochrony," an event-based driving rhythm engages a particular neural frequency as a driven rhythm via resonance.[13]

Yet real-world driving rhythms raise some problems for explanations based on entrainment principles. Everyday events have significant variability; rarely are they isochronous. In fact, real-world events are often unruly, subject to sudden unexpected changes in phase and force. For instance, a soothing lullaby sung by a mother to her infant can be suddenly perturbed by the injection of a loud sound from a malfunctioning washing machine. This not only causes an unscheduled pause in the mother's song, it also inserts a disturbing forceful sound into the melody. But, even the normal unruliness of timing within an ongoing environmental events adds irregularity to their time structures. For instance, certain timing variations in a mother's lullaby can hamper the phase coupling with an ongoing neural oscillation (of the infant) with unusually lengthened (and/or shorten) T values. The point is this: in uncountable ways, real-world events exhibit timing variations in driving rhythms that place demands on a listener's tunable brain as it continually aims to track these events.

For these reasons, studies of exogenous entrainment typically rely on carefully constructed events with controlled deviations from isochrony. Laboratory studies introduce one or two changes to an isochronous event in order to glimpse the momentary responses of an attender's driven rhythm. Ideally, we need to examine how a hypothetical neural oscillation reacts to a perturbation in an otherwise regular event. For instance, compare the isochronous event in Figure 4.1A with the two quasi-isochronous events in this figure. The irregular rhythm in Row B has minor timing variations in T values (jitter), whereas the driving rhythm in Row C is essentially isochronous, containing only a single temporally perturbing item, a *probe*.

In different ways, these three rhythms figure into controlled studies of anticipatory and reactive attending. They help to shed light on people's ability to cope with the timing irregularities prevalent in everyday events. For instance, the quasi-isochrony in Row B is likely to induce weaker driven oscillations than the other two driving rhythms, which exhibit significant isochrony.

Studies in Attending Dynamics: Three Paradigms

This section describes three paradigms used to assess how people cope with regular and irregular events, such as those of Figure 4.1. They are a *perturbation paradigm*, a *temporal context design*, and a *selective attending paradigm*.

The Perturbation Paradigm

The perturbation design was introduced in Chapter 1. Historically, it derives from important biological discoveries surrounding synchrony and entrainment. In psychology, this paradigm aims to study people's synchronization using rhythmic sequences, as depicted in Figure 4.1C, where isochrony prevails, perturbed only by a single probe stimulus, the *probe*. Two examples of this phenomenon, shown in Figure 4.3A,B, include both expectancy and reactive pulses to illustrate the phase correction activities of a hypothetical limit cycle oscillation. Here, anticipatory expectancy pulses are putatively induced by the opening sequential context of stimulus time markers

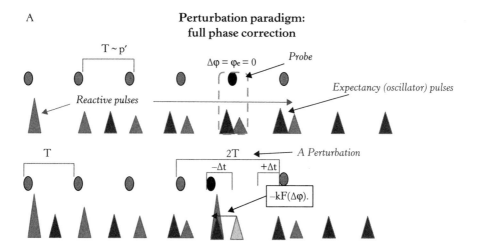

A

Perturbation paradigm:
full phase correction

One embedded probe introduces two successive time changes

Δt   = time deviation; T is the onset-to-onset inter-marker time span.

◄─── = Complete attention shift; full phase correction from $-kF(\Delta\varphi)$.

△ = Violated expectancy: silent pulse

B

Perturbation paradigm:
partial correction

One embedded probe introduces two successive time changes

$\Delta\varphi = \Delta t/T$ ranges from $-.50$ to $+.50$; $\Delta\varphi = \varphi_e = 0$ is the expected phase.

Δt = time deviation; T is the onset-to-onset inter-marker time span.

$-kF(\Delta\varphi) = (\Delta\varphi_n - \Delta\varphi_{n+1})$ is partial phase correction (◄─) on cycle n, manifest on n + 1.

△ = violated expectancy: silent pulse.

FIGURE 4.3 Outline of a perturbation paradigm (dots), reactive pulses (medium gray triangles), and entraining expectancy pulses (dark gray triangles). Top row in panels **A** and **B** show a probe at a contextually expected time. Bottom row shows full phase correction in panel **A** and partial correction in panel **B**.

(ovals) whereas the reactive pulses follow each sound marker.

In perturbation designs, we are concerned with how an entraining rhythm reacts to a single perturbing probe (black dot). When the probe occurs at an expected time (*top row*), its phase difference, Δφ, from the expected phase, φe is zero; hence, no phase resetting happens (*top row* panels A,B). According to Dynamic Attending Theory (DAT), φe values are determined by an internalized prior context. The bottom row of Figure 4.3A illustrates a probe with unexpected timing ($\Delta\varphi > 0$). This promptly generates an automatic phase correction that shifts the violated expectancy pulse. In theory, a strong 'push' from a probe can produce full phase correction; that is, this phase shift matches the deviant interval as shown. By contrast, Figure 3.4B illustrates partial phase correction, where the corrected violated expectancy pulse, not fully corrected, is manifest after a shortened period in next expectancy pulse.

Any phase correction is the result of the competing powers of two opposing forces. On the one hand, the strength of a perturbing stimulus automatically 'pushes' an expectancy pulse to align with the probe's time (Figure 4.3A, *bottom*), essentially capturing attending ($\Delta\varphi$ is large). On the other hand, the strength of an entraining oscillation (contextually induced) "pulls" an expectancy pulse to align with its intrinsic period (p), leading to partial or no phase correction. Whenever there is no phase correction, the oscillator continues to express its unaltered *expectancy* ($\Delta\varphi \sim 0$). Finally, a phase change between two cycles (n, $n + 1$) reflects a phase correction following a function designated as $-k\,F\,(\Delta\varphi) = (\Delta\varphi n - \Delta\varphi n+1)$, where **k** is a coupling strength parameter. (The $-\mathbf{k}\,F\,(\Delta\varphi)$ ranges from -50 to $.50$, where 0.0 is a null change.) A phase change, $\Delta\varphi$, is a complete correction when $\Delta\varphi = -\mathbf{k}F\,(\Delta\varphi)$; a partial change illustrates an inequality (e.g., $\Delta\varphi < -\mathbf{k}\,F\,(\Delta\varphi)$). Figure 4.3A (*bottom row*) shows a complete phase correction, whereas Figure 4.3B (*bottom row*) shows a partial phase correction.

Temporal Context Designs

A variant of the perturbation paradigm allows assessment of the impact of temporal context on people's performance. For instance, we might record an individual's response to a probe placed in either a regular context (Figure 4.1C) or in an irregular context (Figure 4.1B). This paradigm was also introduced in Chapter 2, where the dependent variable either assessed one's time judgment performance in different temporal contexts,[14] or it gauged people's ability to perceive or judge the properties of probes/targets embedded within different contexts.

The Selective Attending Paradigm

The third paradigm, also discussed in Chapter 2, is the popular selective attending task. It is important because it assesses people's voluntary control of attending. People are explicitly told to attend to one event (a relevant driving rhythm)

and ignore another (a specified irrelevant driving rhythm). Thus, the independent variable involves instructions such as "attend only to high tones in a series of high and low tones and detect a timbre change in the high-tone stream."[15]

Notice that elements of the perturbation paradigm creep into this design. This is because, to assess focal attending to an ongoing event, targets are planted within both relevant and irrelevant event streams in order to gauge a person's ability to selectively attend to the relevant rhythm. It turns out that instructions do affect performance, but this effect is modulated by rhythmic regularities of a context.[16,17,18,19] Such discoveries prefigure a major issue confronting studies of attending; namely, the degree to which involuntary (contextual stimulus rhythms) and voluntary (instructions) factors affect people's ability to track events in real time.

Summary of Events and Driving Rhythms

Major points in this section are:

- Exogenous entrainment is defined by stable phase-locking.
- Exogenous entrainment is established by regular and forceful driving rhythms.
- Three paradigms designed to study entrained attending are perturbation, temporal context, and selective attending. All are variants of the perturbation design.

BACKGROUND: ORIGINS OF ANIMATE ENTRAINMENTS

In the second half of the twentieth century, Pittendrigh, Aschoff, and others broke new ground with revolutionary ways to think about internalized circadian rhythms of animate creatures in their environments (see Box 4.1).[20,21,22,23] This was a critical turning point in experimental biology; it revised thinking about light–dark cycles by viewing them as driving rhythms. It also introduced new terms such as "biological entrainment," "driving rhythms," and *"zeitgebers"* that evoked the concept of isochrony. Amidst great debates over innate, internalized rhythms, new designs, including especially the perturbation paradigm, emerged to study timing relationships between driving and driven rhythms. This led to the now famous *phase response curves* (PRCs) introduced by Pittendrigh. These were exciting times, and classic studies of circadian entrainment with *Drosophila*, rats, squirrels, and other animals supported novel ideas about entrainment wherein the observable

BOX 4.1
VARIETIES OF BIOLOGICAL PRCS

Classic entrainment research began with Aschoff[83] and Pittendrigh,[84] although DeCoursey[85] is rightly credited for her original PRC work. Winfree[86] described various PRCs that do not resemble those of Figure 4.4. Thus, a type 1 PRC involves motor phase corrections to powerful probes with high objective salience (intensity, duration) where PRCs exhibit significant negative slopes (e.g., Figure 4.4). However, with very strong probes, overcorrections lead to slope negativities exceeding −1.0. This yields a type 0 PRC, indicating an unstable oscillator. With type 0 PRCs, a driven oscillation can encounter a perturbation of a particular salience at a particular phase point (a *critical point*) that drastically weakens or eliminates the oscillation's amplitude and/or leads to arrhythmias. Winfree's discovery of type 1 versus type 0 PRCs is a remarkable one in the history of biological research on entrainment that remains a source of much debate. Implications of type 0 PRCs for the present context remain unclear. But they raise interesting issues surrounding how entrainment is "turned off," among other things.

activities of animals were phase-locked to slow, regular, light–dark circadian periodicities.

The perturbation paradigm was central to this theoretical movement. A key independent variable for PRCs is the relative time of a probe stimulus, $\Delta\varphi_s$, given an ongoing internalized circadian rhythm. Dependent variables were motor responses that revealed observable phase corrections (partial or complete) to a perturbing probe stimulus. For instance, even today, a typical PRC study takes place in a darkened environment where a probe (e.g., a light flash) occurs at different phase points relative to a free-running, internalized circadian rhythm of an animal. Next, an animal's adjusted response times to various probe times are registered to address questions such as "How do animals respond to a light flash at an expected time (e.g., 7 AM, dawn) versus at various (potentially) perturbing times for a bright light—that is, unexpected times (e.g., 11 PM)?" Classically, the answer depended on two properties of the probe: its relative time and its force (e.g., light intensity).

Or—a more familiar example? Circadian rhythms are one of the main rhythms that structure the lives of animate creatures, including humans. Consider how our bodies automatically adapt to these rhythms as we travel the globe. For example, Bill (of the preceding chapter) who lives in Los Angeles where his expected wake-up time is 8 AM (Pacific Time) flies to New York. On his first night in New York, he awakens at 5 AM (local time) leading to a sense of a phase difference, $\Delta\varphi$, given his expected

(phase) wake-time, φ_e. This is a 3-hour disparity, $\Delta\varphi = -3/24 = -.125$. Bill's got jet lag. Yet, without conscious control, his body automatically begins to adapt to jet lag. Initially, his corrected phase is partial, so he awakens the next morning at 6 AM ($\Delta\varphi = -.0833$). But, after a few days, more partial phase corrections occur, and, happily, Bill falls into synchrony with New York time ($\Delta\varphi = 0$). The downside is that Bill is destined to experience a reversed diet of jet lag on his return to LA.

The Phase Response Curve
Regardless of the animal, PRC curves are informative. Historically, PRCs are the definitive plots of entrainment. They summarize how animals adapt to temporally disrupting stimuli, both large and small. A PRC plots an animal's phase correction as a function of probe timing. That is, $\Delta\varphi$ is an independent variable that reflects the temporal manipulations of a deviant probe. The dependent variable, $-kF(\Delta\varphi)$, reflects the degree of phase correction. For instance, if an unexpected probe arrives early with a $\Delta\varphi$ of −.10, in theory an adjustment to this probe might range from 0 (no phase correction) to .06 (partial correction) or to .10 (full phase correction). A PRC curve plots an observed relationship between $\Delta\varphi$ and $-kF(\Delta\varphi)$ over a range of phase values. Six examples of PRC curves appear in Figure 4.4. A glance at this figure reveals that three major factors influence PRCs: probe timing, $\Delta\varphi$; probe force, **K** (i.e., salience); and driven rhythm strength.

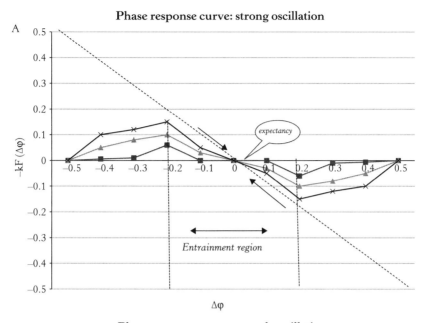

FIGURE 4.4 Phase response curves (PRCs) for three different levels of time marker salience. In these curves, phase deviation of a probe is plotted on abscissa and the correct response to it on the ordinate. Panel **A** shows PRCs for a strong entraining oscillation; panel **B** shows parallel PRCs for a weak entraining oscillation.

Probe Timing

Animals find adjusting to some perturbations easier than others. Thus, not all probe timings, $\Delta\varphi$, provoke complete phase corrections. Overall, perfect adaptation is shown by the straight dotted line in Figure 4.4A where $-\mathbf{k}F(\Delta\varphi) = \Delta\varphi$ (for $\Delta\varphi$ values). This rarely happens. Comparing ideal performance with actual PRCs (for three probe salience lines) clarifies that full phase corrections are not common. However, such corrections do occur with probes occurring near an expected phase point, φ_e (i.e., $\varphi_e = \Delta\varphi = 0$). Indeed, if a probe arrives at the expected time, it is "on-time," and no phase correction is necessary ($-\mathbf{k}F$ ($\Delta\varphi = 0$). Also, slightly early or slightly late probes (relative to φ_e) create minor perturbations that are easily accommodated. Generally, small to modest deviation magnitudes of $\Delta\varphi$, namely those less than 20% of an induced circadian period ($0 \leq l\Delta\varphi l \leq .20$), lead to partial phase corrections. But very deviant probes are extremely perturbing; they fluster individuals, as reflected by partial corrections, which fall far short of the ideal expressed by the dashed PRC lines in Figure 4.4. Finally, note that two extreme outcomes are labeled *capture* and *expectancy* points in PRCs. Respectively, these points refer to corrective responses to probes that are quite unexpected versus responses to other probes that are very expected.

Probe Salience

Effects of probe salience also appear in Figure 4.4. PRCs differ in function probe salience due, in part, to the coupling parameter, $\mathbf{k}$ (three PRC salience lines). A salient probe creates high $\mathbf{k}$ values; salient probes characterize greater driving rhythm force and, hence, stronger coupling. Thus, phase corrections that match a deviant probe are more likely to be complete as $\mathbf{k}$ increases (see Box 4.1). For instance, for $\Delta\varphi = -.10$, a low-salience probe (bar line) yields no phase adjustment, whereas stronger probes with medium (triangle line) or high (x line) driving forces yield partial and complete phase corrections, respectively. Finally, a caveat is in order. Probe salience is relative; a probe is salient if brighter or louder (or the like) from a *prevailing context*. In sum, phase correction is positively correlated with probe salience.

Oscillator Strength

A third, less recognized factor is interesting. This involves oscillator strength. It is also shown to affect PRC curves in Figure 4.4A,B. The strength of an entraining neural oscillation is important in phase-locking. Strength is likely linked to an oscillator's amplitude as well as to other factors. Basically, the measure of an oscillator's inner strength is found in its power in countering the impact of external probe salience. When an oscillation "bumps" into an ill-timed (i.e., unexpected) probe, it usually automatically phase corrects. However, stronger oscillations are *less responsive* to a perturbing probe than are weaker driven oscillations.

At first blush, reduced responsiveness of a strong oscillation may seem counterintuitive. Yet the rationale proposed here is straightforward and interesting. Stronger oscillations stay closer to "home base"—to their intrinsic periods–than do weaker ones. Effectively, they are less "flustered" by an unexpected probe.[24] Notice the reduced PRC range of phase corrections in Figure 4.4A (strong oscillation) relative to that of Figure 4.4B (weak oscillation). Strong oscillations are more stable, hence less variable in phase-locking than are weak ones.

Basically, strong oscillations resist the effects of pushes or pokes from a perturbing probe. This is part of a *push–pull* juxtaposition where the pushing strength (i.e., salience) of a driving rhythm opposes the pulling strength of the driven oscillation. A strong external probe with high salience "pushes" a system toward aligning with it during phase correction, whereas a strong internal oscillation "pulls" back toward alignment with its intrinsic period. This push–pull dynamic in an entrainment dance will weave in and out of future chapters.

Oscillator strength increases as driving rhythm regularity increases, but it may also depend on to-be-discovered physiological factors (including some derived from learning suggested in later chapters). Returning to Bill's circadian oscillation, oscillator strength may explain why his jet lag in New York was so pronounced: his internalized (driven) circadian rhythm was strong not only due to innate factors but also due to well-established lifetime regularities that strengthen internalized circadian rhythms.

The Entrainment Region

A final point relates to a critical feature of all PRC curves. In Figure 4.4, all curves have similar shapes. All show similar response tendencies for on-time, early ($-\Delta\varphi$), and late ($+\Delta\varphi$) probes. Importantly, all have similar *entrainment regions*.

A PRC addresses a subset of $\Delta\varphi$ values for which adaptive behaviors are especially effective (vertical dashed lines). This represents a category of time deviations that allow "manageable" perturbations; namely, ones leading to fairly good phase correction. For instance, in Figure 4.4B a highly salient probe (x line) garners full phase corrections for all $\Delta\varphi$ values in the entrainment region. Within the phase entrainment region, the dotted PRC line has a negative slope (-1.00) indicating complete phase corrections. Shallower PRC trajectories in this region express partial phase corrections. Arrows are directed to a point attractor at a phase of zero.

Summary of Phase Response Curves

Although PRCs may seem removed from our daily lives, in fact, they describe the way we effortlessly stay "in touch" with our dynamic environment. They are tools for understanding involuntary coping skills, quietly operating to modulate phase fluctuations in various rhythmic contexts. To clearly see the effects of their work, consider a more familiar setting, one involving a fast acoustic driving rhythm (i.e., not a slow visual circadian rhythm). Among other things, the gist of PRCs implies that any unexpected noise while listening intently to a regular event—such as a song, for instance—will invite a response predicted by a PRC curve.

Imagine, for instance, that in shuffling through the computer's playlist you happen on Marvin Gaye's classic version of *I Heard It Through the Grapevine*. As you settle into listening, you find yourself automatically tapping to expected beats. This is the essence of participatory attending: your cortical oscillation becomes phase-locked to this rhythm so that you feel "part" of this unfolding event. Then, suddenly, the telltale signal of your ringtone sounds, disrupting this tapping behavior. The preceding scenario specifies three factors that should affect the timing of your tapping at this point: (1) the *time of the ring* (probe timing) relative to an induced (expected) beat ($\Delta\varphi$); (2) the loudness of the ring (probe salience, **k**), and (3) the strength of an ongoing internal oscillation beat, i.e., your internal beat (oscillator amplitude). Consequently, instead of tapping to the next beat, your tap is likely to automatically happen a bit earlier if the ring preceded the prior tap, especially if it is a loud ring. On the other hand, if the ring is soft and you are really invested in this tune, as reflected by a strong internal oscillation, then you will experience only a slight tapping change due to driven rhythm strength. In this case, you successfully "tune out" the perturbing ring and stick with Marvin Gaye's beats.

Major points of this section center on classic aspects of biological entrainment:

- Exogenous entrainment is studied using perturbation paradigms: An external sequence (a driving rhythm) contains a stimulus probe with deviant timing. Relative time changes of probe phase, $\Delta\varphi$, provide an independent variable for a PRC. The dependent variable is a phase-corrective

response, **k** $F(\Delta\varphi)$, of an entraining rhythm (an internal oscillation).
- PRCs show that overt phase corrections (motor acts) are more likely to be complete corrections with small than with large temporal perturbations, $\Delta\varphi$.
- PRCs also show that observable phase corrections increase with the salience/force of a perturbing probe but decrease with increases in driven rhythm strength.

ENERGY PROFILES OF REAL-TIME ATTENDING

Entrainment approaches offer powerful tools that can be exploited to understand attending dynamics. And PRCs depict a wonderful lawfulness in the adaptivity of creatures as they "tune in" to rhythmic events. This section extends these ideas to activity that is less observable than motor behavior but not less important: attending.

Attending, like motor behavior, occurs in real time. Although not as observable as overt motor responses, attending also depends on an entraining oscillation. But, unlike motor responses, *attending is hypothesized to depend also on temporally allocated energy, supplied by entraining oscillations, at moments of coincidence with a probe.* A coincidence *in time* of peak attending energy with a stimulus is an important condition for effective attending. In short, to perceive a changing stimulus, one must boost attending "at the right time."

This argument links attending with a new dependent variable. In a perturbation paradigm, instead of recording time changes in PRC curves, attending is typically evaluated by gauging one's accuracy in perceiving a probe. Accuracy increases as more attending energy falls on a to-be-identified probe stimulus. The coincidence of an internal energy pulse with an external probe is illustrated by a dashed rectangle in Figure 4.3A,B, where a significant overlap of expected pulse energy with probe (dot) is shown. By contrast, overlapping energy for unexpected probes is reduced when energy depends on reactive pluses and partial phase corrections. Finally, note some times expected pulses fall on silent periods; these lighter gray pulses realize the continuity of expectancy pulses through silences to create *silent pulses* (cf. Figure 3.4A,B).

This is a new conceptualization of attending. It features a previously unrecognized role for the amplitude of a driven oscillator as an index of attending energy. And it is grounded by a constraint that attending energy is conditionally allocated in time. The PRC framework determines timing constraints. A driven oscillation's amplitude and phase operate jointly to project peaks of attending energy at expected time points during anticipatory attending. Conversely, probe stimuli happening at unexpected times can command reactive attending energy of an expectancy pulse is shifted (phase corrected) to join a reactive pulse. The latter creates an after-the-fact boost in energy; as such, it literally describes a "capture" scenario where attending involuntarily shifts to align with unexpectedly early probes. Finally, probe identification accuracy depends on the total amount of energy coinciding with a probe stimulus "when" it occurs. The key factor is whether or not sufficient attending energy occurs at the "right" time to identify a probe.

Targeting Attending Energy: Canonical Attending Energy Profiles

Attending is a central concept in psychology because it refers to a vital ability, namely our capacity for orienting to and perceiving environmental stimuli. Simply put, we operate more efficiently if we attend to critical happenings in our environment. For instance, we must attend to a changing traffic light "when" it occurs to avoid a collision. This is also the case in laboratory tasks: successful performance in perception tasks occurs when people "pay attention" at the time a to-be-judged stimulus appears.[25]

Let us return to Figure 4.3 A,B to illustrate how people direct and redirect attending energy in time. In this perturbation paradigm, each of four driving–driven dyads constitutes row of sounds (gray/black ovals) containing one probe (fifth, black, oval) to which a hypothetical individual must attend (dark gray pulses). Each panel (A,B) outlines two types of trials. One type (*top rows*) has a probe which is timed to "fit into" preceding isochronous context, whereas the other type (*bottom rows*) embeds a an 'ill-timed' probe. The opening isochronous context should induce a strong temporal expectancy in a participant's tunable brain. This expectancy is carried by the driven oscillation with phase-sensitive (expectancy) peaks (dark gray triangles). Although initially, expectancy pulses are out of phase with sounds ($\Delta\varphi \neq 0$), as exogenous entrainment takes hold, phase corrections shift these pulses to precede sounds in panels A and B. Theoretically, during this process, reactive pulses (medium gray triangles) dwindle in strength (i.e., repetition suppression) whereas expectancy pulses grow in strength due to contextual regularity. (Note: as shown, a driven oscillator's manifest periods, $p' \sim p$, gravitate to the

inter-onset-time, T). And, during entrainment, the expected phase (φ_e) comes to match probe stimulus timing φ_s ($\varphi_e \rightarrow \varphi_s$; hence $\Delta\varphi_s \rightarrow 0$). These corrective phase changes constitute the "tuning" of an oscillator to successive stimulus time intervals, including those of a deviant (probe) item. During this process, different degrees of overlapping energy arise respectively from partial and complete phase correction (e.g., significant overlap appears in dashed boxes). Thus, more effective attending results from complete than from partial phase corrections because the former involves greater aggregated energy at the "right" time. In this way, exogenous entrainment realizes involuntary attending.

Canonical *attending energy profiles* (AEPs) are derived from PRCs. Involuntary attending reflects the baseline (default) amplitude levels of a driven oscillation. Amplitude is a considered a major feature in entrainments. Here amplitude reflects the aggregated activity of many synchronizing oscillations (technically these profiles of amplitude changes correspond to *potentials* in a dynamical systems framework). In DAT, an AEP is treated as a source of attending strength for a single functional driven rhythm.[26] Timing of peak neural energy depends on successful phase corrections to individual items in an unfolding sequence, including a probe item. Thus, an AEP can focus upon energies allocated to a probe, given a perturbation paradigm. As with a PRC, the AEP depends on relative probe time, $\Delta\varphi$, as the independent variable. But, importantly, the critical dependent variable for AEPs is not phase correction (as with PRCs); instead, it is the degree of successfully targeted internal energy conditional on phase corrections. This dependent measure correlates with the accuracy of probe identification; driven rhythm energy is predicted to be greater for complete than partial phase corrections.

Eight canonical AEPs appear in Figure 4.5. Four AEPs reflect involuntary energy curves (thick line) whereas others suggest voluntary AEP curves (thin line) with higher energy levels. The former apply to attention tasks resting on perturbation paradigms whereas the latter are suited to selective attending tasks. The remainder of this section focuses on involuntary AEPs; the following section considers voluntary attending.

Involuntary Attending: Expectancy and Capture AEPs

The "dynamics" in DAT involve the exogenous entrainment of cortical oscillations. Using a perturbation paradigm, both the amplitude of

Attending energy profiles, AEP

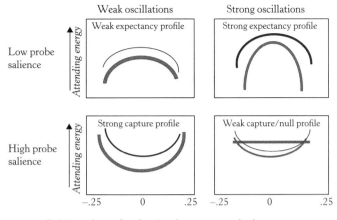

FIGURE 4.5 Attending energy profiles (AEP). Each of four conditions plots the profile of energy levels from coinciding amplitudes with a probe stimulus in a perturbation paradigm. Maximum energy is allocated to temporally expected probes when the probe is of low salience (an expectancy profile) especially with a strong oscillation. Maximum energy is allocated to a deviant probe when it is highly salient (a capture profile), especially with a weak oscillation.

a driven cortical oscillation and the salience of some perturbing probe shape an AEP. But, as already noted, these two factors have opposing impacts on phase corrections that arise from their pull–push contest. This opposition results in two familiar attentional phenomena: expectancy and capture.

These phenomena are reflected in the two different involuntary AEPs shown as thicker curves in Figure 4.5. One, an *expectancy profile* (*top row*), has maximal collective energy aimed at probes occurring at expected points in time in this paradigm. The other, a *capture profile* (*bottom row*), shows maximal energy redirected to an ill-timed probe. Note, both types of profiles are qualified by oscillator strength.

A strong AEP expectancy profile predicts best performance for expected probes (Figure 4.5, *top right*). All else equal, a strong driven oscillation leads to an expectancy AEP with a sharp inverted U shape. This highlights a persisting expectancy pulse operating within an entrainment region. The pulse delivers maximum peak energies at expected probe times ($\varphi_e = \varphi_s$), which boosts energy allocated to each temporally expected item. Thus, while both AEPs in the top row of this figure have expectancy profiles, the signature expectancy more profile is pronounced for a strong oscillation.

A strong AEP capture profile offers a contrast to the strong expectancy profile. The capture profile happens when a highly salient probe

outside the entrainment region overcomes a weak driven oscillation (Figure 4.5, *bottom left*). Here, a clear U-profile emerges, leading to predictions that the best performance will happen with a distinctively ill-timed probe. Capture profiles are most pronounced with highly salient probes because these probes are literally "attention getters"; they effectively redirect (i.e., "push") energy toward ill-timed probes occurring outside an entrainment region. This process entails a weak driven oscillation with unreliable expectancy pulses (poor anticipatory attending). In turn, a salient, ill-timed probe can then "grab" attending (Figure 4.5, *bottom left*). These rapid corrections "push" an expectancy pulse close to the onset time of the unexpected probe and its reactive pulse. Together, these pulses create collected energy (reactive-plus-expectancy pulses). Indeed, this is the famed "surprise" effect instilled by such probes. (A comment: a deviant probe [e.g., $-\Delta\varphi = .20$] that is also very salient can detour a weakly scheduled attending pulse, redirecting an expectancy pulse in time [$-\mathbf{k}F(\Delta\varphi) = -.20$]; see the x line in Figure 4.4B).

The AEPs reflect interactions between probe salience and driven oscillator strength. Low-salience probes yield strong expectancy profiles and weak capture profiles, whereas the reverse is true of high-salience probes. Why is this? The reasons are simple: a strong oscillation is tightly tethered to its intrinsic period. Thus, it shows a clear expectancy profile with low-salience stimuli because these probes fail to force (push) the oscillation from its favored phase ($\Delta\varphi = 0$). AEP profiles inherit this feature from PRCs, where low-salience probes lack the force to "push" a strong oscillation away from its home base. Conversely, a high-salience probe can force a weak, malleable, oscillation into a phase change (cf. Figure 4.4B, x-line; Figure 4.5, *bottom left*).

In sum, canonical AEPs draw on exogenous entrainment to explain involuntary allocations of attending energy. Both expectancy and capture AEPs engage anticipatory and reactive attending. However, anticipatory attending is more prominent in expectancy profiles, whereas reactive attending dominates capture profiles. Finally, all AEPs are grounded in exogenous entrainment; this section explained the role of three major factors: probe timing (from PRCs), probe salience, and oscillator strength.

Evidence for AEPs

This portrait of AEPs leads to several testable predictions about the effects of exogenous attending on involuntary attending in perturbation paradigms. The following section provides some evidence favoring these predictions.

Observed Expectancy Profiles

The AEP profiles generate predictions about people's accuracy in judging expected and unexpected probe stimuli. For instance, a strong expectancy profile predicts best identifications of probes with low salience that appear at expected points in time (Figure 4.5, *top right*).

Observed AEPs confirm this prediction. Listeners asked to identify the pitch of a temporally variable probe embedded in an otherwise isochronous melody are more accurate (d′) in their pitch judgments for "on-time" probe tones than for ones unexpectedly early or late (Figure 4.6).[27] Other studies show similar outcomes.[28,29]

Observed capture profiles have also been reported using these tasks. These AEPs occur when a sequential context is likely to induce a weak driven oscillation (Figure 4.5, *bottom left*).[30] Such AEPs are interesting because they arise from the impact of a salient stimulus that provokes in a perceiver a "double-take" in reaction to a surprising stimulus, which then results in heightened identification accuracy (i.e., expectancy-plus-reactive pulses). This is a defining aspect of the attentional capture since its introduction by Yantis and Jonides[31] (cf. Folk and Gibson for an overview[32]). In visual attention tasks, a sudden stimulus causes an immediate reorienting of a viewer's attention. Similarly, in the

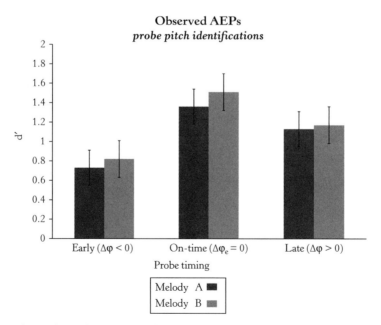

FIGURE 4.6 An observed attending energy profile (AEP) based on listener's pitch identifications of early, on-time, and late probe tones.

An adapted portion of figure 6a in Mari Riess Jones, Heather Moynihan Johnston, and Jennifer Puente, "Effects of Auditory Pattern Structure on Anticipatory and Reactive Attending," *Cognitive Psychology* 53, no. 1 (August 2006): 59–96, doi:10.1016/j.cogpsych.2006.01.003.

auditory domain, a U-shaped capture profile again rises from a realigned (i.e., phase-corrected) expectancy pulse that joins with a reactive pulse to deliver a double dose of attending energy to a surprising probe sound. Confirmation of both strong and weak capture profiles in probe identification tasks is found in a series of studies by Ralph Barnes and Heather Johnston.[33]

Summary of Attending Energy Profiles

In a dynamic context, AEPs express allotments of neural energy that are directed or redirected to temporally align with the occurrence of a to-be-judged probe item. In a perturbation paradigm, performance depends on AEPs that reflect energy levels for variously timed probes. Both probe timing and salience affect AEP shape; the strength of an exogenously entraining oscillation also plays a qualifying role. Strong oscillations, induced by a regular temporal context, are more likely to create AEP shapes of expectancy profiles, whereas weak oscillations are more likely to supply capture profiles. Major points of this section are:

- Baseline levels of oscillator energy reflect default amplitudes of an exogenously entraining neural oscillation.
- Entraining oscillations can support well-timed attending to temporally expected items. Temporally unexpected items invite oscillator phase corrections that contribute to collective attending energy coincident with a to-be-identified item (probe). Timed attending energy determines perceptual accuracy of item identification.
- AEPs (based on PRCs) assume two different generic shapes—expectancy or capture profiles—depending on the timing and salience of a probe and the strength of an entraining oscillation.
- Evidence supports AEP predictions about expectancy and capture profiles.

A GENERAL ATTENDING HYPOTHESIS

This final section broadens the discussion of attending to focus more on voluntary attending. Typically, voluntary attending is studied using selective attending paradigms. In these tasks, instructions typically encourage people to consciously narrow their attentional focus to one of several ongoing events. This reflects our common orientation to surroundings; we are often focused on some goal while we wade through multiple, simultaneously active but irrelevant stimuli in our environment. And we "pay attention" to some events and not others. Without some capacity to ignore unimportant background noise in order to track other, critical, information our species would not have survived. Although less critical to species survival, more mundane examples of selective attending testify to its ubiquity in our daily lives. For instance, in watching a tennis match we consciously shift our focus between one of the two players as we visually track the back and forth of ball motions while at the same time trying to ignore a guy behind us who is noisily eating popcorn. Selective focusing is also evident in many listening behaviors involving speech and music. For example, in listening to a symphony, we may find ourselves focusing on the melodic sounds of a flute, not on the accompanying violins. And, of course, selective attending is most famously portrayed in the classic Cocktail Party effect. In this social context, a listener focuses intentionally on the utterances of one speaker while ignoring those of others. Selective attending is typically taken to reflect a voluntary ability to "tune in" to and follow some extended event while simultaneously "tuning out" concurrent irrelevant stimuli.

Voluntary Attending

Laboratory settings designed to study voluntary attending use carefully controlled selective attending tasks to assess how people's intentions shape their ability to follow a task-relevant event (e.g., a flute or a single speaker). Typically, people are explicitly told to attend to one relevant event and ignore a co-occurring irrelevant one. Note, however, that DAT assumes that both relevant and irrelevant events provide exogenous driving rhythms, meaning that both events automatically entrain a listener's attending, thus forming different exogenous dyads. In other words, voluntary attending is not alone; the automaticity of exogenous entrainment is ever-present. By definition, exogenous attending is hard to escape. Once an environmental event happens, at some default level of attending energy, some ongoing internal oscillation automatically latches on to it.

Voluntary attending, as noted, is *not* automatic. However, in the present view, voluntary attending entails a boost of attending energy that piggybacks on the automaticity of exogenous entrainment. This results from a person's intended increases in the amplitude of the driven rhythm (or rhythms) at times granted by exogenous entrainments. Such intentions are realized internally with the allocation of more AEP energy levels for relevant events and/or less energy for irrelevant events.[34] As shown by thinner AEP curves in Figure 4.5, energy may be voluntarily heightened (or suppressed) for a single probe (in an event). In general, voluntary attending adds energy to exogenously (thicker) driven AEP profiles.

Voluntary AEPs

The canonical AEPs of Figure 4.5 are necessarily idealized because voluntary attending is flexible. Indeed, flexibility is a hallmark of voluntary attending.[35] The AEPs, like PRCs, are snapshots in time. Thus, in selective attending tasks, attending is voluntarily directed to one or another item in an unfolding sequence. For instance, a listener may voluntarily shift focal attending from one word to the next while tracking a phrase uttered by a speaker. Or, reviving the fabled Cocktail Party context, a hypothetical listener may be interested in getting the answer to a question posed to the speaker; in this case, she may voluntarily concentrate (i.e., heighten the amplitude of a driven oscillation) on one anticipated time point in the speaker's utterance. Voluntary AEPs reflect this timed flexibility in attending as momentary additions and/or subtractions of energy directed to certain items of an extended event. In short, given baseline energy limits provided by exogenous entrainment, the shape of an AEP is malleable, changing due to intentional factors. This flexibility leads to predictions of a variety of voluntary AEPs.

There is a catch. For a voluntary boost of energy to be effective, it must be appropriately timed. And this timing is automatically scheduled by exogenous entrainment. That a voluntary AEP depends on involuntary aspects of entrainment is evident in Figure 4.5, which suggests an underlying correlation between voluntary and involuntary profiles. This correlation arises because both voluntary and involuntary AEPs draw on a common PRC format. Yet the flexible nature of voluntary attending obscures this correlation. For instance, the classic AEP expectancy profile as a perfectly inverted U based on involuntary attending does not always happen. This is because if an expected probe fails to occur, people often consciously begin to anticipate its arrival at a later time, yielding a voluntary AEP in the form of an asymmetric expectancy profile.[36]

Voluntary flexibly is not license to deny the role of exogenous entrainment as a platform for voluntary attending. To see this, consider again the Cocktail Party scene. When selectively listening to one of several speakers at a cocktail party, at any moment while concentrating on one speaker, a listener may decide to heighten attending at an interesting point in the speaker's utterance. However, if then this speaker suddenly changes the rate and/ or rhythm of his speech, the listener is doomed to miss this point.[37] Such an outcome underlies the response, "*excuse me . . . could you say that again?*" It acknowledges the fundamental operations of exogenous entrainment that limit AEP shapes.

Voluntary attending is directly affected by the amplitude of a driven oscillation. In theory, factors that affect amplitude changes include task relevance and one's intentions. For example, Rimmele and colleagues found that cortical phase tracking (through MEG) of natural speech was enhanced by instructions to attend to it, but this was not the case with speech that was modified by removal of its fine time structure. However, when told to simply ignore this speech, then similar low-level, automatic neural tracking occurred in both types of speech.[38] This demonstrates the persisting automaticity of involuntary attending. Other factors associated with involuntary attending also indirectly affect voluntary attending. These involve the ongoing phase properties of an entraining oscillation which serve as a platform or baseline level of energy for voluntary attending. Involuntary attending ensures that boosts in attending energy occur at the "right" time. Thus, listeners voluntarily increase the amplitude of an exogenously entraining oscillation at this time. Importantly, this strategy succeeds only with a listener's unwitting reliance on the automaticity of phase-locked timing.

A Basic Proposal: The General Attending Hypothesis

The prominence of voluntary factors in selective attending is undeniable. Yet the preceding discussion implies that such prominence features a grounding role for involuntary factors. Voluntary and involuntary factors simultaneously impact real-time attending. This is formalized as one of the two major hypotheses of DAT: the *general attending hypothesis*:

Dynamic attending is governed by cortical oscillations that become involuntarily phase-entrained to event time structure and, by timed amplitude elevations of one or several active, exogenously driven neural oscillation(s), elevations created by voluntary factors. Specifically:

- *Involuntary attending is based on exogenous entrainment in which the driven oscillator(s) is (are) governed by external driving rhythm* properties (regularity, force). Automatic phase adaptation to driving rhythm schedules peak amplitude(s) at specific phase points in ongoing event-based driving rhythms (relevant or irrelevant).

- Voluntary attending is constrained by exogenous entrainments that support attending to relevant driving rhythms. Voluntary elevation (or suppression) of amplitude(s) of relevant driven oscillation(s) operates on times scheduled by exogenous entrainments involving driving rhythms of relevant events.

This hypothesis expands a definition of selective attending offered by Schroeder and colleagues, which describes voluntary attending as "a neural process by which the brain enhances the representation of task-relevant inputs at the expense of irrelevant inputs."[39][p. 172] The general attending hypothesis differs from this proposal in its explicit incorporation of a fundamental role for event-driven involuntary attending as one source of the timing of brain "enhancements." It recognizes exogenous entrainment as an enabler of voluntary attending that provides (1) baseline energy levels and (2) scheduled times of voluntary energy boosts (enhancements). Finally, with respect to voluntary attending, this DAT hypothesis dovetails with Schroeder's neural hypothesis of selective dynamic attending.[40,41,42,43,44,45,46]

An Example Study from Laboratories of Charles Schroeder, Peter Lakatos, and Colleagues

One of the clearest demonstrations of dynamic brain activity underlying voluntary attending comes from inspiring and prolific research by Peter Lakatos and Charles Schroeder and their colleagues.[47,48,49,50,51] One study nicely highlights the neurodynamics of attending.

In 2008, Lakatos, Schroeder, and colleagues[52] discovered brain activities underlying selective attending using a simplified Cocktail Party paradigm.[53] They presented two concurrent sequences of items to participants (humans, monkeys) consisting of a sequence of auditory beeps that was interleaved with a sequence of light flashes. The result was two concurrent visual/auditory driving rhythms with identical rates.[54] Following familiarization with modality cues, all participants selectively tracked one (cued) of the two, quasi-isochronous, driving rhythms. Each participant had to detect a probe (a modified item) in the

relevant (i.e., cued) sequence.[55] Both sequences had slow (delta range), slightly irregular, driving rhythms. Participations selectively attended (A) either to an Auditory (AA) or Visual (AV) sequence. Subdural brain responses (i.e., across several cortical layers) to successive items were recorded for relevant and irrelevant sequences. Recordings measured oscillators' amplitude and phase corrections (inter-trial-coherence [ITC] measures) of cortical oscillations, thereby gauging exogenous entrainments at two time scales: low-frequency delta rhythms and high-frequency gamma rhythms[56] (see Box 4.2).

Theoretically, what should we expect from such experiments?

Dynamic attending approaches appeal to entrainment concepts.[57] Specifically, the general attending hypothesis offers several tunable brain predictions. First, this hypothesis holds that both of the quasi-isochronous stimulus driving rhythms (relevant, irrelevant) will automatically entrain a weak driven oscillation.[58] It also maintains that listeners told to selectively attend to the relevant sequence will strengthen this driven oscillation (i.e., relative to the irrelevant sequence) by voluntarily boosting its overall amplitude (energy). In turn, the stronger oscillation, tuned to the relevant sequence, will show less responsiveness to driving rhythm irregularities than the weaker driven rhythm tuned to the irrelevant sequence (regardless of modality). In general, weaker tracking of the irrelevant sequence by the driven oscillation following this sequence will be characterized by greater responsivity to disruptions, i.e., to "pushes" from its irregularly timed items than evident in the tracking of the stronger oscillation with the relevant sequence. Consequently, the stronger oscillations (from voluntary instructions) should have lower phase variance scores. Pertinent AEPs for weak versus strong oscillator predictions appear in Figure 4.5 (*top row*).

Five major findings from paradigms designed to test this hypotheses support dynamic attending approaches:

- *Driven oscillator amplitudes*: Amplitudes of recorded (delta) oscillations were higher in task-relevant conditions, encouraging voluntary entrainment to the relevant (vs. irrelevant) driving rhythm regardless of modality. Importantly, amplitude elevation for relevant events depended on baseline amplitude levels indexed by involuntary attending to irrelevant rhythms. This supports the idea that exogenous

---

BOX 4.2
ASSESSING ATTENDING: PHASE AND AMPLITUDE OF DRIVEN OSCILLATIONS

Direct measures of oscillation activity concern momentary phase and amplitude values. Unfortunately, ideal neural indices of these properties are elusive. As Makeig cautions, correct identification of independent oscillator properties is an important first measurement step. And the EEGLAB of Delorme and Makeig[87] is such a starting point.

Phase behavior is variously measured. Techniques directly or indirectly reflect recorded neural activities. A tricky issue concerns metrics reflecting the independence of oscillator phase and amplitude. Phase-locking value (PLV)[88]gauges inter-trial variability of phase differences independently of amplitude variations (A), but it applies only to certain experimental designs. This restriction may also hold for other phase-related measures (e.g., time-locking and inter-trial-coherence [ITC]). Also, most phase-locking measures *average* the variance of phase differences over trials (or time). That is, they do not track instantaneous phase changes of a real-time profile given by adaptive acts of a single oscillation (but see Lachaux et al.[89]). With multiple, interacting oscillators, assessment of network phase-coupling patterns becomes important but difficult to gauge.[90] Newer metrics (e.g., the multivariate phase-coupling estimate [PCE]), begin to address these problems.[91] Finally, no single measure of phase behavior is without limitations.

Amplitude of neural oscillations is *directly* recorded for low-frequency oscillations in sensory cortex layers (e.g., supra-granular, granular, and infra-granular layers in primary auditory [A1] or visual [V] cortex). This requires invasive electrode techniques used with monkeys[92] or compliant patients. Other measures *indirectly* tap into amplitude.[93,94] Thus, a modulation index (MI) reflects distributions of oscillator amplitudes as a function of phase. More direct amplitude measures for EEG and electrocorticography (ECoG) recordings rely on current flow across cell membranes from sources in different cortical layers into cell sinks (e.g., current source density [CSD]). This calibrates the flow of electrical current and positive charges across cell membranes and into a cell.

---

entrainment functions as a platform for voluntary boosts of attending energy.[59,60]

- *Driven oscillator phases*: The oscillation entraining to the relevant driving rhythm revealed lower variance of phase changes than the oscillation entraining to the irrelevant sequence.[61,62,63] In speech, most power occurs in the range of 4 to 7 Hz, where phase-locking is strongest.[64]

- *Exogenous entrainments*: Significant time-locking to item sequences appeared in both irrelevant as well as relevant driving rhythms.[65]

- *Driving rhythm regularity*: A study by Besle et al.[66] indicates that heightened driving rhythm regularity improves coupling of slow (delta) oscillations in both relevant and irrelevant driving rhythms.[67] This supports a long-standing DAT prediction regarding rhythmic regularity and exogenous entrainments.[68,69]

- *Cross-frequency coupling (CFC)*: Recorded slow and fast oscillations revealed endogenous CFC coupling (cf. Chapter 3). Slow delta oscillations elicited by onset-to-onset time intervals between successive items synchronized with fast gamma oscillations elicited by time structure within individual items.[70]

Finally, How Does Voluntary Attending Really Work?

Preceding sections offer a plausible way to tackle selective attending, but puzzles remain. Missing is a mechanism that spells out how instructions, goals, and intentions directly enhance the amplitudes of specific cortical oscillations. When told to "pay attention" to something, what happens in the conscious tunable brain that ramps up amplitudes of certain oscillations? We really don't know.

Two Candidate Mechanisms

At least two explanatory avenues open up. One enlists a new attentional entrainment mechanism; the other appeals to motor activity.

From an entrainment perspective, Large[71,72] proposes a model that includes Andronov-Hopf bifurcations wherein a control parameter manages the amplitude of a driven oscillation. An oscillation's amplitude is suppressed when values of this parameter fall below a critical (bifurcation) point; however, with higher parameter values, oscillator magnitudes grow. One option, then, assumes that such a control parameter is sensitive to instructions, task demands, and one's intentions.

A motor approach to this puzzle addresses goal-directed actions. Thus, an initial goal, conceived as a "how-to" construct, is linked to heightened activity in motor and/or premotor cortices. For instance, the concept of *active sensing*[73] envisions exploratory motor activities in some environment that translate into the voluntary governing of a "where" and "when" of attending. Others hypothesize that voluntary control affects (possibly by imagery) overt motor activity that stimulates sensory oscillations.[74,75] Also, Grahn suggests that motor oscillations can voluntarily align with active sensory oscillations (endogenous entrainment) via a neural network.[76,77,78] To be sure, links between attending/sensory responses and motor behavior are sensitive to voluntary control, but many questions remain unanswered.

Summary of Dynamic Attending Hypotheses

In summary, dynamic attending hypotheses about involuntary and voluntary attending find support in recent neuroscience studies. Taken together, emerging studies fit neatly into the narrative of the general attending hypothesis developed in this chapter. Current trends in neuroscience research are also converging with views of dynamic attending sketched here, wherein exogenous entrainment provides a platform that allows an attender to voluntarily engage in selective attending.[79,80,81,82] In this view, selective attending entails heighten amplitudes of relevant entraining oscillations. This story suggests how we might vary the intensity of our attentional focus on a melody that we are automatically tracking while also ignoring another, co-occurring event.

Major points of this section are:

- When perturbation paradigms are embedded within selective attending tasks, voluntary factors selectively affect perceivers' recorded amplitudes of cortical oscillations that are entraining to the relevant external sequence (containing a probe).
- Following explicit task demands, stronger (recorded) oscillations revealed lower phase variance from less responsivity to fluctuations of their driving rhythms than evident in the weaker entraining oscillations which showed greater responsivities to their respective driving rhythms.
- Focal attending relies on both voluntary and involuntary factors to target attending energy to a driving rhythm.
- A General Attending hypothesis addresses this and related findings.

CHAPTER SUMMARY

The concept of attending is both mysterious and commanding. This chapter describes attention in dynamic terms as a real-time activity that involves a participatory interaction of an individual's internal (neural) oscillation with an external (event) rhythm. This exogenous entrainment is participatory in that it rests on a shaping of cortical oscillations by external event rhythms. This chapter aims to introduce basic concepts pertinent to entrainment dynamics and its related adaptive behaviors.

As we interact with events in our surroundings, at any moment in time we are engaging some level of attending energy. This energy is correlated with amplitudes of cortical (driven) oscillations which "keep time" with an external event, even a fluctuating external event spattered with rhythmic perturbations. Moreover, the amplitude of this driven oscillation at given moment in time determines our degree of attentional participation in this external event.

This chapter grounds predictions about attending in established discoveries about entrainment and phase corrections. Historically, biological entrainment arrived on the scene fighting against mighty skepticism. Yet PRCs are now widely accepted as gauges of the disruptive consequences of a single, temporal deviant item (a probe) in an ongoing driving rhythm. PRC curves also supply a foundation for predicting the accuracy of identifying a disruptive probe in attention tasks where performance depends on the amount of attending energy allocated in a timely manner to the probe. This chapter also introduces analogous attending energy curves: AEPs make a debut. AEPs depict attending energy allocated in time to temporally expected and unexpected items for both involuntary and voluntary attending.

Finally, a new hypothesis distinguishes contributions of involuntary and voluntary factors on attending. According to the general attending hypothesis, involuntary attending consists of exogenous entrainment that carries low levels of attending energy associated with a driven oscillation that is based on the force and regularity of its external driving rhythm. In addition, it stipulates that voluntary attending yields selectively higher levels of attending energy carried by a relevant entraining oscillation. Thus, voluntary attending remains rooted to the automaticity of exogenous entrainments; it "rides" on the automaticity of exogenous entrainment. In sum, voluntary attending is constrained by exogenous entrainment which supplies baseline levels of energy as well as scheduled timing of voluntary boosts of attending energy.

NOTES

1. There is also a more complex situation in endogenous entrainment where both driving and driven oscillations adapt to each other, but discussion of this is for another time.

2. Lewis T. Stevens, "On the Time-Sense," *Mind*, no. 43 (1886): 393–404.

3. J. Devin McAuley, "Tempo and Rhythm," in *Music Perception*, eds. Mari Riess Jones, Richard R. Fay, and Arthur N. Popper, Springer Handbook of Auditory Research 36 (New York: Springer, 2010), 165–99, doi:10.1007/978-1-4419-6114-3_6.

4. J. Devin McAuley and Mari Riess Jones, "Modeling Effects of Rhythmic Context on Perceived Duration: A Comparison of Interval and Entrainment Approaches to Short-Interval Timing," *Journal of Experimental Psychology: Human Perception and Performance* 29, no. 6 (2003): 1102.

5. Christoph S. Herrmann, Ingo Fründ, and Daniel Lenz, "Human Gamma-Band Activity: A Review on Cognitive and Behavioral Correlates and Network Models," *Neuroscience & Biobehavioral Reviews* 34, no. 7 (June 2010): 981–92, doi:10.1016/j.neubiorev.2009.09.001.

6. Mari Riess Jones et al., "Temporal Aspects of Stimulus-Driven Attending in Dynamic Arrays," *Psychological Science* 13, no. 4 (2002): 313–39.

7. Mari Riess Jones, Heather Moynihan Johnston, and Jennifer Puente, "Effects of Auditory Pattern Structure on Anticipatory and Reactive Attending," *Cognitive Psychology* 53, no. 1 (August 2006): 59–96, doi:10.1016/j.cogpsych.2006.01.003.

8. Herrmann, Fründ, and Lenz, "Human Gamma-Band Activity."

9. Catherine Tallon-Baudry and Olivier Bertrand, "Oscillatory Gamma Activity in Humans and Its Role in Object Representation," *Trends in Cognitive Sciences* 3, no. 4 (April 1, 1999): 151–62, doi:10.1016/S1364-6613(99)01299-1.

10. Catherine Tallon-Baudry et al., "Stimulus Specificity of Phase-Locked and Non-Phase-Locked 40 Hz Visual Responses in Human," *Journal of Neuroscience* 16, no. 13 (July 1, 1996): 4240–49.

11. Takako Fujioka et al., "Internalized Timing of Isochronous Sounds Is Represented in Neuromagnetic Beta Oscillations," *Journal of Neuroscience* 32, no. 5 (February 1, 2012): 1791–802, doi:10.1523/JNEUROSCI.4107-11.2012.

12. Edward W. Large and Joel S. Snyder, "Pulse and Meter as Neural Resonance," *Annals of the New York Academy of Sciences* 1169, no. 1 (July 1, 2009): 46–57, doi:10.1111/j.1749-6632.2009.04550.x.

13. Resonance is manifest as an increased amplitude of a vibrating unit by an external force vibrating at this unit's intrinsic frequency.

14. Edward W. Large and Mari Riess Jones, "The Dynamics of Attending: How People Track Time-Varying Events," *Psychological Review* 106, no. 1 (1999): 119–59, doi:10.1037/0033-295X.106.1.119.

15. James Mosher Klein and Mari Riess Jones, "Effects of Attentional Set and Rhythmic Complexity on Attending," *Perception & Psychophysics* 58, no. 1 (January 1996): 34–46, doi:10.3758/BF03205473.

16. Mari Riess Jones et al., "Tests of Attentional Flexibility in Listening to Polyrhythmic Patterns," *Journal of Experimental Psychology: Human Perception and Performance* 21, no. 2 (1995): 293–307, doi:10.1037/0096-1523.21.2.293.

17. Mosher Klein and Riess Jones, "Effects of Attentional Set and Rhythmic Complexity on Attending."

18. Amandine Penel and Mari Riess Jones, "Speeded Detection of a Tone Embedded in a Quasi-Isochronous Sequence: Effects of a Task-Irrelevant Temporal Irregularity," *Music Perception: An Interdisciplinary Journal* 22, no. 3 (March 2005): 371–88, doi:10.1525/mp.2005.22.3.371.

19. Peter Lakatos et al., "Entrainment of Neuronal Oscillations as a Mechanism of Attentional Selection," *Science* 320, no. 5872 (April 4, 2008): 110–13, doi:10.1126/science.1154735.

20. Colin S. Pittendrigh, *Circadian Systems: Entrainment* (New York: Springer, 1981), http://link.springer.com.proxy.library.ucsb.edu:2048/chapter/10.1007/978-1-4615-6552-9_7.

21. Colin S. Pittendrigh, "Circadian Rhythms and the Circadian Organization of Living Systems," *Cold Spring Harbor Symposia on Quantitative Biology* 25 (January 1, 1960): 159–84, doi:10.1101/SQB.1960.025.01.015.

22. Colin S. Pittendrigh and Dorothea H. Minis, "The Entrainment of Circadian Oscillations by Light and Their Role as Photoperiodic Clocks," *The American Naturalist* 98, no. 902 (1964): 261–94.

23. Juregen Aschoff, "Comparative Physiology: Diurnal Rhythms," *Annual Review of Physiology* 25, no. 1 (1963): 581–600.

24. This might be a theoretical vehicle for expressing skill.

25. Mari Riess Jones, Heather Moynihan Johnston, and Jennifer Puente, "Effects of Auditory Pattern Structure on Anticipatory and Reactive Attending," *Cognitive Psychology* 53, no. 1 (August 2006): 59–96, doi:10.1016/j.cogpsych.2006.01.003.

26. Daniel J. Calderone et al., "Entrainment of Neural Oscillations as a Modifiable Substrate of Attention," *Trends in Cognitive Sciences* 18, no. 6 (June 2014): 300–09, doi:10.1016/j.tics.2014.02.005.

27. Riess Jones, Moynihan Johnston, and Puente, "Effects of Auditory Pattern Structure on Anticipatory and Reactive Attending."

28. Jones et al., "Temporal Aspects of Stimulus-Driven Attending in Dynamic Arrays."

29. Nicolas Escoffier, Darren Yeo Jian Sheng, and Annett Schirmer, "Unattended Musical Beats Enhance Visual Processing," *Acta Psychologica* 135, no. 1 (September 2010): 12–16, doi:10.1016/j.actpsy.2010.04.005.

30. Penel and Jones, "Speeded Detection of a Tone Embedded in a Quasi-Isochronous Sequence."

31. Steven Yantis and John Jonides, "Abrupt Visual Onsets and Selective Attention: Voluntary Versus Automatic Allocation," *Journal of Experimental Psychology: Human Perception and Performance* 16, no. 1 (1990): 121–34, doi:10.1037/0096-1523.16.1.121.

32. Charles L. Folk and Bradley S. Gibson, "Attraction, Distraction and Action: Multiple Perspectives on Attentional Capture," accessed February 11, 2016, https://books-google-com.proxy.library.ucsb.edu:9443/books?hl=enandlr=andid=U02MSlawf8kCandoi=fndandpg=PP1anddq=+Folk+and+Gibson,+2001++Attraction++distraction++andots=dVrE6R6ZrFandsig=D0QpFVaYJG3wDv11e764dFpE1S8#v=onepageandq=Folk%20and%20Gibson%2C%202001%20%20Attraction%20%20distractionandf=false.

33. Ralph Barnes and Heather Johnston, "The Role of Timing Deviations and Target Position Uncertainty on Temporal Attending in a Serial Auditory Pitch Discrimination Task," *The Quarterly Journal of Experimental Psychology* 63, no. 2 (February 1, 2010): 341–55, doi:10.1080/17470210902925312.

34. These mechanisms may include neural inhibitions.

35. Riess Jones et al., "Tests of Attentional Flexibility in Listening to Polyrhythmic Patterns."

36. J. Devin McAuley and Gary R. Kidd, "Effect of Deviations from Temporal Expectations on Tempo Discrimination of Isochronous Tone Sequences," *Journal of Experimental Psychology: Human Perception and Performance* 24, no. 6 (1998): 1786.

37. Devin McAuley and Gary R. Kidd, "Effect of Deviations from Temporal Expectations on Tempo Discrimination of Isochronous Tone Sequences.," *Journal of Experimental Psychology: Human Perception and Performance* 24, no. 6 (1998): 1786.

38. Johanna M. Rimmele et al., "The Effects of Selective Attention and Speech Acoustics on Neural Speech-Tracking in a Multi-Talker Scene," *Cortex* 68 (July 2015): 144–54, doi:10.1016/j.cortex.2014.12.014.

39. Charles E Schroeder et al., "Dynamics of Active Sensing and Perceptual Selection," *Current Opinion in Neurobiology* 20, no. 2 (April 2010): 172–76, doi:10.1016/j.conb.2010.02.010.

40. Nai Ding and Jonathan Z. Simon, "Emergence of Neural Encoding of Auditory Objects While Listening to Competing Speakers," *Proceedings of the National Academy of Sciences* 109, no. 29 (July 17, 2012): 11854–59, doi:10.1073/pnas.1205381109.

41. Elana M. Zion Golumbic et al., "Mechanisms Underlying Selective Neuronal Tracking of Attended Speech at a 'Cocktail Party,'" *Neuron* 77, no. 5 (March 6, 2013): 980–91, doi:10.1016/j.neuron.2012.12.037.

42. Herrmann, Fründ, and Lenz, "Human Gamma-Band Activity."

43. Charles E. Schroeder and Peter Lakatos, "Low-Frequency Neuronal Oscillations as Instruments of Sensory Selection," *Trends in Neurosciences* 32, no. 1 (January 2009): 9–18, doi:10.1016/j.tins.2008.09.012.

44. Zion Golumbic et al., "Mechanisms Underlying Selective Neuronal Tracking of Attended Speech at a 'Cocktail Party.'"

45. Peter Lakatos et al., "The Leading Sense: Supramodal Control of Neurophysiological Context by Attention," *Neuron* 64, no. 3 (November 12, 2009): 419–30, doi:10.1016/j.neuron.2009.10.014.

46. B. Morillon and C. E. Schroeder, "Neuronal Oscillations as a Mechanistic Substrate of Auditory Temporal Prediction," *Annals of the New York Academy of Sciences* 1337 (March 2015): 26–31, doi: 10.1111/nyas.12629, accessed February 12, 2016, http://onlinelibrary.wiley.com.proxy.library.ucsb.edu:2048/doi/10.1111/nyas.12629/full.

47. Schroeder and Lakatos, "Low-Frequency Neuronal Oscillations as Instruments of Sensory Selection."

48. Lakatos et al., "Entrainment of Neuronal Oscillations as a Mechanism of Attentional Selection."

49. Zion Golumbic et al., "Mechanisms Underlying Selective Neuronal Tracking of Attended Speech at a 'Cocktail Party.'"

50. Ding and Simon, "Emergence of Neural Encoding of Auditory Objects While Listening to Competing Speakers."

51. Lakatos et al., "Entrainment of Neuronal Oscillations as a Mechanism of Attentional Selection."

52. Lakatos et al., "Entrainment of Neuronal Oscillations as a Mechanism of Attentional Selection."

53. Schroeder and Lakatos, "Low-Frequency Neuronal Oscillations as Instruments of Sensory Selection."

54. Mean periods were 650 ms; i.e., delta range frequencies, held for both modalities.

55. Note that this part of the task resembles a perturbation paradigm.

56. Using a current source density (CSD) measure.

57. Lakatos et al., "Entrainment of Neuronal Oscillations as a Mechanism of Attentional Selection."

58. Driven oscillations are weak due to mildly irregular driving rhythms.

59. Lakatos et al., "Entrainment of Neuronal Oscillations as a Mechanism of Attentional Selection."

60. Schroeder and Lakatos, "Low-Frequency Neuronal Oscillations as Instruments of Sensory Selection."

61. Lakatos et al., "Entrainment of Neuronal Oscillations as a Mechanism of Attentional Selection."

62. Schroeder and Lakatos, "Low-Frequency Neuronal Oscillations as Instruments of Sensory Selection."

63. Huan Luo, Zuxiang Liu, and David Poeppel, "Auditory Cortex Tracks Both Auditory and Visual Stimulus Dynamics Using Low-Frequency Neuronal Phase Modulation," *PLoS Biol* 8, no. 8 (August 10, 2010): e1000445, doi:10.1371/journal.pbio.1000445.

64. J. E. Peelle, J. Gross, and M. H. Davis, "Phase-Locked Responses to Speech in Human Auditory Cortex Are Enhanced During Comprehension," *Cerebral Cortex* 23, no. 6 (June 1, 2013): 1378–87, doi:10.1093/cercor/bhs118.

65. Lakatos et al., "Entrainment of Neuronal Oscillations as a Mechanism of Attentional Selection."

66. Julien Besle et al., "Tuning of the Human Neocortex to the Temporal Dynamics of Attended Events," *The Journal of Neuroscience* 31, no. 9 (March 2, 2011): 3176–85, doi:10.1523/JNEUROSCI.4518-10.2011.

67. Benjamin Morillon, Charles E. Schroeder, and Valentin Wyart, "Motor Contributions to the Temporal Precision of Auditory Attention," *Nature Communications* 5 (October 15, 2014): 5255, doi:10.1038/ncomms6255.

68. Large and Jones, "The Dynamics of Attending."

69. Mari R. Jones, "Time, Our Lost Dimension: Toward a New Theory of Perception, Attention, and Memory," *Psychological Review* 83, no. 5 (1976): 323.

70. Schroeder and Lakatos, "Low-Frequency Neuronal Oscillations as Instruments of Sensory Selection."

71. Edward W. Large, Felix V. Almonte, and Marc J. Velasco, "A Canonical Model for Gradient Frequency Neural Networks," *Physica D: Nonlinear Phenomena* 239, no. 12 (June 15, 2010): 905–11, doi:10.1016/j.physd.2009.11.015.

72. Edward W. Large, "Neurodynamics of Music," in *Music Perception*, eds. Mari Riess Jones, Richard R. Fay, and Arthur N. Popper, Springer Handbook of Auditory Research 36 (New York: Springer, 2010), 201–31, doi:10.1007/978-1-4419-6114-3_7.

73. Schroeder et al., "Dynamics of Active Sensing and Perceptual Selection."

74. Morillon, Schroeder, and Wyart, "Motor Contributions to the Temporal Precision of Auditory Attention."

75. Aniruddh D. Patel and John R. Iversen, "The Evolutionary Neuroscience of Musical Beat Perception: The Action Simulation for Auditory Prediction (ASAP) Hypothesis," *Frontiers in Systems Neuroscience* 8, no. 57 (2014): 10–3389.

76. Jessica A. Grahn, "The Role of the Basal Ganglia in Beat Perception," *Annals of the New York Academy of Sciences* 1169, no. 1 (July 1, 2009): 35–45, doi:10.1111/j.1749-6632.2009.04553.x.

77. Jessica A. Grahn and J. Devin McAuley, "Neural Bases of Individual Differences in Beat Perception," *NeuroImage* 47, no. 4 (October 1, 2009): 1894–903, doi:10.1016/j.neuroimage.2009.04.039.

78. Jessica A. Grahn and James B. Rowe, "Finding and Feeling the Musical Beat: Striatal Dissociations between Detection and Prediction of Regularity," *Cerebral Cortex* 23, no. 4 (April 11, 2012): 913–21, doi:10.1093/cercor/bhs083.

79. David Poeppel, "The Neuroanatomic and Neurophysiological Infrastructure for Speech and Language," *Current Opinion in Neurobiology* 28 (October 2014): 142–49, doi:10.1016/j.conb.2014.07.005.

80. Catia M. Sameiro-Barbosa and Eveline Geiser, "Sensory Entrainment Mechanisms in Auditory Perception: Neural Synchronization Cortico-Striatal Activation," *Frontiers in Neuroscience* 10 (August 10, 2016), doi:10.3389/fnins.2016.00361.

81. Calderone et al., "Entrainment of Neural Oscillations as a Modifiable Substrate of Attention."

82. Peelle, Gross, and Davis, "Phase-Locked Responses to Speech in Human Auditory Cortex Are Enhanced During Comprehension."

83. Jürgen Aschoff, "Circadian Rhythms in Man," *Science* 148, no. 3676 (1965): 1427–32.

84. Pittendrigh, "Circadian Rhythms and the Circadian Organization of Living Systems."

85. P. J. DeCoursey, "Phase Control of Activity in a Rodent," *Cold Spring Harbor Symposia on Quantitative Biology* 25, no. 0 (January 1, 1960): 49–55, doi:10.1101/SQB.1960.025.01.006.

86. Arthur T. Winfree, *The Geometry of Biological Time*, vol. 12 (New York: Springer Science & Business Media, 2001), https://books-google-com.proxy.library.ucsb.edu:9443/books?hl=enandlr=andid=5YktgBuoglACandoi=fndandpg=PR7anddq=Winfree++2001+++Geometry+of+Biological+Time+andots=T5zW0uk5Lsandsig=NGlVW53OEsWmyFHgvb8s4e3cYZg.

87. Arnaud Delorme and Scott Makeig, "EEGLAB: An Open Source Toolbox for Analysis of Single-Trial EEG Dynamics Including Independent Component Analysis," *Journal of Neuroscience Methods* 134, no. 1 (March 2004): 9–21, doi:10.1016/j.jneumeth.2003.10.009.

88. Jean-Philippe Lachaux et al., "Measuring Phase Synchrony in Brain Signals," *Human Brain Mapping* 8, no. 4 (1999): 194–208.

89. J. P. Lachaux, D. Rudrauf, and P. Kahane, "Intracranial EEG and Human Brain Mapping," *Journal of Physiology-Paris* 97, no. 4–6 (July 2003): 613–28, doi:10.1016/j.jphysparis.2004.01.018.

90. Jean-Philippe Lachaux, Mario Chavez, and Antoine Lutz, "A Simple Measure of Correlation across Time, Frequency and Space between Continuous Brain Signals," *Journal of Neuroscience Methods* 123, no. 2 (March 2003): 175–88, doi:10.1016/S0165-0270(02)00358-8.

91. R. T. Canolty et al., "Multivariate Phase Amplitude Cross-Frequency Coupling in Neurophysiological Signals," *IEEE Transactions on Biomedical Engineering* 59, no. 1 (January 2012): 8–11, doi:10.1109/TBME.2011.2172439.

92. Lakatos et al., "Entrainment of Neuronal Oscillations as a Mechanism of Attentional Selection."

93. A. B. L. Tort et al., "Measuring Phase-Amplitude Coupling Between Neuronal Oscillations of Different Frequencies," *Journal of Neurophysiology* 104, no. 2 (August 1, 2010): 1195–210, doi:10.1152/jn.00106.2010.

94. Tolga Esat Özkurt and Alfons Schnitzler, "A Critical Note on the Definition of Phase–Amplitude Cross-Frequency Coupling," *Journal of Neuroscience Methods* 201, no. 2 (October 2011): 438–43, doi:10.1016/j.jneumeth.2011.08.014.

5

The Temporal Niche

An Aging Hypothesis

An ecological niche is conventionally defined by geographical features. Along with available environmental resources and other habitat properties, geographical surrounds are considered to further species survival. Typically, this concept appeals to a circumscribed spatial region that in multiple ways facilitates the resilience of a particular species. In some cases, a niche includes other inhabitants as sources of food, mating, or competition. Yet conspecifics communicate with each other, often through sounds; in this way, they introduce species-specific time patterns into their niche. Although it may seem odd to focus on sound patterns in discussing ecological niches, it is not unreasonable to assert that species survival depends on effective communications among conspecifics in order to find food, to mate, and to warn of danger and/or competitors. The sights and sounds of other living things create essential communicative time patterns. These time patterns introduce dynamism into the concept of an ecological niche. Essentially they define events created by friends and foes that inhabit a common environment.

Nevertheless, traditionally the label "niche" evokes stationarity, suggesting a carved-out region in three-dimensional space. Rarely recognized as a source of survival is the fourth dimension, time. Yet it is relevant. Temporal constraints on intraspecies communications contribute to shaping an ecological niche. Acoustic signals of a given species share rates and rhythms that distinguish them from other species. For example, communicative signals generated by humans comprise event rhythms faster than the lingering songs of whales but slower than the navigating sounds of bats. Communication means these signals are heard and understood by other conspecifics. Another way of saying this is to say that members of the same species share categorically similar rhythmic events in their communicative activities. Conspecifics are bound in time.

This revives the topic of dynamic attending. As portrayed, it addresses communicative exchanges as a time-bound activity involving synchronicity between the neural oscillations of one individual and dynamic events created by another. Synchrony is at the heart of interactions among conspecifics. In short, attending is critical to conspecific survival. At an elementary level, it links a young infant, who must attend and learn, to the communicative signals of its caretakers.

This chapter takes the concept of ecological niche further. It explores the possibility that, even within a species, the ability to communicate is critically shaped by age—namely, a growth function. Remember those growth curves of Chapter 3? Well, growth does not stop with maturity; our brains follow a growth curve throughout our life spans.

The concept of a temporal niche holds that the nature of attending dynamics changes with age. Broadly defined, a temporal niche is a privileged set of event time structures that fosters conspecific communication by circumscribed rates and rhythms. For instance, we favor events of certain rates (and rhythms) at different stages in life. Perhaps this explains the gravitation of young people to fast-paced rock concerts whereas older people populate the halls of slower paced symphonies. In certain ways, this idea taps into the old adage that we slow down with age. It also implies that environmental events will have a natural *age-specific salience* within a species:

> *A temporal niche is defined as a collection of environmental time structures (i.e., driving rhythms) that is most compatible with the natural, age-specific biological time patterns of a species. Compatibility here refers to constraints on biological tendencies favoring specific rates and time patterns.*

Our environment is not static. It harbors various rhythmic events characterized by elementary time patterns, both fast and slow. Although we may be unaware of the subtle hold some events levy on our behaviors, these events nonetheless *can* tacitly influence our behavior, and their impact changes with age. Age-related changes are manifest in biases that show up in preferential orienting to some events and not others; they are also evident in the spontaneous activities of certain endogenous brain rhythms (i.e., neural oscillations). Evidence from preceding chapters lends strength to an assumption that humans are bequeathed, at birth, with primitive configurations of such oscillations, configurations that support early, selective orienting behaviors even in infants. Thus, at any moment, an infant (or an adult) can automatically react to a novel event by the selective resonance of certain neural oscillation in reaction to this event's vibrations. This is because this vibrating time structure happens to "fit" neatly into an individual's temporal niche, whereas faster or slower events do not. Moreover, it is likely that maturational forces influence such preferential orienting, hence such biases shift with age. This chapter discusses this preferential orienting and the way it changes over the life span.

CHAPTER GOALS

A primary goal of this chapter involves defining a temporal niche. This entails developing an *aging hypothesis* that posits certain inborn temporal biases which change with age.[1] Briefly, this hypothesis proposes age-related slowing: very young children selectively resonate to fast events, and, with maturation, they become increasingly sensitive to slower events. The particular temporal objects that drive participatory attending change systematically with age.

A second goal pursues maturational stages of attending. The aging hypothesis implies that attending changes over a life span. However, both resonance and entrainment are universal principles that influence attending in special ways across the life span. Although resonance is resonance at any age, its efficacy may shift with growth. Similarly, from an entrainment perspective, attractors are also operative throughout the life span, although simpler attractors may be more prevalent than complex ones early in life. One aim is to flesh out these details of an aging hypothesis which posit that certain driving/driven features of a temporal niche change with age.

A third goal involves distinguishing the aging hypothesis from the general attending hypothesis (Chapter 4). Together, these two hypotheses form the backbone of Dynamic Attending Theory (DAT) theorizing. Both hypotheses address attending, including selective attending. However, respectively, they speak to different determinants of selective attending. Briefly, the general attending hypothesis addresses external influences on attending involving driving rhythm properties (e.g., force, regularity) and task demands, whereas the aging hypothesis is concerned with internal constraints of driven rhythm strength, including innate biases. Nevertheless, because both express ever-present influences on attending, this chapter also aims to explain how the two hypotheses "fit together."

Finally, this chapter develops the construct of "temporal niche" mainly as it applies to event rate. However, the temporal niche also involves special rhythmic relationships expressed by innate attractors. Whereas sensitivity to event rate may change with age, the relative power of attractors is innate, with basic preferences favoring simple over complex attractors regardless of age. This is important because it implies that even early in life the appeal of the simple harmonies of attractors plays a critical role in infants' early reactions to speech sounds, especially vowels.

The main focus in this chapter is on event rate and our differential sensitivity to it over the life span. By definition, a temporal niche implies limits. Thus, there are many things to which humans cannot respond. For instance, we cannot hear the communications of bats because their signaling frequencies are too high. And, unlike elephants, we cannot sense a forthcoming earthquake because the relevant vibrations are too slow for us to experience. These events are either too fast or too slow for our species-specific temporal niche. However, it also the case that other species may communicate via different innate attractors than humans, hence they operate in very different temporal niches.

IN THE BEGINNING: THE FAST-DRIVING INFANT

The idea of age-related slowing in attending explains why infants so rapidly learn speech. Even older children, who seem to buzz about in a fast-driving world of their own making, fit into this theoretical account, as do their observing grandparents who own a different, slower niche and shake their heads as they watch little children zip around. Infants are naturally "tuned in" to the fast time spans of acoustic rhythms, whereas older attenders are "tuned in" to slower rhythms. This section offers snapshots of infants' behaviors to support this proposal.

Let's begin at or before birth. Does anything important happen in human communication in the first weeks of life? This chapter suggests the answer is "yes." Infants are designed to tune in to rapidly changing aspects of their surroundings. This contributes to their shockingly fast mastery of speech during the first year of life. Infants rely selectively on inborn neural time structures to differentially guide attending to relatively fast and rhythmically simple speech sounds, whereas older listeners settle into slower ambient sound patterns. According to an *aging hypothesis*, special neural structures enable engagements that bias infants toward certain event rates even in the first weeks of life. This hypothesis implies that events in our world which appear "too fast" to be accommodated by adults will nonetheless "tap into" the tunable brains of young infants just fine. It offers glimpses of the temporal niche of newborns.

Let us begin, then, with a focus on infants' early vocalizations. Although various arguments can be made about the systematic relationships between the way an infant's auditory environment changes during the first year of life, the present argument focuses on infants' shifts in attending from very fast events to slower ones. Hence, we begin by diving into a fast-paced acoustic environment that describes an infant's world. Human vocalizations that contribute to this environment comprise multiple frequency components, as shown in Table 5.1. Although frequency components are outlined in this table, it is important to keep in mind that, in the time domain, each frequency reflects a waveform. For example, Figure 5.1[2] shows how a complex sound, C, embeds three different, co-occurring, simple waveforms S_1, S_2, and S_3 (i.e., with sine wave isochrony), where waveform periods are inversely related to frequency. Essentially, waveforms tell this story. A time domain expression shows how combining component waveforms yields a more elaborate amplitude envelop. It also reveals that each contributing waveform qualifies as a simple stimulus driving rhythm. These distinctions hold for more complex speech sounds, such as the phonemes of Table 5.1. This point is important because entrainment deals with waveforms of components and their interrelations (see Box 5.1 for relevant terminology).

Rhythmic components of produced phonemes vary with a speaker's age and gender. Therefore, to study age-related attending, at least with acoustic events, it is essential to examine these components.

TABLE 5.1 VOCALIZATIONS OF A SINGLE PHONEME AS A FUNCTION OF GENDER AND AGE: TRUE VERSUS QUASI-VOWELS

		ɛ	ɛ	ɛ	ɛ	ɛ
Adult male	True vowel					
Formants	F	130 (F0)	530 (F1)	1840 (F2)	2480 (F3)	
Integer	N	1	4	14	19	
Harmonics	nF0	130	520	1820	2470	
Deviation (Hz)		0	10	20	10	
Adult female[a]	True vowel					
Formants	F	250 (F0)	684 (F1)	2612 (F2)	3352 (F3)	
Integer	N	1	3	10	13	
Harmonics	nF0	250	750	2500	3250	
Deviation (Hz)		0	66	112	102	
Infant[b]	Quasi-vowel					
Formants	F**	300 (F0)	1004 (F1**)	3012 (F2**)	4154 (F3**)	
Integer	N	1	3	10	13	
Harmonics	nF0	300	900	3000	3900	
Deviation (Hz)		0	104	12	254	

Frequencies (Hz) of male adults are from Bakan (1996, pg. 358) for the phoneme category /ɛ /.
[a]Frequencies of female adults' fundamental; F0 is scaled slightly higher than Bakan's average to coordinate with Figure 3.1.
[b]Frequencies of infants are scaled up from Bakan's measures on older children to reflect a very young infant range with variable formants (Oller's Phonation stage.) Deviation is the difference (in Hz) between a formant frequency and its nearest harmonic. Attractors correspond to nF0:F0 where n = 1, 2, 3, etc.

BOX 5.1
TIME STRUCTURE IN VOCALIZATIONS: FREQUENCY VERSUS TIME DOMAIN DESCRIPTIONS

This briefly reviews time and frequency domain terminology. A *frequency domain* description (also termed *spectral analysis*) of speech units focuses on the average rate of a periodicity, given in Hertz (Hz). However, sometimes waveform descriptions more vividly capture synchronous aspects between frequency components that change from moment to moment. Also, waveform descriptions (in milliseconds, or cycles) further our discussions of entraining activities of micro- or macro-driving rhythms in an entrainment approach.

FREQUENCY DOMAIN DESCRIPTIONS OF ACOUSTIC EVENTS: PHONEME EXAMPLES

A few examples of frequency domain descriptions of rhythms in speech vocalizations appear in Table 5.1. These summarize contrasting spectral properties of quasi- and true vowels for different speakers (age, gender for /ɛ/). Typically, formant relationships are summarized as frequency ratios (e.g., F2:F1), which are useful in differentiating phoneme categories.

A true vowel contains a group of frequencies, as in Table 5.1 Also shown are quasi-vowels uttered by a hypothetical (very young) infant. These contain only harmonically related frequency components; formants (F**) are missing. This table illustrates Oller's idea in showing that infants' early vocalizations (quasi-vowels) rely on harmonic frequencies, not formant frequencies. Table 5.1 shows estimates of missing formants for a quasi-vowel using an infant's harmonic frequency ratios (i.e., missing F2 and F3 values are multiples of the infant's fundamental, F0 (300 Hz). Hence an F2:F1 harmonic ratio of 3.33 is not a bad approximation to the corresponding adult true vowel formant ratio (e.g., F2:F1 = 3.78). Quasi-vowels are harmonically "purer" driving rhythms within an infant's temporal niche. Support for this analysis and Oller's hypothesis is found in his detailed analysis of the vocalizations of very young infants with phonemes (e.g., /ə/, /i/, or /u/).

TIME DOMAIN DESCRIPTIONS OF ACOUSTIC EVENTS: WAVEFORM EXAMPLES

Figure 5.1 presents waveforms of three pure tones, all with periods under 50 ms; these are fast *simple micro-rhythms*. Figure 5.1 depicts these micro-rhythms as continuous sine waves: S1, S2, S3. Assuming they are harmonically related ($n = 1, 2, 3$, for nF0) they combine to form a *complex micro-rhythm*: C1 or C2. However, if S3 were a nonharmonic, in a produced vowel it would be a formant waveform. Together, properties associated with simple micro-rhythms collectively are referred to as the *fine time structure* of a compound (complex) rhythm. Once a compound rhythm is formed, its recurrence establishes its own rate, which is termed the *repetition rate*.

In their capacity as *micro-driving rhythms*, component waveforms instill resonance and entrainment in listeners. For young listeners, this opens a window onto one of the most astounding aspects of human development: namely, infants' ready talent for perceptual learning of speech. Infants seem to effortlessly (indeed, often with joy) assimilate important features of the speech sounds washing over them. They don't have to enroll in a 'new baby school' that teaches them phonemes;

they naturally 'soak-up' phoneme knowledge from ambient sounds.

Aspects of the view presented here are not inconsistent with processes for which there is substantial evidence. At least with young infants, one proposal of Oller is consistent with some ideas developed here.[3] Oller stresses the import of raw acoustic properties for understanding the development of speech skills. In an analysis of stages of learning, he presents the idea that, in their first

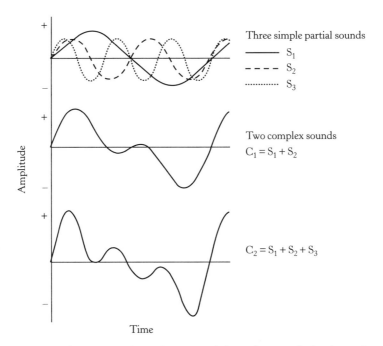

FIGURE 5.1 Time domain descriptions of sounds. Top panel shows three simple (sine) waveforms (S1, S2, S3) as components (partials) of a complex period wave with same initial phase. Generally summed components' shapes of complex waves differ as a function of components' amplitudes, frequencies, and starting phases. One complex waveform, C1, adds two components, S1 and S2 (middle panel); C2 (bottom panel) adds all three components (see Box 5.1 for details).

Adapted from figure 5.4 in C. E. Speaks, *Introduction to Sound: Acoustics for Hearing and Speech Science* (2nd edition; 1998)

year of life, infants progress through stages defined by slowing event rates.

Very Young Infants and Fast Driving Rhythms

A temporal niche, defined by DAT, reflects special event time properties. In human communications, a niche is defined by the rate and rhythm shared by sets of external time patterns (i.e., stimulus waveforms) produced by infants and adults.[4] This section defines these sets for infants as relatively fast and simple acoustic driving rhythms. Assuming these features capture an infant's temporal niche, then, according to the aging hypothesis, this niche expands and changes with maturation.

Early in life, novel acoustic patterns flood the acoustic environment of newborns. They come in the form of the sounds of a mother's voice (even in gestation) and vocalizations of other welcoming adult caretakers. But, not be overlooked are the intermingled vocalizations of infants themselves. Infants' own vocalizations are especially interesting for two reasons. First, they are diagnostic of infants' preferred vocal gestures, and, second, infants' own vocalizations add to acoustic events in

the ambient sound environment they inhabit: they "hear" themselves try out various sounds. In this mix of vocalizations are found those embedded driving rhythms most likely to automatically grab infants' attending.

In the beginning, candidate driving rhythms for early infant entrainments are submerged in the vocalizations of the infants themselves (0–3 months); for example, these sounds may be their own high-frequency squeals. These are sounds rich in higher frequency components; that is, they are fast *micro-rhythms* (i.e., periods << 50 ms). In this stage (resembling Oller's *Phonation stage*), the sound-making of infants differs from that of adults in both rate and relative time structure.

Consider first age-related rate differences. It is well known that young infants create high-pitched, complex sounds with fast fundamental frequencies, F0 (i.e., F0s above 300 Hz), whereas typical adult vocalizations are distinctly slower due to their longer vocal tracts (e.g., F0s around 130–250 Hz). Consequently, infants' rapid vocal rhythms, rooted in the glottal fold changes of F0, have rhythmic periods of 3.5 ms and less. And it also follows that harmonics of complex sounds are still faster micro-rhythms (nF0, n is an integer). Thus, a basic speech sound, such as the phoneme /ɛ/, comprises many co-occurring frequencies, as suggested in Table 5.1 (for adults or infants). These well-established rate differences are generally true for human speech sounds.[5] From a DAT perspective, these productions function for listeners as *micro-driving rhythms* with a potential for entraining a listener's attending at these time scales. In other words, adults produce slower micro-driving rhythms than do infants.

A second age-related distinction involves relationships among vocalized micro-rhythms. Not surprisingly, adult vocalizations are more complex than infants'. But the form of this complexity is interesting. With regard to relative timing, infants' vocalizations tend to be more *harmonious* than adults'.[6] Table 5.1 shows a few component frequencies of the /ɛ/ vowel, including formants and harmonics for infant, male, and female speakers. Relationships among harmonics, based on the glottal rhythm F0, are naturally straightforward (nF0); however, this is not the case for formant frequencies (F1, F2, F3).[7]

Formants play an important role in communication as they facilitate differentiation among critical speech units (e.g., as with vowels of *bit* versus *bet*). In adults' speech, formant frequencies correspond to distinct peaks (in amplitude) in a phoneme's spectral envelope due to the vocal tract's momentary filtering/articulation functions. A mature talker produces a particular phoneme using well-honed vocal tract motor configurations which shape the resulting sound by creating additional, locally resonant frequencies—formants—due, for example, to lips closing versus opening and the like. Even one constriction point in the vocal tract can result in multiple resonant frequencies (formants) which together may yield bandwidths between, for example, 1 and 2 kHz. However, in infants, formants (F**) are not only higher in frequency than in adults, they are also weaker and less stable, resulting in a dominance of harmonic relationships in infants' productions. Furthermore, F0 is less variable in these infants (e.g., a range of 150 Hz), showing minor pitch patterns of up/down (glides). And it turns out that certain formants, which are not harmonically related to F0, are often suspiciously close to a harmonic frequency (nF0).[8] In sum, infants' phoneme vocalizations embed both harmonic and rudimentary formant micro-driving rhythms that are faster, and arguably simpler, than those of adults. By this yardstick, infants and adults operate in different temporal niches, defined by different rates and micro-rhythmic relations.

More About Stages

Age-related vocal stages in produced rates are clearly linked to a young infant's anatomical changes in maturing vocal tract length.[9] Oller also proposed that because young infants, unlike adults, cannot control muscles that modulate the vocal tract, this filtering function is unstable in babies. In other words, adults skillfully change the shape of their vocal tract momentarily using different, refined muscle configurations to specify particular speech sounds via articulatory gestures involving the mouth, tongue, jaw movements, and more. By contrast, an infant's motor inability to produce reliable formant frequencies means that harmonically related micro-rhythms dominate the speech sounds they produce. According to Oller, this differentiates infant from adult sound-making, leading to their productions of *quasi-vowels*.

Quasi-Vowels Versus True Vowels

Oller distinguishes two types of vowel configurations—*quasi-vowels* and *true vowels*—in infants' vocalizations. The spectra of quasi-vowels do not reflect a systematic control of formants by infants; instead, this spectra is more harmonic in character. True vowels of adults are more complex due to the inclusion of strongly articulated formants. Table 5.1 illustrates a true vowel, /ɛ/, for adults (male and female speakers). The hypothetical infant's production shown in this table reflects higher formants that are weaker and less stable than in adults.[10] Interestingly, Kent and Murray found that 3-month-old infants produce a preponderance of such vocalic vowels (/ɛ/, /I/, /ʌ/) in which mean formant frequencies fell into a common F1-F2-F3 pattern across ages, which approximates a 1-3-5 kHz relationship.[11]

According to Oller, infants graduate from producing quasi-vowels to true vowels as they gain motor control in articulating their vocal tracts. Although the nature of formants remains a topic of debate, it is undisputed that formants reflect nonharmonic frequencies that play a major role in defining phoneme categories in speech. Nevertheless, the role of harmonics remains intriguing. On this topic, Baken[12] observes that neither formants nor harmonics can be ignored in speech recognition: "Individual harmonics serve as 'samples' of the vocal tract's resonant responses."[13[p.354]]

A Rhythmic Perspective on Infant's Early Attending

Although preceding sections focused largely on speech production, it is reasonable to conclude that the resulting speech patterns described here contribute to the acoustic environment that infants inhabit. From a DAT perspective, it is helpful to focus upon the time structure of these acoustic patterns using time domain concepts because they highlight entrainment functions. Thus, each produced frequency component is treated as a simple waveform, and, in an entrainment scenario, its periodicity functions as a fast acoustic micro-driving rhythm.

Let us assume, then, that very young infants, including newborns, inhabit a niche populated by fast rates and simple rhythms. In this dynamic environment, infants' attending preferences apply to waveforms that are much different from those enjoyed by the adults who care for these infants. Although infants experience an environment that is rich with potential driving rhythms of various rates, they will nonetheless gravitate to, and resonate with, faster sound patterns.

From this perspective, the special acoustical world of the youngest, wordless listeners presents as a grand mixture of various and fluctuating driving rhythms created by ambient adult speech. Indeed, a means of simplifying this buzzing-busy world that newborns face depends on this notion of selective orienting to preferred driving rhythms. In other words, young infants' attending operates selectively, limited to the confines of their temporal niche of fast rhythms—micro-rhythms. And, as we have seen, the speech of adult caretakers offers infants restricted access to their slower micro-driving rhythms. Mainly, it is the higher frequency components in adult female voices that fall into the admissible realm of driving rhythms preferred by younger infants. Young infants automatically rely on resonant fast neural oscillations to *selectively entrain* neural oscillations to individual waveforms (frequency components). This is exogenous entrainment. Given the phase response curves (PRCs) and attending energy profiles (AEPs) of Chapter 4, flexible entrainments can simultaneously track the various individual, fluctuating, micro-driving rhythms that correspond to higher frequencies, e.g. formants, of adults' voices.[14]

During this early stage, infants will also hear their own vocalizations of largely quasi-vowels. This is important because it affords early learning of the critical harmonic aspects of different phoneme categories. Generally, these young infants track, via exogenous entrainments, individual formant waveforms as well as those of high-frequency harmonics. Furthermore, compelling harmonic relationships between co-occurring harmonic waveforms will reinforce these relationships, which describe self-generated quasi-vowels. This strengthens a young infant's journey into the next stage, where formants become stronger.

Expanding the Temporal Niche: Older Infants

As infants age, two important changes happen. First, with maturation, an infant's tunable brain grows more spontaneous configurations of slower neural oscillations. With age, the temporal niche asymmetrically expands into slower ranges. Older infants gain the ability to resonate to slower vibrations in the adult's voice, such as the fundamental frequency. Second, older infants also refine articulatory motor skills that enable formant productions.[15] This enables an infant's control over her vocal tract, hence her formants.

A puzzle lingers. Not unlike a young bird struggling with song-producing mechanisms, young human infants struggle to transform a quasi-vowel (akin to a bird's "subsong") into true vowels (full song). At this time, around 6 months of age, infants become sensitive to slower waveforms within adult speech (i.e., including adults' F0). Along with refined motor skills, these older infants are on the brink of mastering the hurdle from quasi-vowels to true vowels, which younger infants could not do. Why?

One answer is that perceptual mastery of true vowels happens as older infants begin to refine motor articulations of the vocal tract to incorporate formants. For instance, Oller argues that this adds stable formants into the mixture of produced frequencies.

Quasi-Vowels and Attractors?

Another answer to the question of why infants at this stage master true vowel is more speculative (developed further in Chapter 14, where its relationship to Kuhl's magnet theory is discussed). This explanation draws on DAT hypotheses. It posits that harmonics, *specifically F0:nF0, function as attractors* often, hidden define phoneme categories for attenders exposed to these sounds. By definition, any produced sound with harmonics contains attractor ratios. Hence, each attractor is defined by a mode-locking relationship linking an nF0 component with its slower referent, F0, in an $n:m$ relationship. For instance, the vowel /ɛ /, spoken by an adult male in Table 5.1, has an F0 with a waveform period of 7.70 ms (130 Hz) and a coinciding waveform of the fourth harmonic (520 Hz) with a period of 1.92 ms. Together, these time layers afford to entraining listeners a simple synchrony between two micro-driving rhythms.

Specifically, four cycles of the F0 periods mode-lock with one cycle of this harmonic ($n = 4$), given the n:m attractor of 1:4. Assuming that resonant cortical oscillations follow suit, these harmonic relationships establish in adult listeners simple or complex attractors.[16] Importantly, a listener encountering such a speech sound may find several such attractors, perhaps clearly outlined but more often as hidden attractors, depending on the presence of nearby frequencies of formants with higher amplitudes and wide bandwidths. Yet, whether hidden or not, attractors are ever-present in harmonic sounds.

In this analysis, the fundamental frequency plays a significant role in both the production and the perception of speech sounds of adults. Harmonics and formant frequencies are produced with different source mechanisms (glottal rhythm vs. vocal tract filter). Nevertheless, this approach assumes that these attending listeners respond not to the source, but to ambient energies of the coinciding sound waves. A rhythm is a rhythm regardless of its origin. Accordingly, listeners of certain ages use both types of frequencies as potential micro-driving rhythms.

The aging hypothesis posits attending limits in young infants. Specifically, these listeners cannot entrain effectively to lower frequencies, such as F0, present in adult vocalizations as they are outside the infant's temporal niche. Attending proclivities of these infants gravitate to higher frequencies. In older infants, selective attending involving F0 becomes feasible. As the fundamental frequency of adults comes within perceptual reach, older infants begin to use it as a referent driving rhythm. In turn, the harmonic relationships involving F0 become functional. Specifically, the harmonics of the F0 driving rhythm highlight *deviations from harmonic attractor states* levied by high-energy formant frequencies. That is, an individual speaker produces an F0 that automatically *implies* a set of implied/weak harmonics that serve as *hidden attractors,* from which many (not hidden) formants necessarily deviate. A strong but fluctuating formant frequency, Fj, then yields a momentary ratio (e.g., Fj:nF0) that is specific to that speaker. Importantly, such ratios inevitably deviate from the nearest harmonic ratio (e.g., mF0:F0).[17] Multiple Fj:nF0 ratios may float about this attractor because formants change over time (as well, F0 changes with speakers). Observed Fj:nF0 ratios are not constant. By nature, these observable ratios deviate from relevant attractor ratios. In fact, averaging ratios over time, speaker's

age, F0, and the like tends to obscure the gist of this ratio driven hypothesis. Typically, for a given listener, a momentary formant ratio (vis-á-vis F0) belongs to a category that includes many deviant formant ratios, all of which that *imply a common, nearby, attractor.* Consequently, at a given moment, a speaker's formant, when heard as related to a speaker's F0 by listeners, is a fleeting deviant ratio that merely *approximates the nearest hidden attractor ratio.* (See Chapter 14 for a detailed, but speculative, discussion of infant phoneme learning.)

An Example: Attending in Young and Old Infants

An expanding temporal niche facilitates the perception (and production) of true vowels in older infants. For instance, the produced F0 of 130 Hz of an adult male in Table 5.1 is likely to be out of reach for a very young listener. However, older infants, who operate within a broader niche, can entrain attending to this low-frequency driving rhythm.

Next, imagine this older infant hears his mother produce the vowel phoneme /ɛ/ of Table 5.1 (with a higher F0 of 250 Hz). This infant can now automatically track the fluctuating waveform of an F1 formant of 684 Hz, given exogenous entrainment (i.e., following a PRC). As Table 5.1 shows, this formant does not match the $n = 3$ harmonic (750 Hz). Accordingly, this infant will momentarily experience a deviant F1:F0 ratio of 2.74 (i.e., a period ratio of 4.0:1.46 ms). Following an AEP curve, the strong F1 micro-waveform will capture this infant's attention, momentarily boosting the amplitude of the entraining oscillation. Yet, even in the next moment, the mother could produce a slightly different F1. Although F1:F0 ratios vary, they are not random; all fall within some "pull" range (i.e., entrainment region) of the third harmonic ratio of 3.0 (for 750 Hz) specific to this speaker. Variable token ratios of an attractor rarely match a prototypical 3.0 ratio; rather, they *implicate this as a hidden attractor.* Nevertheless, in this example, the observed F1:F0 ratio of 2.74 is "close enough" to this nearby attractor to instill in a maturing infant a sense of a hidden attractor "pull" (2.74 → 3.00).

Importantly, real-time attending adapts to changing fundamental frequencies and formants that vary within and between speakers. Thus, a vetting of this novel interpretation should avoid averaging stimulus properties over time, speaker age, and F0. Resulting formants of a given phoneme, normalized by a speaker's fundamental frequency, should scatter about certain harmonic ratios. And, although Fj:nF0 ratios will vary, they are predicted to do so within a limited range where observed ratios "point to" this hidden attractor. From Chapter 3, the "pull" of a hidden attractor refers to a trajectory in phase space that "points to" a nearby attractor.

In sum, age-related slowing facilitates an infant's ability to access certain defining attractor relationships. As older infants become more sensitive to lower vowel frequencies, they also become increasingly sensitive to a variety of different frequency ratios involving formants that implicate the same innate attractors.

Age-Related Slowing in the First Year

As infants mature, their brains become increasingly attuned to slower events. Along with their slowing vocal frequencies, their temporal niche continues to widen throughout the first year. This is evident in the preceding section, where vocalized frequencies of infants drop with age. Oller's aptly termed *Expansion stage* (3–8 months) follows. Infant vocalizations show a slowing F0 period from around 2.58 ms to near 3 ms in the first year.[18] Also vocalizations grow more complicated with age as slower frequencies create complex interactions with harmonic components and subharmonics enter the picture.[19] And infants also show greater sensitivity to the slower timing of social turn-taking that characterizes face-to-face interactions with parents.[20]

Developmental timing changes also include infants' productions of longer, speech-like, units. This is evident in a final, *Canonical Babbling* stage (5–10 months), when infants combine true vowels with consonants to create longer syllabic units. This familiar babbling stage is filled with monosyllabic time patterns (e.g., ba ba . . .) as well as longer, polysyllabic rhythms involving pitch contours.[21]

Overall, infants' growing ability to operate at slower rates is reflected in predispositions for slower speech productions, trends well-established in current research. Infants vocalize and orient attending in compliance with common preferred rates that shift with age. Moreover, as infants produce longer, slower sound patterns, they also listen to these events. What parent hasn't discovered her infant in the babbling stage contently absorbed in playing alone as he vocally burbles out different, self-generated phoneme combinations? Surely he enjoys listening to the babbles of phonemes he creates. MacNeilage[22] observed that, during this playful period, babbling rhythms realize durations that correlate with periodic jaw oscillations. Consistent with this idea, he argues that these productions reflect a major temporal frame indicative of infants' general reliance on longer syllable durations (200–300 ms).

Finally, age-related slowing continues beyond the first year. Roy Patterson and colleagues[23] provide a nice interpretation of maturational slowing of vocalizations during childhood, as indexed by a declining F0, due to vocal tract growth. This suggests that body size/weight may contribute to resonance trends. The remainder of this chapter also illustrates that age-related slowing continues over the life span.

Summary of Temporal Niches and Age-Related Slowing

This section provides snapshots of the world inhabited by infants in their first year of life. It focuses on the role of timing during a critical period in life when speech is mastered. The importance of timing during infancy is captured by the concept of a temporal niche. Some have emphasized the bottom-up learning of sequences (e.g., from phonemes to syllables, then words, etc.), whereas others promote top-down learning of various speech categories. The DAT approach does not conflict with such approaches. It merely highlights potential roles for resonance and entrainments at different time scales in coping with multilayered speech signals.

Applied to speech mastery, dynamic attending constructs imply that the age-specific driving rhythm rates will figure into explanations of the attending/learning efficacy of individuals at different developmental stages. The idea is that children shift with age from reliance on fast micro-driving rhythms, as the quasi-vowels of very young infants, to a reliance on slower micro-driving rhythms by older infants who can produce true vowels. As infants mature physically, the time spans of temporal niches for attending grow wider, characterized by increasingly slower rates. Throughout developmental stages of the first year, a steady trend is apparent in which production—and probably attending—increasingly engage slower and longer time frames. The major points of this section are:

- The temporal niche of newborns is defined by fast, simple driving rhythms.
- Infants produce faster (higher frequency) sounds than adults due to their shorter vocal tracts.

- Preferred speech micro-rhythms (rate, rhythm) differ for very young infants versus adults.
- Young infants produce quasi-vowels with fast micro-driving rhythms and simple (harmonic) attractors. Adults produce true vowels with slower micro-driving rhythms and complex formant ratios that define phoneme categories.
- Generally, vocal rhythms (e.g., of F0) slow during the first year, and durations of speech units lengthen from phonemes to phrases.

DYNAMIC ATTENDING, AGING, AND SELECTIVE LISTENING

Attending entails a synchronous interaction of cortical oscillations with event rhythms. It involves a concentrated sensitivity to external events. Yet, in newborns, attending remains rather enigmatic. We really don't know "if" newborns attend in a manner comparable to adults. In fact, it is reasonable to wonder whether infants are even able to engage in something defined in Chapter 4 as "voluntary" attending. This term seems to imply a conscious and willful delegation of attending energy to specified events. And, if infants possess this capacity, it is unclear "what" a hypothetical, perhaps willful, infant will voluntarily attend to.

Some clues to "what" enigmatic infants selectively perceive may be inferred from observations of infants' preferred vocalizations (from the preceding section). It appears that infants' early vocalizations reflect a preference for attending to simple rapid rhythms. More direct evidence for infants' early attentional biases comes from converging research that assesses selective listening in newborns. At birth, and even before, it is clear that the novel world noises that engulf young infants evoke certain tell-tale responses. For instance, if maternity ward contagion is any indication, newborns spontaneously react to hearing high-pitched sounds as they join with other babies in riotous choruses of high-frequency cries. They also favor human vocalizations over comparable synthetic sounds.[24] Even fetuses orient to faster (high-frequency) sounds (e.g., 500 Hz vs. 250 Hz) and they also show preferential listening to their mothers' voices, as well as to rhythmically pulsed sounds.[25,26,27,28]

These discoveries testify to biases in the early orienting of newborns. They reveal a rudimentary but selective attending activity. However, this selectively in attending is involuntary. It reflects an infant's innate sensitivities that favor higher frequency components in speech and not necessarily an infant's voluntary (i.e., thoughtfully guided) attending. The latter fits into the idea of a special temporal niche that affects infants' attending. This section pursues this idea by developing an aging hypothesis.

The *aging hypothesis* embodies the concept of a temporal niche by featuring a role for age-dependent selective attending. However, this hypothesis cannot be fully understood without considering the other major hypothesis about selective attending, namely the *general attending hypothesis* introduced in Chapter 4. Together, these two hypotheses are central to explaining selective attending. For involuntary attending, these hypotheses operate in tandem, whereas, for voluntary attending, both allow for intentions/goals to affect oscillator strength. The general attending hypothesis concentrates on exogenous entrainments, particularly on driving rhythm properties (e.g., regularity, force), whereas the aging hypothesis concentrates on limits on exogenous entrainments arising from driven rhythm capacities (oscillator strength and attractor ratios). Together, these two hypotheses offer a more complete theory of dynamic attending. For reasons of scope, alternative selective attention views are not discussed.[29]

Finally, this age-based theory of attending delivers an evolutionary advantage. The temporal niche of very young infants ensures that these little, rather helpless creatures nonetheless "hit the ground running" when it matters: They arrive equipped with selectively stronger neural oscillations designed to engage relatively fast sounds produced by communicating care-takers. "Fast" is not a handicap to these young listeners. This talent enhances the potential for species survival.

A Unifying Concept: Dominant Oscillations

The aging hypothesis together with the general attending hypothesis echo a long-standing divide in thinking about human behavior. This refers to the vaunted nature–nurture debate. At one extreme are theories presenting a "totally wired" view of attention/perception that attributes certain attentional phenomena to innate processes whereas, at the other extreme, are approaches that present a "blank slate" description that assumes no inborn constraints, attributing all behavior to repeated exposure to environmental stimuli. Alternatively, it is possible to find elements of the former in the aging hypothesis, which emphasize innate resonant capacities with respect to rates of latent driven rhythms and innate attractor relations. Conversely, elements of a blank slate stance emerge from the general attending hypothesis because it emphasizes salience and repetition of external stimuli as a driving rhythm in entrainment activities, which may promote learning.

But, in fact, the engagement of both resonance and entrainment takes this discussion in a different direction. That is, together, these two hypotheses co-constrain each other, leading to an interactionist approach to the nature–nurture debate. The present view implies listeners are neither totally wired nor do they arrive in the world as blank slates. The truth is somewhere in between.

In the present view, interactions between environmental and innate determinants of attending feature a new concept: dominant oscillations. *Dominant oscillations are neural oscillations with amplitudes exceeding the amplitudes of locally surrounding oscillations (e.g., in a power spectrum). Dominant oscillations are important because they dictate selective attending.* As a consequence, selective attending is carried by one or several dominant oscillations as they resonate to certain event rhythms but not to others. This might happen, for instance, if young infants preferentially allocate relatively high amplitudes to those driven rhythms that are "tuned in" to certain higher frequency harmonics of vowels, thus selectively ignoring lower frequency formants (cf. Table 5.1). These infants, then, tend to "hear" quasi-vowels, not the true vowels in adult voices that implicate different dominant oscillations.

The concept of dominant oscillations is a unifying one. Any driven oscillator that has a locally higher amplitude will carry more attending weight than nearby active oscillations with lower amplitudes. In short, the stronger, high amplitude, oscillation functions as a dominant micro-rhythm. Such an increase in amplitude can arise either from innate responsivity of the aging hypothesis, and/or from voluntary factors described by the general attending hypothesis, or both. An oscillator's energy increment can depend on a preference for driven rhythms of a certain rate or attractor (the aging hypothesis), and/or it can result from a driving rhythm constraint, such as the regularity or force of an external event (the general attending hypothesis).

Regardless of the originating hypothesis, *a dominant oscillator governs selective attending.* Intuitively, this means that a listener may be captivated by simple harmonies in a sound, or merely by the fact that it is loud (i.e., it creates a strong driving rhythm force), or both. The point is that there are different routes for creating a dominant oscillation. In brief, innate and/or environmental factors (including task demands), determine the strength of a dominant oscillation.

Figure 5.2 provides a simplified sketch of joint actions involving these two major hypotheses as they feed into one hypothetical, common driven oscillation. Although these hypotheses can operate in conflict, this figure showcases supplementary activities wherein they concurrently add energy to build a dominant oscillation. The aging hypothesis initially boosts amplitude by resonance (with an attractor corollary discussed shortly). The general attending hypothesis then boosts oscillator

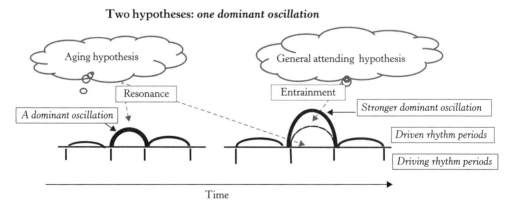

Two hypotheses: *one dominant oscillation*

FIGURE 5.2 Simplified schematic illustrating hypothesized coordination of *aging* and *general attending* hypotheses to create a single dominant oscillation. Initially, the aging hypothesis singles out (from three active oscillations; dark gray) one dominant oscillation via heightened resonance. This is followed in time with further boosts of this oscillation's amplitude given entrainment principles, stipulated for voluntary or involuntary attending, by the general attending hypothesis (Chapter 4).

amplitude still higher, granting this oscillation a dominant role if other oscillations (not shown) become active. This schematic does not address complex interactions; it merely offers a backdrop for topics central to this and other chapters.

The Aging Hypothesis and Primitive Oscillator Configurations

The aging hypotheses suggests that infants tend to "tune in" to fast events, and, with age, this orientation shifts to rate biases for increasingly slower event rates (age-related slowing). This idea is now formalized as follows:

> *Aging Hypothesis. The dominant oscillations in youth resonate to relatively fast event rates whereas the dominant oscillations in aging individuals resonate to increasingly slower events. In the tunable brain, this dominance reflects an increase in the number of active cortical oscillations with intrinsic periods specific to some point on a cortical growth curve. The result is changes in the resonating capacity of primitive oscillator configurations such that those dominant oscillations with longer periods become increasingly prevalent with age. Essentially dominant oscillations determine the nature of a temporal niche.*

People's preferred event rates change over a life span as periods of dominant oscillations shift following age-specific resonance capacities. The temporal niche of a newborn supports orienting to fast event rhythms due to fast dominant oscillations, whereas the temporal niches of older children and adults increasingly favor orienting to slower driving rhythms due to a growing prevalence of dominant oscillations with longer periods.

These predictions about aging depend heavily on the *resonance principle: the amplitude of a neural oscillation automatically increases as an event's driving frequency approximates the oscillation's intrinsic frequency.* Furthermore, as more oscillations with the same intrinsic rate (frequency) become simultaneously active, this pooled resonance results in a greater (aggregated) amplitude for a driven rhythm with this rate.

Resonance, Driven Rhythm Strength, and Aging

The resonance principle predicts age-related slowing. Notably, this paves a way for exogenous entrainment activity at each age level because entrainment depends on active, vibrating oscillations. Basically, resonance occurs between two periodic processes, for example, an external event rhythm and an internal neural oscillation. Resonance heightens the amplitude of the neural oscillation when the two frequencies are similar. As such, it has an excitatory role. Resonance initially "charges up" amplitudes of harmonically related neural oscillations. This creates an *oscillator flurry* in that it will also boost amplitudes of harmonically related oscillations.

The primacy of resonance is suggested in Figure 5.2, which shows that resonance from an external event first boosts the amplitude of (at least) one neural oscillation with a frequency of the event (i.e., a resonant frequency). However, once a driven oscillation is awakened via resonance with an external driving rhythm, then exogenous entrainment between rhythms begins. In this way entrainment is served by resonance because entrainment requires two or more simultaneously active periodicities.

Entrainment, then, proceeds to phase-align and fine-tune activated oscillations. As already stipulated, in addition to driven rhythm strength, entrainment is governed by two main factors: ever-present attractors and a phase-coupling parameter (cf. the PRC curves in Chapter 4). These considerations mandate a corollary to the aging hypothesis that addresses age-related changes in entrainment.

An Aging Hypothesis Entrainment Corollary

Over a life span, entrainment capacity is governed by synchronies of entraining oscillations constrained by three factors: innate attractors, phase-locking strength, and driven oscillation strength.

- *Innate attractors* retain their inherent power over the life span such that simple attractors are consistently more compelling than complex ones, regardless of age.
- *Phase-locking strength changes with age.* Effective coupling parameter values change curvilinearly with age, with strongest coupling parameter values associated with the middle years (18–40).
- *Driven oscillations tend to be weaker in infants than in adults.* Weaker entraining oscillations are more responsive to perturbing stimuli (all else equal); hence, infants tend to be stimulus-driven.

Among other things, this corollary features a life-long role for attractors. The relative impact of simple and complex attractors in governing entrainment does not change over the life span. By contrast, an individuals' overall capacity for synchronizing to events, whether attractors are simple or complex, is reduced for the very young and the very old due age–related changes. This predicts declines in the effective strength of phase-coupling parameters for these age groups.[30] Consequently, young adults should perform certain rhythmic tasks with greater precision and stability than other age groups, regardless of rhythmic rate.

Intuitively, the entrainment corollary of the aging hypothesis may not surprise readers as it is obvious that young adults, who populate rock concerts and dance clubs, are pretty good at tracking a beat. But this corollary also implies that in more controlled (and perhaps more boring) laboratory tasks that require sensory and/or motor synchronizations, young adults will outperform other age groups. In fact, this corollary predicts a nonlinear function over the life span for tasks based on one's phase-locking competence: weaker coupling parameters (e.g., effective **k** values of PRC curves), hence poorer performance, are predicted for the very young and very old relative to young adults. Informally, this means that we arrive in the world a bit wobbly, and we leave it somewhat wobbly as well.

Age-Related Changes in Driven (Oscillator) Rhythms: Any Evidence?

The crux of the aging hypothesis is its proposal that latent growth changes in brain dynamics lead to specific age-related activities of driven oscillations. This is an unusual proposal. A reader may rightly ask if there is evidence for the claim that fast cortical waveforms (high-frequency oscillations) are dominant in infants, whereas slow ones prevail in older adults. For both technical and theoretical reasons, evidence is sparse. Technical reasons concern difficulties in measuring the resonant responses of neural oscillations of the human brain (not to mention infant brains) which may involve invasive recording techniques involving neurons buried deep in cortical brain regions. Theoretical reasons relate to the fact that few, if any, governing frameworks have articulated a developmental approach that motivates such research.

Furthermore, we are only beginning to learn about the brains of newborns. Yet a few promising findings pertain to the aging hypothesis. Minimally, these show that infants' cortical oscillations cannot be dismissed as random noise indifferent to interactions with other active oscillations.[31,32] Certain primitive oscillations are present at birth, and, with maturation, they grow or shrink depending on spurts or declines in growth over a life span (Chapter 3). Also, there is evidence that fast, high-energy cortical oscillations are active early in life, especially in sensory brain rhythms.[33,34,35] Others find disproportionately greater EEG power (plus bursting activity) in the high-frequency neural activity of newborns, which declines over the next 6 months as lower frequencies grow in power.[36,37]

From a different angle, Strogatz's conception of brain *hubs*[38,39] inspired Fransson and colleagues[40] to search for neural correlates in a young infant's brain (cf. Chapter 3). (Recall that a brain hub is a ringed oscillator configuration associated with spatial proximities.) Using functional magnetic resonance imaging (fMRI), they found larger hubs in adult than in infant brains. Also, hubs in adult brains were distributed over multiple brain regions, whereas in infant brains they were sparse and concentrated in sensory and motor regions. These findings support the idea of "starter" brain configurations that are incomplete versions of mature oscillator configurations. They also imply that early brain activity centers on elementary (involuntary) levels of sensory/motor activity, not on higher, possibly voluntary control levels.

In conclusion, the brain dynamics of infants appear to be neither highly structured nor entirely random. Unlike adults, infants have a brain structure that is constrained in both number and kinds of oscillator configurations at work. Perhaps unsurprisingly, infants start life with brains full of oscillations mainly equipped to react to sensory stimulation.

The Aging Hypothesis at Work: An Example

A proposed function of the aging hypothesis can be illustrated by a thought experiment involving an infant presented with a phoneme. Figure 5.3A shows, in light gray bars, a cluster of component harmonic frequencies in a bland complex sound (admittedly this schematic of a phoneme cluster is unrealistic as a depiction of a real e.g. vowel because it lacks formants and signature amplitude changes). Also shown are hypothesized resonating neural oscillations (dark gray bars) in the sensory brain regions of an ideal newborn infant. The aging hypothesis maintains that primitive oscillator clusters are readily recruited in this case because this infant

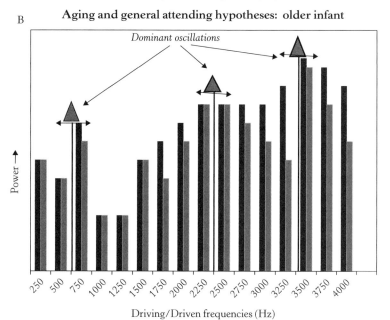

A   **Aging hypothesis predictions: young infant**

Dominant oscillations →

Power →

Driving/Driven frequencies (Hz)

B   **Aging and general attending hypotheses: older infant**

Dominant oscillations

Power →

Driving/Driven frequencies (Hz)

FIGURE 5.3 In panel **A**, bars indicate hypothetical power spectra capture relative strengths of driving (light gray) and driven (dark gray) rhythms for component frequencies of an arbitrary complex sound with a flat driving rhythm spectrum. It illustrates that a young infant's attending biases (dark gray) nonetheless favor higher frequencies. Panel **B** shows an older infant responding to a complex sound resembling an adult's vocalization of /ɛ/. High-energy formant frequencies (narrow vertical lines) are shown as eliciting dominant oscillations that add energy to neighboring harmonics (dark gray).

automatically favors reliance on configurations of oscillations linked together with simple attractors (here, activity is harmonically organized from 250 Hz and 4,000 Hz). Although these infants will respond to formant frequencies, this idealization suggests infants' initial weak predispostions. The aging hypothesis implies that young infants have a naturally strong resonant bias for higher stimulus frequencies, ones generally higher than the F2 formants in adult vocalizations (e.g., Table

5.1). Figure 5.3A shows higher amplitudes that characterize dominant oscillations resonating to certain higher harmonic frequencies. Heightened amplitudes depend on biases for certain internal oscillations (dark gray bars) and not external stimuli (light gray bars).

The aging hypothesis also speaks to entrainment via a corollary. The entrainment corollary predicts that once an oscillation resonates to a given micro-driving rhythm in a speech sound, infants then encounter opportunities for entraining to other frequency components within this complex sound (e.g., /ɛ/). For infants, this is exogenous entrainment governed by simple attractors (e.g., n:m = 1:1, 1:2, etc.) and by phase-coupling strength. However, phase corrections are also predicted to be relatively weak in young and old individuals, according to this corollary. Consequently, young infants are bathed in sounds that afford multiple driving rhythms, but it is the faster and simpler driving rhythms that selectively draw and tenuously hold their attending. These driving rhythms determine dominant oscillations.

The General Attending Hypothesis and Selective Attending

The general attending hypothesis takes this story further. Instead of focusing on predispositions for certain driven rhythms, this hypothesis focuses on properties of external driving rhythms. As with the aging hypothesis, the general attending hypothesis holds that selective listening depends on the activity of dominant oscillations. However, this hypothesis concentrates on entrainment (rather than resonance). It distinguishes between voluntary attending, where the strength of an entraining oscillator derives from a listener's conscious intentions to boost oscillator strength, and involuntary attending, where the strength of an entraining oscillation depends on the regularity and force of a driving rhythms. In this chapter, the focus remains on aspects of involuntary attending based on entrainment by certain driving rhythm properties described in Chapter 4.

To recap, the general attending hypothesis (rephrased for dominant oscillations) states that:

> *Dynamic attending to an event is automatically governed by multiple exogenous entrainments from which a few dominant oscillations emerge to instantiate selective attending. Regardless of age, selective attending involuntarily rides on local timed elevations of oscillator energy (i.e., relative height) resulting from the force and/or temporal regularity of relevant external driving rhythms.*

This hypothesis grants priority to certain stimulus properties of a driving rhythm, such as its force and/or regularity, as the basis for strengthening a driven oscillation (i.e., increasing its potential). Here, a forceful driving rhythm is assumed to recruit more neural oscillations, leading collectively to a stronger driven amplitude. Thus, one automatically "pays attention" to the louder, but annoying, speaker in crowd. This tendency to be captured by an unexpected component is heightened in younger infants due to their relatively weak driven oscillations. Generally, this means that powerful but nonharmonic speech sounds, such as formants, can capture infants' attending. This feature is formalized in the AEP capture curves described in Chapter 4. Of course, sounds with compelling regularities will also automatically engage attending; these too are formalized in the AEP expectancy curves of Chapter 4. Thus, dominance can be achieved by attentional capture by a formant or by anticipation of an harmonic. The main point is that, in both cases, there is a selective boost in amplitudes of the resonating neural oscillations linked to this driving micro-rhythm.

Combining Predictions of the Aging and General Attending Hypotheses

Normally, the aging hypothesis and the general attending hypothesis are both busy "at work" as we confront everyday events in our environment. Together, they highlight input from different factors that affect attending dynamics. The "brew" that results from this mix reveals the emergence of one or several dominant oscillations that blend influences of innate and environmental factors. The aging hypothesis identifies factors that innately regulate oscillator strength, such as the age-specific rate of a resonant driving rhythm (given a simple attractor). The general attending hypothesis identifies driving rhythm properties, such as rhythmic regularity and force, regardless of age-specific frequencies.

These two hypothesis jointly predict selective attending biases by identifying dominant oscillations that operate in real speech sounds. The schematic of Figure 5.2 suggests abstractly how these hypotheses supplement each other in heightening the amplitude of the same driven rhythm. However, in other situations, the two hypotheses may strengthen different driven rhythms and lead to competing dominant oscillations. A range of options for automatic boosts in selective attending opens up in this framework. Ultimately, selective attending depends on the oscillator configuration that delivers the strongest dominant oscillations.

Joint Influences on Selective Attending: Examples

The portrait arising from a marriage of two hypotheses blends their predictions. To illustrate, consider infants listening to complex sounds. Figure 5.3A showed selective attending of very young infant (with a narrow temporal niche) based mainly on the aging hypothesis. But what happens if an older infant (with a wider temporal niche) listens to the phoneme /ɛ/ spoken by a female, as outlined in Figure 5.3B? Both the aging hypothesis and the general attending hypothesis apply; their joint predictions answer this question next.

The aging hypothesis applied to the older infant of panel B predicts that selective attending (dark gray bars) is based on a wider temporal niche than that available to the younger infant portrayed in panel A. Also, certain lower frequencies are now accessible to the older infant, hence more attending energy is allocated to slower frequency components.

The general attending hypothesis also weighs in on the older infant's attending. It implies that stimulus properties of certain micro-driving rhythms in this phoneme also selectively direct attending energy due to their force and regularity. Let this power spectrum reflect the vocalizations of a hypothetical adult female. As outlined, it projects a few relatively intense frequency components as this speaker utters /ɛ/. Specifically, certain defining harmonics (dark gray) and formants (thin vertical lines) are more powerful than surrounding micro-rhythms. Significantly, formant frequencies are usually more forceful than their nearest harmonic. For this reason, the general attending hypothesis posits that formants readily contribute to the creation of dominant neural oscillations, as in Figure 5.3B. The basic idea is that certain salient stimuli evoke elevations in the amplitude of driven rhythms that create dominant oscillations.

In sum, two major DAT hypotheses combine to spell out predictions about a listener's involuntary (but selective) attending to a complex sound (e.g., a speech sound). In this portrayal, the aging hypothesis paves the way by outlining resonance constraints that immediately constrain attending. Next, the general attending hypothesis adds

strength to activated (resonating) oscillations, strength deriving from driving rhythm properties of force and regularity. This further shapes selective attending as it is realized by dominant oscillations.

Summary of Dynamic Attending and Selective Attending

The ambient sounds of our world supply multiple driving rhythms that fluctuate over time. Most critical are the communicative sounds of speech and music because these engage participatory attending. Many of these driving rhythms are micro-rhythms based on tiny periods (milliseconds or less) embedded in the more complex sounds of speech and music. Selective attending to one or several micro-rhythms in a complex sound is involuntary, depending on factors identified by two hypotheses: the aging hypothesis and the general attending hypothesis. Both envision selective attending as an interaction of cortical oscillations with subsets of micro-driving rhythms of a more complex sound.

This chapter has focused on the aging hypothesis, which holds that age-related biases involving resonance favor selective attending based on the rates of certain driving rhythms (a temporal niche). This predicts age-related slowing. The general attending hypothesis adds two more factors that affect selective attending: namely, driving rhythm force and regularity. Together, these three driving rhythm factors (rate, regularity, and force) jointly contribute to the emergence of dominant oscillations that involuntarily determine selective attending.

Major point in this section are:

- Two DAT hypotheses about involuntary attending are the aging hypothesis and general attending hypothesis. The former, introduced in this chapter, addresses age-related constraints on selective attending based on innate resonance biases for event rate (the temporal niche). The latter, introduced in Chapter 4, identifies two driving rhythm entrainment factors—force and regularity—that contribute to driven rhythm attending energy.
- The aging hypothesis posits that infants' resonate selectively to relatively fast, and simple (versus complex attractors) sounds that define their temporal niche. With age, the temporal niche widens to include slower driving rhythms.

- The aging hypothesis corollary assumes that entrainment (phase-locking) also varies with age; in addition, young listeners have weaker driven oscillations than do older ones.
- Dominant oscillations determine selective attending; these oscillations gain joint strength from the aging and general hypotheses.

THE LIFE SPAN: THE AGING HYPOTHESIS OVER A RANGE OF AGES

It is not uncommon to remark on the impatience of young children. An example is found in the quintessential folklore of the "family trip" wherein, half-way through a trip, young children begin to scream "Are we there yet?" Conversely, a common perspective on our senior citizens—often offered by seniors themselves—is that they operate on a slower "clock." Although the metaphor of a mechanical clock is misleading, is there some merit to these age-related stereotypes? According to the aging hypothesis, the answer is "yes."

Yet perhaps the aging hypothesis is wrong.

Are aging hypothesis ideas about inborn biases and age-related slowing too speculative? If dismissed, then the most obvious alternative is to assume that newborns, overwhelmed by the booming and buzzing of novel noises, soldier on to massively learn "what goes with what" oblivious of whether the sounds they must master embed fast or slow rhythms. And, if the aging hypothesis is wrong, then perhaps older listeners will *benefit* from years of exposure to fast speech patterns, implying that seniors should excel, due to overlearning, at tracking fast stimulus events. In short, without assumptions of innate biases and age-related slowing, seniors would rarely ask a young enthusiastic speaker to "please . . . speak more slowly."

This final section tackles the merits of the aging hypothesis by fleshing out concepts about age-related modulations of cortical structure. It also considers converging evidence consistent with such aging concepts and predictions of life span changes, beginning with newborns and ending with seniors.

Life Span Changes in Primitive Brain Configurations

In newborns, spontaneous fluctuations in cortical brain activity show complex time series properties, often characteristic of the chaotic (e.g., 1/f) noise of a primitive dynamical system.[41,42] Also, self-organizing brain oscillations progress from initial states that manifest numerous connections among different cortical regions in newborns to maturational pruning of brain connections around 3 months of age in some brain regions. Thereafter, the cortical oscillations of a self-tuning brain manifest increases in connectivity, leading to new spatial-temporal configurations of cortical units. Given early reorganizations, it is possible that primitive oscillator configurations operative in the first 3 months of life provide "starter" configurations that survive this pruning. Although ready at birth, primitive configurations are incomplete. According to the aging hypothesis, these primitive configurations lack spontaneous oscillations with longer periods, which are sparse in newborns' brains. Conversely, other incomplete neural configurations are postulated by growth curves near the end of a life span. That is, with aging, fast brain oscillations begin to disappear over the years, leaving in elderly brains a prevalence of dominant oscillations with relatively long periods. Together, configurations of slow oscillations form "ending" configurations. Between the age extremes of starter and ending configurations are neural configurations predicted to fulfill the aging hypothesis about age-related slowing over the life span.

Very Young Infants "Like" Very Fast Micro-Rhythms

At the beginning of life, young infants are hypothesized to operative with primitive, incomplete oscillatory configurations that have survived the third-month cortical pruning. These configurations are dominated by fast oscillations, assuming that nature equips newborns with a fast track to rapid perceptual learning the first year of life. And it appears that infants ride this track with zest. The first step in this process involves selective attending to (to-be-learned) critical nuggets of adult speech, such as phonemes. Even newborns are not passive recipients of the ambient sounds they encounter nor are they overwhelmed by their novelty. Rather, infants operate contentedly with a brain selectively "tuned" to orient to the higher frequency sound components of speech. And it helps that infants begin life with a predisposition to be responsive to novel stimuli due to relative weak oscillations; they are designed to engage in exogenous attending. Bluntly put, young infants do not attend to the world of sounds in the same way as do adults. Infants inhabit a different temporal niche. And, rather than being overwhelmed by these novel sounds, these little creatures may enjoy the game of discovering how preferred, but novel, sound frequencies fit together.

The aging hypothesis has generality across age and culture because it is rooted in universal mechanisms of resonance and entrainment. The following paragraphs return to the youngest infants examined in the beginning of this chapter. However, instead of focusing on their gestural vocalizations, this section returns to observations about infants' early orienting of attending. If the brains of young listeners are really "tuned" to resonate to faster rhythms, as proposed, then, even when passive, their brain recordings should reveal selective, automatic orienting to fast micro-rhythms.

One aim is to pin down the attending biases of very young infants described by the temporal niche concept. The world of sound in which infants engage is one we adults have long forgotten. Newborns' attending is captured by changes happening over tiny time spans. Just as cats see a different world than do we, snatching at the speedy motions of a tiny spider that we barely notice, so, too, human newborns tune into a different world, snatching at tiny changes in spectral frequencies of sounds that we no longer "hear." To clarify, infants with immature brains are neither more skilled or more discriminative than adults in reaction to fast sound patterns. There is evidence that neither is true.[43,44,45] The issue is not whether infants perform better or worse than adults. Young infants are often perceptually less acute than adults. Instead, the basic idea is simpler: infants are initially wired to automatically resonate to faster, not slower, rhythmic events.

To explain age-related differences in preferential orienting, the aging hypothesis implies that, relative to the preferred resonant frequency range of adults, preferred resonant frequencies of young infants occupy a higher frequency range. It is well established that adults' optimal frequency range centers on 1 kHz (a 200 Hz–2 kHz range, indexed by manifest perceptual responses to pure tones). In light of this, the aging hypothesis implies that the temporal niche of young infants is centered *above* 1 kHz.

Supporting evidence comes from studies that expose very young infants to a range of acoustic micro-rhythms. Newer methodologies allow theoretical inferences to be made about the automaticity of infants' responses because these techniques pick up specific neural reactions to the fine time structure of sounds even in sleeping infants.[46] Using both music-like and speech-like sounds, this research confirms the claim that infants' preferential neural reactions are automatic and aimed at higher spectral frequencies.

Music-Like Sounds

Newborns are more sensitive to pure tones with frequencies over 500 Hz than to lower ones. Also, they are keener at differentiating tones with frequencies in the high formant frequency range (i.e., 1–3 kHz) than with ones of lower frequencies (i.e., near adult F0's).[47] Related outcomes use a wide range of tone frequencies with event-related potential (ERP) mismatch negativity responses. Young infants turn out to be most sensitive to frequency changes in tones higher than 1 kHz[48] (1–4 kHz). In a similar vein, newborns' ERPs differentiate "up" from "down" frequency relationships only for high-frequency tones (above 520 Hz), especially those near the frequencies of adult vowel formants.[49] Taken together, these findings suggest that when newborns are presented with pure tones, they involuntarily orient toward sounds with higher frequencies (i.e., faster micro-rhythms). And, while adults' preferred frequency range for pure tones is centered on 1 kHz, very young infants prefer a range of higher frequencies, close to the range of formants in adult speech.

Speech-Like Sounds

Arguably, speech-like sounds provide a better glimpse of selective listening tendencies because, unlike pure tones, they are complex micro-rhythms containing multiple frequency components. Therefore, selective attending can be monitored by recording which of several frequency components in phoneme-like nuggets engages an infant's attending. It turns out that even very young infants show automatic and heightened sensitivity to the faster micro-rhythmic components. Interestingly, again the preferred frequency components are in the high-frequency range of adult formants (e.g., for females this is 650 Hz to 3.4 kHz; Table 5.1). Also in line with these findings, Dehaene-Lambertz and Pena[50] used ERPs to reveal that newborns readily distinguish between spoken phonemes (e.g., /pa/ from /ta/) on the basis of their higher frequency components. Others, using magnetoencephalography (MEG) data, find that newborns distinguish phonemes /a/ from /i/ (equated for F0), which they accomplished largely by relying on high formant frequencies.[51] Taken together, these findings support a proposal that infants are "tuned" to master speech by first tackling higher frequency components (harmonics, formants). Only with maturation do infants begin to focus on slower speech components.

Collectively, emerging research implies that, at the beginning of a life, neonates readily "tune in" to and differentiate complex micro-rhythms on the basis of a sound's higher frequency components. And this behavior appears to be automatic. Indeed, underscoring such automaticity, babies appear to "play with" differentiating higher frequency harmonics and formants, even in their sleep. Telkemeyer and colleagues[52] found that sleeping newborns showed most neural sensitivity to spectral frequencies in the higher frequency speech-formant range (1–1.5 kHz).[53] Finally, Cone and Garnis[54] convincing established that newborns indeed differ from adults in their predisposition for higher frequencies of speech-like sounds. Using sounds containing four carrier frequencies (500 Hz–4 kHz; ASSR), they found that the infant threshold for carrier frequencies of 500 Hz was 20 dB higher than the adult thresholds, whereas their thresholds for the faster carrier frequencies (1.5, 2.5 kHz) were *significantly lower* than those of adults! This is most compelling evidence that newborns are biased toward faster micro-rhythms, whereas adults are not.

Summary of the Aging Hypothesis over the Life Span

Very young infants operate with dominant cortical oscillations "tuned" to higher sound frequencies, whereas adults do not. These infants immediately master the very fast frequency components of complex sounds even in their sleep. Thus, this research on selective attending dovetails with that on the development of infant vocalizations outlined early in this chapter. Together, such evidence supports predictions of the aging hypothesis involving age-related slowing and a widening temporal niche. Both infants and adults are moderately tuned to a range of overlapping micro-rhythms, but the temporal niche of neonates centers this range in higher frequencies, near the formants of adults (1–3 kHz), whereas the favored niche for adults is lower (e.g., 200 Hz to 1–1.5 kHz).

CYCLING OVER THE LIFE SPAN WITH SLOWER MACRO-RHYTHMS

The aging hypothesis addresses attending across the life span. However, preceding discussions focused on individuals' responses to timing variations in micro-rhythms (e.g., frequency components) with an emphasis on differences between infants and young adults. In contrast, this section leaps ahead to focus on the timing variations of macro-rhythms and the manner in which people of all ages respond to changes in the rate of such rhythms. To test this, people of different ages perform the same set of tasks designed to probe their responses to isochronous sequences in which rhythmic rate is varied. The aim is to examine age-related trends over the life span, trends specific to the same set of event macro-rhythm rates across different event rates in all tasks.

The aging hypothesis offers two predictions about life span changes. One prediction concerns the involuntary age-related slowing (i.e., period lengthening) of driven oscillations due to changing resonance sensitivities. The second prediction derives from the entrainment corollary of the aging hypothesis, which postulates curvilinear changes in phase-locking ability over the life span. To assess both predictions, Devin McAuley and colleagues[55] presented a number of tasks to listeners ranging in age from 4.5 to 95 years. Some tasks gauged listeners' rate preferences, others assessed spontaneous motor tempo (SMT), and still other tasks assessed phase-locking abilities in a synchronized tapping task. Importantly, all tasks required listeners to respond to the same isochronous tone sequences with rates varying from fast (T = 150 ms) to very slow (T = 1,709 ms).

Predictions About Age-Related Slowing over the Life Span

Age-related slowing predictions rest on the idea that, with age, increasingly more neural oscillations with intrinsically slower periods serve as dominant oscillations. In turn, this leads people to preferentially orient to slower rates with age. Figure 5.4 illustrates this prediction as a monotonic trend in the period lengthening of dominant oscillations with age.[56]

This prediction was evaluated by assessing age-related changes in the performance of several tasks (dependent measures varied with task: tempo ratings, tapping accuracy, spontaneous motor tapping [i.e., SMT], etc.). Results across tasks converged to support predictions of the aging hypothesis. For instance, the tapping task revealed monotonic slowing of spontaneous taps consistent with the idea that dominant internal oscillations with increasingly longer periods become more prevalent with age. Thus, young children spontaneously tapped faster than young adults, and seniors were consistently the slowest tappers. Also in a perception task, younger children expressed greater preferences for faster sequence rates than did all older age groups. After

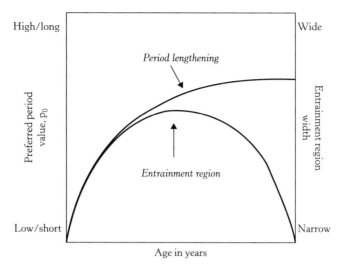

FIGURE 5.4 Two conceptual trends predicted by the aging hypothesis. Lengthening of the period (Po) of a dominant oscillation with age following the resonance principle. Also, the entrainment corollary predicts that coupling strength (hence the width of an entrainment region) is optimal in the middle age range.

Reprinted from figure 1 in J. Devin McAuley et al. (2006) in *Journal of Experimental Psychology: General* volume 135: 365).

listening to each tempo, children rated their preference by locating a toy turtle on a scale (strong dislike to strong like). In one amusing, but telling incident, an expressive 5-year-old "rated" slower rhythms so low that he literally threw the toy turtle past the "strongly dislike" end of the scale! Older adults were more constrained, yet they too had little patience with unpreferred rates, which (predictably) turned out to be the faster rates—namely, the ones children loved. Occasionally seniors, irritated by faster rates, simply stopped listening to the rhythms enjoyed by young children. And when asked to spontaneously tap their preferred tempo (SMT), older adults tapped nearly twice as slowly as the youngest listeners. All tasks supported the predicted monotonic trend in Figure 5.4 for period slowing over the life span.[57,58]

As Time Goes By

On reflection, these discoveries lend credence to general observations of lapsed time. As time goes by, people often do have different estimates of the same lapsed time. Children are typically impatient with long time intervals; to them time is "passing too slowly," whereas, at the other end of the life span scale, a converse concern is expressed by seniors that "time seems to pass too quickly." In conventional studies of time estimation, such contrasting impressions of the same elapsed time are explained by hypothesizing an internal mechanical clock that "runs" faster in some individuals or in certain situations than in others.

Although in DAT, internal clocks are not mechanical, it is possible to explain this phenomenon in a parallel fashion. Specifically, the number of elapsed cycles of dominant oscillator that fill some to-be-judged time span should determine a listener's judgment about this elapsed time. This sheds light on classic family trip episodes, mentioned earlier, where children, halfway through the trip, cry out over the "unbearable length" of elapsed time. In this case, although children and adults experience the same objective trip time, children, who operate with faster dominant oscillations, have experienced many more cycles of their (fast) dominant oscillation than have their parents who, in theory, operate with slower dominant oscillations. Thus, the same elapsed time in the car seems longer to children than to adults.

Predictions About Phase-Locking over the Life Span

The second major prediction of the aging hypothesis involves its entrainment corollary. This addresses age-related changes in phase-locking skills. This aspect of the aging hypothesis implies that entrainment coupling parameters change systematically, with the strongest phase-locking capacity associated with young adults. This is a task-specific prediction. It holds that young to middle-aged adults excel over younger and older age groups primarily in tasks featuring phase synchrony of attending and/or motor activity with respect to an external event. Figure 5.4 shows this prediction as

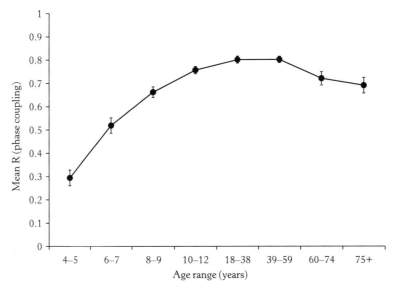

FIGURE 5.5 A measure of phase coupling performance (in a tapping task) is R (for a Rayleigh test; $0 \le R \le 1.00$). This figure shows that coupling performance is best for middle-aged listeners (unpublished data).

a quadratic trend in phase-coupling strength with age, where peak performance occurs around the ages of 18–40 years.

This account implies that phase-locking performance in tapping tasks follows a curvilinear function over the life span, where the best tappers are young adults. Support for this idea is shown in Figure 5.5, where a measure of phase-coupling shows that very young and very old age groups performed significantly more poorly in a tapping task than did middle-aged tappers.

Entrainment: Motor, Attending, or Both?

Dynamic attending theory maintains that the phase-locking abilities of entraining neural oscillations should have a widespread effect on attending. Although the synchronized tapping data of Figure 5.5 illustrate that overt motor tapping conforms to the aging hypotheses, theoretically, a similar function should hold for non-motor tasks. The rationale is straightforward: just as we must time an overt response to a sound, so, too, we must precisely guide attending in time to allocate attending energy to a target event. Following DAT, phase-locking skills are not limited to motor acts, such as tapping, they also apply to sequential attending and even to time discrimination.[59,60] In other words, time discrimination tasks will also show the age-specific effects of Figures 5.4 and 5.5.

Converging Evidence: It's Complicated

The aging hypothesis distinguishes two age-related trends. One is overall age-related slowing (due to resonance); the other is a curvilinear function based on phase-locking capacity (due to entrainment). Although some behavioral studies confirm this distinction, teasing apart these two neural trends can be complicated.

The good news is that current research on issues surrounding neural synchrony is increasing. The bad news: it is necessarily confined to probing nonprimate brains. Nevertheless, Wang and colleagues intriguingly show that some neurons in marmosets are specialized to respond to synchrony and/or rate, whereas others are not.[61,62] Also pertinent are studies of humans' developmental trends in neural responses to period versus phase properties. A study of Cho et al.[63] offers some rather complex neural support for age-related distinctions of period and phase sensitivity (for listeners 8–16 years) using fast isochronous click trains.[64]

In sum, a dynamic attending account leads to life span distinctions between the course of dominant oscillator periods and the potential these oscillations hold for instilling successful phase-locking as a function of age. A monotonic trend in period-slowing with age, which happens in some tasks (SMT, preference rating) is explained by the resonance principle. By contrast, a different, curvilinear trend over the life span describes phase-locking skills in tasks requiring synchrony (motor, attentional); it is attributable to the entrainment principle. Together, both resonance and entrainment principles operate over the life span.

Summary of the Aging Hypothesis and Life Span Predictions

In landmark research, Esther Thelen documented maturing stereotypes of overt motor rhythms in infants throughout the first year of life.[65] So, too, Oller finds maturational changes at smaller produced rhythmic time scales in vocalized sounds in the first year of life. Although these innate tendencies chart observable motor rhythms, it is not unreasonable to consider that covert but systematic maturational changes of other sorts co-occur early in life and even beyond the first years of life. Indeed, discoveries of brain activities consistent with the aging hypothesis about attending mirror developmental changes in infant vocalizations. They suggest that infants display early orienting preferences for high-frequency sound components.

The aging hypothesis embodies maturational attending changes associated with timing, as summarized by a temporal niche proposal. It extends the thrust of maturational sensitivities to event timing that covers a life span. This hypothesis proposes systematic age-related changes in overt measures of attending as well as in recordings of cortical correlates. The aging hypothesis rests on the resonance principle to explain involuntary age-specific orienting biases in the form of age-related slowing. It also engages a corollary that speaks to maturational changes of phase-locking in entrainment. These shifts in phase-locking behavior are attributed to the changing adaptivity levels of cortical oscillations over the life span, peaking in young adulthood. In turn, these changes derive from entrainment parameters. Together, these aspects of the aging hypothesis predict different life span trends in attending behaviors. Evidence favoring one or both of these trends is described in this section, with the following major points:

- The temporal niche for humans depends on rhythmic rate; it widens asymmetrically with age.
- The aging hypothesis successfully predicts age-specific biases for rates of (simple) rhythms over a life span. Human infants involuntarily resonate (i.e., orient) to faster rates and adults to slower rates.
- An aging hypothesis corollary stipulates that age-specific phase-locking ability

peaks in young adults; it is based on changing values of a relevant entrainment parameter.

CHAPTER SUMMARY

Our sense of timing is relative. The same event rate that seems slow in one context can feel fast in another. Furthermore, what seems slow (or fast) changes with age. This is captured in the concept of a temporal niche, which evolves with age. A temporal niche is a collection of event rhythms (candidate driving rhythms) most compatible, via resonance, with a person's ongoing active (dominant) attending oscillations. Infants, who operate within a resonance-constrained temporal niche, favor fast events; they find the speedy pace of fast events "just fine," whereas older listeners, who operate with slower entraining rhythms, find the same event "too fast." We function within a temporal niche that shifts, asymmetrically broadening with age.

This chapter links the temporal niche concept to an aging hypothesis. This hypothesis features an innate reliance on the resonance principle that explains selective orienting to events of certain rates. Selectivity is due to the involuntary, age-specific resonance tendencies of cortical oscillations. It is hypothesized that the period of dominant oscillations slows with age, with support deriving from infants and children who orient to (prefer) relatively fast event rhythms in contrast to older individuals who operate with dominant oscillations of slower rates. An entrainment corollary of the aging hypothesis posits systematic changes in entrainment parameters over the life span. Supporting this are findings that young adults are more skillful at synchronizing to event rhythms than are younger and older individuals.

More generally, entrainment principles share with resonance principles the status of being universal and automatic. Entrainments do not create a temporal niche; instead, they ride on the resonating oscillations associated with a temporal niche. Entrainment is governed by attractors as well as by event-based driving rhythm properties, such as force and regularity, where the latter figure in the general attending hypothesis. Together, these two hypotheses create a picture of selective attending as one involving heightened amplitude(s) of driven cortical oscillations, namely dominant oscillations. Finally, attending is a dynamic activity involving interactions between neural oscillations and environmental events. Selective attending happens when certain events in this environment receive heightened attending energy (relative to others) conveyed by oscillations of higher amplitudes.

Returning to the broader perspective of ecological niches outlined at the beginning of this chapter, these attending dynamics hold implications for understanding the limits to which we can change our temporal niche within a more expansive interpretation of both the environment and the creatures that inhabit it. If, as conceived here, our environment is aptly described by four dimensions, including time, then the dynamics of our interactions within this habitat afford natural constraints which we, as theorists, should take seriously. It implies that we can change our environmental habitats. This is obvious in recent changes in climate. However, less obvious are ways in which our communicative environment is changing. That is, as we introduce machine-made driving rhythms that realize ever increasing rates (computers, cell phones, etc.), we are unwittingly speeding up this environment. In light of a main theme of this chapter, we can infer that our contemporary environment is being transformed into habitats that suit one age group (young adults) at the expense of other age groups (seniors). This topic is revisited in Chapter 15.

NOTES

1. Mari R. Jones, "Time, Our Lost Dimension: Toward a New Theory of Perception, Attention, and Memory," *Psychological Review* 83, no. 5 (1976): 323.

2. Charles E. Speaks, *Introduction to Sound: Acoustics for the Hearing and Speech Sciences.* (Singular Publishing Group, 1992), Second Edition. San Diego, California. http://psycnet.apa.org/psycinfo/1994-97721-000.

3. D. K. Oller, *The Emergence of the Speech Capacity.* (Mahwah, NJ: Lawrence Erlbaum, 2000).

4. The author is grateful for the insightful comments of Laura Dilley in this section.

5. For a deeper explication of growth factors, see Patterson and colleagues.

6. "Complex" and "complexity" here refer to the nature of interactions summarized by the relative time ratios of simple components as estimates of attractor ratios. This differs from a conventional distinction between simple and complex waveforms in sound; see Box 5.1.

7. Throughout all chapters, conventional notation of a fundamental stimulus frequency is F0, its harmonics are nF0 and generic stimulus frequencies are noted as F. Corresponding oscillator frequencies are italized.

8. The contour pitch patterns reported by Kent and Murray mirror those described as tempo response curves for slower time patterns in Chapter 8.

9. Roy D. Patterson, Etienne Gaudrain, and Thomas C. Walters, "The Perception of Family and Register in Musical Tones," in *Music Perception*, eds. Mari Riess Jones, Richard R. Fay, and Arthur N. Popper, Springer Handbook of Auditory Research 36 (New York: Springer, 2010), 13–50, doi:10.1007/978-1-4419-6114-3_2.

10. Presumably in Oller's Phonation stage.

11. Raymond D. Kent and Ann D. Murray, "Acoustic Features of Infant Vocalic Utterances at 3, 6, and 9 Months," *Journal of the Acoustical Society of America* 72, no. 2 (August 1982): 353–65, doi:10.1121/1.388089.

12. R. J. Baken, *Clinical Measurement of Speech and Voice* (San Diego, CA: Singular Publishing Group, 1996).

13. Taken from the first edition of Bakan's book; p. 354.

14. Related to determinants of P-centers discussed in later chapters.

15. This is Oller's primitive articulary stage.

16. Endogenous entrainment of these two activated oscillations is a precursor to the concept of oscillator clusters developed in later chapters.

17. Although F0 also varies over time, this is less common and less pronounced. See also tempo response curves on this topic in Chapter 8.

18. Hartmut Rothgänger, "Analysis of the Sounds of the Child in the First Year of Age and a Comparison to the Language," *Early Human Development* 75, no. 1–2 (December 2003): 55–69, doi:10.1016/j.earlhumdev.2003.09.003.

19. Gwen E. Gustafson and James A. Green, "On the Importance of Fundamental Frequency and Other Acoustic Features in Cry Perception and Infant Development," *Child Development* 60, no. 4 (1989): 772–80, doi:10.2307/1131017.

20. Patricia K. Kuhl, "Is Speech Learning 'Gated' by the Social Brain?" *Developmental Science* 10, no. 1 (January 1, 2007): 110–20, doi:10.1111/j.1467-7687.2007.00572.x.

21. David Snow, "Polysyllabic Units in the Vocalizations of Children from 0;6 to 1;11: Intonation-Groups, Tones and Rhythms," *Journal of Child Language* 34, no. 04 (November 2007): 765–797, doi:10.1017/S030500090700815X.

22. Peter F. MacNeilage, "The Frame/Content Theory of Evolution of Speech Production," *Behavioral and Brain Sciences* 21, no. 04 (August 1998): 499–511, doi:null.

23. Roy D. Patterson, Etienne Gaudrain, and Thomas C. Walters, "The Perception of Family and Register in Musical Tones," in *Music Perception* (Springer, 2010), 13–50, http://link.springer.com.proxy.library.ucsb.edu:2048/chapter/10.1007/978-1-4419-6114-3_2.

24. Athena Vouloumanos et al., "The Tuning of Human Neonates' Preference for Speech," *Child Development* 81, no. 2 (March 1, 2010): 517–27, doi:10.1111/j.1467-8624.2009.01412.x.

25. A. J. DeCasper and W. P. Fifer, "Of Human Bonding: Newborns Prefer Their Mothers' Voices," *Science* 208, no. 4448 (June 6, 1980): 1174–76, doi:10.1126/science.7375928.

26. Anthony J. DeCasper and Melanie J. Spence, "Prenatal Maternal Speech Influences Newborns' Perception of Speech Sounds," *Infant Behavior and Development* 9, no. 2 (April 1, 1986): 133–50, doi:10.1016/0163-6383(86)90025-1.

27. Peter G. Hepper and S. Shahidullah, "The Development of Fetal Hearing," *Fetal and Maternal Medicine Review* 6, no. 03 (August 1994): 167–79, doi:10.1017/S0965539500001108.

28. B. S. Kisilevsky et al., "Fetal Sensitivity to Properties of Maternal Speech and Language," *Infant Behavior and Development* 32, no. 1 (January 2009): 59–71, doi:10.1016/j.infbeh.2008.10.002.

29. For example, critical band constraints on micro-rhythms are not discussed.

30. A caveat is that for the same fixed coupling parameter, younger individuals are more stimulus-oriented (weak driven oscillations) than are older individuals. But they will typically have lower effective K values than adults.

31. "Rhythms of the Brain - György Buzsáki - Google Books," accessed February Oxford University Press, Inc., New York, New York, 2006. https://books-google-com.proxy.library.ucsb.edu:9443/books?hl=enandlr=andid=ldz58irprjYCandoi=fndandpg=PA4anddq=Buzsaki,+2006andots=Q1X836eGASandsig=pvOzjx2ylzrNmQwOmG-Ed1XIPbQ#v=onepageandq=Buzsaki%2C%202006andf=false.

32. Fumitaka Homae et al., "Development of Global Cortical Networks in Early Infancy," *Journal of Neuroscience* 30, no. 14 (April 7, 2010): 4877–82, doi:10.1523/JNEUROSCI.5618-09.2010.

33. Ivica Kostović and Nataša Jovanov-Milošević, "The Development of Cerebral Connections During the First 20–45 Weeks' Gestation," *Seminars in Fetal and Neonatal Medicine*, 11, no. 6 (December 2006): 415–22, doi:10.1016/j.siny.2006.07.001.

34. Zdravko Petanjek et al., "Lifespan Alterations of Basal Dendritic Trees of Pyramidal Neurons in the Human Prefrontal Cortex: A Layer-Specific Pattern," *Cerebral Cortex* 18, no. 4 (April 1, 2008): 915–29, doi:10.1093/cercor/bhm124.

35. Sophie Vanvooren et al., "Theta, Beta and Gamma Rate Modulations in the Developing Auditory System," *Hearing Research* 327 (September 2015): 153–62, doi:10.1016/j.heares.2015.06.011.

36. M. B. Sterman et al., "Quantitative Analysis of Infant EEG Development During Quiet Sleep," *Electroencephalography and Clinical Neurophysiology* 43, no. 3 (September 1, 1977): 371–85, doi:10.1016/0013-4694(77)90260-7.

37. M. M. Myers et al., "Developmental Profiles of Infant EEG: Overlap with Transient Cortical Circuits," *Clinical Neurophysiology* 123, no. 8 (August 2012): 1502–11, doi:10.1016/j.clinph.2011.11.264.

38. Duncan J. Watts and Steven H. Strogatz, "Collective Dynamics of 'Small-World' Networks," *Nature* 393, no. 6684 (June 4, 1998): 440–42, doi:10.1038/30918.

39. Steven H. Strogatz, "Exploring Complex Networks," *Nature* 410, no. 6825 (March 8, 2001): 268–76, doi:10.1038/35065725.

40. Peter Fransson et al., "The Functional Architecture of the Infant Brain as Revealed by Resting-State FMRI," *Cerebral Cortex* 21, no. 1 (January 1, 2011): 145–54, doi:10.1093/cercor/bhq071.

41. György Buzsáki, *Rhythms of the Brain* (New York: Oxford University Press, 2006), https://books-google-com.proxy.library.ucsb.edu:9443/books?hl=enandlr=andid=ldz58irprjYCandoi=fndandpg=PA4anddq=Buzaki+++Rhythms+of+the+brain+andots=Q1Ya5ZcGDXandsig=GcvM82ZD1Q25nWclKSJ7bdfog84.

42. Fumitaka Homae et al., "Development of Global Cortical Networks in Early Infancy."

43. Nikolai Novitski et al., "Neonatal Frequency Discrimination in 250–4000-Hz Range: Electrophysiological Evidence," *Clinical Neurophysiology* 118, no. 2 (February 2007): 412–19, doi:10.1016/j.clinph.2006.10.008.

44. Barbara Cone and Angela Garinis, "Auditory Steady-State Responses and Speech Feature Discrimination in Infants," *Journal of the American Academy of Audiology* 20, no. 10 (November 1, 2009): 629–43, doi:10.3766/jaaa.20.10.5.

45. Nicole A. Folland et al., "Processing Simultaneous Auditory Objects: Infants' Ability to Detect Mistuning in Harmonic Complexes," *Journal of the Acoustical Society of America* 131, no. 1 (January 1, 2012): 993–97, doi:10.1121/1.3651254.

46. Specifically, electrical brainstem recording of auditory steady-state response (ASSR) measures.

47. Yvonne S. Sininger, Carolina Abdala, and Barbara Cone-Wesson, "Auditory Threshold Sensitivity of the Human Neonate as Measured by the Auditory Brainstem Response," *Hearing Research* 104, no. 1–2 (February 1997): 27–38, doi:10.1016/S0378-5955(96)00178-5.

48. Novitski et al., "Neonatal Frequency Discrimination in 250–4000-Hz Range."

49. Vanessa Carral et al., "A Kind of Auditory 'Primitive Intelligence' Already Present at Birth," *European Journal of Neuroscience* 21, no. 11 (June 1, 2005): 3201–04, doi:10.1111/j.1460-9568.2005.04144.x.

50. G. Dehaene-Lambertz and M. Pena, "Electrophysiological Evidence for Automatic Phonetic Processing in Neonates," *NeuroReport* 12, no. 14 (2001), http://journals.lww.com/neuroreport/Fulltext/2001/10080/Electrophysiological_evidence_for_automatic.34.aspx.

51. A. Kujala, M. Houtilainen, M. Hotakainen et al., "Speech-Sound Discrimination in Neonates as Measured with MEG," *NeuroReport* 15, no. 13 (September 15, 2004): 2089–92, accessed February 18, 2016, http://journals.lww.com/neuroreport/Fulltext/2004/09150/Speech_sound_discrimination_in_neonates_as.18.aspx.

52. Silke Telkemeyer et al., "Sensitivity of Newborn Auditory Cortex to the Temporal Structure of Sounds," *Journal of Neuroscience* 29, no. 47 (November 25, 2009): 14726–33, doi:10.1523/JNEUROSCI.1246-09.2009.

53. These modulations were strongest in the left hemisphere with FM modulations of a 25 ms period, indicating infant sensitivities to fine time structures of 1 ms period embedded in the slower modulating period.

54. Barbara Cone and Angela Garinis, "Auditory Steady-State Responses and Speech Feature Discrimination in Infants," *Journal of the American Academy of Audiology* 20, no. 10 (November 1, 2009): 629–43, doi:10.3766/jaaa.20.10.5.

55. J. Devin McAuley et al., "The Time of Our Lives: Life Span Development of Timing and Event Tracking," *Journal of Experimental Psychology: General* 135, no. 3 (2006): 348–67, doi:10.1037/0096-3445.135.3.348.

56. McAuley et al., "The Time of Our Lives."

57. W. Jay Dowling et al., "Melody Recognition at Fast and Slow Tempos: Effects of Age, Experience, and Familiarity," *Perception & Psychophysics* 70, no. 3 (April 2008): 496–502, doi:10.3758/PP.70.3.496.

58. Carolyn Drake, Amandine Penel, and Emmanuel Bigand, "Tapping in Time with Mechanically and Expressively Performed Music," *Music Perception: An Interdisciplinary Journal* 18, no. 1 (October 1, 2000): 1–23, doi:10.2307/40285899.

59. Edward W. Large and Mari Riess Jones, "The Dynamics of Attending: How People Track Time-Varying Events," *Psychological Review* 106, no. 1 (1999): 119–59, doi:10.1037/0033-295X.106.1.119.

60. J. Devin McAuley and Mari Riess Jones, "Modeling Effects of Rhythmic Context on Perceived Duration: A Comparison of Interval and Entrainment Approaches to Short-Interval Timing," *Journal of Experimental Psychology: Human Perception and Performance* 29, no. 6 (2003): 1102.

61. Daniel Bendor and Xiaoqin Wang, "Neural Coding of Periodicity in Marmoset Auditory Cortex," *Journal of Neurophysiology* 103, no. 4 (April 1, 2010): 1809–22, doi:10.1152/jn.00281.2009.

62. X. Wang et al., "Neural Coding of Temporal Information in Auditory Thalamus and Cortex," *Neuroscience* 154, no. 1 (June 12, 2008): 294–303, doi:10.1016/j.neuroscience.2008.03.065.

63. Raymond Y. Cho et al., "Development of Sensory Gamma Oscillations and Cross-Frequency Coupling from Childhood to Early Adulthood," *Cerebral Cortex*, December 10, 2015, Issue 6, (June 1, 2015): 1509–1518, doi:10.1093/cercor/bht341.

64. These results, however, are qualified and quite complicated.

65. Esther Thelen, "Rhythmical Stereotypies in Normal Human Infants," *Animal Behaviour* 27 (August 1, 1979): 699–715, doi:10.1016/0003-3472(79)90006-X.

6

Tuning in to Very Fast Events

Pitch Perception

The concept of a temporal niche, introduced in the preceding chapter, advanced the idea that, as people age, they tune in to increasingly slower sets of privileged event-based driving rhythms. Adults involuntarily react to a wide range of low-frequency sounds, whereas infants preferentially orient more narrowly to sounds of higher frequencies. This idea raises questions about "what" listeners of different ages actually experience as they tune in to certain sounds. In particular, how do they follow, in real time, the fast events we know elicit pitch perception?

This chapter addresses this broad question while acknowledging constraints involving the temporal niche. According to the aging hypothesis (i.e., its corollary), one constraint holds that our sensitivity to privileged time relationships, i.e., powerful attractors that persist over the life span. Other constraints involve age-related sensitivities surrounding event rate and phase-locking. This chapter builds on the first constraint. It considers how people of all ages use attractor relationships to entrain to certain fast acoustic patterns that determine pitch percepts.

Attending redux. First, let's review the relationship between perception and attending from a dynamic attending perspective. As suggested by phase response curves (PRCs) and attending energy profiles (AEPs) from an earlier chapter, attending is linked to the amplitude of a driven oscillation. Regardless of the time scale of an entraining oscillation, attending energy depends on the amplitude of an entraining oscillation. In this chapter, this means that complex sounds comprising many frequencies will afford multiple fast driving rhythms for such entraining oscillations. Moreover, in a collection of driven oscillations, those periodicities with most energy govern attending. Typically, time scales pertinent to pitch perception are in the range of milliseconds or even fractions of milliseconds. This means that attending associated with listeners' responses to complex sounds, i.e., sounds that embed many driving rhythms in these ranges, is largely involuntary. As such, attending is inseparable from perception.

This chapter proposes that listeners can automatically entrain to fast driving micro-rhythms that comprise everyday sounds. And as they do so, amplitudes of correlated driven oscillations contribute to the perceptual sharpness of such sounds. As amplitudes of entraining oscillations increase, so does one's attending energy directed to a particular sound. Thus, even at the fast time scales of frequencies of musical tones or speech phonemes, the heightened energy of one or several fast entraining oscillations is diagnostic of heightened attending, hence improved perception.

So, what exactly *is* a fast event? In this approach fast events are sounds based on very fast rhythms, namely micro-rhythms. They are associated with relatively high frequencies (e.g., often exceeding the high gamma frequencies of 70-80 Hz). Indeed, periods of these driving rhythms are typically less than 10 ms. Although some might argue that such micro-rhythms are too fast to effectively entrain a corresponding driven oscillation, in theory *entrainment is not rate limited*. However, what is limited are current methods for recording possible activities of proposed driven oscillations that qualify as very fast brain rhythms (i.e., form scalp EEG or intracranial EEG recordings). Reliable recordings of normal oscillatory activities faster than 100 Hz (i.e., for periods less than 10 ms) are difficult to achieve.

Nevertheless, this chapter builds on the hypothesis that fast events support phase-locking behaviors. Moreover, the attending associated with a fast driving/driven dyad is never an all-or-none affair. Rather attending differs in degree as a function of the momentary energy of an engaged driven rhythm. And, as with attending to slow events, attending to fast events involves voluntary and involuntary forces. Although some may deny any role for attending at these time scales by reserving the term 'perception' for describing involuntary responses to fast events (e.g., for small time scales of pitch), the DAT approach outlined in this (and the preceding) chapter assumes that a listener's perception of these events reflects the momentary impact of involuntary as well as voluntary attending on the experience of perceiving.

Basically, pitch perception depends on automatic attending at very fast time scales. For instance, given a pure tone of 200 Hz, with a micro-driving rhythm period of 5 ms, this tone affords entrainment of a resonant neural correlation of the same period. Moreover, in a context of other competing pure tones, this tone may draw a listener's attending if its entraining oscillation is dominant. That is, if the amplitude of a waveform, with a period of 5 ms, is high relative to amplitudes of competing (pure tone) waveforms, then this favors a listener's percept of this sound which determines the dominant periodicity (cf. preceding chapter regarding dominant oscillations). In short, in episodes of entrainment involving fast micro-time levels, attending becomes perceiving.

Attractors also figure in explanations of perception of fast events. Following the corollary of the aging hypothesis, attractors are available anchors that express prototypical time relationships. Attractors command synchrony between a produced event and a listener's internal response to this event. From preceding chapters, it is clear that attractor synchrony will differ in complexity. For instance, simple attractors, such as $n:m$ = 1:1 or 1:2, function prominently in infants' early reliance on harmonically based synchronies of quasi-vowels in speech. In this chapter, where we consider adults' synchronizations to very fast events, issues of attractor complexity play a more prominent role.

Perceptual puzzles. This chapter addresses several puzzles involving pitch percepts of complex sounds. To preview, one such sound is outlined in Table 6.1. This is a complex sound rich in multiple harmonic components. Each component is a frequency with a waveform that provides a micro-driving rhythm. Moreover, in this example sound, all component micro-rhythms are harmonically related to the same referent driving rhythm, namely the fundamental frequency (F0 = 200 Hz).

A major puzzle facing theories of pitch perception surrounds a well-known finding. It turns out that a complex sound, with multiple harmonic frequencies, is heard to have the pitch of only the fundamental frequency. And, surprisingly, this is true even when the fundamental frequency is missing![1] Now, that's a puzzle. Clearly, these harmonics have some impact because sounds with anharmonic components deliver less clear pitch percepts. And everyday sounds such as lawn mowers, automobile engine noise, and bubbling water, which lack harmonic components, invite still less clear percepts of a given pitch.

This chapter considers explanations of such findings. It turns out that pitch perception of complex sounds is often affected by relative timings among component frequencies, also termed *partials*. Thus, a partial is a micro-rhythm. For example, Table 6.1 shows partials nestled inside complex sounds. Each complex sound has partials that are harmonic components, listed in the left-most column. Partials that are nested in such complex sounds not only affect the perceptual clarity of the pitch of these sounds, they also contribute to a listener's sense of sound quality or consonance. By contrast, if people encounter only a single partial, i.e., as a pure tone, this stimulus is judged along a subjective continuum. For instance, a very fast pure tone will seem higher in pitch than a pure tone with a lower frequency (i.e., one with a slower micro-rhythm). However, in the context of multiple, co-occuring, pure tones (now partials), as in Table 6.1, the relationships between these micro-rhythms 'take charge'. Relationships among partials in complex tones affect a listener's perception of the pitch of such tones.

Finally, communicative sounds of music and speech are populated by various captivating micro-rhythmic relationships. Opinions differ on precisely how frequencies of partials come together to influence listeners' percepts of pitch and of consonance. Nevertheless, in this story, few debate the import of frequency components, including the fundamental frequency.

Attractor timing and the temporal niche. This chapter focuses on the harmonic relations of complex sounds under the assumption that they "call up" innate attractors. The dynamic framework of proceeding chapters described attractors as special micro-time relationships that are accessible to an individual over the life span. More precisely:

> An attractor corresponds to a stable endogenous state specified by an ideal time relationship between periods of separate waveforms corresponding to driving and driven rhythms. This relationship satisfies a general commensurate property of mode-locking in which synchrony of two rhythms, with periods, pi and pj, is determined by a common product when multiplied, respectively, by integers n and m, as in n (pi) = m (pj). This attractor constraint

TABLE 6.1 COMPLEX TONES

A complex tone 15 ms with multiple harmonics (F0 = 200 Hz)

Harmonics n	Three 5 ms segments			Total T cycles	T1:Tn	Tn:Tn + 1
200 Hz 1	1 (5.0) = 5	1 (5.0) = 5	1 (5.0) = 5	3	1:1[b]	2.1[b]
400 Hz 2	2 (2.5) = 5	2 (2.5) = 5	2 (2.5) = 5	**6**	**2:1[b]**	3:2[b]
600 Hz 3	3 (1.67) = 5	3 (1.67) =5	3 (1.67) = 5	**9**[a]	**3:1[b]**	4:3[b]
800 Hz 4	4 (1.25) = 5	4 (1.25) = 5	4 (1.25) = 5	**12**[a]	**4:1[b]**	5.4 [b]
1,000 Hz 5	5 (1.0) = 5	5 (1.00) = 5	5 (1.00) = 5	**15**[a]	**5:1**	~ 10:8
.						
.						
2,000 Hz 10	10 (.50) = 5	10 (.50) = 5	10 (.50) = 5	30	10:1	10:9
2,200 Hz 11	11 (.454)~5	11 (.454) ~ 5	11 (.454) ~ 5	33	11:1	11:10
2,400 Hz 12	12 (.416)~5	12(.416) ~ 5	12(.416) ~ 5	36	1:12	12:11

This complex sound lasts for three segments of 5 ms. A 5 ms cycle is the period of F0: 5 ms = (1/F0) 1,000 ms.
For nth harmonic, the first harmonic is n = 1, for F0 = 200 Hz.
T1 is the stimulus period of F0; p1 ' is notation of an oscillation locked to T1.
Partial time spans, Tn, contribute to cycles (columns 2–4); oscillator correlates of Tn have period, pn~Tn. The p1 is a F0 period of 5 ms (columns 2–4); pn is the period of a resonant oscillation of harmonic partial, Tn.
[a] Indicates cycle totals exceeding 8.
[b] Indicates relatively simple attractors (columns 6, 7).
Bold items in columns 5 and 6 define the dominance region

extends to phase relationships. A generalized mode-locking phase relationship conforms to the algorithm: n (φi) = m (φj).

Attractors are ever-present internal entrainment states. They are the heart of synchrony. In a tunable brain, attractors express an intriguing potential that compels two different rhythms (e.g., cortical oscillations) to "fall into step" (i.e., to synchronize) based on special time relations (of periods, phases; Chapter 3). This creates a gravity-like pull; namely, an "attractor pull" (cf. Figure 3.4).

Consider, for example, a simple case of attractors involving two different pure tones presented simultaneously. Let this create a two-tone chord comprising middle C and C′ (an octave above C). For a listener, each tone supplies an external driving rhythm that elicits resonance in a

neural correlate of the listener's tunable brain (i.e., selectively heightens the resonating oscillator's amplitude). For each tone in the chord, this then sets the stage for exogenous entrainment between the driving and driven rhythms. Assuming then the two driven oscillations of these tones then also engage in endogenously entrainment, the listener will experience this tone pair as a distinctly harmonious chord. This experience arises from the fact that the endogenous entrainment of these oscillations is governed by a strong attractor that "commands" a palpable "pull" between the two activated neural oscillations. Specifically, this attractor expresses an *n:m* chord relationship of 2:1.

Next, let's generalize these ideas. Imagine that instead of an octave ratio, a two-tone chord expresses a different relationship, as depicted in Figure 6.1A (*n:m* = 3:2; i.e., a chord formed

A   **A two-tone chord**

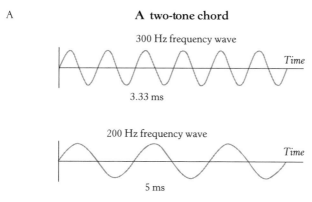

B   Entrainments: Exogenous and endogenous

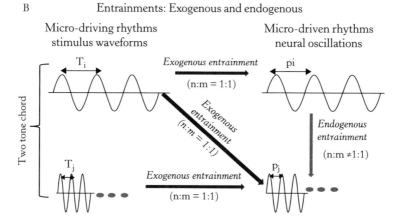

FIGURE 6.1 (**A**) Sinewave components of a two-tone chord. The faster, 300 Hz, waveform has a period of 3.33 ms; the slower, 200 Hz, one has a period of 5 ms. (**B**) How entrainments emerge in chords. Here, two exogenous entrainment configurations are governed by simple (n:m = 1:1) and more complex (*n* ≠ 1:1) attractors. Also shown is endogenous mode-locking involving two oscillations with periods related by a more complex attractor ratio (e.g., n:m ≠1:1, e.g., 3:2).

by second and third harmonics of Table 6.1). Although musically this ratio connotes a perfect fifth ratio, a DAT analysis applies to waveforms of *any* two harmonics of a complex sound. Figure 6.1B illustrates a general case involving two types of fast entrainments: exogenous (dark gray connections) and endogenous entrainments (light gray connections). Each tone in this chord provides a stimulus micro-driving rhythm (respective time periods: T_i, T_j). And each driving rhythm immediately activates a resonant oscillator period, $p_i \neq p_j$ (e.g., $p_i \sim T_i$). Together, in this example, two such two activated oscillations form a compelling endogenous dyad (e.g., an octave or perfect fifth). More generally, any pair of two tones (or any complex sound) can implicate an attractor, either a simple (e.g., $n{:}m = 1{:}1$, $2{:}1$ ...) or a complex (e.g., $n{:}m = 8{:}5$, $1{:}12$, etc.) attractor.

Figure 6.1B shows that attractors govern both exogenous and endogenous entrainment couplings. As their label implies, attractors express idealized time relationships that *literally attract* nearby (possibly deviant) dyadic relationships. In turn, the attractors implicated during entrainment influence "what" we perceive as pitch. How this happens is the topic of this chapter.

CHAPTER GOALS

This chapter has two goals. The first involves extending dynamic attending theory to tackle phenomena surrounding perception of very fast acoustic events. Of special interest are fast events defined by complex relationships. Of special interest are the communicative sounds of music and speech. Two perceptual phenomena are of particular interest: pitch perception and consonance judgments.

A second goal aims to contrast Dynamic Attending Theory (DAT) explanations of pitch perception and consonance, expressed in the *aging* and *general attending hypotheses*, with those of successful theories that do not incorporate entrainment ideas.

BACKGROUND: PAST AND PRESENT THEORIES OF PITCH PERCEPTION

Although the sound of a friend's voice is easy to recognize, opinions differ on why this is so. There is little debate about the importance of the fundamental frequency in adults' capacity to recognize the complex sounds of speech and music. But the absolute frequency of the fundamental is not the only factor determining voice recognition; if that were the case, we would suffer from severe, sometimes comical, perceptual confusions of speakers. Such vocalizations, by their complex nature, deliver informative complex sounds. Nevertheless, discussions about absolute versus relative pitch judgments remain unsettled, as Patel notes in an insightful review.[2][pp.46–48]

Topics central to this chapter are related to pitch perception of complex sounds, which comprise not only a fundamental frequency, but also numerous fast partials (i.e., time scales in milliseconds or less). At first glance, simply the speed of frequency components might seem to thwart a goal of coherent communication. For instance, all the partials of complex tones in Table 6.1 have frequencies that exceed 180 Hz (i.e., the high gamma range). Yet, surprisingly, we effortlessly meet such communicative goals in our ordinary conversations. We readily follow the utterance of a colleague, instantly picking up syllables with embedded phonemes as they occur. Perhaps more surprising, given these brief time scales, we even anticipate forthcoming items, sometimes annoyingly finishing another's sentence. Certainly, explanations based on absolute time limits of processing would make such skills implausible. So, how do we effortlessly "process" complex sounds at seemingly lightning speeds?

Perhaps this puzzle is resolved by assuming that expertise with fast partials is established early in life, when our attending is putatively oriented to fast micro-driving rhythms. This must be part of the story; however, it fails to explain adults' ability to detect the pitch of novel fast sounds. As this chapter shows, our ability to cope, in the moment, with fleeting, unfamiliar, complex sounds presents knotty problems that have fascinated scholars for decades. Among the knottiest of problems is understanding precisely *how* partials affect pitch percepts of complex sounds. Historically, this topic stretches back to Helmholtz. Still today, theorists struggle with it, using contemporary tasks that require people to judge the pitch of a complex sound ("Is sound A higher or lower than sound B?" Or, "Does this complex sound match a pure tone of a fixed frequency?"). Contemporary theories are numerous (see excellent reviews by de Cheveigné,[3] Moore,[4] and Oxenham[5]). In fact, the creative diversity of these theories sends a clear message: no one theory has emerged as a clear winner.

Generally, pitch perception theories belong to one of two categories. In one category, *place theories* emphasize mechanisms associated with the locus of spectral frequencies (i.e., partials, fundamental) on the basilar membrane; these frequencies include partials and the fundamental frequency. The other category includes *time theories*, which are grounded in the timing properties of components in a complex sounds. As these labels imply, relevant theoretical categories build on either frequency (spectra) domain properties or time domain properties. Most begin by analyzing a sound's impact on the basilar membrane, a cochlear membrane that spirals inward from a base in the inner ear toward the cochlear apex. All theories aim to understand how the many partials comprising a complex sound affect a listener's ultimate percept of the sound's pitch. The following sections cannot do justice to the vast literature on this topic; rather, they focus selectively on a few instructive issues pertinent to attending to fast events.

Place Theories

Place theories build on two assertions regarding the basilar membrane.[6] First, complex tones with high-frequency components are heard as higher because they stimulate places on the basilar membrane near the cochlear base where this membrane is narrow and stiff. Conversely, lower frequency components resonate at specific places along this membrane near its wider, less stiff apex end. Thus, this spiraling membrane gradient offers natural, place-specific, filters for incoming frequencies, including those of partials.

Second, critical bandwidths surround an activated place on the basilar membrane (bandwidths estimates are ~12% of input frequency). These bandwidths serve as peripheral filters; that is, as *critical bands*. Although partial frequencies contribute to pitch perception of a complex sound, higher frequency partials have wider critical bandwidths than lower frequency partials. This means the precise "place" of high-frequency partials is difficult to resolve.[7,8] Specifically, poor frequency resolution among high-frequency partials is attributed to *overlapping critical bands*. Therefore, place theories predict best pitch perception for complex sounds containing low-frequency harmonic partials since the critical bands of these partials do not overlap.

One challenge for place theories comes with findings that listeners often judge the pitch of a complex sound as equivalent to its fundamental frequency component (F0) even when this component is missing (i.e., when it is impossible to stimulate a special place on the basilar membrane). This well-known phenomenon is referred to as the case of the *missing fundamental*. The reported percept of a missing F0 is termed a *virtual pitch*.

Time Theories

Time theories of pitch perception emphasize temporal properties of complex sounds. One approach focuses on the *fine time structure* created by unresolved (i.e., overlapping) partials, namely, the higher frequency components of a complex sound. Waveforms of the latter components are assumed to sum (e.g., a Fourier-like summation) to yield a temporal envelope; fine time structure then, is defined as time spans that pop up in this envelop.[9] Figure 6.2A shows an envelope's fine time structure with three time spans, t1, t2, t3 (as arrows).

Schouten,[10] an early champion of time theory, argued that the pitch of a complex sound depends on the fine time structure of a sound's envelop; this involves the distribution of time spans, ti, in a sound's fine time structure temporal envelope. Specifically, it is, the joint activity of unresolved, high-frequency components leads to a temporal envelope which carries distinctive time spans that influence a listener's pitch.

But classic time theories also faced problems. In particular, they incorrectly predicted that sounds with different fine time structures should lead to different pitch perceptions. Figure 6.2

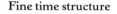

Fine time structure

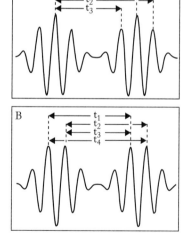

FIGURE 6.2 Illustration of fine time structure of two complex sounds. Bottom panel is an inverted waveform of that in the top panel. In both, fine time structure refers to the set of time intervals, ti, between peaks of frequency components (e.g., t_1, t_2 ... etc.).

Reprinted from Frederic L. Wightman, "Pitch and Stimulus Fine Structure," *The Journal of the Acoustical Society of America* 54, no. 2 (1973): 397, doi:10.1121/1.1913591.

illustrates this point. Note that the fine structure of the sound in Figure 6.2A clearly *differs* from that of Figure 6.2B, implying that listeners will hear these sounds as differing in pitch. In fact, people report that both sounds have the same pitch (i.e., panel B is the inverted waveform of panel A). This and related research confirms that classic time theories grant too much weight to fine time structure.[11,12]

Contemporary time theories take a different path. A common approach decomposes a complex sound into a series of discrete time intervals marked by a series of brief clicks of varying intensity. The resulting fast sound pattern conveys a pitch. These theories explain this by assuming that pitch percepts depend on a rate code. For instance, a series of brief time intervals, T_i values, between successive clicks might be 10 ms, 12 ms, 10 ms, 11 ms, 8 ms, 10 ms, and so forth. Indeed, people do report hearing a distinct pitch correlated with average rate.[13,14] Thus, one current explanation of pitch perception assumes that people rely on a *rate code* based on an average discrete interval. For instance, in the preceding example, the mode T_i interval is 10 ms; as a rate code, this statistic correctly predicts the reported pitch of 100 Hz.

These approaches suggest that the brain computes a distribution of independent interspike time intervals. That is, the brain does not directly respond to such sequences as if they are quasi-isochronous driving rhythm.[15] Instead, Cariani developed a time theory based on an elaborate network of rate codes.[16,17] Aspects of this approach also emerge in various contemporary pitch perception theories.

Summary of Place and Time

Historically, a central problem for pitch perception theories concerns the powerful role played by the fundamental frequency. Although pitch perception of complex sounds is influenced by partials, it remains unclear exactly how partials shape perception that is dominated by the fundamental component. Place theories of pitch perception have failed to explain pitch perception of complex sounds because they ignored the role of unresolved high-frequency harmonics on pitch perception. Early time theories also ran into trouble by heavily weighting the fine time structure of unresolved harmonic partials. As Oxenham's review neatly concludes: "Place models predict performance with unresolved harmonics that is too poor, and temporal models predict performance that is too good."[18[p.6]]

A PITCH PERCEPTION THEORY: TIME AS SMALL INTERVALS

This section concentrates on a contemporary time domain approach to pitch perception developed by Brian Moore. Moore's psychoacoustic theory extends earlier time domain theories, overcoming traditional obstacles to become a highly prominent approach to pitch perception.[19] Because this approach has successfully tackled challenges confronted by earlier approaches, it is a useful yardstick for assessing the potential of entrainment theory in this realm.

This pitch perception theory addresses why we hear the pitch of a complex tone as linked to its fundamental frequency. After all, these sounds, by definition, contain many frequencies—so why is the fundamental so dominant? Moore's time theory supplies one answer. It relies on the unifying role of a common denominator found in both place and time theories. Specifically, in complex sounds, stimulus time intervals are contributed by both low- and high-frequency components.

Figure 6.3 summarizes Moore's theory in five stages. Following an input filtering stage (stage 1), which differentiates resolved (low-frequency) partials from unresolved (high-frequency) partials, stage 2 involves a neural transduction for all inputs (resolved, unresolved) that expresses them as time

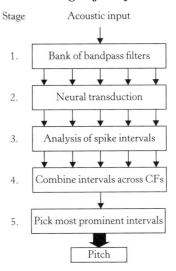

A Time theory of pitch perception
Five stages of analysis

Stage	Acoustic input
1.	Bank of bandpass filters
2.	Neural transduction
3.	Analysis of spike intervals
4.	Combine intervals across CFs
5.	Pick most prominent intervals
	Pitch

FIGURE 6.3 A stage scheme of Brian Moore's theory of pitch perception.

Reprinted from. B. C. J. Moore, *An Introduction to the Psychology of Hearing* (Amsterdam: Brill, 2012; figure 6.8).

intervals in the brain as outlined by interspike time intervals. Importantly, in stage 3, the resolved low frequency partials elicit internalized time spans based on their frequencies, whereas the unresolved high-frequency partials contribute to a fine time structure envelope that can be decomposed into different time spans (e.g., as in Figure 6.2). In stage 4, Moore persuasively argues that pitch perception is based on a collection of internal estimates of the period of the fundamental frequency. This stage summarizes the distribution of time spans from both low and high-frequency partials. Finally, stage 5 provides a criterion for producing a pitch judgment based on the most common overall time spans estimate (i.e., the mode T) as a basis for reporting the fundamental frequency.

An Example

To flesh out Moore's theory, let's return to the complex sound of Table 6.1. It has a fundamental frequency, F0, of 200 Hz and 12 harmonics ranging from 400 Hz all the way to higher partials of 2,200 or 2,400 Hz (left column of Table 6.1). This F0 determines a stimulus time interval of 5 ms. Other harmonics also contribute various shorter time spans, Tj. For instance, lower resolved frequency harmonics (e.g., 400 or 600 Hz) have T intervals from characteristic frequencies: here, 2.5 ms and 1.67 ms, respectively. A different story holds for the high-frequency unresolved components, however. These unresolved components combine to create a fine time structure that delivers a modest number of internalized time spans (i.e., Ti values not listed in Table 6.1).[20]

Finally, discrete time spans provide estimates of the interval of F0 following an algorithm: $T1 = nTj$, where Tj represents the estimated spike interval of a resolved nth harmonic. However, unresolved harmonic partials (above 2 kHz) produce few estimates of T1 (for F0) from the fine time structure. Consequently, higher harmonics of a complex sound have less impact on the final pitch code than do lower ones.[21] In Stages 3 and 4, the brain analyzes and compares estimates of the interval, T1, of F0 from all interspike intervals (i.e., resolved plus unresolved frequencies).[22,23] In the last stage, stage 5, the brain picks the most common (i.e., the mode) of collected neural estimates of T1. In this example, the mode interval underlying F0 is 5 ms.

As with most pitch theories, Moore's theory honors the role of the fundamental frequency. In this view, a sound's pitch gains prominence as a function of accessible interspike time estimates of the F0 interval. However, this theory is unusual for its incorporation of *both* low (resolved) and high (unresolved) frequencies of a complex sound. Consequently, it correctly predicts that listeners' should perceive a complex harmonic sound to have the pitch of F0 based largely on a greater impact of low (resolved) frequencies.

Finally, Moore's theory assumes that listeners judge a sound's pitch based on the most frequent interspike interval in a distribution of interval estimates of the F0. This assumption allows a deft explanation of *virtual pitch*. Virtual pitch refers to a puzzle posed by a well-known phenomenon that has baffled theorists for decades. "Virtual pitch" concerns observations that people, when presented with complex harmonic sounds lacking a fundamental frequency (e.g., 200 Hz in Table 6.1), nevertheless report hearing this missing fundamental as the sound's pitch. Moore neatly explains this as a consequence of estimating T1 in a harmonic sound as the mode interval. This statistical estimate does not change if F0 is removed. For instance, in Table 6.1, the T1 estimate of 5 ms remains the mode of collected T1 estimates even without estimates from a F0 of 200 Hz. With this brief sound, columns 2, 3, and 4 illustrate the prominence of various harmonic estimates of T1 (= 5 ms).

In sum, Moore's theory depicts listeners who rely on distributions of discrete time intervals comprising a complex sounds. Listeners extract from all partials (resolvable and unresolvable) brief interspike intervals, yielding a distribution of neural time spans that all estimate the time span of the fundamental frequency. However, estimates from low-frequency partials are predicted to be more reliable estimates than those of high-frequency partials due to poor resolution in the latter. Finally, this theory correctly predicts both virtual pitch as well as other established findings that harmonious complex sounds lead to stronger pitch percepts than do nonharmonious ones.

Main points of this section are:

- Historically, pitch perception theories fall into two broad categories: place theories and time theories.
- Place theories focus on peripheral neural activity at places along the basilar membrane as the basis for pitch perception. But they fail to explain phenomena surrounding virtual pitch.
- Early time theories focused exclusively on fine time structure determinants of pitch percepts. But they failed to explain findings

that low-frequency harmonics in a complex sound have a strong impact on pitch perception.

- Contemporary time theories, including Moore's, feature estimates (i.e., time codes) arising from collections of independent time intervals from both low- and high-frequency partials of complex sounds.
- Moore's theory extends weighted codes to address virtual pitch.

PITCH PERCEPTION FROM A DYNAMIC PERSPECTIVE

An alternative theory of pitch perception features entrainment concepts. Unlike Moore's model, this is not a psychoacoustic theory. Instead, it draws on dynamic attending principles, extending these to the small time spans of stimulus frequencies that populate sounds in speech and music. In this view, entrainment principles are not limited by time scale: entrainment happens with fast as well as slow events. Moreover, assuming that attending depends on the amplitude of a driven rhythm, descriptions of involuntary attending show that, at fast time scales, it is experienced as perceiving.

Of course, people's ability to effortlessly track rapid micro-time patterns in music and speech is rather remarkable. To explain this, this section has two parts. The first part describes entrainments involving fast acoustic events that determine pitch perception. The second part offers supporting evidence for this view.

Dynamics of Attending to Fast Events: Pitch Perception

A dynamic attending perspective to pitch perception appeals to neural correlates capable of entraining to micro-driving rhythms within complex sounds. Basically, it considers how we tune into fast events. Originally, dynamic attending theory addressed attending to events unfolding at the slower rates of melodies and phrases.[24,25,26] However, since this time, DAT has been adapted to fast time scales of complex sounds by Edward Large and his colleagues.[27,28,29]

It may seem foolhardy to add another psychoacoustic perspective on pitch perception to a field where many viable, distinguished views on this topic already flourish. However, certain aspects of DAT differentiate it from other pitch perception theories. In particular, although it focuses on the time domain, DAT does not formalize complex sounds as collections of independent (i.e., discrete) time intervals, as outlined in Figure 6.3. Rather,

complex sounds are viewed as comprising many different micro-driving rhythms, each capable of entraining a resonant neural oscillation as its dyadic partner. That is, a stimulus driving rhythm has recurring periods, T. Here, T denotes a period not a discrete time span. In fact, any stimulus sequence of discrete time spans is *directly responded to by a listener's tunable brain as a driving rhythm, not as a collection of independent intervals that is statistically summarized as a mode.*

Both the aging hypothesis and the general attending hypothesis suggest factors that influence responses to driving rhythms, even fast driving rhythms with small periods. The aging hypothesis (Chapter 5) spells out innate predispositions involving preferred rates of individual driving rhythms as well as preferred relationships among such driving rhythms. Specifically, it stipulates age-specific rates of preferred driven rhythms (with resonance) as well as innate preferences for simple (vs. complex) rhythmic relationships. The general attending hypothesis (Chapter 4) applies to properties of a driving rhythm involving its force and its regularity. Although these two hypotheses suggest a variety of factors that affect pitch perception, the following paragraphs concentrate on two factors: namely, rates of preferred micro-driving rhythms and rhythmic ratios associated with attractor complexity.

Fast-Tracking Entrainments for Fast Events: Does Entrainment Keep Pace?

Misconceptions about entrainment are not uncommon. One holds that entrainment is a lumbering, slow activity. This is a misconception because entrainment rides on *relative, not absolute,* time.[30] If entrainment works only with slow events with periods of, for example, 1 second then, of course, entrainment cannot address how people perceive pitch nor how people "keep pace" with fast-paced phonemes in speech, among many other things. However, entrainment principles apply over a wide range of different rates. In fact, in theory coupling in entrainment is *rate resistant*; it "runs" on the relative time of attractors. As we have seen, an attractor is a special *ratio* of two periodicities: a driving rhythm period, T, synchronizes with the period, p, of a driven rhythm based on their ratio, *not* their absolute values.

Entrainment also reflects adaptive behavior. This is evident whenever a driven rhythm adjusts its phase and/or period to synchronize with a driving rhythm. Regardless of the absolute rate of a driving rhythm, the goal of synchrony depends on the number of adaptive driving rhythm iterations (cycles) required for stable coupling with a given driven rhythm. The "tuning in" of a driven with a driving rhythm rides on relative, not absolute, cycle time, quantified as the ratio of *an oscillation's period, p, relative to a driving periodic stimulus cycle, T; namely, a T:p ratio.*

The T:p ratio gauges time-to-asymptotic synchrony (i.e., stability) for a simple or complex attractor.[31,32] Thus, if a driving rhythm has a period of T = 5 ms and a resonant neural rhythm has an intrinsic period, p, of 2.5 ms, this yields an implicit T:p attractor ratio of 2:1. This is a simple attractor, conveying high asymptotic stability relative to a more complex attractor ratio. For instance, with Tn = 5 ms, let an entraining oscillation have a period, p, of .50 ms. This T: p of 10:1 is a more complex ratio involving an internal harmonic oscillation of 2,000 Hz (in Table 6.1). Generally, asymptotic stability during an entrainment episode depends on (1) attractor complexity and (2) the number of available driving rhythm cycles in an entraining episode.

Speedy Entrainments

Granada and Herzel demonstrated entrainment to arbitrarily fast rhythms using the simplest of attractor relationships (T:p = 1.0; i.e., *n:m* = 1:1). They discovered that, for this simple attractor, an entrainment episode requires *at most* eight cycles of a driving rhythm to achieve asymptotic stability. This is important. It means that regardless of the absolute rate of a driving rhythm, given this attractor, stable entrainment happens with only eight or fewer opportunities for phase/period adjustments.

This discovery confirms that limits on entrainment are independent of the absolute time of a driving rhythm's period. They depend only on relative time. This is pertinent to understanding perception of fast events. Specifically, with complex sounds, the partials are not conceived as sequences of discrete, unrelated time spans; rather, each partial is a micro-driving rhythm and is gauged relative to another micro-rhythm.

Table 6.1 provides a brief, 15 ms complex tone full of instructive examples. Frequencies in these fast ranges are those found in ones of music and speech. Each of the many harmonics, Tn, in column 1 is a micro-driving rhythm. Following convention, the first harmonic ($n = 1$) represents F0 (with period, T1 = 5 ms). As an external (stimulus) driving rhythm, T1 elicits a resonant internal period, $p_1 \sim 5$ ms. The attractor n:m, governing entrainment, then is 1:1 (a T:p ratio of 1.0).

Given the preceding algorithm, it takes, *at most,* eight cycles of p_1 to stably phase-lock p_1 with T1. However, Table 6.1 shows that this 15 ms sound allows only three cycles of p_1 (column 5). By contrast, the fifth harmonic activates a faster rhythm with a frequency of 1 kHz and a period, p_5, of 1 ms. Now, the relationship between this faster oscillation and the F0 driving rhythm (T1 = 5 ms) results in a driving: driven dyad with a T:p ratio of 5:1. Table 6.1 indicates that it requires nine oscillator cycles to match a single T1 driving rhythm cycle. This affords more opportunities for stable phase-locking. Furthermore, over the course of a 15 ms entraining episode, a total of 15 cycles of this driven oscillation occur (column 5). Although asymptotic entrainment may require at least eight cycles with this attractor, it is clear that entrainment with T1 is faster for this oscillation than with other, slower driven oscillations (e.g., only six cycles happen with T2 = 2.5 ms, for 400 Hz). More generally, Table 6.1 shows that harmonic partials with simple attractors, based on T1:Tn (column 6), are likely to deliver fewer entrainment cycles than those based on more complex attractors. At first blush, this may seem odd.

Importantly, the above outcomes highlight a theoretical puzzle involving two opposing features of complex sounds. The puzzle is evident in columns 5 and 6 in Table 6.1. The first factor, in column 5, concerns total cycles based on driven rhythm rate ($p_n \sim Tn$). Increasing the speed of an entraining periodicity relative to its driving period adds more entraining cycles, thereby speeding entrainment (indexed in column 5). The second factor involves attractor stability (indexed in column 6). Simpler attractors provide more stability. As harmonics of this sound increase in frequency, their oscillatory periods implicate more complex attractors (vis-á-vis a T1 driving rhythm). A special set of harmonics contains components with reasonable total cycles (six or more) plus stable attractors (2:1–5:1) (bold in Table 6.1, columns 5, 6). The set corresponds to a *dominance region.* In psychoacoustics, a dominance region refers to harmonics most powerful in determining F0 pitch percepts. In a nutshell, although very-high-frequency components offer more entrainment opportunities than lower ones, they also induce driven rhythms that create difficult, less stable attractors.

Virtual Pitch and Related Percepts

Another puzzle involves virtual pitch. Explanations of this phenomenon also draw on Table 6.1. If this harmonically complex sound is presented to a listener for only a very brief period (e.g., 15 ms), as shown, then the first harmonic, T1, and its entraining oscillation will produce weak entrainment because it is based on only three cycles of p_1 (= 5 ms). Consequently, we might imagine that people will fail to perceive the pitch of this sound as F0. This reasoning holds that the driving rhythm is weaker (fewer cycles) than other components in this sound (see column 5).

Yet, as previously described, listeners typically report hearing the pitch of such a complex sound as its fundamental harmonic, not that of other seemingly stronger harmonics. Even if F0 is removed from this sound, people continue to report hearing it as a virtual pitch. One explanation, offered by Moore, appeals to the statistical mode of the distribution of discrete time spans of harmonic partials.

Can entrainment theory also explain this phenomenon? It can. However, this explanation rests on different concepts, ones involving attractors and their stabilities. Columns 6 and 7 of Table 6.1 show relevant time relations among micro-rhythm periods, T1:Tn and Tn:Tn + 1, that set the stage for entrainments. In particular, oscillations activated by harmonics in the dominance region (n = 2–5), are simply related to the period of F0; that is, p_1 (of T1). Driven rhythms of these low-frequency harmonics endogenously interact due to their compelling time ratios (column 6); they also interact with other harmonics (see footnote in Table 6.1 for ratios of column 7).

Concretely, imagine that this brief complex sound has a weak F0 due to three cycles (of 5 ms) within the 15 ms. But it happens to be accompanied by a stronger second harmonic: 400 Hz (T2 = 2.5 ms). This faster micro-rhythm readily entrains an oscillation with period p_2, half the F0 period, p_1 (i.e., $p_1 = n$ (p_2) = 2(2.5) = 5 ms). These commensurate oscillations, jointly aroused by different low-frequency driving rhythms (n = 3–5), strengthen endogenous entrainments. Strengthening includes activating a weak (or missing) fundamental frequency oscillation (period p_1). In this fashion, an entrainment approach also addresses virtual pitch perception.

By contrast, virtual pitch does not happen if a sound's partials involve only high-frequency harmonics (n = 10–12); such oscillator interactions do not happen. Although these partials generate more rapid entrainments than those sparked by low-frequency partials (n = 1–5), high-frequency components implicate complex, less stable attractors. They do not belong to the dominance region, rendering virtual pitch perception

unlikely. These differences between low and high frequencies increase as the duration of a sound increases.[33]

The Dynamic Attending Theory and Pitch Perception

This section pulls together preceding ideas about fast entrainment, placing them within a larger DAT framework. According to DAT, the pitch of a complex sound depends on the period of F0 plus periods of other, simply related, harmonics. Although popular psychoacoustic theories of pitch perception also feature a prominent role for the fundamental frequency and related harmonics, DAT views these relationships through a different lens. An overarching difference, highlighted in preceding sections, involves the conception of time. In psychoacoustic theories, stimulus timing is cast as discrete *time intervals*, Ti; by contrast, in DAT, the Ti notation reflects a recurring *period of a stimulus driving rhythm*.

Key concepts in the DAT framework derive from this concept of time. They involve periods of resonant neural driven rhythms, as well as attractors and mode-locking, all introduced in prior chapters. Also returning in this chapter is the concept of dominant oscillations that figure in explanations of a pitch construct known as the *dominance region*.[34,35]

Attractors: Simple and Complex Mode-Locking

A fundamental DAT idea holds that relationships among harmonic partials of a complex sound elicit attractor states in perceivers/attenders. Simpler attractors rest on small integer, rational time ratios: n:m = 1:1, 2:1, 3:1, 3:2 and so forth, whereas complex ones do not (i.e., n:m = 8:5, 10:1, 7:5, etc.).[36] Moreover, simple attractors exert a more powerful "pull" on one's perception than do complex ones.

To review the role of these concepts in this chapter, let's return to Figure 6.1B. This figure depicts pure tones comprising a two tone-chord, each functioning as a micro-driving rhythm, one slower than the other (i.e., here, stimulus partials are recurring time spans: Ti, Tj). Each partial immediately entrains exogenously (dark gray) with a corresponding (resonant) neural oscillation of the same periodicity, governed by a simple attractor (n:m = 1:1). A more complex attractor is also shown (n:m ≠ 1:1); it, too, governs exogenous entrainment coupling, now between the slow external (Ti) waveform and a faster internal neural waveform (pi). The latter connection shows commensurate mode-locking where n:m ≠ 1:1 (diagonal dark gray line).

These basic ideas were in play in describing pitch perception of the complex sound of Table 6.1. However, such a sound has more harmonic partials activating more related oscillations. Consequently, it affords more opportunities for multiple endogenous entrainments among the activated oscillations. The sound of Figure 6.1B showed one such endogenous coupling involving engagement of a fast neural oscillation by a slower one. This implies a complex attractor, n:m ≠ 1:1 (see light gray vertical line). As with exogenous entrainments, endogenous entrainments are also governed by attractors. Thus, in this example underlying attractors might express the time ratios of 2:1, 3:1, or 3: 2 of Figure 6.1A, for instance. The main point is that an underlying attractor has innate power to facilitate various mode-locking orders of synchrony evident in both exogenous and endogenous entrainments.

Nevertheless, complex sounds of speech and music entail a panoply of frequency components (and neural correlates). As the more complex sound of Table 6.1 suggests, a typical harmonic sound can include multiple micro-driving rhythms, thus affording a wide range of opportunities for both exogenous and endogenous entrainments. Even the complex sound in Table 6.1 simplifies this story. That is, the time relationships in column 6 of this table focus only on Tn and T1, where Tn is any harmonic (*n*) and T1 is the fundamental period. Yet many other relations among partials are possible, as suggested in column 7 (e.g., Tn:Tn + 1). Clearly, opportunities for oscillator interactions via phase-locking escalate rapidly in such sounds.

So, let's bring in a new, simplifying theoretical construct: the *oscillator cluster*. An oscillator cluster is defined as a set of simultaneously active neural oscillations wherein member oscillations endogenously engage to one another. For instance, ratios in columns 6 and 7 (Table 6.1) relate all partials to the fundamental (Tn:T1) or to a neighboring partial (Tn:Tn + 1). In theory, a set of related micro-driving rhythms spawns a large cluster of related neural oscillations with corresponding periodicities. Member oscillations of a cluster become linked, via endogenous entrainment, to the same referent oscillation, here with a period of $p_R = p_1$. In other words, this is a *pitch oscillator cluster* which consists of many active oscillations, all coupled to a common referent oscillation, with a period, p_R, that matches the fundamental's period, p_1.

More About Oscillator Clusters

The idea of a pitch oscillator cluster is suggested graphically in Figure 6.4. In this figure, a listener's responses to a complex sound appear as pulses (light gray triangles). Periods of harmonic oscillations to partials appear in left column. In the top panel (Figure 6.4A) are consonant micro-rhythms with hypothetical widths of entrainment regions shown for each partial within the consonant sound. Also shown are mode-locking relations between the fundamental (5.0 ms) and periods of other partials. Panel B shows a dissonant complex sound. Both panels contain micro-driving rhythms that afford exogenous entrainment of driven oscillations. Consequently, both panels show sets of exogenously activated oscillations wherein member oscillations may endogenously entrain to form *oscillator clusters*.

Notice that the emergent clusters depicted in these two panels differ. Consonant sounds have multiple attractor ratios (right column) that relate *all oscillator periods* in this cluster to the same fundamental period. By contrast, dissonant sounds do not exhibit this property. This difference is apparent in the alignments of micro-rhythms that distinguish the two oscillator clusters in Figure 6.4 A versus B.

For the present, let's focus on the consonant pitch oscillator cluster of panel A. Endogenous mode-locking states between oscillations are activated largely by the harmonic waveforms of a dominance region (oscillator periods, p_n, of leftmost column). As endogenous oscillator couplings increase in number so does cluster size. This figure outlines a hypothetical *pitch oscillator cluster* which arises from fast and stable endogenous entrainments among oscillations activated by five lower harmonics of a complex sound (Table 6.1).

In this pitch oscillator cluster, the fundamental periodicity (*top row*) is the slowest oscillation with a referent period, p_R, of 5 ms (i.e., $p_R = p_1$). Members of this cluster endogenously mode-lock with this referent oscillation.[37] Together, the internal oscillations of exogenous dyads become synchronously glued to the fundamental periodicity by mode-locking relations ranging from n:m of 1:1 to n:m of 5:1 (rightmost column). Note that excluded from this cluster are mode-locking states with complex attractors that derive from high-frequency partials (e.g., n:m attractors of 10:1 or 11:1).

Limits on Mode-Locking of Attending

Attractor complexity affects mode-locking efficiency in attending dynamics. The impact of complexity is correlated with the width of an attractor's entrainment region. Complex attractors are less

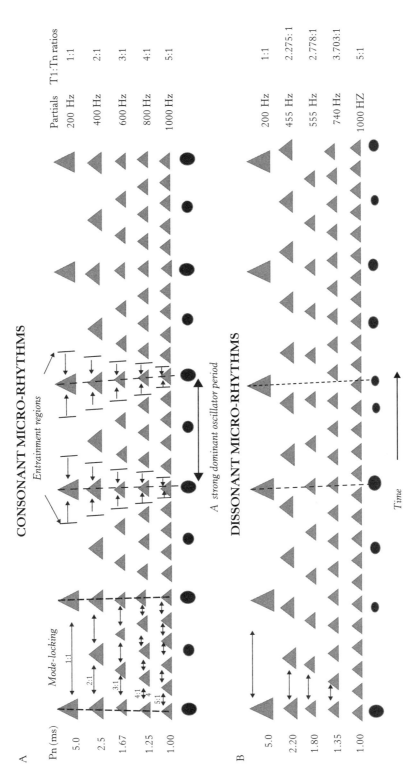

FIGURE 6.4 (**A**) Five consonant harmonic micro-driving components (partials) of complex sound are outlined, including the fundament, F0, of 200 Hz (top row). Gray triangles express the internal pulses of driven periods (i.e., oscillator periods, p_n, on left) for each driving rhythm partial (frequencies on far right). Mode-locking relationships (n:m per partial) range from n:m = 1:1 to 1:5 (left) with F0 (stimulus period, T0). Width of entrainment regions (black V's) increases with simpler n:m relations. (**B**) Dissonant versions of frequency components in **A**. Rate ratios of these components are not commensurate (T1:Tn in far right).

stable, having less "pull" power than simpler attractors. This lower stability is manifest in narrower entrainment regions, as shown graphically in Figure 6.4A. Mode-locking differs with endogenous n:m relations (i.e., between p_R and other oscillator periods) for the five harmonic partials shown (on left). Entrainment region limits appear for each attractor. For example, the second harmonic ($n = 2$), with a driving rhythm period of 2.5 ms, observes an octave relationship (1:2) with a 5 ms referent period of F0. In turn, this implicates a simple attractor with a relatively wide entrainment region.

In sum, this account of consonant complex sounds and pitch oscillator clusters implies that contributions of lower frequency partials are necessarily more influential on pitch perception than those of higher frequency partials. In the latter clusters, reduced stability derives from narrower entrainment regions of complex attractors. Consequently, although high-frequency harmonics deliver more cycles (per T1) than low-frequency harmonics, they also create more complex, less stable attractors. Note that this explanation of the low potency in high-frequency harmonics does not appeal to the notion of poor resolution, which is a more common explanation in conventional theories of pitch perception.

The Rise of a Dominant Oscillation

Ultimately, the percept of the pitch of a complex sound depends on a listener's sensitivity to its fundamental frequency. In DAT, this sensitivity depends on the rise of a dominant oscillation (cf. Chapter 5), one with a relatively high driven rhythm amplitude. The strength of a dominant oscillation derives not only from its driving rhythm force; it also depends on coordinated synchrony of mode-locking activity from multiple oscillations within a pitch oscillator cluster.[38] That is, coinciding energy pulses comes from simultaneously active oscillations of a pitch oscillator cluster; together these pulses contribute to forming a dominant oscillation of F0. This is shown in Figure 6.4A (cf. large black dots). Accordingly, in this example, a listener experiences a dominant oscillation with a 5 ms period from aligned energies of low-frequency partials ($n < 5$).

To sum up, a dynamic attending portrait envisions listeners involuntarily tuning in to multiple micro-rhythms of complex sounds. Automatic entrainments depend on rhythmic properties rather than statistical properties of discrete time interval distributions. This involves rhythms of various time scales, even very fast rhythms of harmonics. Moreover, people are naturally sensitive to the relative timing of these various micro-rhythms, especially those expressing simpler attractors. When attractor ratios are simple, synchrony between driving and driven rhythms arises from standard mode-locking among neural oscillations; this entrainment mode glues together oscillations within an oscillator cluster. All of this happens effortlessly because synchrony is a guiding rule. The end result is formation of a pitch oscillator cluster which delivers a pitch percept based on the activity of a dominant oscillation within this cluster.

The Canonical Entrainment Model of Edward Large: Mode-Locking with Fast Events

Ideas described informally in the preceding paragraphs attain rigor in entrainment models developed by Edward Large and his colleagues.[39] They propose a canonical entrainment model based on the assumption that the auditory system is inherently nonlinear. Drawing on dynamical systems constructs involving weakly coupled networks of neural oscillations (inhibitory, excitatory), they describe entrainments that lead to various pitch percepts. Although mathematically complex, this DAT model is elegant.[40,41,42] It describes various nonlinear exogenous couplings among different driving and driven periodicities. Importantly, it neatly predicts a range of mode-locked perceptual responses to the multiple frequencies embedded in the fast, complex sounds of music.

In this model, pitch perception is influenced by attractor complexity, formalized by the width of an entrainment region surrounding an attractor state. Figure 6.5 shows V-shaped entrainment regions for driving–driven dyads with different attractor ratios; these entrainment regions are termed *Arnold tongues*. In this figure, the symbol *fo* reflects the frequency of an internal oscillation capable of entraining exogenously to four different external driving rhythms, denoted by *f*.[43,44]

Importantly, two factors predict the effectiveness of entrainment states. Both influence the width of an entrainment region surrounding an attractor. First, an entrainment region narrows as the force of a driving rhythm declines (**c**, ordinate), as shown in this figure. Second, also shown is the narrowing of an entrainment region with increasing attractor complexity (abscissa). Phase-locking is most effective with a wide entraining region about the attractor frequency ratio with *f/fo* = 1.00 (i.e., n:m = 1:1), which is the simplest

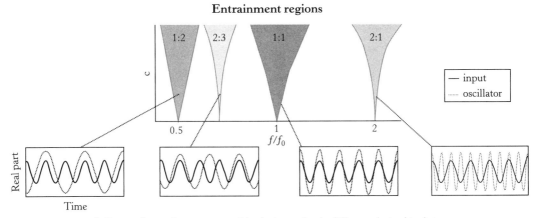

Ordinate reflects a force parameter (c); abscissa scales the different relationships between an oscillator, with frequency fo, that mode-locks with four rhythms of different input frequencies.

FIGURE 6.5 Top shows mode-locking in an Arnold tongue regime. Entrainment regions change with the frequency ratio, *f/fo*. An oscillation active with a fundamental *fo*, can synchronously mode-lock to each of four different partial frequencies in a complex sound.

Reprinted from figure 1 in Karl D. Lerud et al., "Mode-Locking Neurodynamics Predict Human Auditory Brainstem Responses to Musical Intervals," *Hearing Research* 308 (February 2014): 41–49, doi:10.1016/j.heares.2013.09.010.

attractor. However, couplings involving a less simple attractor (e.g., 2:3) operate in a narrower entrainment region and so on. This correlation of attractor complexity with entrainment region width reflects standard dynamical system formalizations involving the stability of attractors, as discussed in preceding sections.

Of course, most complex sounds will not offer external frequencies that conform precisely to the *f/fo* = 1.00. Rather, ordinary sounds typically implicate attractors with approximate ratios (e.g., 1.10 or .90) that approach an idealized attractor state. Nevertheless, through an entrainment lens, such "deviations" are perceived within a wide entrainment region. Thus, with a simple n:m = 1:1 attractor, the attractor "pull" on such deviations leads a listener to perceive such deviant micro-rhythms as "close enough" to be a unison. Categorically, "very good" approximations are often prototype instances. Effectively, the entrainment region that surrounds an attractor documents a flexibility inherent in dynamical systems. Each region tolerates deviations from an attractor, allowing corrections of period and/or phase especially with simple attractors.

Two major entrainment hypotheses underlie behaviors illustrated in Figure 6.5. First, under the umbrella of the aging hypothesis, innate attractor states operate over one's life span. Regardless of age, the relative timing of complex attractor states

specifies greater phase coupling stability with simple than with complex attractors. Second, following the general attending hypothesis, greater driving rhythm force increases driving–driven coupling (*c* on ordinate). At any age, increases in driving rhythm strength lead to wider entrainment regions for all attractors. This constraint figured in PRCs (see Chapter 4); it speaks to the salience of a coupling parameter (i.e., *c* ~ **k** in PRCs).

Summary of Fast Events and Small Time Scales

This section details how dynamic attending applies to fast events, based on small time scales. Even with these events, concepts of rhythm and synchrony remain viable. Although sounds might last only fractions of a second, they can arouse an army of different micro-driving rhythms. This is because entrainment is rate-resistant, transcending the "speed limits" often applied to percepts of fast events. Relative, not absolute, time rules! Finally, the foundations of DAT, summarized in aging and the general hypotheses, remain relevant to explanations of people's reactions to fast events.

Evidence for Dynamic Attending in Adult Pitch Perception

A wealth of research reveals that people's perceptions of complex tones are influenced by the harmonic structure of these tones. The richness of harmonic partials in such a tone motivates listeners to peg its overall pitch using its lowest frequency. Theoretically, the fundamental frequency plays a leading role in explaining pitch perception of complex sounds. This section briefly highlights major phenomena in research on adult pitch perception that fit into DAT. It sketches how DAT tackles a few pitch perception puzzles.

Pitch perception predictions of DAT address the behaviors of average listeners. These are people like Bill, who has once again wandered into a popular psychoacoustic laboratory to volunteer as a participant in another experiment (for money, of course). An obliging experimenter happily explains a basic *pitch matching* task to Bill. In this task, on each of series of trials, Bill hears two tones, a standard, usually a pure tone, and a comparison, which is a complex tone. Bill's job is simple: on each trial, he judges whether or not the two tones seem identical in pitch. The job of the experimenter is to creatively vary the properties of these sounds over trials and record Bill's responses.

Pitch Matching: The Role of Dominant Oscillations

In pitch matching tasks, people often orient to certain partials within one of the two presented sounds. Some tasks encourage this selective attending, as when a single pure tone occurs first (i.e., as a standard). Such a standard can prime a listener to hear this component even when buried in a following comparison (i.e., people can "hear out" several individual partials of complex sounds[45,46,47]). Moreover, with fast events, listeners like Bill may engage in voluntary attending by selectively allocating attending energy to certain dominant partials of a complex sound.

Theoretically, a pitch matching task encourages a listener to rely on two dominant oscillations arising, respectively, from standard and comparison sounds. Furthermore, if these dominant oscillations have the same frequency, then the listener (e.g., Bill) should judge the standard and comparison as identical in pitch.

Central Findings in Pitch Matching Tasks

A few central findings from these tasks illustrate how DAT accommodates this research.

The Missing Fundamental

Virtual (or residue) pitch is the pitch reported for a complex comparison sound (e.g., sounds in Table 6.1 or Figure 6.4) when the fundamental frequency (F0 = 200 Hz) is missing. Thus, if Bill performs a matching task in which a complex comparison sound contains several lower harmonics but not the fundamental, he is likely to report its virtual pitch. That is, the pure tone standard exhibiting the frequency of the missing F0, is deemed a good match to this comparison which lacks the F0.

At first glance, this seems impossible. In this example, the comparison is missing the micro-driving rhythm, with period T1 of F0 (e.g., 5 ms, in Table 6.1). Gone also are links between F0 and other partials (i.e., in column 6 of Table 6.1, T1:Tn). In other words, grounds for attractors, implied by other ratios involving T1, are also missing. Nevertheless, Bill and others report hearing the virtual pitch.

A DAT explanation, prefigured in preceding sections, relies on the impact of other attractor time ratios implicated in a comparison that command a pitch oscillator cluster. These time relations appear in column 7 of Table 6.1, and in Figure 6.4. Together, several harmonic ratios of $Tn:Tn' + 1$ spark mode-locking that activates a pitch oscillator cluster (e.g., from attractor driving ratios of 3:2, 4:3, and 5:4; see footnote to column 7).

Generally, DAT holds that mode-locking activities among low-frequency oscillations ($n = 2$–5) stimulate a *pitch oscillator cluster*. And from this cluster emerges a *dominant oscillation with a period of missing foundation*: $p_1 = pR = 5$ ms (Figure 6.4A). This is illustrated in Figure 6.4A by simply eliminating the top row, thus simulating a missing F0 (i.e., the 5 ms period). The period of a dominant oscillation (large black dots) is minimally affected; low-frequency components collectively revive a missing p_1 as the period of a dominant oscillation which guides Bill's judgment. Specifically, the dominant period evoked by this complex comparison sound is perceived by Bill to have the same F0 period (5 ms) as the pure tone standard of 200 Hz. Accordingly, Bill's response confirms long-standing evidence that virtual pitch depends on the presence of lower harmonics.[48,49,50]

The Dominance Region

Traditionally, in psychoacoustic studies a dominance region involving low-frequency harmonics has been shown to reliably cause listeners to report a particular pitch. This is related to the missing fundamental because, together, low-frequency harmonics ($n = 3, 4, 5$) enhance perception of F0 when this micro-driving rhythm is missing in a complex sound.[51,52,53,54] DAT also correctly predicts a related finding. That is, when F0 is present in a complex sound, a listener's judgment of this sound's pitch is less stable when low harmonics (of the dominance region) are absent than when they are present.

Unresolved Frequencies

A complex sound containing only unresolved (i.e., high) harmonics elicits weak virtual pitch percepts.[55,56,57] Although poor resolution among higher frequencies is commonly attributed to overlapping basilar membrane filters, DAT offers a different explanation. It holds that weak virtual pitch percepts arise from the failed endogenous coupling of oscillations related to complex attractors. Partials with higher frequencies (2 kHz or more) implicate complex attractors with vanishingly narrow entrainment regions. Hence unstable dyads are responsible for weak virtual pitch percepts.

Irregular Frequency Components

Irregularity of fast micro-rhythmic components degrades pitch percepts.[58,59,60,61,62] Converging evidence from monkeys also shows that timing irregularities perturb the neural synchrony associated with pitch.[63,64] According to DAT, greater regularity of any micro-driving rhythm facilitates phase-locking with a driven oscillation and thereby enhances pitch perception.

Cortical Activity

Cortical correlates of dominant oscillations manifest as neural rhythms, not distributions of discrete intervals. Evidence for this DAT claim appears in recordings of the primary auditory cortex of monkeys (evoked potentials, current source density [CSD] analysis).[65] Also, phase-locking to pure tones appears in the inferior colliculus and auditory thalamus of guinea pigs.[66,67] Other functional magnetic resonance imaging (fMRI) findings indicate that anterior regions of the human auditory cortex selectively react to the pitch of spectrally resolved harmonic components (vs. nonresolved frequencies or nonharmonics).[68]

In sum, the universality of entrainment suggests that it should happen whenever conditions for synchrony exist, whether in the auditory nerve, the brainstem, and/or auditory cortex, even at fast rhythmic rates. Dynamic attending constructs are time-scaled, based on relative not absolute time; thus, they apply to fast as well as slow micro-driving rhythms. Moreover, driving rhythms of neural oscillations can be either external or internal (as oscillations). Whether the resulting entrainments are exogenous or endogenous, they depend on attractor complexity as this figures into pitch perception.

Summary of Different Views of Adult Pitch Perception

Prominent psychoacoustic theories bequeath us a wealth of knowledge about adult pitch perception. They explain phenomena such as virtual pitch and dominance regions. Yet these theories also draw on assumptions about pure and complex sounds that overlook their most essential nature: rhythmicity. Instead, a pitch percept is often conceived as an estimated interval code resulting from a listeners' extraction (ironically, from a stimulus rhythm) of a collection of discrete (independent) time intervals. Arguably, it seems more parsimonious to assume that listeners directly respond to—well—the rhythm itself.

Yet, in spite of critical differences, the highly successful time theory developed by Brian Moore (2013) shares instructive commonalities with DAT. Both approaches are wedded to the time domain and both maintain that the pitch of complex sounds depends on integer time relationships among harmonic partials. Also both theories specify neural correlates of individual sound frequencies.

The differences with a dynamic attending account are also instructive. First, unlike DAT, the neural correlates of stimulus rhythms in Moore's theory (Figure 6.3) are not conceived as adaptive neural periodicities with limit cycle properties. Second, Moore's approach is grounded in statistical properties of time intervals, not in principles of rhythmic resonance and entrainment endorsed by DAT. Also, Moore's model does not appeal to attractors nor to mode-locking synchronies, meaning that DAT concepts of endogenous entrainment and cluster formations are not paralleled in Moore's theory. Finally, these theories specify respectively different determinants of a listener's pitch judgment. In Moore's theory, a pitch judgment (stage 5) relies on a brain's counting mechanism that "compares/selects" within a collection of estimated time intervals. In this stage, the most common time interval determines a pitch percept. By contrast, DAT assumes that at the time of a pitch judgment listeners simply rely on the momentary period of an emergent dominant oscillation. Ideally, these theoretical differences may stimulate useful discussions.

PITCH PERCEPTION IN INFANTS

Can infants' perceive the pitch of a complex sound? They might. We know that babies master phonemes in speech by 6 months of age. Also, evidence favoring the aging hypothesis has shown that infants selectively orient to the higher frequency components of complex sounds.[69] But do infants show a similar sensitivity to the lower frequencies so critical to pitch perception of complex sounds? Certainly Oller's proposal of quasi-vowels (which infants hear) argues that infants possess an early sensitivity to harmonic relationships. And infants tend to operate with weaker neural oscillations than adults, meaning they are more stimulus driven (i.e., responsive to novel stimulation). On the other hand, the temporal niche concept in the aging hypothesis suggests that young infants are not especially tuned into lower frequencies of complex sounds. So, perhaps we should not leap to the conclusion that young infants experience low-frequency components of complex sounds as the source of pitch perception in the same way adults do.

Yet even marmosets show sensitivity to pitch when the fundamental frequency of a complex sound is missing. So isn't it possible that young human infants also hear virtual pitch? A quick answer to such questions is: "We don't know, yet."

Here is what we do know. We know that 6-month-old infants are sensitive to relative timing of harmonic partials in complex sounds because they respond to mistunings of embedded harmonics.[70,71] Also, sleeping newborns automatically react to differences between nonharmonic and harmonic frequencies (above 500 Hz) in complex tones.[72,73] Thus, newborns can involuntarily differentiate certain harmonics of complex sounds. Moreover, the latter findings also suggest that newborns are sensitive to violations of simpler harmonic ratios. In short, infants can "hear out" some individual frequencies of complex sounds as well as react to the relative timing that is characteristic of attractor ratios. Taking this a step further, it remains possible that young infants are capable of developing rudimentary oscillator clusters and perhaps able to rely on the strongest oscillation within such clusters (i.e., a dominant oscillation), which determines pitch perception.

Nevertheless, this research does not answer one "big" question: "Do young infants hear the virtual pitch of a missing fundamental frequency?" He and Trainor directly addressed this question.[74] They presented complex tones with missing fundamentals (500 Hz or less) to young infants (3 and 4 months old). Using electroencephalograms (EEGs) and mismatch negativity responses (MMN), they concluded that older infants and adults perceived the virtual pitch of missing

fundamentals, but interestingly the youngest infants did not. This is despite the fact that 3-month-old infants *did* respond to harmonics *above* the frequency of the missing fundamental. (Importantly, this study did not asses infants' sensitivity to lower harmonic frequencies.)

The failure of the youngest infants to perceive virtual pitch invites several explanations. One maintains that these infants are "stimulus-bound" (i.e., they are unable to exploit attractors relevant to virtual pitch). Consistent with the idea that infants operate with relatively weak latent oscillations in a push–pull contest between an attractor "pull" and a stimulus driving rhythm's "push," the latter wins. Alternatively, situations with repeated co-occurrence of harmonics with a given fundamental frequency (e.g., in vowels, quasi-vowels) prompted Terhart to suggest that these relationships are learned.[75,76] So, possibly, 3-month-olds have not yet learned these relationships.

A third explanation stems from the aging hypothesis; it appeals to temporal niche constraints. If very young infants are selectively sensitive to higher frequency driving rhythms (approximately 1 kHz or greater), then they should not be able to resonate to relatively low harmonics (i.e., to probe frequencies below about 500 Hz, used to test for virtual pitch in the He and Trainor study). This implies that an infant's mastery of phonemes may depend on his facility in incorporating lower frequency oscillations into a growing pitch cluster.

Summary of Infant Perception

Sounds that afford percepts of pitch involve very small micro-time periods ranging from .1 ms to 10 ms. Yet, amazingly, both adults and infants can track these tiny time intervals in complex tones. According to DAT, young listeners rely on the same pitch perception mechanisms used by adults—namely, resonance and entrainment—to tune into the micro-rhythms of complex sounds but with different aging constraints. From a DAT perspective, a listener's tunable brain reacts by simultaneously tracking multiple micro-driving rhythms (partials) embedded in complex sounds. Such sets of external driving rhythms lead, via exogenous entrainments, to corresponding sets of oscillations which eventually grow into oscillator clusters. Harmonic relationships among micro-driving rhythms implicate attractors and motivate active sets of related cortical oscillations in a listener's tunable brain. In turn, certain pitch oscillator clusters embed a strong (dominant) neural oscillation (from cortical mode-locking) that determines pitch perception.

Synchrony is a guiding principle even when tracking fast events. This is evident in endogenous mode-locking configurations of oscillator clusters, which are governed by attractors (the aging hypothesis). In addition, stimulus properties (driving rhythm force and micro-rhythm regularity) contribute to mode-locking synchronies (the general attending hypothesis). Ultimately, an emergent, dominant oscillation determines the pitch a listener reports. Finally, although infants are sensitive to harmonics in complex sounds, the jury is out on whether or not this sensitivity extends to "hearing" a missing fundamental.

The following points are noteworthy:

- Contrary to time theories that posit discrete time spans as determinants of pitch percepts, a dynamic approach to pitch perception relies on micro-driving rhythms that activate/entrain correlated neural oscillations.
- Together, multiple driven oscillations endogenously entrain to form pitch oscillator clusters.
- Applied to fast events, dynamic attending concepts predict listeners' performance in various pitch matching tasks.
- DAT maintains that pitch percepts depend on the dominant (referent) oscillation of a pitch oscillator cluster.
- Adult pitch perception of a complex (harmonic) tone depends largely on its fundamental frequency and lower frequency harmonics (i.e., in a dominance region).
- Infants older than 3 months exhibit pitch perception, including virtual pitch perception.

PERCEIVING CONSONANCE

To most, a consonant sound is one that is "pleasing." Virtually everyone recognizes such a sound as "good" or "pleasant." For this reason, the striking consonance in vocal harmony of four-part chords in barbershop quartets, popular in earlier decades, remains widely recognized today. As well, the powerful sonority of opera singers testifies to the thrilling aspects of voices honed to maximize harmony. Even a more mundane sound, such as a cat's purr, is pleasantly soothing for its engagement of many harmonics having a fundamental frequency of around 25 Hz. Conversely, the dissonance of cat's hiss or growl derives from a loss of harmony. Dissonant sounds elicit negative reactions, involving tension or unease.

Despite seeming unanimity in our categorical reactions to consonance and dissonance, there is less theoretical agreement surrounding the origins of consonance. But, before pursuing this topic, it is useful to clarify that consonance in this context *does not* refer to tonality percepts—that is, compatibilities in a musical key (e.g., tones "in" or "out" of an established key).[77,78,79] Tonality issues are discussed in later chapters. Here, "consonance" and "dissonance" refer to the qualitative impact of a set of simultaneously occurring frequencies found in any complex sound, musical or not.

One way to formalize the consonance–dissonance distinction was previewed in Figure 6.4, where dissonant sounds implicate fewer simple attractors than consonant sounds. In fact, DAT assumes that attractors play a major role in consonance perceptions. This section explores these ideas by focusing on the *temporal texture* of complex sounds. Temporal texture refers to the joint impact of all micro-driving rhythms of a complex sound. Indeed, the interrelationships of many oscillations, elicited by multiple micro-driving rhythms, can lead to neural nonlinearities that affect sound quality (see Box 6.1). As examples in Figure 6.4 suggest, there is something about a sound's temporal texture *as a whole* (i.e., its timbre) that moves us to judge it as consonant.

Attending Dynamics and Temporal Texture

To understand people's responses to temporal texture, let's return to the confines of laboratory paradigms. Two paradigms for studying this topic are popular. One, a two-choice categorization task, requires a listener to assign various complex sounds to one of two categories: consonant or dissonant. The other task simply requires listeners to rate the degree of perceived consonance of a complex sound. People find both tasks easy. Moreover, both provide substantial agreement about what "seems" consonant versus dissonant.

Categorizing Consonance

Consonance percepts are typically addressed using "laboratory" versions of complex sounds. Although Figure 6.4 illustrates two such sounds, it is common to use simpler complex sounds with only two partials, as initially illustrated by the chord of Figure 6.1. Such sounds limit the number of internal interactions elicited by the partials in consonance judgment tasks. Again, the opening examples in Figure 6.1 are useful; rates (periods) of just two partials can be systematically varied

> # BOX 6.1
> ## NONLINEARITIES: DIFFERENCE TONES
>
> The tricky but important topic of nonlinearities is often associated with consonance versus dissonance. In psychoacoustics, nonlinearity refers to certain kinds of interactions among partials which involve *difference tones*, purported to influence perception. Nonlinearity refers to interactions based on (but not limited to) certain famous difference tones, namely a frequency difference such as F_2-F_1, or the cubic difference tone, $2F_1-F_2$. Although difference tones present problems for some perception theories, this is not the case for DAT. This is because nonlinearity actually reflects mode-locking states. For instance, in Table 6.1, the difference between harmonics $n = 5$ and $n = 4$ (1,000–800 Hz) is typically cast as a 200 Hz difference tone, with a 5 ms period. However, the Tn:Tn + 1 ratio of these frequencies, 1.25, is a common attractor ratio (i.e., n:m = 5:4) (column 7; Table 6.1). This entrainment relationship reinforces a pitch percept based on the fundamental frequency. Nonlinearities are central to entrainment models of pitch perception. In fact, eliminating nonlinearities for the sake of parsimony is "throwing out the baby with the bathwater."

to assess the impact of different rate ratios on perceived consonance.[80]

From a dynamic attending perspective, each tone in a chord-like pair functions as a fast micro-driving rhythm which engages a matching neural oscillation (e.g., Figure 6.1B). A consonant percept then depends on the nature of internal (cortical) synchrony as instilled by the consequential endogenous interaction of the two activated oscillations. Of particular interest is the internal rate ratio between two oscillations (each induced by a different stimulus period). The resulting endogenous dyad has a ratio of oscillator periods: $p_1:p_2$. According to DAT, as this ratio approximates a simple attractor, it expresses a mode-locking order with compelling synchronicity. In turn, this synchrony heightens one's sense of consonance. This topic is developed in subsequent paragraphs.

Two-Tone Chords: An Example

In a remarkable review of the consonance literature, Schellenberg and Trehub derived a *simplicity index* based on the rate ratios of partials in two-tone chords. The aim was to understand consonance percepts.[81] Table 6.2 (column 3) shows ratios of their tone pairs (within one octave).[82,83] Interestingly, simplicity ratings (column 6) correlate highly with attractor complexity measures from an entrainment framework; as such, they capture mode-locking efficiency. Thus, the simplest rate ratios are those with attractors of n:m = 1:1 and 2:1 (unison and octave). The perfect fifth chord (3:2) has the next highest simplicity

score, and so on, with the dreaded tritone interval (45:32) earning the lowest score. Clearly, such ratios correspond to attractors of varying complexity. As such, they predict corresponding differences in mode-locking synchronization of interacting oscillations. Finally, we might assume that all these attractors levy an innate influence on listeners, a position consistent with Pack's proposal of innate harmonicity.[84]

In music, the consonance or dissonance of certain pitch intervals takes on special meanings. Thus, the perfect fifth is a prominent pleasing interval that forms the bottom interval in the three- and four-tone chords of rock music (especially for the guitar). Its prominence is well-established in classical music, with a famous example in the final chord of Mozart's Requiem. By contrast, the dissonant tritone interval (from an augmented fourth) in Western music allegedly delivers a harsh texture, suggesting the presence of "evil" (cf. Liszt's *Dante Sonata* and the song *Black Sabbath* by Black Sabbath).

However, attractor impact is not limited to music. It describes differences in vocal textures as well. Rough speaking, voices arise from pitch oscillator clusters involving many complex attractors and attractor deviations. The topic of attractors opens a broad spectrum of time relationships in complex sounds. For instance, Figure 6.4A shows a complex sound with many converging harmonics and numerous simplicity ratios, confirming high consonance. By contrast, the absence of simple ratios in panel B

TABLE 6.2 RATE (FREQUENCY) RATIOS FOR MUSICAL CHORDS

Interval Size (in Semitones) With corresponding Interval Name, Justly Tunes Frequency Ratio, Sum of Integers in the Ratio, Logarithm of the Sum, and Inverse of the Logarithm

Interval Size	Interval	Frequency Ratio	Sum of Integers	Logarithm of Sum	Reciprocal of Logarithm
0	unison	1:1	2	0.693	1.443
1	minor second	16:15	31	3.434	0.291
2	major second	9:8	17	2.833	0.353
3	minor third	6:5	11	2.398	0.417
4	major third	5:4	9	2.1977	0.455
5	perfect fourth	4:3	7	1.946	0.514
6	tritone	45:32	77	4.344	0.230
7	perfect fifth	3:2	5	1.609	0.621
8	minor sixth	8:5	13	2.565	0.390
9	major sixth	5:3	8	2.079	0.481
10	minor seventh	16:9	25	3.219	0.311
11	major seventh	15:8	23	3.135	0.319
12	octave	2:1	3	1.099	0.910

Note—The reciprocal of the logarithm of the sum of integers is used as the index of simplicity of frequency ratios.
From Schellenberg & Trehub, 1994

evokes dissonance. In general, panel A will induce a pleasing temporal texture due to overall synchrony among coordinated oscillations; all partials "beat together." In short, jointly, they produce a strong dominant oscillation along with a rich temporal texture.

Temporal Texture in Consonance– Dissonance Mixtures

Most everyday sounds offer temporal textures that mix various time relationships. For example, phoneme categories combine distinctive harmonic and nonharmonic (formant) frequencies. To neatly pluck out certain harmonic components within complex sounds of speech and music requires a trained ear. For instance, musicians are more sensitive than others to the implications of higher harmonics and nonlinear components of two-tone chords.[85,86,87]

Ordinary sounds are rarely neatly packaged as two-tone chords or even as harmonically complex sounds (e.g., Table 6.1). While possibly hiding attractors, everyday sounds are messier than harmonically crafted sounds or laboratory sounds. Therefore, it is reasonable to consider the role of other complex, even strange (i.e., chaotic or noisy) relationships within everyday sounds. Arguably, some (ill-termed) consonant phonemes, such as strident fricatives (e.g., /s/), evoke nonlinear dynamics. Betty Tuller[88] and colleagues favor such a dynamical orientation.

This line of thinking implies that everyday sounds inevitably vary in consonance. Rather than coarse categories of consonance and dissonance, perhaps a consonance–dissonance continuum exists involving a range different attractors, including so-called *strange attractors*. Also blends of consonance with dissonance invite considering new metrics, perhaps resembling the HNR metric, which involves a harmonic-to-noise ratio.[89] The HNR, developed to assess animal sounds, might also apply to human communications. Finally, metrics that calibrate approximations to attractors may shed light on sound categories of daily life: "Is my cat purring or growling?", or "Is that sound a delivery truck or a visitor's car, or a lawn mower?" or "Did that guy say 'bit' or 'bet?'"

Consonance Controversies

The concept of consonance has a distinguished history, one infused with debates over its "true" meaning. Indeed, the idea that simple frequency ratios contribute to consonance is hardly new. In some form, time ratios have been part of dialogues surrounding consonance extending as far back as Pythagoras, through Rameau and Stumpf and the grandfather of psychoacoustics, Helmholtz, to current views on this topic (cf. Terhardt for a brief history).[90,91,92,93] Yet consonance controversies continue. For instance, an influential contemporary view denies a role for harmonic ratios, which are dismissed as spurious correlates of the true cause of dissonance. Instead, the claim is that consonance is simply the absence of dissonance. In turn, dissonance is caused by beat frequencies that interfere with peripheral (basilar membrane) activity.[94]

Recently, such peripheral explanations of consonance have come under scrutiny. One reason for this is that beat frequencies, the presumed cause of dissonance, appear to have less impact on consonance judgments than do harmonic relations.[95,96,97,98] Also, distinctive neural correlates of consonance (vs. dissonance) were discovered in populations of auditory nerve fibers and cortical gamma band activity (EEG) in the right auditory cortex, with parallel neural correlates of consonance in speech and musical domains.[99,100] Together, such findings favor a central (cortical) explanation of consonance rather than a peripheral one.

Finally, others have weighed in on this controversy, tipping the scales still further from a peripheral dissonance interpretation and toward treating consonance as a real, centrally located construct. These theorists argue that musical sounds containing harmonically related musical periodicities are simply more appealing than sounds lacking simple harmonic ratios. According to these musical experts, the most consonant musical intervals are those based on small commensurate ratios, as in unison (1:1), octave (2:1), perfect fifth (3:2), and perfect fourth (5:4). Dissonant harmonies arise from more complex ratios, for instance, the major second (9:8), the seventh (16:9, 15:8), and, of course, the most dramatic tritone (augmented fourth: 45:32). Also, consonance judgments of ordinary listeners confirm experts' predictions,[101] as well as dovetailing with the simplicity rankings of Schellenberg and Trehub.[102] Together, such findings reinforce the idea that consonant musical intervals correspond to the rate ratios of simple attractors. Of course, in real musical compositions the range of different attractor ratios offers a variety of tools for an artistic composer with goals of strategically exposing both consonant and dissonant sounds to an audience.

In music, composers use dissonance and consonance to achieve various emotional effects. Western traditions view the tritone as essential in blues and jazz, where they create tension prior to a resolution supplied by simpler pitcher intervals. Without the latter resolution, musicians and filmmakers often turn to prolonged bouts of dissonance to provoke unsettling feelings, whether through an endless tritone underlying Ozzy Osbourne's bemoaning appearance of a demon or through excerpts from Bartok's *Music for Strings, Percussion and Celesta* accompanying Jack Nicholson wild activity in *The Shining*. Dissonant time ratios stir up uncanny effects for listeners.

Is Consonance Perception Universal?

A broader issue concerns whether or not consonance and dissonance are universal experiences. Do they cross age groups? Are they cross-cultural? How universal? Could they apply to other species?

Aging and Consonant Perception

A DAT approach to consonance prompts a strong prediction from the aging hypothesis. Specifically, it posits that consonance–dissonance distinctions are universal because they represent differences among basic attractor categories. Moreover, these attractor-based distinctions should persist over a life span and across cultures.

Consistent with this prediction, Sandra Trehub and colleagues showed that infants, like adults, respond differentially to consonant versus dissonant sounds consistent with an attractor ratio simplicity index (Table 6.2).[103,104,105] Also, young infants are differentially sensitive to consonant sounds.[106,107] Two-tone chords presented to infants (as young as 3 months) contained either consonant (3:2 or 4:3) or dissonant (45:32) pairs. In each chord, a slight frequency deviation appeared in the higher tone. Infants were best in detecting the deviation with the simplest rate ratio (3:2) and worst with the most complex ratio (45:32). Newborns, too, differentiate consonant from dissonant music.[108] These discoveries imply that the power of attractors is present at birth.

At the other end of the life span spectrum, the aging hypothesis maintains that older adults should also differentiate temporal textures featuring simple attractor relations (consonance) from those with complex ones (dissonance). Bones and Plack[109] compared consonant judgments of two-tone chords by older (over 40 years) and younger (under 40 years) adults (all nonmusicians). Both groups were sensitive to attractor differences, favoring a consonant perfect fifth over a dissonant tritone intervals. However, aging effects in listeners' pitch tracking were also evident in frequency-following responses (FFRs) in brainstem oscillatory responses. Consistent with the aging hypothesis, older listeners showed poorer neural mode-locking than young adults largely with higher harmonics.

In sum, consistent with the aging hypothesis, young and old listeners are sensitive to consonance differences that reflect attractor complexities. More complex attractors lead to poorer performance than simple ones in both young and old listeners.

Consonance Across Species: A Second Take on Universality

Principles of resonance and entrainment have a universal status that remains to be validated. Although the premise of universal consonance across species has not been widely examined, an inspiring attack on this topic appears in the prolific writings of W. Tecumseh Fitch and colleagues.[110,111,112,113] By focusing on synchronies in chorusing of various species, Fitch observes that low-order synchronies of 1:1 and 2:1 describe group signaling sounds in species of insects and frogs. And, in postulating a continuum of dynamical systems from simple limit cycles to strange attractors of chaos, Fitch notes that communicative sounds in most species involve sound signals that include simple attractor states, states that can momentarily shift (i.e., a transition via bifurcation) to more complex states including chaotic (strange) attractors. For instance, as with the purrs of our pet cat, the "coos" of a macaque monkey can be simply described by harmonics. And, in both species, these orderly sound signals can be rapidly transformed (via bifurcations) when an animal suddenly growls, hisses, or screeches. Such momentary state changes inject noisy (i.e., dissonant) components into an animal's vocalizations. Whereas coos and purrs readily implicate simpler attractors, screeching and hissing growls require chaotic attractors. Even in human speech signals, a consonance continuum of entrainment states ranges from speech sounds that instill consonance via simple attractors (e.g., in open vowels) to sounds sparking the complex and/or chaotic attractors (in strident fricatives) of dissonance.

Duets in the communications of certain species are fascinating. Among these, the bird duets of the South American honeros are champions.[114] Synchronies in these communications exhibit an enthralling exercise of mode-locking using a consonant n:m attractors. Also, Japanese monkeys, chimpanzees as well as sparrows and starlings prefer consonance in sound-making.[115] Even newly hatched chicks show enhanced visual imprinting to objects paired with consonant (vs. dissonant)

sounds.[116] And it is rather touching to discover that even the lowly rat discriminates consonant from dissonant chords.[117] Finally, neural correlates of consonance versus dissonance distinctions are found in both humans and monkeys.[118,119]

Across species, the prevalence of commensurate time ratios supports attractor universality. So what does this imply about temporal niches? A temporal niche refers to a species-specific range of functional driving rhythms. Rhythms may be effective due to their rate and/or their rhythms (i.e., ratios of favored attractors). That is, niche constraints can include species-specific criteria for certain kinds of attractors. For instance, simple attractors may be a requisite criterion for temporal niches across a broad range of species, while complex attractors are likely to be more specialized.

As speculation, what is universal across species boundaries may be the *concept of attractors*, not the specific attractors. This implies that the communications of many animals are not only rate-specific, but their temporal niches are also constrained by species-specific attractor rhythms.

Summary of Consonance and Dissonance

Consonant controversies remain. Nevertheless, mounting evidence favors explanations of consonance–dissonance judgments rooted in the temporal texture of communicative sound patterns. Specifically, sounds that embed various harmonic ratios are heard as more sonorous/consonant, whereas sounds lacking these harmonies tend to be dissonant. Moreover, these distinctions have central neural correlates in periodic activity within the brainstem and auditory cortex. According to DAT, listeners' sensitivity to external micro-driving rhythms implicate a role for attractors in activating neural oscillations with periods related by attractor ratios. Evidence consistent with this view comes with consonance judgments of adults and infants, as well as in neural activities across many species. This evidence reinforces assumptions that principles of resonance and entrainment are universal. Major points of this section are:

- Theories of perceived consonance of a sound as a lack of dissonance due to disruptive peripheral processing fail to explain listeners' sensitivity to attractor ratios in complex sounds and neural activity responsive to consonant relationships.

- Adult listeners judge complex sounds as consonant if temporal textures implicate multiple, relatively simple attractors.
- Universality of consonant–dissonant percepts is supported by findings that human newborns and other species differentiate consonant from dissonant sounds.
- Dynamic attending hypotheses about aging and general stimulus properties find support in listeners' judgments about pitch and consonance.

CHAPTER SUMMARY

This chapter addresses how we tune into fast sound events that lead us to experience the pitch and consonance of complex sounds. Complex sounds comprise many fast rhythms that shape our response to these sounds. Unlike pure tones, complex sounds are everywhere in our environment, where they form the building blocks of speech and music.

This chapter describes two viable but contrasting frameworks for understanding pitch perception. One well-established psychoacoustic approach postulates that pitch perception of complex sounds depends on staged processing of collections of discrete (interspike), independent time intervals from different harmonic components of a complex sound. The other approach extend DAT concepts to describe listeners' response to micro-driving rhythms of complex sounds. In the latter view, complex sounds present sets of micro-driving rhythms which enable listeners to automatically entrain attending to fast sound frequencies. Clusters of co-occurring (neural) micro-driven rhythms respond to (i.e., synchronize with) the corresponding micro-driving rhythms of complex sounds. Two operative hypotheses (aging and general attending) contribute to predictions about various phenomena associated with percepts of the pitch and consonance of complex sounds.

A goal of this chapter was to demonstrate that entrainment principles can successfully address phenomena surrounding pitch perception. Broadly speaking, applications of DAT hypotheses (aging and general attending hypotheses) show that these principles operate across a range of fast-driving rhythm rates, regardless of the absolute timing of such rates.

Finally, this chapter not only extends the explanatory potential of entrainment mechanisms to fast events, it also explains percepts of different age groups and species. The essence of this theory is that rhythmic synchrony, at any time scale, is a unifying primitive that explains how animate creatures connect with their environment. Creatures that occupy this environment neither produce nor perceive arbitrary collections of independent time spans. Rather, the world that we and other species create and inhabit is rhythmical. It is a dynamic world full of interacting rhythmical organisms.

NOTES

1. A complex sound, which contains multiple partials, is not to be confused with a complex attractor.

2. Aniruddh D. Patel, *Music, Language, and the Brain* (New York: Oxford University Press, 2010), https://books-google-com.proxy.library.ucsb.edu:9443/books?hl=enandlr=andid=qekVDAAAQBAJandoi=fndandpg=PR9anddq=A.++Patel,+2008+++Music,+language+and+the+brainandots=sPXEJrG8Kkandsig=SzEm4C3Zg3Y43jzFO97Vt1ocJ-Y.

3. Alain De Cheveigne, "Pitch Perception Models," in *Pitch* edited by Plack C.J., Fay R.R., Oxenham A.J., Popper A.N. (New York: Springer, 2005), 169–233. http://link.springer.com.proxy.library.ucsb.edu:2048/chapter/10.1007/0-387-28958-5_6.

4. B. C. J. Moore, *An Introduction to the Psychology of Hearing*, Netherlands: Brill, 2012.

5. Andrew J. Oxenham, "Revisiting Place and Temporal Theories of Pitch," *Acoustical Science and Technology/Edited by the Acoustical Society of Japan* 34, no. 6 (2013): 388–96.

6. Ernst Terhardt, "Calculating Virtual Pitch," *Hearing Research* 1, no. 2 (March 1979): 155–82, doi:10.1016/0378-5955(79)90025-X.

7. Georg Von Békésy and Ernest Glen Wever, *Experiments in Hearing*, vol. 8 (New York: McGraw-Hill, 1960), http://www.abdi-ecommerce10.com/asa/images/product/medium/0-88318-6306.pdf.

8. Brian C. J. Moore, Robert W. Peters, and Brian R. Glasberg, "Auditory Filter Shapes at Low Center Frequencies," *Journal of the Acoustical Society of America* 88, no. 1 (July 1, 1990): 132–40, doi:10.1121/1.399960.

9. Brian C. J. Moore and Hedwig E. Gockel, "Resolvability of Components in Complex Tones and Implications for Theories of Pitch Perception," *Hearing Research*, Annual Reviews 2011, 276, no. 1–2 (June 2011): 88–97, doi:10.1016/j.heares.2011.01.003.

10. J. F. Schouten, "The Residue Revisited," *Frequency Analysis and Periodicity Detection in Hearing*, 1970, 41–54.

11. Moore and Gockel, "Resolvability of Components in Complex Tones and Implications for Theories of Pitch Perception."

12. Moore, *An Introduction to the Psychology of Hearing*.

13. Robert P. Carlyon et al., "Temporal Pitch Mechanisms in Acoustic and Electric Hearing," *Journal of the Acoustical Society of America* 112, no. 2 (August 2002): 621–33, doi:10.1121/1.1488660.

14. Astrid van Wieringen et al., "Pitch of Amplitude-Modulated Irregular-Rate Stimuli in Acoustic and Electric Hearing," *Journal of the Acoustical Society of America* 114, no. 3 (September 2003): 1516–28, doi:10.1121/1.1577551.

15. P. A. Cariani and B. Delgutte, "Neural Correlates of the Pitch of Complex Tones. I. Pitch and Pitch Salience," *Journal of Neurophysiology* 76, no. 3 (September 1, 1996): 1698–716.

16. Kumaresan Ramdas, Vijay Kumar Peddinti, and Peter Cariani, "Auditory-Inspired Pitch Extraction Using a Synchrony Capture Filterbank for Speech Signals," *Journal of the Acoustical Society of America* 135, no. 4 (April 1, 2014): 2426, doi:10.1121/1.4878068.

17. P. A. Cariani, "Neural Timing Nets," *Neural Networks* 14, no. 6–7 (July 9, 2001): 737–53, doi:10.1016/S0893-6080(01)00056-9.

18. Oxenham, "Revisiting Place and Temporal Theories of Pitch."

19. Moore, *An Introduction to the Psychology of Hearing.*

20. Fine time structure intervals are less predictable and less common than others.

21. In fact, when $n \geq 10$, the nTj estimates of T0 in Table 6.1 *don't work.*

22. In this respect, Moore's theory resembles Cariani's rate code, but Moore's theory is more comprehensive.

23. Moore, *An Introduction to the Psychology of Hearing.*

24. Mari R. Jones, "Time, Our Lost Dimension: Toward a New Theory of Perception, Attention, and Memory," *Psychological Review* 83, no. 5 (1976): 323.

25. Mari R. Jones and Marilyn Boltz, "Dynamic Attending and Responses to Time," *Psychological Review* 96, no. 3 (1989): 459–91, doi:10.1037/0033-295X.96.3.459.

26. Edward W. Large and Mari Riess Jones, "The Dynamics of Attending: How People Track Time-Varying Events," *Psychological Review* 106, no. 1 (1999): 119–59, doi:10.1037/0033-295X.106.1.119.

27. Edward W. Large and John F. Kolen, "Resonance and the Perception of Musical Meter," *Connection Science* 6, no. 2–3 (1994): 177–208.

28. Edward W. Large, "Neurodynamics of Music," in *Music Perception*, eds. Mari Riess Jones, Richard R. Fay, and Arthur N. Popper, 36 (New York: Springer, 2010), 201–31, doi:10.1007/978-1-4419-6114-3_7.

29. Edward W. Large and Felix V. Almonte, "Neurodynamics, Tonality, and the Auditory Brainstem Response," *Annals of the New York Academy of Sciences* 1252, no. 1 (April 1, 2012): E1–7, doi:10.1111/j.1749-6632.2012.06594.x.

30. Phase-locking constraints over a life span refer to DAT hypotheses about coupling strength changes with age.

31. Adrián E. Granada and Hanspeter Herzel, "How to Achieve Fast Entrainment? The Timescale to Synchronization," *PLoS ONE* 4, no. 9 (September 23, 2009): e7057, doi:10.1371/journal.pone.0007057.

32. Recall that, if this ratio is the golden mean, then synchrony fails.

33. Hedwig E. Gockel et al., "Effect of Duration on the Frequency Discrimination of Individual Partials in a Complex Tone and on the Discrimination of Fundamental Frequency," *Journal of the Acoustical Society of America* 121, no. 1 (January 1, 2007): 373–82, doi:10.1121/1.2382476.

34. Roelof J. Ritsma, "Frequencies Dominant in the Perception of the Pitch of Complex Sounds," *Journal of the Acoustical Society of America* 42, no. 1 (July 1, 1967): 191–98, doi:10.1121/1.1910550.

35. A dominance region is a set of low-frequency harmonics (e.g., 400–1,000 Hz in Table 6.1) that levy a powerful impact on pitch perception.

36. In dynamical systems, attractor complexity is formalized in the construct of a devil's staircase.

37. They may also entrain to each other. For simplicity, this is not shown.

38. This is correlated with the repetition rate of a complex sound.

39. Karl D. Lerud et al., "Mode-Locking Neurodynamics Predict Human Auditory Brainstem Responses to Musical Intervals," *Hearing Research* 308 (February 2014): 41–49, doi:10.1016/j.heares.2013.09.010.

40. Frank C. Hoppensteadt and Eugene M. Izhikevich, "Synaptic Organizations and Dynamical Properties of Weakly Connected Neural Oscillators," *Biological Cybernetics* 75, no. 2 (August 1996): 117–27, doi:10.1007/s004220050279.

41. Edward W. Large, Felix V. Almonte, and Marc J. Velasco, "A Canonical Model for Gradient Frequency Neural Networks," *Physica D: Nonlinear Phenomena* 239, no. 12 (June 15, 2010): 905–11, doi:10.1016/j.physd.2009.11.015.

42. Large, "Neurodynamics of Music."

43. Lerud et al., "Mode-Locking Neurodynamics Predict Human Auditory Brainstem Responses to Musical Intervals."

44. This is adapted from Lerud et al., note 37.

45. G. S. Ohm, "Ueber Die Definition Des Tones, Nebst Daran Geknüpfter Theorie Der Sirene Und Ähnlicher Tonbildender Vorrichtungen," *Annalen Der Physik* 135, no. 8 (January 1, 1843): 513–65, doi:10.1002/andp.18431350802.

46. R. Plomp and H. J. M. Steeneken, "Interference Between Two Simple Tones," *Journal of the Acoustical Society of America* 43, no. 4 (April 1, 1968): 883–84, doi:10.1121/1.1910916.

47. Brian C. J. Moore et al., "Effects of Level and Frequency on the Audibility of Partials in Inharmonic Complex Tones," *Journal of the Acoustical Society of America* 120, no. 2 (August 1, 2006): 934–44, doi:10.1121/1.2216906.

48. Moore, *An Introduction to the Psychology of Hearing*.

49. Christopher J. Plack and Andrew J. Oxenham, "The Psychophysics of Pitch," in *Pitch*, ed. Christopher J. Plack et al., Springer Handbook of Auditory Research 24 (New York: Springer, 2005), 7–55, doi:10.1007/0-387-28958-5_2.

50. William A. Yost, "Pitch Perception," *Attention, Perception, and Psychophysics* 71, no. 8 (November 2009): 1701–15, doi:10.3758/APP.71.8.1701.

51. Roelof J. Ritsma, "Periodicity Detection," *Frequency Analysis and Periodicity Detection in Hearing. Sijthoff*, 1970, 250–63.

52. Ritsma, "Frequencies Dominant in the Perception of the Pitch of Complex Sounds."

53. R. Plomp, "Pitch of Complex Tones," *Journal of the Acoustical Society of America* 41, no. 6 (1967): 1526, doi:10.1121/1.1910515.

54. Roy D. Patterson, "Residue Pitch as a Function of Component Spacing," *Journal of the Acoustical Society of America* 59, no. 6 (1976): 1450, doi:10.1121/1.381034.

55. Moore, *An Introduction to the Psychology of Hearing*.

56. Plack and Oxenham, "The Psychophysics of Pitch."

57. Yost, "Pitch Perception."

58. Timothy D. Griffiths et al., "Direct Recordings of Pitch Responses from Human Auditory Cortex," *Current Biology* 20, no. 12 (June 22, 2010): 1128–32, doi:10.1016/j.cub.2010.04.044.

59. D. Bendor and X. Wang, "Neural Coding of Periodicity in Marmoset Auditory Cortex," *Journal of Neurophysiology* 103, no. 4 (April 1, 2010): 1809–22, doi:10.1152/jn.00281.2009.

60. William A. Yost et al., "Pitch Strength of Regular-Interval Click Trains with Different Length 'Runs' of Regular Intervals," *Journal of the Acoustical Society of America* 117, no. 5 (May 1, 2005): 3054–68, doi:10.1121/1.1863712.

61. Sundeep Teki, Manon Grube, and Timothy D. Griffiths, "A Unified Model of Time Perception Accounts for Duration-Based and Beat-Based Timing Mechanisms," *Frontiers in Integrative Neuroscience* 5 (2012): 90, doi:10.3389/fnint.2011.00090.

62. Timothy D. Griffiths et al., "Analysis of Temporal Structure in Sound by the Human Brain," *Nature Neuroscience* 1, no. 5 (September 1998): 422–27, doi:10.1038/1637.

63. Bendor and Wang, "Neural Coding of Periodicity in Marmoset Auditory Cortex."

64. X. Wang et al., "Neural Coding of Temporal Information in Auditory Thalamus and Cortex," *Neuroscience*, 154, no. 1 (June 12, 2008): 294–303, doi:10.1016/j.neuroscience.2008.03.065.

65. Yonatan I. Fishman, Mitchell Steinschneider, and Christophe Micheyl, "Neural Representation of Concurrent Harmonic Sounds in Monkey Primary Auditory Cortex: Implications for Models of Auditory Scene Analysis," *The Journal of Neuroscience* 34, no.

37 (September 10, 2014): 12425–43, doi:10.1523/JNEUROSCI.0025-14.2014.

66. Liang-Fa Liu, Alan R. Palmer, and Mark N. Wallace, "Phase-Locked Responses to Pure Tones in the Inferior Colliculus," *Journal of Neurophysiology* 95, no. 3 (March 1, 2006): 1926–35, doi:10.1152/jn.00497.2005.

67. M. N. Wallace, L. A. Anderson, and A. R. Palmer, "Phase-Locked Responses to Pure Tones in the Auditory Thalamus," *Journal of Neurophysiology* 98, no. 4 (August 1, 2007): 1941–52, doi:10.1152/jn.00697.2007.

68. Sam Norman-Haignere, Nancy Kanwisher, and Josh H. McDermott, "Cortical Pitch Regions in Humans Respond Primarily to Resolved Harmonics and Are Located in Specific Tonotopic Regions of Anterior Auditory Cortex," *The Journal of Neuroscience* 33, no. 50 (December 11, 2013): 19451–69, doi:10.1523/JNEUROSCI.2880-13.2013.

69. C. Marie and L. J. Trainor, "Development of Simultaneous Pitch Encoding: Infants Show a High Voice Superiority Effect," *Cerebral Cortex* 23, no. 3 (March 1, 2013): 660–69, doi:10.1093/cercor/bhs050.

70. Nicole A. Folland et al., "Processing Simultaneous Auditory Objects: Infants' Ability to Detect Mistuning in Harmonic Complexes," *The Journal of the Acoustical Society of America* 131, no. 1 (2012): 993–7.

71. Laurel J. Trainor and Kathleen A. Corrigall, *Music Acquisition and Effects of Musical Experience* (New York: Springer, 2010), http://link.springer.com.proxy.library.ucsb.edu:2048/chapter/10.1007/978-1-4419-6114-3_4.

72. This was indexed by cortical mismatch negativity.

73. Elena Kushnerenko et al., "Maturation of the Auditory Change Detection Response in Infants: A Longitudinal ERP Study," *NeuroReport* 13, no. 15 (2002), http://journals.lww.com/neuroreport/Fulltext/2002/10280/Maturation_of_the_auditory_change_detection.2.aspx.

74. Chao He and Laurel J. Trainor, "Finding the Pitch of the Missing Fundamental in Infants," *Journal of Neuroscience* 29, no. 24 (June 17, 2009): 7718–8822, doi:10.1523/JNEUROSCI.0157-09.2009.

75. Terhardt, "Calculating Virtual Pitch."

76. Ernst Terhardt, "Pitch, Consonance, and Harmony," *Journal of the Acoustical Society of America* 55, no. 5 (May 1, 1974): 1061–69, doi:10.1121/1.1914648.

77. W. Jay Dowling and Dane L. Harwood, *Music Cognition* Academic Press, Inc. (London) LTD (1986).

78. Akio Kameoka and Mamoru Kuriyagawa, "Consonance Theory Part II: Consonance of Complex Tones and Its Calculation Method," *Journal of the Acoustical Society of America* 45, no. 6 (June 1, 1969): 1460–69, doi:10.1121/1.1911624.

79. R. Plomp and W. J. M. Levelt, "Tonal Consonance and Critical Bandwidth," *Journal of the*

Acoustical Society of America 38, no. 4 (October 1, 1965): 548–60, doi:10.1121/1.1909741.

80. More generally, these have periods Ti and Tj in Figure 6.1A,B.

81. E. Glenn Schellenberg and Sandra E. Trehub, "Frequency Ratios and the Perception of Tone Patterns," *Psychonomic Bulletin and Review* 1, no. 2 (June 1994): 191–201, doi:10.3758/BFO3200773.

82. Following the *Just* musical scale; see Backus (note 83) for scale descriptions.

83. John Backus and John W. Coltman, "The Acoustical Foundations of Music," *Physics Today* 23 (1970): 69, doi:10.1063/1.3022122.

84. Christopher J. Plack, "Musical Consonance: The Importance of Harmonicity," *Current Biology* 20, no. 11 (June 8, 2010): R476–78, doi:10.1016/j.cub.2010.03.044.

85. Kyung Myun Lee et al., "Selective Subcortical Enhancement of Musical Intervals in Musicians," *Journal of Neuroscience* 29, no. 18 (May 6, 2009): 5832–40, doi:10.1523/JNEUROSCI.6133-08.2009.

86. Gavin M. Bidelman and Ananthanarayan Krishnan, "Neural Correlates of Consonance, Dissonance, and the Hierarchy of Musical Pitch in the Human Brainstem," *Journal of Neuroscience* 29, no. 42 (October 21, 2009): 13165–71, doi:10.1523/JNEUROSCI.3900-09.2009.

87. Oliver Bones et al., "Phase Locked Neural Activity in the Human Brainstem Predicts Preference for Musical Consonance," *Neuropsychologia* 58 (May 2014): 23–32, doi:10.1016/j.neuropsychologia.2014.03.011.

88. Betty Tuller et al., *Nonlinear Dynamics in Speech Perception* (Berlin/Heidelberg: Springer, 2010), http://link.springer.com.proxy.library.ucsb.edu:2048/chapter/10.1007/978-3-642-16262-6_6.

89. Eiji Yumoto, Wilbur J. Gould, and Thomas Baer, "Harmonics-to-noise Ratio as an Index of the Degree of Hoarseness," *Journal of the Acoustical Society of America* 71, no. 6 (June 1, 1982): 1544–50, doi:10.1121/1.387808.

90. Terhardt, "Pitch, Consonance, and Harmony."

91. Terhardt, "Pitch, Consonance, and Harmony."

92. Plomp and Levelt, "Tonal Consonance and Critical Bandwidth."

93. Paul Boomsliter and Warren Creel, "The Long Pattern Hypothesis in Harmony and Hearing," *Journal of Music Theory* 5, no. 1 (1961): 2–31, doi:10.2307/842868.

94. Plomp and Levelt, "Tonal Consonance and Critical Bandwidth."

95. Marion Cousineau, Josh H. McDermott, and Isabelle Peretz, "The Basis of Musical Consonance as Revealed by Congenital Amusia," *Proceedings of the National Academy of Sciences* 109, no. 48 (November 27, 2012): 19858–63, doi:10.1073/pnas.1207989109.

96. Josh H. McDermott, Andriana J. Lehr, and Andrew J. Oxenham, "Individual Differences Reveal the Basis of Consonance," *Current Biology* 20, no. 11 (June 8, 2010): 1035–41, doi:10.1016/j.cub.2010.04.019.

97. Christopher J. Plack, "Musical Consonance: The Importance of Harmonicity," *Current Biology* 20, no. 11 (June 8, 2010): R476–78, doi:10.1016/j.cub.2010.03.044.

98. Oliver Bones and Christopher J. Plack, "Subcortical Representation of Musical Dyads: Individual Differences and Neural Generators," *Hearing Research* 323 (May 2015): 9–21, doi:10.1016/j.heares.2015.01.009.

99. Gavin M. Bidelman and Michael G. Heinz, "Auditory-Nerve Responses Predict Pitch Attributes Related to Musical Consonance-Dissonance for Normal and Impaired Hearing," *Journal of the Acoustical Society of America* 130, no. 3 (September 1, 2011): 1488–502, doi:10.1121/1.3605559.

100. Gavin M. Bidelman, Jackson T. Gandour, and Ananthanarayan Krishnan, "Cross-Domain Effects of Music and Language Experience on the Representation of Pitch in the Human Auditory Brainstem," *Journal of Cognitive Neuroscience* 23, no. 2 (November 19, 2009): 425–34, doi:10.1162/jocn.2009.21362.

101. McDermott, Lehr, and Oxenham, "Individual Differences Reveal the Basis of Consonance."

102. Schellenberg and Trehub, "Frequency Ratios and the Perception of Tone Patterns."

103. Schellenberg and Trehum, "Frequency Ratios and the Perception of Tone Patterns."

104. E. Glenn Schellenberg and Sandra E. Trehub, "Natural Musical Intervals: Evidence From Infant Listeners," *Psychological Science* 7, no. 5 (September 1, 1996): 272–77, doi:10.1111/j.1467-9280.1996.tb00373.x.

105. Sandra E. Trehub, Leigh A. Thorpe, and Laurel J. Trainor, "Infants' Perception of Good and Bad Melodies," *Psychomusicology: A Journal of Research in Music Cognition* 9, no. 1 (1990): 5–19, doi:10.1037/h0094162.

106. Schellenberg and Trehub, "Natural Musical Intervals."

107. Laurel J. Trainor, Christine D. Tsang, and Vivian H. W. Cheung, "Preference for Sensory Consonance in 2- and 4-Month-Old Infants," *Music Perception: An Interdisciplinary Journal* 20, no. 2 (December 1, 2002): 187–94, doi:10.1525/mp.2002.20.2.187.

108. Daniela Perani et al., "Functional Specializations for Music Processing in the Human Newborn Brain," *Proceedings of the National Academy of Sciences* 107, no. 10 (March 9, 2010): 4758–63, doi:10.1073/pnas.0909074107.

109. Oliver Bones and Christopher J. Plack, "Losing the Music: Aging Affects the Perception and Subcortical Neural Representation of Musical Harmony," *Journal of Neuroscience* 35, no. 9 (March 4, 2015): 4071–80, doi:10.1523/JNEUROSCI.3214-14.2015.

110. Silvia P Gennari et al., "Motion Events in Language and Cognition," *Cognition* 83, no. 1 (February 2002): 49–79, doi:10.1016/S0010-0277(01)00166-4.

111. W. Tecumseh Fitch, Jürgen Neubauer, and Hanspeter Herzel, "Calls out of Chaos: The Adaptive

Significance of Nonlinear Phenomena in Mammalian Vocal Production," *Animal Behaviour* 63, no. 3 (March 2002): 407–18, doi:10.1006/anbe.2001.1912.

112. W. Tecumseh Fitch, "Toward a Computational Framework for Cognitive Biology: Unifying Approaches from Cognitive Neuroscience and Comparative Cognition," *Physics of Life Reviews* 11, no. 3 (September 2014): 329–64, doi:10.1016/j.plrev.2014.04.005.

113. Hugo Merchant et al., "Finding the Beat: A Neural Perspective Across Humans and Non-Human Primates," *Philosophical Transactions of the Royal Society B* 370, no. 1664 (March 19, 2015): 20140093, doi:10.1098/rstb.2014.0093.

114. Rodrigo Laje and Gabriel B. Mindlin, "Highly Structured Duets in the Song of the South American Hornero," *Physical Review Letters* 91, no. 25 (December 19, 2003): 258104, doi:10.1103/PhysRevLett.91.258104.

115. Tasuku Sugimoto et al., "Preference for Consonant Music over Dissonant Music by an Infant Chimpanzee," *Primates* 51, no. 1 (July 22, 2009): 7–12, doi:10.1007/s10329-009-0160-3.

116. Cinzia Chiandetti and Giorgio Vallortigara, "Chicks Like Consonant Music," *Psychological Science* 22, no. 10 (October 1, 2011): 1270–73, doi:10.1177/0956797611418244.

117. Paola Crespo-Bojorque and Juan M. Toro, "The Use of Interval Ratios in Consonance Perception by Rats (*Rattus norvegicus*) and Humans (*Homo sapiens*)," *Journal of Comparative Psychology* 129, no. 1 (2015): 42.

118. Yonatan I. Fishman et al., "Consonance and Dissonance of Musical Chords: Neural Correlates in Auditory Cortex of Monkeys and Humans," *Journal of Neurophysiology* 86, no. 6 (December 1, 2001): 2761–88.

119. Daniela Sammler et al., "Music and Emotion: Electrophysiological Correlates of the Processing of Pleasant and Unpleasant Music," *Psychophysiology* 44, no. 2 (March 1, 2007): 293–304, doi:10.1111/j.1469-8986.2007.00497.x.

7

Tuning in to Slow Events

Conversational speech seems to rattle along at a fairly fast pace. Nevertheless, the timing of syllables and words in human utterances actually spells out many rhythms that are much slower than the micro-rhythms of pitch perception. Similarly, musical events commonly deliver tones at rates based on intertone intervals ranging from 200 ms to more than 800 ms. In other words, in contrast to the fast micro-rhythms of individual sounds in speech and music discussed in the preceding chapter, relatively slow rhythms are also found to populate the speech and musical domains. This chapter examines how we interact with slow rhythms—macro-rhythms.

Our interactions with slow events are interesting for other reasons. As this chapter shows, often slow rhythms are variably timed in ways that do not meet the isochrony qualifications often associated with faster rhythms (e.g., partials) in the preceding chapter. Instead, the slow events introduced in this chapter project non-isochronous but coherent *time patterns*. These sequences form familiar, often appealing time patterns such as the short-short-long *anapest rhythm* or the *long-short-short* of a dactyl rhythm,[1] and so on. Most readers need no introduction to these rhythmic patterns, which will be termed *coherent time patterns*. However, they may need an explanation of another new term introduced in this chapter, namely *fuzzy rhythm*.

As its label implies, a fuzzy rhythm is a time pattern that is not quite "right." To illustrate, let us return to the simplest of time patterns, the isochronous rhythm. A fuzzy isochronous rhythm is often found in phrases as, "How are you?" or in the unsteady "rap, rap, rap" knocking on a door, finally, it occurs as an expressive series of timed bass drum hits, such as in the first measures of *Iron Man* (by Black Sabbath).[2] These are vastly different events. Nevertheless, all share the same *underlying* time pattern: specifically, a highly regular isochrony. All these examples convey a strong, in some cases gripping, sense of isochrony which is not obvious in their surface structures. Nevertheless, careful

analysis of their acoustic signals will reveal that fluctuating temporal deviations blur the surface timing of these examples. Just as formant deviates from a hidden harmonic, so too does the fuzzy time surface structure literally "hide" the underlying precision of isochrony. In both cases, attractor relationships are buried under moderate surface irregularities. With slow rhythms, the idea of fuzziness generalizes from quasi-isochornous time patterns to variations in time patterns. Thus, an idealized anapest rhythm might be 300-300-600 ms, but this is often hidden beneath various fuzzy versions of this short-short-long time pattern, of which 330-290-620 ms is only one.

Fuzzy rhythms contain superficial irregularities that deviate from a simpler, hidden relative time format. They are modest temporal modulations of an ideal time pattern. The ideal pattern functions as a *prototype time pattern*, and it is defined by special time relationships, namely attractor ratios. Simply put, *fuzzy rhythms* are blurred instances of an ideal prototype that defines a rhythmic category. They may seem slightly "off" an implied beat here or there, but these minor variations may be heard as signatures, or expressive ornaments, that all "point to" a hidden attractor state.

In an entrainment framework, fuzzy rhythms in a phase space can be viewed as occupying a spot on a trajectory in the entrainment region of a particular attractor that specifies a prototypical rhythm. That is, a prototype is a stimulus rhythm with no superficial timing deviations from its defining attractor. Fuzzy rhythms, by their ostensible irregularities, literally hide defining attractors. This chapter proposes ways that entrained attending deals with such irregularities while exploiting hidden attractors that are prevalent in macro-rhythms of speech and music.

Categories of macro-rhythmic patterns are also addressed in this chapter. Some categories are defined by the simple prototypes of isochrony, whereas others feature prototypes that express the tantalizing time patterns of familiar, but non-isochronous, rhythms. All these categories cut across the domains of music and speech.

Two important entrainment hypotheses continue to be relevant in this chapter. Respectively, these are the general attending hypothesis and the aging hypothesis. The general attending hypothesis, which emphasizes driving rhythm properties of force and regularity, provides a rationale for describing exogenous entrainments to certain forceful stimulus rhythms. The aging hypothesis emphasizes the innate power of attractors. It describes the power of mode-locking within individual time patterns that last over a lifespan. That is, the aging hypothesis implies that simpler rhythmic time patterns lead to perceptually compelling rhythmic forms regardless of a listener's age.

CHAPTER GOALS

A primary goal of this chapter entails extending the entrainment approach to attending in a fashion that addresses how people track a wide range of events with different rates and time patterns. Too often, entrainment explanations are not pursued due to mistaken beliefs that they "work" only with slow isochronous rhythms. The preceding chapter discounts the belief that entrainment cannot handle fast events. This chapter aims to discredit the belief that entrainment is only possible with slow rhythms that preserve isochrony.

This chapter has two major parts. The first part considers entrained attending to slow complex rhythms that embed *multiple isochronous rhythms* of different rates; it also addresses fuzzy versions of isochronous rhythms, termed "quasi-isochronous rhythms." This part of the chapter focuses on listeners' development of temporal expectancies based on entrainments that conform to a *traditional mode-locking* protocol.

The second half of this chapter tackles entrainments with *coherent,* but *non-isochronous,* rhythmic patterns. This topic covers a range of familiar time patterns that populate music and speech, including time patterns such as dactyl, anapest, and so on. Here, relevant entrainment principles draw on an important new concept: the *transient mode-locking protocol.* This concept counters the mistaken belief that entrainment "works" only for isochronous time patterns. In short, this chapter proposes a major theoretical distinction between traditional and transient mode-locking protocols. In turn, this results in distinctly different kinds of prototypical rhythmic categories.

An overview of chapter topics appears in Table 7.1. In this table, column 1 distinguishes between two kinds of prototypes: isochronous versus coherent time patterns. Each prototype has fuzzy variations, as suggested in column 2 (quasi-isochrony vs. quasi-rhythms). Most important are entrainment (mode-locking) differences associated with these prototypes. Column 3 distinguishes traditional from transient entrainment protocols. Finally, column 4 stipulates attractor differences associated with these two protocols. Isochronous categories involve constant attractors (over time); here, traditional entrainments lead to a single global attractor. By contrast, categories of coherent time patterns involve changing local attractors (over time); here, transient mode-locking leads to several local attractors. This table prefigures issues discussed in this chapter.

A major chapter goal involves unpacking differences between traditional and transient mode-locking protocols of attending. A related goal addresses the nature of resulting attractor differences. As suggested in Table 7.1, attractors underlying the category of isochronous rhythms are global attractors whereas categories of non-isochronous time pattern attractors are described by a series of local attractors.

TABLE 7.1 PROTOTYPE RHYTHMS AND FUZZY RHYTHMS

Prototype Rhythm (T values; ms)	Fuzzy Rhythm (T values; ms)	Mode-locking	Attractors
Isochronous (600-600-600 . . .)	Quasi-Isochrony (595-620-581 . . .)	Traditional↓ *Oscillator cluster*	n:m = constant *A global attractor*
Coherent Non-isochronous (300-300-600 . . .)	Quasi-rhythm (330-290-620 . . .)	Transient↓ *Attractor profile*	n:m = varies *Local attractors*

BACKGROUND

Psychological studies of time and rhythmic patterns trace back to classic work of Paul Fraisse.[3] Fraisse explored people's responses to simple time patterns in which the time relationships between successive time intervals, Ti, varied. Listeners heard patterns ranging from strictly isochronous sequences to distinctly non-isochronous patterns containing two or three very different time spans. For instance, listeners had to reproduce (by tapping) a coherent but non-isochronous prototypical rhythm with a *short-short-long* time pattern (300-300-600 ms) and also several fuzzy versions of it (e.g., example T values of 330-290--620 ms in column 2 of Table 7.1). Fraisse discovered that people inevitably distort fuzzy rhythms in the direction of the closest prototype. For instance, the preceding fuzzy rhythm might be tapped as 305-299-610 ms, thereby moving it closer to the category prototype. In short, distortions of a fuzzy time pattern are unidirectional, reflecting a "pull" towards the simple short-short-long pattern of the prototype (where short:long is 2:1). Also, Fraisse found that, when reproducing quasi-isochronous rhythms, a listener's strongest distortions were based on gravitations to 1:1 time ratios (row 2 of Table 7.1), whereas with various non-isochronous rhythms (e.g., row 3, Table 7.1) the strongest distortions involved a pull toward time ratios implied by a 1:2 relationship. Related biases, discovered by Dirk Povel, include ratios of 1/3 and ¼.[4]

In sum, historically, the exploration of rhythm perception extends beyond isochronous time patterns. Indeed, certain time patterns are so compelling that classic studies find people distort fuzzy rhythmic patterns to regularize them in the direction of certain prototypes. Although this early research was not designed to study entrainment, it turns out to fit neatly into an entrainment story featuring attractor ratios. The remainder of this chapter uses isochronous and non-isochronous time patterns to pursue this line of thought.

FORMS OF ISOCHRONY: TRADITIONAL MODE-LOCKING

Isochrony undeniably exerts a strong force on people's responses to an acoustic event, as recognized by some theories of speech timing.[5] This section explores a listener's real-time attending to varieties of isochronous rhythms. It documents how a temporally regular series of sounds functions as a driving rhythm for an entraining oscillation that carries temporal expectancies. The idea is that driving–driven dyads supply periodic attending in a stable entrainment state; in turn, this motivates listeners to anticipate onsets of future sounds. Not surprisingly, the most effective phase-locking between a driven oscillation and its driving rhythm occurs when the two rhythms have the same periods; that is, one implicating a simple governing attractor of n:m = 1:1, the hallmark of isochronous entrainments. This section concentrates on listeners' performance with driving rhythms that are either isochronous, that represent a combination of several isochronous rhythms, or that are fuzzy versions of these prototypical rhythms. In other words, it considers a wide variety of isochronous-like rhythms, as suggested in row 2 of Figure 7.1.

Varieties of Isochrony

A prototypical isochronous rhythm is the simplest of all stimulus time patterns. Figure 7.1 presents this pattern (row A) along with various other rhythms in which isochrony plays a critical role. For instance, Row B in this figure shows a quasi-isochronous sequence; this is a fuzzy version of the "pure" isochrony (of row A). The remaining examples (C, D, E) in this figure illustrate other disguises of isochrony in common time patterns. Each of the latter three sequences involves overlapping two isochronous rhythms with different rates (marked respectively by ovals vs. x's).

Prototypes Versus Fuzzy Rhythms

Let's begin with the two driving rhythms in Figure 7.1A versus B. Respectively, these reflect an isochronous prototype and its fuzzy counterpart. Both have the same average rate (mean T is 600 ms), but the fuzzy rhythm in row B has several time spans that deviate from the fixed 600 ms time spans of the prototype. Nevertheless, from an entrainment perspective, a listener hearing each pattern will likely be governed by the same attractor (i.e., n:m = 1:1). That is, both patterns A and B elicit a limit cycle oscillation with a latent period near p = 600 ms. An event that matches the prototype (row A) presents no perturbing (deviant) time intervals. However, while the event with a fuzzy rhythm (as in row B) invites a similar latent period of a driven oscillation (i.e., with p = 600 ms), this oscillation will automatically confront deviations from 600 ms. Specifically this driven oscillation will engage in momentary phase-corrective activities in response to a deviant time span. An entrainment approach focuses on *in-the-moment reactions* to perturbing (i.e., deviant) time spans.

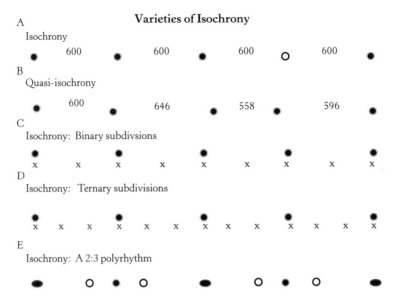

FIGURE 7.1 (A) A single isochronous driving rhythm with a fixed period, T, of 600 ms. (B) A quasi-isochronous (fuzzy) driving rhythm with an average period of 600 ms. (C) Two isochronous rhythms (⬤) implicating a 2:1 period ratio. (D) Two isochronous rhythms implying a 3:1 periodic relationship. (E) Two isochronous rhythms with a 2:3 periodic relationship.

In this respect, this analysis differs from statistical descriptions of rhythms that average time spans over the course of an event. What happens in real time is really important.

Momentary phase corrections by a driven oscillation figure into the phase response curves (PRCs) discussed in earlier chapters. In the present examples, these corrective actions on the part of entraining oscillation bring into play a fleeting manifest driven frequency (Ω) based on momentary period corrections of the entraining oscillation. Specifically, an internal oscillation entraining to pattern B can have a *momentary manifest period, denoted p′, which differs from latent period, p, of this oscillator* (p′ ≠ p ~ 600 ms). Although fleeting, manifest periods are important. They briefly substitute the oscillator's latent ratio, p/T, for an observable ratio: p′/T. Nevertheless, as such a stimulus rhythm unfolds, it evokes successive momentary responses of an entraining oscillation that are governed by a constant but hidden attractor.

This account is consistent with PRCs of Chapter 4. A salient perturbing time marker momentarily (and automatically) pushes an adaptive oscillation away from an attractor state such that it then briefly aligns its focal energy (its attending energy profile [AEP]) with the deviant sound (i.e., as a reactive pulse). Imagine this corrective action in terms of a rubber band; once the stimulus push

of perturbing force is removed, a rubber band snaps back to a resting state. Similarly, a perturbation only briefly captures attending. A strong internal attractor exerts an opposing force to this external perturbation, a force that pulls the system back to its stable attractor state (i.e., restoring p′ to p). Thus, a listener who is presented with a quasi-isochronous rhythm, as in row B, will usually find it is "good enough" as a stand-in for its prototype (row A) because both share the same attractor (n:m = 1:1). In other words, within entrainment limits, people hear these two rhythms as belonging to a common rhythmic category defined by the same attractor.

Expectancies and Capture

A skeptic of the preceding narrative may argue that people cope with temporal deviations of fuzzy rhythms voluntarily, by simply ignoring them. In short, this entrainment scenario is deemed lacking in parsimony or it is far-fetched (or both). However, this criticism ignores the fact that, routinely, people *do* respond involuntarily, *in the moment*, to temporal fluctuations. Moreover, this automaticity is adaptive; it allows a listener to instantly and effortlessly adjust to (partially or completely) timing deviations. For instance, in this quasi-isochronous rhythm, the timing deviations are (at least) partially accommodated for subjectively because an attender automatically adjusts a manifest period, p', of an entraining oscillation. As the rhythm unfolds, such corrective activities are governed by three factors: the strength of persisting neural oscillation, the salience of a perturbation, and the simplicity of a nearby attractor (here, n:m = 1:1).

Theoretically, the "pure" isochrony of Figure 7.1A readily promotes entrained attending. A variety of laboratory findings using tapping tasks confirm the power of regular stimulus timing in shaping the precision of a listener's tapping. But there is a catch. While "pure" isochrony is compelling, it is rare in ordinary soundscapes. In fact, when we do encounter a persisting isochronous rhythm, as when a neighbor repeatedly hammers at a fixed rate or a rock band drives a strong, monotonous beat, there comes a point when undecorated isochrony becomes boring, annoying, or both. Moreover, any claim that a prototypical isochronous pattern (as in Figure 7.1A) adequately describes speech timing patterns or even musical rhythms is dubious. Much contrary evidence documents the prevalence of temporal variability in natural acoustic signals. Fuzzy rhythms abound.

Fuzzy Rhythms and Hidden Attractors: A Paradox

The juxtaposition of prototypical isochrony with fuzzy isochrony raises a paradox. This is evident in speech timing, which is quite variable, arguably cluttered with fuzzy rhythms. Yet, paradoxically, people often claim to hear speech as rhythmical. Similarly, in music, the lead-in drum hits in *Iron Man*, for instance, are commonly experienced as highly regular (confirmed by timely bobbing of fans' heads), but, in reality, the actual sound signal is—yes, a *fuzzy rhythm*.

This paradox is resolved if we recognize that listeners "hear through" a fuzzy rhythm to intuit governing hidden attractor(s) that define a prototype. Listeners sense the hidden attractor in a fuzzy rhythm. In turn, this promotes a feeling of regularity that resembles pure isochrony while also offering temporal nuances that modulate the steely regularity of isochrony. Indeed, creatively placed irregularities in fuzzy rhythms of music and speech constitute what is termed *expressive timing*, implying an actual enhancement of the impact of an underlying attractor. Finally, fuzzy rhythms exemplify quasi-rhythms that motivate listeners to report their "sense" of an underlying rhythm. And, they are right. Prototypical and fuzzy versions of isochrony have the same attractor.

Attractors hide in fuzzy rhythms. Consequently, attractors surreptitiously control listeners' responses to events due to surface irregularities. Even discriminable time deviations do not necessarily disrupt entrained attending if supra-threshold changes remain within the limits of an attractor's entrainment region. Generally, a listener's real-time tracking of fuzzy rhythms depends on temporal expectancies guided by a hidden attractor. Such attractors supply entrainment regions that allow, yet limit, adaptive responses to perturbing sounds. (John Michon must be credited for the original analyses of isochronous perturbations.[6]) Adapting attending to a deviant sound that delivers a surprising, but artfully placed, expectancy violation can happen if the unexpected time change does not exceed 15–20% of an entraining oscillation's period.

Latent Versus Manifest Oscillator Periods

There is still more to this story. An important part of the narrative involves how fuzzy rhythms affect a listener's expectancies. A temporal expectancy is carried by the period of an entraining oscillation. But, what period? To this point, we have identified two different periods of an entraining oscillation, its latent period, p, and its manifest form, p' (i.e., of Ω). Which one carries a listener's expectancy?

Figure 7.2 shows the neural activity of an entraining oscillation as a listener attunes to a series of sounds created by either an isochronous rhythm or its fuzzy counterpart. Driving rhythms are not shown in Figure 7.2 in order to focus on the two forms of the internal (driven) oscillation: latent and manifest.

Panel A shows internal oscillator activity responding to an external isochronous rhythm, whereas panel B shows internal responses to a quasi-isochronous rhythm. Both share the same latent oscillation with a resting period of p = 600 ms. Moreover, with the isochronous driving rhythm, $p' = p = 600$ ms. That is, the stable latent period matches its manifest period (as in finger tapping, event-related potentials [ERPs], etc.). Clearly, in panel A, a listener's expected period is not in question: it is based on $p = p'$.

Matters are less clear with the fuzzy (quasi-isochronous) rhythm of panel B. Fleeting values of the manifest period, p', result from ongoing phase corrective activities of an entraining limit cycle oscillation. Entraining region constraints now enter the picture, as illustrated in Figure 7.2B. These regions suggest limits of adaptive corrections. Notice that all but one of the corrected oscillator peaks

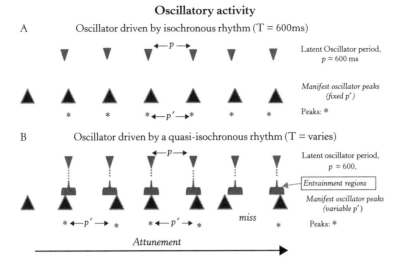

FIGURE 7.2 Peak energies of two different oscillations are shown. (**A**) Latent and manifest for an isochronous driving rhythm (not shown) with p = p′ of 600 ms. (**B**) Two different oscillations for a hypothetical quasi-isochronous driving rhythm (not shown) are latent and manifest where p ≠ p′. Also shown are hypothesized entrainment regions within which a deviant p′ might reside (as p′/Tj).

land in their respective entrainment region. In panel B, the latent expectancy, p, does not change but the manifest one, p′, does.

To sum up, fuzzy rhythms share an attractor with their prototype. Consequently, both prototype rhythms and fuzzy rhythms levy a distinct impact on listeners' momentary responses to these rhythms. However, the intrinsic period of a listener's driven oscillation delivers a steady expectancy in both cases, whereas manifest periods lead to observable expectancies that are more flexible and adaptive. Thus, hidden-plus-manifest expectancies may be a more realistic picture of our routine encounters with the rhythms that surround us and how we cope with them.

A Paradox: Rhythmic Irregularities Yet Still a Sense of Rhythm?

A quandary remains regarding listeners' ability to actually *sense* some hidden regularity in a fuzzy rhythm. This "sense" reflects the persistence of an entraining latent oscillation. The manifest period, p′, of this oscillation momentarily shrinks and expands as the oscillation respectively adapts to shortened or lengthened deviant time spans. By contrast, the *latent period of an entraining oscillation, p, does not change.*

In addition to anecdotal reports, some experimental evidence supports this double expectancy interpretation. For instance, Schmidt-Kassow and

Kotz[7] presented listeners with quasi-isochronous speech rhythms (stress markers with deviations around 17%), but they still responded to these rhythms as if they preserved an underlying regularity. Despite the fact that EPRs reflected changes (P600) to stress markers (indexing p′), participants still responded to these sequences as if they preserved a hidden temporal regularity (e.g., a constant p).

Paradox Resolved: Latent and Manifest Periods of Driven Rhythm

Several factors contribute to the stability of an entraining oscillator. First, from earlier chapters, we know that a strong driven oscillation is more stable than a weak oscillation, meaning that it is less responsive to deviant timing. Strong driven rhythms exhibit restrained adaptive reactions to perturbations. This is evident in a lower variance of observable (i.e., produced) time intervals that assess p′.

In contrast to strong driven rhythms, strong driving rhythms deliver an opposite effect on performance. A strong stimulus driving rhythm, for example, adds force to adaptive behaviors during entrainment. Basically, forceful stimulus time markers can capture our attending. Effectively, in a push–pull tension, salient stimulus time markers "push" a driven oscillation to adjust to a stimulus driving rhythm, creating corresponding changes in p′ (as in PRCs). In terms of dependent measures, increases in driving marker strength (K) increase the variance of produced time intervals, p'.

All else equal, a stable oscillatory period is a good candidate for guiding a listener's expectancies and for instilling in her a steady sense of an underlying rhythm. Despite vagaries of surface timing, a stable driven oscillation supplied by a strong oscillation contributes to a listener's sense of a "hidden regularity" in quasi-isochronous patterns. And, as $p' \rightarrow p$, a listener's sense of hidden regularities increases. In short, in speech or music, when a strong internal (driven) rhythm is combined with weak and/or irregular external driving rhythm, this leads to listeners reporting that a surface time pattern is *more regular than it actually is*.

Driven Versus Driving Rhythm Strength: An Example

Consider the following scenario. Bill is listening to his English professor discuss Chaucer. He is a bit bored. Nevertheless, he follows this droning lecture via entrainment using expectancies from a weak driven oscillation. These weak expectancies lead Bill to nod vaguely in time with the teacher's soft, somewhat irregular, phrasing. However, suddenly, the professor (noting Bill's glazed eyes) begins to speak louder, adding a few calculated pauses. To Bill's ears, these salient time markers force his attention into more a precise tracking of the professor's somewhat more regular phrasings. Especially, his entraining oscillation is responsive to the louder markers of time spans in this utterance because they increase with the professor's driving rhythm strength; stronger time markers increase phase-locking of Bill's ongoing driven oscillation. Consequently, Bill's driven oscillation automatically undergoes changes in its manifest period, p', as it adapts to successive pauses in this new driving rhythm, but Bill's latent oscillator period, p, remains unchanged.

Originally, Bill's oscillation operated with a manifest period, p', close to its resting period, p. However, as a weak oscillation, a strong external driving rhythm readily pushes it away from the default expectancy period, p, to a manifest period, p', more aligned with the speaker's stronger driving rhythm. This is an adaptive change of the manifest period, p'. A new value of p' is installed that matches deviant pauses in the upgraded lecture. Effectively, the heightened strength of the professor's new driving rhythm wins over the lesser strength of Bill's original driven rhythm. So, the professor also wins Bill's attention.

Quasi-Isochrony and Temporal Expectancies

Temporal expectancies need no introduction at this point.[8,9,10] They arise from listeners' automatic reliance on contextually induced self-sustaining oscillations that prepare a listener for the "when" of future happenings. And the strength of this driven neural oscillation is important. But a question about driven rhythms lingers concerning respective roles of an oscillator's two periods: latent and manifest. Put bluntly: Does a temporal expectancy reflect activity of p or p'? Both are active during entrainment. So which is the "real" expectancy?

The answer is the latent period, p. It is the logical candidate for capturing a listener's inner premonitions of regularity within a fuzzy rhythm. It is also the best determinant of temporal expectancies because an oscillation's intrinsic (i.e., latent) period does not change over time. The stability of p is its sustaining quality. By definition, an expectancy persists over time, whereas manifest oscillator periods appear only when a temporal expectancy is violated. As shown in Figure 7.2, p' changes over time, only assuming its intrinsic form when an expectancy is confirmed: $p' = p$.

Latent and manifest periods operate simultaneously as a listener tracks an event, but they serve different functions. The oscillator's intrinsic period realizes persisting periodic energy pulses that determine temporal expectancies, whereas its manifest period reflects transitory allocations of attending energy for phase corrections when expectancies are violated. An invariant intrinsic period prepares listeners for "when" future sounds may occur. As such, it is fallible; it can be wrong. By contrast, manifest periods are transitory, reorienting attending when a latent expectancy is wrong.

Modeling Attending to Quasi-Isochrony

This theoretical approach was formalized by Edward Large, who designed a single oscillator model to capture how temporal expectancies operate in time-change detection tasks.[11] Assuming that rhythmic context entrains an oscillation with an intrinsic period of p, this model focused on the impact of such a context rhythm on entraining an oscillation and its adaptive responses (in phase, period) when its expected period is wrong.

Entrainment regions are also part of this story. Given the limits of the entrainment region of some implied attractor, an oscillation entraining to an external rhythm automatically changes its phase, φ_i, when provoked by a rhythmic irregularity. Among other things, a phase shift temporarily affects the oscillator's manifest period. In this model, phase corrections rely on a sine circle mapping formula of phase changes from one phase at cycle i to the next at cycle i + 1; time spans, Ti, reflect driving rhythm intervals:

$$\varphi_{+1} = \varphi_t + \left(T_{t+1} - T_t\right)/p - KF(\varphi_t),\qquad 7.1$$

where $F(\varphi_i) = -1/2\pi$ [sin $2\pi \varphi$; mod -0.50 to $+0.50$, and **K** is a coupling parameter gauging marker salience; p, this latent period, was approximately 600 ms.

This model was applied to performance in a time-change detection task that required people to detect a single changed (target) time interval planted in an isochronous test rhythm. The test region was surrounded by a rhythmic context that varied in regularity. The model predicts that a listener's ability to detect a time-change target in the test region depends on the expectancy violation created by a target, which should increase with (1) the magnitude of a target interval change (i.e., expectancy violation) and (2) the overall regularity of the surrounding rhythmic context (i.e., oscillator strength). Both predictions were confirmed.[12]

Entrainment Regions Revisited

Dynamic attending theory (DAT) draws on another critical construct introduced in earlier chapters: the *entrainment region*. To see how this works, consider the most elementary case of quasi-isochrony: an isochronous driving rhythm with a single deviant (target) interval. For example, the fifth sound (open oval) in the isochronous rhythm of Figure 7.1A might shift to create a shorter/longer time span relative to other T values in this sequential context. However, as a time pattern, the preceding T values opening this sequence render a dynamic opening context that entrains the driven oscillation with a period, p ~ T. The period, p, reflects a latent expectancy which is violated if a deviant time span suddenly appears. The deviant time is denoted by T'. To cope with this change, a listener may ignore it or adapt, such that p' ~ T'. What happens ultimately depends on the entrainment region associated with this exogenous driving–driven dyad.

An entrainment region is typically pegged to a particular attractor. Figure 7.3 shows a hypothetical entraining region for the simplest attractor, n:m = 1:1 (i.e., p ~ T) along a continuum of driving–driven time ratios (abscissa). On the ordinate is a measure of driving rhythms coupling

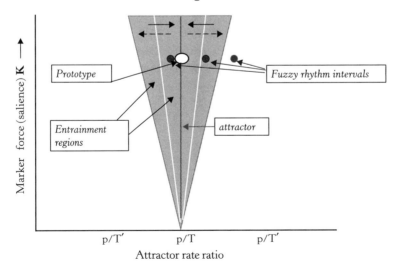

An entrainment region:
Weak and strong oscillations

Prototype

Fuzzy rhythm intervals

Entrainment regions

attractor

Marker force (salience) **K** →

p/T'   p/T   p/T'

Attractor rate ratio

FIGURE 7.3 An entrainment region is shown as a bluish gray V area pink area surrounding a simple vertical attractor line (n:m). Generally, the width of an entrainment region increases with force or salience of a driving rhythm (ordinate) and decreases with the strength of a driven rhythm (white vs. black category boundary limits). Prototypes (e.g., pure isochrony) fall along the attractor line. Categorical instances expressing quasi-isochrony (tokens with p/T') fall inside this entrainment region (dark gray dots). Not shown are corrected (i.e., manifest) periods, p'; however, for complete correction p' ~ T'. Opposing arrows reflect push (dashed) versus pull (solid) effects of perturbations versus attractors.

strength (**k**). Stronger driving rhythms produce a wider range of coupling with deviant time spans. The entrainment region, here V-shaped, is termed an "Arnold tongue;" it made a brief appearance in the preceding chapter. In general, the width of a tongue determines the momentary range of partial corrections allowable in adapting p′ to p. The inner strength of a driven rhythm is also expressed in this figure. Narrower entrainment regions (white lines) apply to stronger driven oscillations whereas wider regions apply with weak driven oscillations (black lines). In other words, this captures the tendency of a strong oscillation to hover close to its latent period and that of a weak oscillation to allow drifting from its latent period, thus becoming more responsive to a perturbing stimulus.

Returning to the exemplar isochronous driven rhythm in Figure 7.1A, a listener experiencing such a sound pattern operates with an expectancy based on p ∼ T (i.e., p/T ∼ 1.0). This signals the simple attractor of n:m = 1:1. Next, Figure 7.3 illustrates a prototypical isochronous stimulus that earns a special location within the Arnold tongue entrainment region: A prototype, **O**, here aligns with its attractor, i.e., vertical line where p = T, hence p/T = 1.0. Along this line are prototypical driving rhythms of various strengths, **k** (ordinate). Also note that as coupling strength, **k**, increases and the entrainment region widens.

Next consider what happens when a driving rhythm is quasi-isochronous. Shown Figure 7.3 are dark gray ovals that illustrate relationships of several disruptive time intervals to a prototype (vertical line). In each case, the gray oval represents a single time change from prior temporal regularity, creating one (or two) deviant time intervals, denoted Tj′. In turn, this leads to a different ratio: p/T′. The three deviant time spans hypothesized in Figure 7.3 reflect different degrees of deviation associated, respectively, with these gray ovals. Within this entrainment region, a deviant close to the prototype (p/T), is likely to be "pulled" toward this attractor, essentially realizing assimilation (p′ ∼ p; see solid arrow). On the other hand, more deviant time changes will reflect corrective changes that reflect the 'push' of a disruptive force. In this case, adaptive changes that shift toward the changed time interval become evident in a driven oscillation's manifest period, p′, as it is pushed away from its latent period, p. That is, an adaptive "push" of the oscillation is rendered by a perturbing stimulus, T′ (dashed arrow) which forces p′ away from p. Such is the gist of a push-pull relationship. These deviations earn render the

otherwise isochronous rhythm the label of a fuzzy rhythm.

Other factors also influence people's responses to fuzzy rhythms. These involve properties of entrainment regions considered in the next sections (summarized in Box 7.1). Note that this builds on distinctions of partial (p′ ≠ T′) and complete (p′ = T′) phase corrections.

Coupling strength, **k**, reflects the salience of a perturbation (i.e., the force of a time marker). A more powerful perturbation levies a stronger corrective push on an oscillation, forcing it away from an attractor and toward alignment with T′. In other words, higher **k** values increase the chances that a listener's attention is captured by a deviant time interval.

Driving Rhythm Regularity/Irregularity

Fuzziness increases with the number of deviations in a driving rhythm. A strictly isochronous driving rhythm corresponds to a prototype stimulus rhythm that matches the attractor: p/T = n/m for all T values (e.g., Figure 7.3A) creating "pure" isochrony and earning a prototypical locus on the vertical attractor line: **o**. By contrast, any irregularity created by one or more T′ values contributes to a quasi-isochronous rhythm, as in Figure 7.1B (e.g., T′ values of 646, 558, 596).[13]

Oscillator Strength

An active oscillation can be weak (white line) or strong (black outline) as in Figure 7.3. A variety of factors contribute to oscillator strength (already discussed). Stronger oscillations have narrow entrainment regions, rendering them less responsive in adapting to a deviant time interval. Essentially, strong oscillations "stay on message": they stay near p.

Traditional Mode-Locking: Various Faces of Isochrony

Distinguishing prototypical rhythms from fuzzy rhythms is important because speech as well as music is filled with fuzzy isochronous rhythms. For instance, the speech phrase 'How are you?" is most simply described in terms of approximate periodic recurrences of hypothetical marker sounds of syllable onsets.[14] So, too, other sound-making activities fit into a rough isochronous format such as a light "rap, rap" on a door. Yet isochrony is disguised in various other forms in speech and music. Sometimes it is hidden in quasi-isochronous rhythms, but it is also commonly obscured by the overlapping presence of

> # BOX 7.1
> ## SUMMARY OF ENTRAINMENT REGION PROPERTIES
>
> Six properties of attunement during entrainment are summarized with reference to the entrainment region of a particular attractor ratio, $n{:}m$:
>
> 1. An *entrainment region*: Limits phase- or mode-locking to a perturbing time interval, T', given a fixed n:m attractor.
> 2. *Coupling strength*, K: Associated with salience of a perturbing time marker in a driving rhythm. Higher **K** values determine a wider entrainment region.
> 3. *Oscillator strength*: Stronger driven oscillations yield narrower entrainment regions (white vs. black outlines in Figure 7.3).
> 4. *Driving rhythm irregularity*: Variable driving rhythms in, for example, fuzzy rhythms contain one or more deviant time intervals. Phase-locking to any deviant time interval is partial or complete in an entrainment region.
> 5. *Manifest periods*: Within entrainment region limits, the manifest period, p' is the changed period of an entraining oscillation (in a fuzzy rhythm) from a deviant p/T' in an entrainment region.
> 6. *Attractor complexity*: Simple attractors have wider entrainment regions than do complex ones; a complexity index on entrainment region width is termed the *devil's staircase*.

other, co-occurring isochronous driving rhythms of different rates. Combinations of multiple isochronous rhythms often yield a time pattern that "seems" non-isochronous due to percepts of emergent groups. A few examples appear in Figure 7.1C–E. These configurations reflect pleasant patterns formed by hierarchical nestings of faster patterns within slower ones. Often they heard as rhythmic groups, but, on closer inspection, it is clear that they derive from combinations of several isochronous rhythms. For instance, in Figure 7C,D, people typically hear such sequences as groups of two (binary) or three (ternary) sounds, respectively. (Note: In this figure, time markers of different rates are indicated by x and o; or for the polyrhythm of panel E, by gray dots).

Other examples of multiple isochronous driving rhythms appeared in the preceding chapter, where many fast rhythms of different rates combined to deliver pitch percepts (e.g., complex consonant vs. dissonant sounds). Complex sounds embed many different isochronous components; this leads to internalized sets of related oscillations (i.e., oscillator clusters; e.g., Table 6.1). Parallel configurations happen with sets of slower isochronous rhythms. Groups of several, simultaneously active oscillations with

different slow periods can endogenously synchronize to form slower, internalized oscillator clusters.

Similar entrainment principles apply for slow- and fast-driving rhythms because entrainment is rate-resistant. Entrainment between co-occurring rhythms with different but fixed rates has been described as *traditional mode-locking*. Traditional mode-locking between a driving and driven rhythm is a protocol based on the unchanging nature of *both* the driving and the driven rhythm. Both members of an entraining pair must be approximately isochronous rhythms. Neither the driving nor the driven rhythm can change significantly over the course of an event. The caveat of "significantly" acknowledges temporal irregularities in T and p within entrainment region limits. Minor fluctuations of fuzzy rhythms fall within the attractor's entrainment region, hence are tolerated. However, significantly large driving rhythms deviations are not tolerated in traditional mode-locking protocols. As a result, entrainments based on traditional mode-locking preserve a particular attractor throughout all cycles of a driving–driven dyad.

Traditional forms of exogenous entrainment involve a series of recurrent fixed time spans, T, that activate a neural oscillation, p (driven oscillations are omitted in this figure). This protocol holds for all examples of Figure 7.1 A–D. However, in some cases (C, D, E), it entails simultaneous activity of two (or more) entraining oscillations entraining to driving rhythms of different rates. In these contexts, the external stimulation varies over time while remaining tethered to a common internal referent. In other situations an external regularity may excite various internal oscillations (e.g., faster harmonics) that phase lock to the slower referent. The latter enables endogenous entrainments among different exogenously entraining oscillations (of different, fixed rate); in turn, *oscillator clusters* develop. A cluster is held together by one or several attractors, all constant throughout a sequence. These are *global attractors* because they do *not change throughout the event*. For example, global attractors of rhythmic clusters arising from pairs of oscillations activated in Figure 7.1C, D, E are n:m = 1:2, 2:3, and 2:3, respectively. Global attractors govern entrainments in events that follow a traditional mode-locking protocol.

Attractor Complexity and Arnold Tongues

Entrainment regions, expressed as Arnold tongues, describe limits on entrainment. However, these limits vary. From the preceding chapter, we have seen that one factor affecting entrainment region width is attractor complexity. The well-established *Arnold tongue regime* is depicted Figure 7.4. Here, different widths of entrainment regions apply to different attractors. Each attractor, expressed as a rate ratio (center vertical lines), is surrounded by a **V** entrainment region. For instance, global attractors of 1:1, 1:2, 1:3, and 2:3 apply, respectively, to patterns A through E of Figure 7.1. Rate ratios serve as complexity scores in Table 6.2. A more sophisticated, but correlated, complexity index derives from the *devil's staircase*.[15] The latter builds on the fact that entrainment region width, hence stability, increases with attractor simplicity, as in Figure 7.4. In short, a wider entrainment region, associated with a simpler *n:m* attractor ratio, specifies greater stability.

For each attractor, a prototype driving rhythm defines a category that includes fuzzy driving rhythms that fluctuate about a prototype. To illustrate, Figure 7.4 shows four entrainment regions of hypothetical fuzzy rhythms with hidden attractor (rate ratios) of 1.0, .33, .50, and .67 (at **O** points). Respectively, these attractors correspond to the five prototypical driving rhythm relations of Figure 7.1A–E. Effectively, each attractor defines a category with a central prototype that is

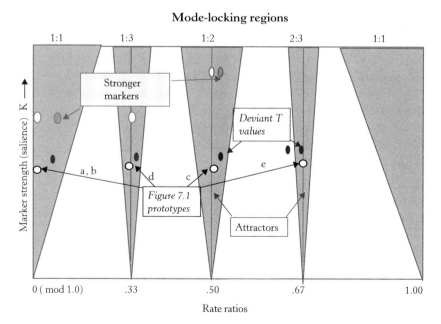

FIGURE 7.4 A schematic of several Arnold tongues, each corresponding to a different attractor (abscissa). Each of the five types of isochrony (A–E) from Figure 7.1 is shown by its respective prototypes (open circles). Also shown are hypothesized deviant (perturbing) time relations (dark gray ovals). Note that stronger marker strength (high **K** values) increases the push of a deviant time intervals (light gray ovals).

surrounded by related fuzzy tokens. Fuzzy versions (dark gray ovals) of each prototype represent a categorical token. In other words, a single deviant T' in a given rhythm functions as a category token (see caption for details). Figure 7.4 displays the generality of entrainment attractors and regions. Most striking is that entrainment regions narrow with attractor complexity, a feature critical to predictions based on attractor complexity, as demonstrated in the preceding chapter on the perception of complex sounds.

Finally, isochrony and its various guises often instill in listeners percepts of groups of sounds. This is suggested in Figure 7.4C–E. For instance, an individual may rely on a slow entraining oscillation with a period that is twice that of period T determing a presented isochronous sequence, as in Figure 7.5A (*top row*). In this case, emergent binary groups draw on a global attractor of 2:1.[16,17] However, the rhythms of Figure 7.4 and 7.5A reflect a small sample of time patterns that we normally encounter. In fact, it is not uncommon to find sequences that include multiple co-occurring isochronous and/or quasi-isochronous driving rhythms that persist throughout an event. As such, opportunities increase for ambiguity and conflicting percepts of rhythmic groupings across listeners. For psychologists familiar with individual differences, this should not be surprising.

Summary of Varieties of Isochrony

Entrainment is a robust and hardy activity. With entrainment, an oscillator survives and adapts to irregularities of fuzzy rhythms. The traditional entrainment protocol is flexible in admitting temporal fluctuations in a single driving rhythm that fool listeners into sensing that a fuzzy rhythm is "really" isochronous. This protocol also persists in rhythms comprising many co-occurring but different isochronous rhythms. And it leads to the following observation: isochrony assumes many guises wherein it continues to offer a range of opportunities for traditional entrainment modes diagnostic of more complex global attractors. Traditional mode-locking identifies specific, global attractors that vary in complexity, as formalized by an Arnold tongue regime.

Major points are:

- Isochrony has many forms in driving rhythms of different fixed rates.
- Quasi-isochrony is fuzzy isochrony featuring modest deviations from isochrony. As driving rhythms, different quasi-isochronous rhythms can implicate the same simple attractor that defines a truly isochronous rhythm: $n{:}m = 1{:}1$.
- Events that include several different, co-occurring rates of driving rhythms invite entrainment mode-locking based on rate ratios which are formalized as attractors with $n{:}m \neq 1{:}1$.
- Traditional mode-locking describes conventional entrainment. It occurs when both the driving and the driven rhythm of a dyad are isochronous or quasi-isochronous.

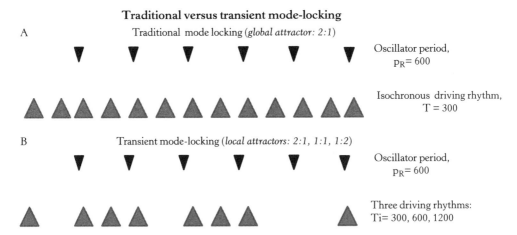

Traditional versus transient mode-locking

A   Traditional mode locking (*global attractor: 2:1*)

Oscillator period, $p_R = 600$

Isochronous driving rhythm, $T = 300$

B   Transient mode-locking (*local attractors: 2:1, 1:1, 1:2*)

Oscillator period, $p_R = 600$

Three driving rhythms: $T_i = 300, 600, 1200$

FIGURE 7.5 Traditional and transient mode-locking. Panel **A** shows traditional mode-locking in which both T and p are constant. Panel **B** shows transient mode-locking in which T is variable but p remains constant.

With a single dyad, this entrainment protocol implicates a single global attractor.

- Multiple, co-occurring isochronous rhythms (of different rates) lead to multiple, co-existing global attractors (cf. Chapter 6).
- Arnold tongue regimes express entrainment region limits as a function of the salience of a time marker, **K**, and attractor complexity.

COHERENT NON-ISOCHRONOUS RHYTHMS: TRANSIENT MODE-LOCKING

The next step of this journey takes us into true time patterns. Many environmental events simply cannot be reduced to fuzzy versions of isochrony. Nor do they neatly fit into a combination of co-occurring isochronous rhythms of different rates. Instead, they belong to distinct rhythmic categories involving patterns of truly different time intervals. Let's term these *coherent non-isochronous rhythms*.

Coherent non-isochronous time patterns are often so captivating, they cannot be ignored. This reality poses a new explanatory hurdle. Most popular time patterns we enjoy simply fail to "neatly" conform to the simple attending protocol just described as traditional mode-locking. Instead, these events have time patterns with external driving rhythms that do not conform to the traditional requirement for an isochronous driving rhythm, namely the specification of a fixed recurring time span, T (i.e., one that does not change

significantly over time). However, our acoustic soundscape is populated with a number of truly non-isochronous yet patently coherent rhythmic patterns which challenge us to invent a workable meaning of the term *coherent*.

What does coherence mean? Webster's dictionary tells us that "coherent" implies stickiness or cohesion, as well as implying a logical connection. So, a certain abstractness accrues to the meaning of coherence. Paraphrasing an old adage, "we know coherence when we feel it." In an attempt to further pin down this concept, let "coherence" apply to a set of attractor relationships implicated by successive, but significantly different time spans within a distinctly non-isochronous stimulus sequence.

Less technically, coherent non-isochronous rhythms are simply those enjoyable time patterns most familiar to us. They captivate us. The opening themes of familiar television shows, for instance, frequently exploit our fondness for certain time patterns. Fans of the TV series *Hawaii Five O* will be happy to learn that its opening moments project a coherent non-isochronous rhythm comprising five (similar) short time intervals followed by two distinctly longer time spans. Other musical examples are plentiful. On a higher plane, the famous beginning of Beethoven's fifth symphony is another compelling example with its short-short-short-long rhythm.[18] Beyond musical examples, compelling time patterns in speech have long intrigued psycholinguists because they are tantalizing

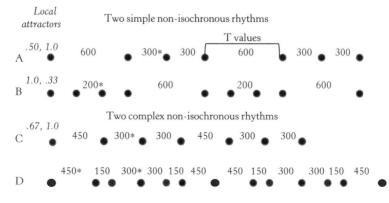

Varieties of non-isochronous rhythms
Four prototypical rhythms with commensurate time ratios

FIGURE 7.6 Four prototypical non-isochronous rhythms. Two of these interweave simple time ratios in panels **A** and **B** (implicating local attractors). Two others form patterns of more complex time relationships in panels **C** and **D**, where the latter affords ambiguity about candidates for most common T value (*).

approximations to certain iconic rhythmic forms such as *long-short* (trochaic), *short-long* (iambic), *long-short-short* (dactyl), and so on. In music, similar coherence is found in the anapest musical phrasing comprising a series of short time spans (quarter or eighth notes) followed by a final, distinctively longer one (a whole note) which is a simple multiple of preceding time spans.

As few visual illustrations of such patterns appear in Figure 7.6 and Figure 7.7 (*bottom*). These stimulus sequences reflect several non-isochronous rhythms that differ significantly from their isochronous counterparts in Figure 7.1. Overall, these rhythms cannot be described as either isochronous or quasi-isochronous time patterns. Instead, all present stimulus time spans, Ti, that change significantly over the course of an event.

This section attempts to explain why such time patterns nonetheless "seem" so coherent that they engage our attending in an entrainment-like fashion. This explanation rests on three main points that differentiate entrainments to non-isochronous time patterns from that of traditional mode-locking evident with strictly isochronous external time patterns, as in the preceding section. These points are:

- *Changing driving rhythms (time spans).* Mode-locking can be transitory. Non-isochronous rhythms contain a series

of time spans that differ significantly, providing a succession of changing driving rhythms. For instance, a pattern may open with two or three time spans, Tj, of 300 ms which are then followed by several different time spans (e.g., of 450 ms and/or 600 ms). Consequently, a listener must flexibly change mode-locking orders to synchronize attending with subsequent time spans. In other words, a given mode-locking state is not fixed over time, as in traditional mode-locking which involves only unchanging isochronous driving rhythms.

- *An unchanging driven rhythm (i.e., a common driven period, p_R).* In traditional mode-locking, the period, p, of an induced oscillation does not drastically change throughout an event. This is also the case with transient mode-locking. Even with non-isochronous time patterns, a sustained driven period reflects the ongoing operation of a stable internal rhythm. This driven rhythm represents a strong oscillation, one that persists as an *internalized referent period, p_R,* over a series of different external driving rhythms in an event. Hence, one way in which this referent emerges as an active oscillation is through stimulation is by one of the several different driving rhythms in a non-isochronous, but

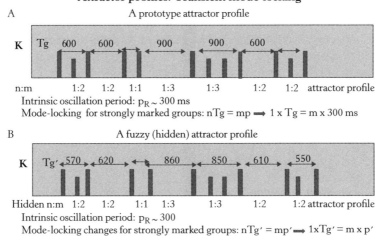

Attractor profiles: Transient mode-locking

A   A prototype attractor profile

K Tg 600   600   900   900   600

n:m   1:2   1:2   1:1   1:3   1:3   1:2   1:2 attractor profile
Intrinsic oscillation period: $p_R \sim 300$ ms
Mode-locking for strongly marked groups: $nTg = mp \Rightarrow 1 \times Tg = m \times 300$ ms

B   A fuzzy (hidden) attractor profile

K Tg' 570 620   860   850   610   550

Hidden n:m 1:2   1:2   1:1   1:3   1:3   1:2   1:2 attractor profile
Intrinsic oscillation period: $p_R \sim 300$
Mode-locking changes for strongly marked groups: $nTg' = mp' \Rightarrow 1 \times Tg' = m \times p'$

FIGURE 7.7 Two attractor profiles illustrate results of transient mode-locking. Panel **A** shows changing driving rhythms, Tg, of group time spans. Within each group, weaker time markers subdivide these time spans to create different n:m ratios. Assuming a referent oscillator period of $p_R \sim 300$ ms, a series of local attractors are implicated that form a prototype attractor profile. In panel **B**, Tg vary as a fuzzy rhythm. Local hidden attractors lead to the same attractor profile as in panel **A**.

coherent, sequence. For instance, in the above example, the Ti of 300 ms may function as a persisting referent. This instills, via resonance, a critical *referent periodicity, p_R*. As an event unfolds, then, subsequent external driving rhythms, as successive time spans, Tj, become fleetingly coupled to this persisting referent period: Tj:p_R.

- *Attractor profile.* Successive Tj driving rhythm time spans, referenced to p_R, lead to a series of local attractor ratios, implicated by Tj:p_R tokens. Thus, instead of *global attractors,* which characterize traditional mode-locking, transient mode-locking yields a series *local attractors.* Together, they form an *attractor profile*: a serial ordering of local attractor ratios.

Transient Mode-Locking

The preceding proposal implies that certain time patterns, containing distinctive driving rhythm changes create a series of driving–driven dyads that deny a traditional entrainment protocol. Instead, this section considers how these coherent time patterns enable *transient mode-locking.* This entrainment protocol features fleeting bouts of entrainment to each successive (local) driving rhythm, all referenced to the same sustaining driven rhythm.

To flesh out transient mode-locking, imagine the following situation: a listener hears a sound pattern containing a series of very different stimulus time spans. One option is that a listener perceives temporal chaos. Oddly enough, this rarely happens. More often listeners are caught up in such sequences, reading into them some inner structure. Traditional mode-locking has trouble explaining this because this conventional entrainment protocol is linked to the premise of the *stationarity of both* driving and driven rhythms.

Transient mode-locking, by contrast, requires stationarity *only for the driven rhythm.* That is, an entraining neural oscillation retains its persisting, unchanging, latent period. A driven rhythm functions as an self-sustaining internal referent periodicity. Transient mode-locking portrays each successive, brief, driving rhythm as "bouncing off" this referent period. More precisely, it features a listener fleetingly phase-locking with each successive time interval in a non-isochronous time pattern. Any sequence containing several novel time intervals, Ti (i indexes ordinal time in sequence), immediately connects (couples) each

successive time span with the persisting temporal expectancy carried by an ongoing referent oscillation (p_R).[19]

So, what activates this referent periodicity? Most obvious candidates are initial and/or common time spans in an unfolding event that invite a resonant p_R. Indeed, there is a certain primacy of beginnings. Transient mode-locking, then, relies on the growing strength of this internal periodicity. As an event unfolds, successive time spans (Ti, Ti + 1, etc.) function as fleeting driving rhythms that briefly connect with the sustaining referent oscillation. In this fashion, this neural oscillation serially phase-locks with successive driving rhythms. According to transient mode-locking: *a listener responds to each successive time span, Ti, in an event by automatically referencing it to a persisting referent period, pR, that behaves as if the external time span reflects a continuing driving rhythm.*

Schematic contrasts of traditional mode-locking versus transient mode-locking, defined in Table 7.1, appear in Figure 7.5A,B. External driving rhythms for both entrainment protocols evoke reactive pulses, shown in light gray, these rhythms engage a driven (oscillator) rhythm shown as dark gray (expectancy) pulses. However, note that with a traditional mode-locking protocol (panel A), two cycles of an isochronous driving rhythm (T = 300 ms) readily fit into a sustaining period of a slower entraining oscillation (p = 600 ms). This stationary driven rhythm is one of many spontaneous, ongoing neural oscillations in a tunable brain. In panel A, it delivers a single 2:1 global attractor, fixed throughout an entrainment episode. By contrast, a transient mode-locking protocol (pane B) parades three different time spans in a non-isochronous time pattern. This driving rhythm pattern lacks stationarity because Ti is a time span of 300, 600, or 1,200 ms. Instead, a listener automatically synchronizes in a transitory fashion to (truncated) driving rhythms. This instantly references each time span to the same ongoing driven oscillation. As a result, given a p_R of 600 ms, transient mode-locking creates a series of *local attractors*: 2:1-1:1-1:2.

In sum, the same oscillator periodicity figures as an internal driven rhythm in both entrainment protocols. Only the outside world changes when shifting from traditional to transient mode-locking of attending. With traditional modes of entrainment, this leads to global attractor states. Alternatively, with the entrainment protocol of transient mode-locking, the result is a series of local attractors within an attractor profile.

Implications of Transient Mode-Locking

Transient mode-locking is a new construct. Consequently, it requires the usual experimental vetting. Nevertheless, it is a reasonable concept which raises interesting questions about vetting avenues. For instance, transient mode-locking rests on the assumption that an ongoing neural oscillation, alerted briefly via resonance, persists and begins to serially develop an attractor profile. Indeed, one can imagine this internal referent as a persisting background beat in music or as a listener's tendency to "hold on to" the talking rate of a particular speaker during a conversation. In these and other contexts, the external stimulation varies over time while remaining tethered to a common internal referent. As such, transient mode-locking has broad implications for understanding our ability to fluently track changing rhythmic soundscapes, especially when other factors are also considered (e.g., k, regularity, attractor complexities, strength of referent oscillation, etc.). A range of issues surrounding this new concept remain to be explored.

One point deserves a final comment. The attractor profile delivered by transient mode-locking is a new idea with novel implications. For instance, this profile instantiates a serial order of local attractors that putatively appeals our inborn sensitivity for abstracted time relationships. Moreover, the form of mode-locking implies that profiles with many simple attractors are preferred over those with many complex attractors. Thus, in Figure 7.5B, the prototypical attractor profile of 2:1-1:1-1:2 comprises only simple attractors. However other, more ambiguous or fuzzy versions of a rhythmic time pattern may motivate listeners to gravitate to simpler (vs. complex) profiles. Thus, the dactyl rhythm (in Figure 7.6A) boasts several simple attractors, whereas rhythms in Figure 7.6C,D lead to more complex attractors. Although in theory all these patterns can promote transient mode-locking of attending, entrainment should be more effective with time patterns based on simpler local attractors (Figure 7.6A,B) than for those with complex local attractors Figure 7.6C,D.

Fuzzy Rhythms and Transient Mode-Locking

Rarefied laboratory contexts usually do not capture the fleeting experiences people have as they interact conversationally with friends, listen to music, engage in the timely back and forth of tennis, or generally respond to other dynamically changing environmental events. However, transient mode-locking comes closer to offering a tool to address these fluid situations than does the traditional mode-locking protocol. This is because it addresses how people automatically adjust attending, in-the-moment, to inevitable changes in ordinary driving rhythms. A variety of idealized non-isochronous time patterns appear in Figure 7.6 (and Figure 7.5B). It is possible to dream up many more.

Again, a reality check is in order. Although the non-isochronous driving rhythms discussed thus far do widen the scope of rhythmic influences on attending, the examples presented in Figure 7.6 remain rather constrained as time patterns. Basically, they are "too pretty" for the messiness of the real world. Clearly, neat dactyl patterns that precisely realize rational time ratios are rare. Yet "dactyl-like" rhythms are quite common in both speech and music across different cultures. Our ordinary environment is filled with natural communicative exchanges checkered with vocalized sound patterns that whisk back and forth between listeners and speakers at varying speaking rates and generally in messy forms. To simplify this point, the actual production of the non-isochronous prototypical rhythm of Figure 7.6A is unlikely to be exactly 600-300-300-600-300-300 (ms). Instead, it will probably arrive as a fuzzy rhythm such as 610-291-330-620-308-340 (ms). And especially in rapid speech, we routinely create utterances containing brief slurs and inadvertent pauses here and there. Yet, these fuzzy time patterns seem to be "good enough" to make sense to a listener. Amazingly, they remain intelligible.

The Return of Fuzzy Rhythms

The ability of listeners to transcend the fuzzy surface structure of a rhythmic event stems from the governing power of attractors hidden beneath surface unruliness. This power is operative in transient mode-locking, where hidden attractors are local attractors. Nevertheless, resulting attractor profiles influence a listener's sense of the inner structure of this event. In spite of superficial irregularities, people often blithely and effortlessly follow seemingly problematic rhythms.

Theoretically, to keep in touch with such patterns listeners rely on internal expectancies carried by an induced referent period, p_R. Consequently, their momentary adaptive responses to any unexpected time span, T', in a stimulus time pattern is based on a rational multiple or subdivision of an oscillation's manifest period, p_R', wherein this referent period is influenced by the nearest hidden attractor. In short, depending on this adaptive activity, fuzzy speech time patterns are often "good enough" to convey a comprehensible utterance.

Of course, it is possible that listeners simply rely directly on superficial surface irregularities without intuiting an inner attractor profile hidden in a fuzzy rhythm. These two extremes have been discussed in earlier chapters as two opposing forces ever-present within a dynamic attending approach. This revives the *push–pull contest* (cf. solid vs. dashed arrows in Figure 7.3). Mnemonically, heavy reliance on external stimulus deviations "pushes" listener's attending to align (fully phase-correct) with a surface perturbation in the driving rhythm. For example, heavily accented speech adds surface changes to the acoustic signal that obscure a hidden attractor profile, rendering comprehension difficult for some listeners. Opposing this, at least in adults, is a strong driven rhythm that "pulls" the system in the opposite direction, toward a hidden attractor (i.e., no phase correction). This listener is not distracted by accent deviations and thus reports very good speech comprehension. Finally, most listeners experience something between these two extremes. This outcome is a "good enough" compromise.

Rhythmic Categories and Attractor Pulls

Prototypes continue to define categories of non-isochronous time patterns. But, with transient mode-locking, a category is defined by a whole set of attractors within an *attractor profile*, i.e., not by a single global attractor as with traditional mode-locking. This rekindles broader issues concerning categorization that are related to prototypes and fuzzy rhythms. The pull of an attractor profiles during transient mode-locking, especially profiles with strong local attractors, will influence how listeners respond to individual instances of a category: namely, fuzzy rhythms that share the same hidden attractor profile.

A graphic illustration of categories of non-isochronous rhythms appears in Figure 7.7. Here, in panel A, one rhythmic category is defined by a series of attractors implied by the succession of group time spans, Tg. In this panel is a prototypical stimulus that implicates a series of local n:m attractors forming an attractor profile. By contrast, in panel B, a fuzzy version of this prototype is shown. It is a token time pattern that implicates the same attractor profile (panel A). Both profiles depend on the persisting activity of the same referent oscillation: $p_R = 300$ ms. Also shown is how marker strength (**k**) figures into such a picture. That is, these examples outline a series of different time

spans based only on the salient (high **K**) markers in these rhythms. These markers highlight the longer time spans of groups, Tg, that cover (embed) shorter spans, Tj. In Figure 7.7A, local attractors are clearly implicated by group time spans (Tg) of 600, 900 ms via Tg:p_R. The resulting attractor profile is a series of simple local attractors that reflect the prototype of panel A. Figure 7.7B shows a fuzzy counterpart of panel A with deviant Tg′/p_R vectors. More generally, in a hypothetical phase space, such deviant rate ratios fall within an entrainment region where they "point to" the same attractor profile that defines the categorical prototype in panel A. In this way, a fuzzy rhythm is judged as a category instance (i.e., a token) of the same category spelled out by the prototypical attractor profile.

Evidence for Transient Mode-Locking and Attractor Profiles

Terms such as "transient mode-locking" and "attractor profile" are admittedly novel. Yet justification for these ideas comes from well-established research which confirms that people naturally prefer certain non-isochronous time patterns. A majority of research on this topic relies on motor tasks. For instance, a typical task requires a listener to synchronously tap to successive time markers in a sequence and then continue tapping once the sequence is removed or to simply reproduce it by tapping. With this topic, we come full circle from the beginning of this chapter, which opened with the classic work of Fraisse[20] and Povel[21] who relied on such tapping tasks to show that people distort tapped intervals in the direction of prototypical time patterns.[22]

More recent research on this topic has been skillfully undertaken by Bruno Repp and colleagues, who replicated classic findings surrounding responses to non-isochronous rhythms.[23] These researchers extended early studies using recycled coherent non-isochronous sequences comprising three distinctly different time intervals. They used both prototype and fuzzy versions of time patterns that implicated three different local attractor ratios (e.g., 1:1, 1:2, 1:3). Confirming classic work, they found reliable tapping differences due to attractor complexity of both the prototypical rhythms and their fuzzy counterparts. Other studies also report steadier tapping to sequences implicating simple (vs. complex) time ratios.[24,25]

Importantly, this research also confirms the "pull" of hidden attractors in its discovery of systematic distortions of fuzzy rhythms in the direction of these attractors. Thus, tapping was relatively difficult with time interval ratios of 3:2 due to stronger biases from a "pull" toward simpler attractor ratios of 2:1 and 1:1. Even skilled tappers had difficulties tapping in synchrony to sequences with hidden attractor profiles involving more complex attractor ratios, especially at fast rates.[26,27] For instance, a complex rhythm with a long-to-short ratio of 1.67 was more likely to be produced as a 1.83 ratio with faster rates (i.e., closer to a 2:1 attractor). Other biases for simpler ratios emerged in tapping to a coherent non-isochronous rhythm with an attractor profile of 3:1-3:1-2:1. People initially reverted to simpler ratios, producing intervals closer to 1:1 attractors.

Given the prevalence of motor tasks in studies of synchrony, it is tempting to conclude that observed preferences for certain rhythmic ratios reflect motor constraints, not attending biases. However, this is questionable in light of other studies that did not use motor tasks. Peter Desain, Henkjan Honing, and colleagues discovered clear evidence for listeners' preference for special time ratios in non-isochronous time patterns.[28,29] Musicians heard brief, typically fuzzy rhythms containing three time spans (e.g., 474-263-263 ms). Their reports showed overwhelming perceptual preferences for simpler time ratios. For example, the most popular response categories involved simple time ratios between successive time spans, as in 1:1:1, 1:2:1, 2:1:1, and 1:1:2.[30] One highly preferred time pattern was the iconic dactyl rhythm (long, short, short, with a 2:1:1 ratio). Interestingly, rhythmic context is also important. When presented with a metrical lead-in context of duple (2:1) or triple (3:1) ratios, listeners greatly preferred subsequent sequences with these ratios. In general, fuzzy versions of prototypical time patterns were reported to be the prototype itself, providing strong support of rhythmic categorization.

Are such biases restricted to musicians? The answer appears to be "no." Nonmusicians show similar perceptual distortions favoring simpler rate ratios (e.g., 1:1).[31,32,33,34,35] In addition, brain activity of nonmusicians, measured by functional magnetic resonance imaging (fMRI), revealed heightened sensitivity to simpler time ratios.[36]

In summary, it seems clear that "coherent," as in coherent non-isochronous time patterns, aptly describes serial time patterns with special attractor ratios. Not only do people prefer simple time ratios over complex ones, but these favored ratios also function in prototypical profiles as anchors for categorizing other (fuzzy) rhythms. In short, rhythmic categories are defined by prototypical attractor profiles.

Alternative Theories

The evidence just reviewed is consistent with entrainment concepts embodied in transient mode-locking. Following DAT, transient mode-locking is hypothesized to produce attractor profiles of varying complexity. Simple versus complex attractor profiles lead to several confirmed predictions about the perceptual distortions that people experience when presented with such patterns. The concept of attractor profiles that hide beneath the surface of a pattern's relative time structure opens new avenues for studies of differential perceptual distortions due to serial profiles of stability.

Nevertheless, two major theories that spawned much of the reviewed research rest on premises that differ fundamentally from those of DAT. Both theories concentrate on the impact of surface time structure on listeners' percepts. One rests on statistical descriptions of the surface time structure, whereas the other applies Gestalt principles to surface timing.

The statistical account draws on Bayesian algorithms.[37] In this view, biases for certain simple ratios reflect expectancies formalized as conditional probabilities involving certain surface time intervals. Specifically, people learn conditional probabilities that reflect the relative frequency of certain contingencies between surface time spans.[38]

Gestalt theory, on the other hand, relies on nativist principles to explain people's percepts of surface timing in rhythms. These principles are expressed in familiar Gestalt "laws" of proximity, continuation, and, more broadly, in the law of *prägnanz* (i.e., good figure). Handel eloquently argues for this view.[39] Applied to a rhythm's surface time structure, Gestalt laws neatly describe certain grouping effects. For instance, the proximity principle implies that percepts of tones separated by small time intervals should lead to their assimilation into a group.[40,41] Similarly, the law of continuation suggests the impact of preceding intervals on people's documented preference for isochrony.[42] The Gestalt law of *prägnanz* is a bit more mysterious but may apply to certain surface time ratios.

Gestalt theory has earned respect for its lasting influence over the past century. At one explanatory level, it "works." Yet, at a more operational level, Gestalt principles remain vague and open to various after-the-fact interpretations. For instance, temporal proximity nicely describes the fact that rhythms with relatively small surface time intervals promote grouping/assimilation percepts. Yet it does not address the fact that proximity *is inherently relative*: what is a small interval in one context may be a large one in another context. Finally, Gestalt principles are more successful in capturing an individual's intuitive response to rhythmical events than in formulating testable hypotheses about relative timing.

Dynamic Attending Theory and the Attraction of Attractors

The theories just described differ from DAT in instructive ways. Among other things, their strict adherence to the surface time structure of time patterns contrasts with DAT's emphasis on relative timing, mode-locking, and hidden attractors.

The role of attractors, especially hidden attractors, leads to predictions of perceptual distortions of surface time intervals. Attractors literally "attract"; that is, they "pull" entrained attending in certain directions. This "pull" reflects the power of synchronicity. A synchronous mode draws one's percepts toward more stable entrainment states. What is new in this chapter is that attractors operate in transient as well as traditional entrainment protocols. Transient mode-locking has the potential of instilling in listeners serial patterns of local attractors (i.e., attractor profiles).

Innateness and Attractors

Attractors capture innate predispositions according to the aging hypothesis. They reflect an automatic pull levied by synchronous goals. Attractors clearly differ in attractive power, as indexed by different widths of their related entrainment regions (e.g., Figure 7.5). These differences hold over the life span. Regardless of age, the most powerful attractors, such as $n{:}m$ = 1:1, 1:2, 1:3, remain so for the very young and old alike. Moreover, because attractors are innate, they are found universally across linguistic and musical cultures.

Issues surrounding innateness are best addressed in studies of listeners who have the least exposure to rhythmic patterns: newborns. Evidence for attractor innateness, reviewed in earlier chapters, indicates that newborns are indeed sensitive to spectral consonance in fast event rhythms. This supports the claim that attractors based on traditional mode-locking operate at the tiny event time scales of pitch and consonance. Assuming that fast event rates tap into the newborn's temporal niche, this also reinforces the aging hypothesis. Moreover, other evidence indicates that young infants also respond to attractors in slower rhythms.

Newborns respond to implied beats in relatively slow rhythmic patterns based on simple duple meter ratios.[43,44] Also, they differentiate similar relative time differences in linguistic stress patterns (disyllabic vs. trisyllabic words).[45] Relevant, too, is classic work of Demany and colleagues on rhythm perception in 2-month-old infants.[46] They found that these infants differentiated among time patterns with commensurate time ratios where component time spans were based on multiples of 100 ms (hence relative times of 1:1, 1:2, 1:3). These infants had no difficulty distinguishing an isochronous series of 100 ms time intervals from a non-isochronous one of 100-200-300-200 ms.[47] More telling, these infants distinguished among different coherent non-isochronous rhythms with the same but reordered time spans that specified different attractor profiles. Finally, older infants (e.g., 6–12 months) exhibit clear sensitivity to iambic and trochaic time patterns in speech rhythms.[48] All of this suggests that rhythm perception, based on commensurate time relations, is innate or emerges very early in life.[49]

Sensitive Infants: The Research of Sandra Trehub

Over the years, Sandra Trehub has brilliantly demonstrated that we often underestimate the perceptual acumen of very young infants.[50,51] With Erin Hannon, she argued for a domain-general approach to infants' early perception of speech and music. In several important studies, they found that infants (6 months old) distinguished among various coherent non-isochronous rhythms (e.g., as in Figure 7.7). At this age, infants are sensitive to certain slower time patterns. Accordingly, these slow rhythms included time patterns with attractors popular in Western folk songs (e.g., 2:1 ratios), as well as other time patterns with more complex local attractors (e.g., 3:2) popular in Balkan folk tunes. Young infants readily detected deviant time changes planted in all time patterns, implying an early general sensitivity to various attractors. Therefore, it is interesting that this culture generality disappeared in older infants and adults.[52] Adults familiar only with Western music failed to spot the same time deviations in complex (Balkan) rhythms that young infants detected.

It appears that, very early in life, infants are equal-opportunity listeners: they can "tune in" to various non-isochronous time patterns, exploiting a native sensitivity to many different attractor profiles. However, this ability vanishes by the end of their first year, apparently overcome by early learning via exposure to native time patterns. This is consistent with the claim that infants arrive in the world prepared to attune to the rhythms of many different attractor profiles. Early orienting of attending then jump-starts a learning process, resulting in speed learning of certain culture-specific attractor profiles.

Underlying this research is an important general assumption. It is that speech and music within a given cultural share similar rhythmic properties.[53] Hannon and Trehub argued that infants are better rhythm learners than adults in these contexts. They exposed 12-month-olds, who at 6 months differentiated 1:2 and 2:3 rhythms but later lost this ability, to Balkan folk music.[54] Interestingly, 12-month-olds who had lost the ability to detect timing violations in Balkan music then regained this ability, but adults did not. Western adults, given similar exposure to Balkan folk tunes, continued to exhibit a Western bias, suggesting that age of exposure is critical.

Innately Guided Learning?

The findings of Trehub and Hannon are important. They imply that we arrive in the world generally equipped to orient to all attractor relationships, not to those specific to a certain culture. This is consistent with the aging hypothesis proposal that attractors are innate.

Nevertheless, hypotheses about innate predispositions remain contentious in psychology. So-called "blank slate" theories place the burden of skill acquisition squarely on exposure frequency, sometimes formalized in conditional probabilities. In other words, infants should exhibit no early biases for privileged time relationships. Alternatively, Jusczyk[55] and others[56] favor a broader perspective, proposing instead *innately guided learning of sound patterns*. Jusczyk argued that infants have inborn domain-general capacities which allow them "to begin to make sense of sound patterns"[57][p.6] These inborn capacities bias infants' attention in ways that prepare them for rapid learning.

Clearly, these views of innate predispositions converge with those of DAT. In both traditional and transient entrainment protocols, attractors (global, local) serve as innate guides to early attending of the time patterns common in speech and music. In turn, this innate capacity facilitates perceptual learning of culture-specific patterns based on certain attractors.

Summary of Non-Isochronous Rhythms

The rhythms we live by are rarely isochronous or even quasi-isochronous. Although the varieties of isochrony discussed early in this chapter are part of the puzzle of environmental timing, also important are varieties of non-isochronous but coherent time patterns. Both kinds of rhythmic events engage our natural tendencies to find special time relationships that facilitate our goal of synchronizing with world events. In this section, the non-isochronous time patterns are shown to promote a transient mode-locking protocol that guides attending to an unfolding environmental event.

Transient mode-locking is premised on the idea that people automatically "tune-in" to non-isochronous events that carry changing driving rhythms. Often these events present as coherent time patterns, as with anapest, dactyl, and other rhythmic configurations of well-formed patterns in speech and music. These patently non-isochronous rhythms compel our attending with their potential for inducing expectancies based on a persisting, internal referent period. Transient mode-locking rests on the assumption that coherent time patterns, which do not present a single, fixed driving rhythm, nonetheless elicit a persisting driven oscillation that fleetingly responds (phase-locks) to a succession of different driving rhythm time intervals. This assumes a resiliency of certain cortical oscillations that step in to fulfill the role of supporting, referent periodicities.

As with traditional mode-locking, transient mode-locking also expresses synchronies following principles of resonance and entrainment (Table 7.1). Traditional mode-locking, discussed in early sections of this chapter, leads readily to the development of endogenous entrainments of simultaneously active oscillations and to the birth of oscillator clusters containing one (or more) global attractors. On the other hand, transient mode-locking, described in this section, leads to the growth of persisting referent oscillation that supports a series of local attractors in an attractor profile. Such profiles function as prototypes of rhythmic categories. Finally, attractors and attractor profiles are assumed to be innate. Major points in this section are:

- Transient mode-locking differs from traditional mode-locking in addressing listeners' momentary synchronies with changing driving rhythms of non-isochronous time patterns.

- Transient mode-locking entails successive, but fleeting, locking of a strong and persisting neural (referent) oscillation to the changing time spans of a non-isochronous driving rhythm.
- Transient mode-locking yields prototypical attractor profiles that define rhythmic categories.
- Support for concepts of rhythmic prototypes and related fuzzy rhythms, based on common attractor profiles, comes from both motor and perceptual tasks.

CHAPTER SUMMARY

A general property of DAT is illustrated in this chapter. It concerns how people *use time* (correctly or incorrectly) to attend to and to keep in touch with the world around them. The theme of "keeping in time" means synchronizing in various forms, as implied by traditional and transient mode-locking. Both protocols ensure connections between a listener (driven rhythms) and his immediate surrounds (driving rhythms). However fleeting, these connections between driving and driven rhythms depend on entrainments that express the way we "connect" (or fail to) with our environment. Specifically, they describe how we synchronize with various external events. At an elementary level, the entrainment protocols featured in this chapter—namely, traditional and transient mode-locking—convey a dazzling capacity to synchronize with changing environmental events. This capacity is a critical and universal one for any species. Losing it implies disorder and disengagement. Retaining it holds the promise of engagement, anticipatory attending, and communicative understanding.

This chapter concentrates on entrainments with macro-rhythms. At one extreme are slow-driving rhythms that are fairly simple in exhibiting "pure" isochrony or modest variations of it (fuzzy isochronies). At the other extreme are slow time patterns that are not isochronous, offering instead a series of different, fleeting driving rhythms. Our interactions with various isochronous event rhythms are described by traditional mode-locking protocols. By contrast, interactions with non-isochronous time patterns call for a new concept: transient mode-locking. This protocol describes mode-locking synchronies that govern attending to events with locally changing driving rhythms. This chapter explores how each mode-locking protocol allows a listener to "use" event timing to arrive at internalized prototypes and rhythmic categories.

The first half of this chapters centers on traditional mode-locking in environmental events that exhibit various forms of isochrony. Often these are fuzzy versions of isochrony (i.e., quasi-isochronous stimulus sequences); also common are events arising from combinations of multiple isochronous driving rhythms. In general, such events instill in listeners an entraining neural oscillation which carries an expectancy based on the oscillation's latent period. This mode-locking protocol builds on the stationarity of both driving and driven rhythms throughout an event. It is governed by global attractors.

The second half of this chapter broadens the picture to include environmental patterns that are neither isochronous nor quasi-isochronous. Truly non-isochronous time patterns (i.e., as in iambic and dactyl time patterns) require extending entrainment principles to describe attending to non-isochronous rhythms. Unlike external driving rhythms in traditional mode-locking, the driving rhythms of coherent time patterns are not isochronous. Instead, they comprise coherent arrangements of changing time spans (i.e., truncated driving rhythms) that promote in listeners a different form of mode-locking: transient mode-locking.

Transient mode-locking is a new concept. It assumes that mode-locking order shifts with changes in successive time spans. A motivating assumption underlying transient mode-locking holds that a strong referent oscillation persists throughout such an event. Consequently, mode-locking opportunities (n:m) change as successive time spans of a time pattern are encountered. This leads to another new construct, the attractor profile. An attractor profile is an internalized serial pattern of local attractors. Finally, attractors, whether global or local, are assumed to be innate and responsible for early biases in infants as well as for the lasting biases observed in adults.

NOTES

1. These are poetic definitions of rhythmic time patterns.
2. When scored as quarter notes.
3. Paul Fraisse, *The Psychology of Time* (Oxford, England: Harper & Row, 1963).
4. Jeffery J. Summers, Richard Bell, and Bruce D. Burns, "Perceptual and Motor Factors in the Imitation of Simple Temporal Patterns," *Psychological Research* 51, no. 1 (June 1989): 23–27, doi:10.1007/BF00309272.

5. Ilse Lehiste, "Isochrony Reconsidered," *Journal of Phonetics* 5, no. 3 (1977): 253–63.

6. John Albertus Michon, *Timing in Temporal Tracking*, dissertation summary (Soesterberg, Netherlands: Instituut voor Zintuigfysiologie RVO-TNO, 1967), http://www.jamichon.nl/jam_writings/1967_ttt_psyfor.pdf.

7. Maren Schmidt-Kassow and Sonja A. Kotz, "Attention and Perceptual Regularity in Speech," *NeuroReport* 20, no. 18 (December 2009): 1643–47, doi:10.1097/WNR.0b013e328333b0c6.

8. Edward W. Large and Mari Riess Jones, "The Dynamics of Attending: How People Track Time-Varying Events," *Psychological Review* 106, no. 1 (1999): 119–59, doi:10.1037/0033-295X.106.1.119.

9. Mari Riess Jones, Heather Moynihan Johnston, and Jennifer Puente, "Effects of Auditory Pattern Structure on Anticipatory and Reactive Attending," *Cognitive Psychology* 53, no. 1 (August 2006): 59–96, doi:10.1016/j.cogpsych.2006.01.003.

10. J. Devin McAuley and Mari Riess Jones, "Modeling Effects of Rhythmic Context on Perceived Duration: A Comparison of Interval and Entrainment Approaches to Short-Interval Timing," *Journal of Experimental Psychology: Human Perception and Performance* 29, no. 6 (2003): 1102.

11. Edward W. Large and Mari Riess Jones, "The Dynamics of Attending: How People Track Time-Varying Events," *Psychological Review* 106, no. 1 (1999): 119–59, doi:10.1037/0033-295X.106.1.119.

12. Large and Jones, "The Dynamics of Attending: How People Track Time-Varying Events."

13. Note: If a manifest period, p′, actually matches T′ (as with small deviations) then p′/T′ resembles the attractor; e.g., if p′ adapts to a T′ of 596 ms in Figure 7.1B, then p′/T′ → p/T = 1.00).

14. Functional markers of syllables in speech (e.g., vowel onsets, stress vs. P-centers, etc.) are considered in later chapters to be tailored to speech timing.

15. Arkady Pikovsky, Michael Rosenblum, and Jürgen Kurths, *Synchronization: A Universal Concept in Nonlinear Sciences*, vol. 12 (Cambridge University Press, 2003), Cambridge, United Kingdom, https://books-google.

16. X. Pablos Martin et al., "Perceptual Biases for Rhythm: The Mismatch Negativity Latency Indexes the Privileged Status of Binary vs Non-Binary Interval Ratios," *Clinical Neurophysiology* 118, no. 12 (December 2007): 2709–15, doi:10.1016/j.clinph.2007.08.019.

17. R. Brochard et al., "The 'Ticktock' of Our Internal Clock: Direct Brain Evidence of Subjective Accents in Isochronous Sequences," *Psychological Science* 14, no. 4 (July 1, 2003): 362–66, doi:10.1111/1467-9280.24441.

18. Other examples abound in Beethoven's music, as in the opening of the second movement of his Seventh Symphony.

19. A referent oscillation is not *necessarily* the most dominant oscillation, but often it is. In this tableau, the opening parts of an event become important.

20. Fraisse, *The Psychology of Time.*

21. Dirk-Jan Povel and Peter Essens, "Perception of Temporal Patterns," *Music Perception: An Interdisciplinary Journal* 2, no. 4 (1985): 411–40.

22. From a DAT perspective, a produced motor time interval is based on the manifest period, p′, of driven oscillation.

23. Bruno H. Repp, Justin London, and Peter E. Keller, "Systematic Distortions in Musicians' Reproduction of Cyclic Three-Interval Rhythms," *Music Perception: An Interdisciplinary Journal* 30, no. 3 (February 1, 2013): 291–305, doi:10.1525/mp.2012.30.3.291.

24. Jeffery J. Summers, Simon R. Hawkins, and Helen Mayers, "Imitation and Production of Interval Ratios," *Perception & Psychophysics* 39, no. 6 (November 1986): 437–44, doi:10.3758/BF03207072.

25. Geoffrey L. Collier and Charles E. Wright, "Temporal Rescaling of Simple and Complex Ratios in Rhythmic Tapping," *Journal of Experimental Psychology: Human Perception and Performance* 21, no. 3 (1995): 602–27, doi:10.1037/0096-1523.21.3.602.

26. Joel S. Snyder et al., "Synchronization and Continuation Tapping to Complex Meters," *Music Perception* 24, no. 2 (December 2006): 135–46, doi:10.1525/mp.2006.24.2.135.

27. Also, faster tempi exaggerated these tendencies. For instance, in studies of Repp and colleagues, a complex rhythm with a long-to-short ratio of 1.67 was more likely to be produced as a 1.83 ratio (i.e., closer to 2:1) with faster rates.

28. Peter Desain and Henkjan Honing, "The Formation of Rhythmic Categories and Metric Priming," *Perception* 32, no. 3 (March 1, 2003): 341–65, doi:10.1068/p3370.

29. Makiko Sadakata, Peter Desain, and Henkjan Honing, "The Bayesian Way to Relate Rhythm Perception and Production," *Music Perception: An Interdisciplinary Journal* 23, no. 3 (2006): 269–88, doi:10.1525/mp.2006.23.3.269.

30. These are *surface time ratios* $T_1:T_2:T_3$, *not* $T_j:p_i$ ratios, but they readily convert to attractor profile estimates.

31. Gert Ten Hoopen et al., "Time-Shrinking and Categorical Temporal Ratio Perception," *Music Perception: An Interdisciplinary Journal* 24, no. 1 (September 1, 2006): 1–22, doi:10.1525/mp.2006.24.1.1.

32. Gert ten Hoopen et al., "Auditory Isochrony: Time Shrinking and Temporal Patterns," *Perception* 24, no. 5 (May 1, 1995): 577–93, doi:10.1068/p240577.

33. Ryota Miyauchi and Yoshitaka Nakajima, "The Category of 1:1 Ratio Caused by Assimilation of Two Neighboring Empty Time Intervals," *Human Movement Science* 26, no. 5 (October 2007): 717–27, doi:10.1016/j.humov.2007.07.008.

34. Yoshitaka Nakajima et al., "Time-Shrinking: A Discontinuity in the Perception of Auditory Temporal

Patterns," *Perception & Psychophysics* 51, no. 5 (September 1992): 504–07, doi:10.3758/BF03211646.

35. Yoshitaka Nakajima et al., "Time-Shrinking: The Process of Unilateral Temporal Assimilation," *Perception* 33, no. 9 (September 1, 2004): 1061–79, doi:10.1068/p5061.

36. Katsuyuki Sakai et al., "Neural Representation of a Rhythm Depends on Its Interval Ratio," *Journal of Neuroscience* 19, no. 22 (1999): 10074–81.

37. Sadakata, Desain, and Honing, "The Bayesian Way to Relate Rhythm Perception and Production."

38. Pieter-Jan Maes, "Sensorimotor Grounding of Musical Embodiment and the Role of Prediction: A Review," *Frontiers in Psychology* 7 (March 4, 2016), 1–10, doi:10.3389/fpsyg.2016.00308.

39. Stephen Handel, *Listening: An Introduction to the Perception of Auditory Events*, vol. xii (Cambridge, MA: MIT Press, 1993).

40. Takayuki Sasaki et al., "Time-Shrinking, Its Propagation, and Gestalt Principles," *Perception & Psychophysics* 64, no. 6 (August 2002): 919–31, doi:10.3758/BF03196796.

41. Yoshitaka Nakajima et al., "Time-Shrinking: The Process of Unilateral Temporal Assimilation," *Perception* 33, no. 9 (September 1, 2004): 1061–79, doi:10.1068/p5061.

42. Gert ten Hoopen et al., "Auditory Isochrony: Time Shrinking and Temporal Patterns," *Perception* 24, no. 5 (May 1, 1995): 577–93, doi:10.1068/p240577.

43. István Winkler et al., "Newborn Infants Detect the Beat in Music," *Proceedings of the National Academy of Sciences* 106, no. 7 (February 17, 2009): 2468–71, doi:10.1073/pnas.0809035106.

44. Henkjan Honing et al., "Is Beat Induction Innate or Learned?" *Annals of the New York Academy of Sciences* 1169, no. 1 (July 1, 2009): 93–96, doi:10.1111/j.1749-6632.2009.04761.x.

45. Alessandra Sansavini, Josiane Bertoncini, and Giuliana Giovanelli, "Newborns Discriminate the Rhythm of Multisyllabic Stressed Words," *Developmental Psychology* 33, no. 1 (1997): 3–11, doi:10.1037/0012-1649.33.1.3.

46. Laurent Demany, Beryl Mckenzie, and Eliane Vurpillot, "Rhythm Perception in Early Infancy,"

Nature 266, no. 5604 (April 21, 1977): 718–19, doi:10.1038/266718a0.

47. Actually, the base interval was 97 ms.

48. James L. Morgan and Jenny R. Saffran, "Emerging Integration of Sequential and Suprasegmental Information in Preverbal Speech Segmentation," *Child Development* 66, no. 4 (August 1, 1995): 911–36, doi:10.1111/j.1467-8624.1995.tb00913.x.

49. Hsing-Wu Chang and Sandra E. Trehub, "Auditory Processing of Relational Information by Young Infants," *Journal of Experimental Child Psychology* 24, no. 2 (October 1977): 324–31, doi:10.1016/0022-0965(77)90010-8.

50. Erin E. Hannon and Sandra E. Trehub, "Metrical Categories in Infancy and Adulthood," *Psychological Science* 16, no. 1 (January 1, 2005): 48–55, doi:10.1111/j.0956-7976.2005.00779.x.

51. E. E. Hannon and S. E. Trehub, "Tuning in to Musical Rhythms: Infants Learn More Readily than Adults," *Proceedings of the National Academy of Sciences* 102, no. 35 (August 30, 2005): 12639–43, doi:10.1073/pnas.0504254102.

52. Among adults, only listeners familiar with both musical cultures detected deviant timing in simple and complex (attractor) rhythms. Adults familiar only with Western music failed to spot the time deviations in complex (Balkan) rhythms that young infants detected.

53. Aniruddh D. Patel, John R. Iversen, and Jason C. Rosenberg, "Comparing the Rhythm and Melody of Speech and Music: The Case of British English and French," *Journal of the Acoustical Society of America* 119, no. 5 (2006): 3034, doi:10.1121/1.2179657.

54. Hannon and Trehub, "Tuning in to Musical Rhythms: Infants Learn More Readily than Adults."

55. P. W. Jusczyk, *Language, Speech, and Communication. The Discovery of Spoken Language* (Cambridge, MA: MIT Press, 1997).

56. P. Marler, "Song Learning: The Interface between Behaviour and Neuroethology," *Philosophical Transactions of the Royal Society B: Biological Sciences* 329, no. 1253 (August 29, 1990): 109–14, doi:10.1098/rstb.1990.0155.

57. Jusczyk, *Language, Speech, and Communication. The Discovery of Spoken Language.*

8

Parallelism

Expectancy and Production Profiles

The ability to "keep time" refers to the momentary tracking of a dynamic environmental event. Sometimes our natural tendencies for "keeping" time are apparent as we tap a foot "in time" with a tune heard on the radio. But synchronies of attending are less obvious. For example, a common teaching ploy to ascertain if a student has been attending happens when a teacher suddenly announces "Bill, what would you do in this case?" Put on the spot, Bill may belatedly try to mentally "replay" parts of the teacher's preceding remarks after the fact (assuming he *was* attending).

But "replaying" a past speech event does not equate with the original act of attending, which entails keeping time mentally with an event *as it is produced*. Yet psychologists rarely tackle dynamics of this "in-the-moment" attending, relying instead on memory tasks that focus on a "replay." This invites concepts such as phonological loops, rehearsal buffers, codes, and the like. This chapter, by contrast, invites a focus on in-the-moment attending.

As social animals, the events we produce during social exchanges reveal our continuous reliance on back-and-forth, in-the-moment communicative signals. Social roles are played out in speaker–listener interactions that bear intriguing resemblance to "call-and-answer" exchanges in other species. We regularly switch speaker/listener roles during conversations, alternatively producing an utterance then listening to a reply. It is evident when one produces conventional exchanges such as "Hello, how are you?" then listens to the answer: "Fine, thanks." Call-and-answer interactions observe rhythmical conventions.[1] These conventions acknowledge time-tracking sensitivities that abide in both partners who seamlessly switch between producing and attending. Moreover, this activity not only depends on the synchronicity essential to "keeping time," it also hints at a mirroring, or parallelism, between the time structures involved in producing an event and those involved in attending to it. Arguably, this parallelism suggests that role changes (i.e., talker vs. listener) do not necessitate fundamental changes in the mechanisms underlying production and attending.

The idea of parallelism between production and attending is explored in this chapter. Certain unspoken rules of engagement are similar during exchanges in communicative duets. Speakers and listeners are playing the same game with somewhat similar rules. This chapter proposes that a deep commonality obtains between synchronized attending to an event, which relies on driven rhythm expectancies, and well-timed productions of the same event that generates driving rhythms.

CHAPTER GOALS

This chapter addresses three goals. One goal tackles similarities between expectancies about events and productions that create communicative events, as captured in the concept of parallelism. The first two sections, respectively, develop expectancy and production profiles with this in mind.

A second goal involves unpacking parallel features in production and attending arising from involuntary and voluntary factors. This revives the general attending hypothesis, which features both involuntary and voluntary attending components. This chapter fleshes out distinctions between involuntary and voluntary factors that affect how we produce various acoustic signals (musical or speech-like) and their counterparts in expectancies that mirror these productions.

A third goal, addressed in a final section, offers empirical validations of concepts of productions and expectancies and their parallelism, including voluntary and involuntary contributions to parallelism.

EXPECTANCY PROFILES: CREATING ANTICIPATORY DRIVEN RHYTHMS

In Chapter 7, expectancies were equated with the latent period (p) of an entraining oscillation. Such expectancies are internalized, but fallible, anticipations or "guesses" about "when" something will happen in the future as some event unfolds. However, such a periodicity may also function in producing such an event. That is, underlying expectancies can prepare a speaker or musician to generate certain expected actions. But, during a production, other factors may intervene that lead to incorporation of a new type of manifest period (also described in Chapter 7). That is, manifest periods (p′) have been described as internal corrective responses to violations of latent expectancies (p), often arising from irregularities of fuzzy driving rhythms. In an attempt to relate constructs of production and perceptions, this chapter develops a new version of p′ that figures in overt responses i.e., production, namely, **r**p′. Finally, continuing themes from Chapter 7, this chapter proposes a parallelism between expectancies formed by listeners and productions created by speakers and musicians.

Expectancy Profiles: Attractor Profiles and Timing

Expectancy is broad concept. In this chapter, it is fleshed out using two factors that contribute to a person's expectancy. One factor is an internalized attractor profile, introduced in Chapter 7. Another factor, also from Chapter 7, is tethered to this profile; it involves a driven rhythm's ongoing referent period. That is, as we have seen, an attractor profile, which reflects a serial ordering of local attractors, depends on the nature of a prevailing referent oscillation. However, practically, serial ordering is somewhat vague in that it does not specify exactly "when" each local attractor in a profile will happen. Here the referent oscillation (of a profile) plays an important role. An attractor profile is abstract, but, when combined with the rate of a strong internal referent oscillation, it becomes real. Finally, an internal attractor profile of some event depends on both a series of local (i) attractors of this event and the rate with which local attractors unfold in real time. More formally, from a listener's perspective, an expectancy is based on both a reliance on an underlying attractor profile (i.e., an ordered series of *mi:ni* ratios, and an implied rate (i.e., an index of p, which is supplied by the referent oscillation).

An Example Expectancy

Consider a very detailed example, spelled out in Figure 8.1. It illustrates momentary expectancies involving the phrase, "Take this book." This figure is schematized as a realistic fuzzy rhythm involving three different external (marked) time spans, Ti (600-540-660 ms; **i** indexes serial location, i = 1, 2, 3). As a produced fuzzy rhythm, these time spans realize a timing irregularity that *hides* an underlying series of attractors for the *mi:ni* attractor profile of **1:1-1:1-1:1.** In short, this speech production hides an isochrony. As such, it will induce in listeners correlated, i.e., parallel, expectancies (from Chapter 7). Despite surface irregularities, this phrase projects to listeners a sense of an underlying regularity in a listener. The hidden attractor profile motivates listeners to anticipate isochrony in the phrase "Take this book."

Nevertheless, irregularities in this production cannot be ignored. We must also specify how listeners handle timing irregularities, *in the moment*. In theory, speech irregularities create violations of a listener's expectancies that are based on the latent entraining oscillation. To this point, such violations have been described as a triggers to listeners who rapidly, and *automatically*, correct their expectancies, where the expectancies are carried by a driven rhythm with period p. Following phase response curves (PRCs), the resulting phase shifts lead to momentary p modifications expressed by p′. Specifically, by incorporating involuntarily corrected expectancies over time, an *involuntary expectancy profile develops*; it is denoted **IEi** (Ti).

Figure 8.1 traces the development of successive, and corrected, expectancies, p′, experienced by a listener hearing the production "Take this book." To detail this, consider the three word time spans Ti where i varies for 600, 540, 660 ms.[2] Notice that both latent, p (black lines), and manifest, p′ (lighter gray) are shown in this figure. Oscillator periods function as expectancies for each word's time span, Ti (from Chapter 7). In this case, the manifest (corrected) periods, p′ are respectively 600, 564, and 654 ms. This figure, then, expresses an internalized series of corrected time spans (manifest periods) that form neither an isochronous sequence nor one that matches the three external time spans. Hence, this example illustrates adaptive attending adjustments of a hypothetical listener to a fuzzy speech rhythm. It reflects 'good enough' attending/perceiving of this phrase.

Figure 8.1 (*lower panel*) details the resulting involuntary expectancy over time (i) as: **I Ei (Ti))** = *mi:ni* pi′. This formula incorporates

A fuzzy rhythm
Two expectancy profiles

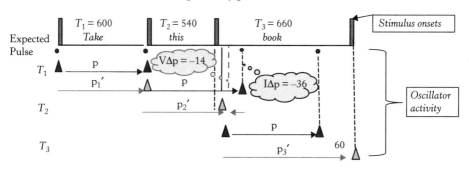

	T_1	T_2	T_3	
Terms		Period and phase properties		Formulae
Intrinsic period (ms)	600	600	600	p
Manifest period (I Ei)	600	564	654	$p_i' = p + \Delta pi$
Phase shift (PS)	0	−60	+90	$t_{onset} - t_{expected\ pulse}$
Phase correction (PCR):	0	−36	+54	$PCR_i = -F(\varphi_{i-1}) = I\Delta p$
New phase (φ_i):	0	−.06	.09	$\varphi_i = (1 - PCR_i)/p$
I Expectancy, I Ei (T_i):	600	564	654	$(m_i/n_i)p_i'$
V Expectancy, V Ei (T_i)	600	550	660	$(m_i/n_i)[p + f(I\Delta pi + V\Delta\ pi]$

FIGURE 8.1 An introduction to terminology of expectancy profiles of a fuzzy rhythm. A pattern of three time spans: Ti of 600, 540, and 660 illustrates hypothesized adaptations by a listener to T_1, T_2, and T_3. The T_1 establishes an initial expectancy of p = p′ = 600 ms (p is darker horizontal line; p′ lighter gray horizontal line). The p_2′ adapts (shortens) to T_2 (shortening), then (expanding) to T_3. Terms (below) provide formulas for involuntary expectancies, I E(Ti), and involuntary expectancies, V E(Ti); see also Box 8.1.

both momentary attractors plus an adjusted index of sequence rate (i.e., pi′, where pi′ can differ from p; i.e., pi′ = Δp).

A major theme in this chapter involves the parallelism between a listener and a producer as this is reflected in corrected expectancies of a listener relative to the produced timing of a speaker or performer. This idea is captured by comparing a speaker's timed production of the phrase "Take this book" (Figure 8.1, *top line*: 600-540-660 ms) with the momentary attractor profile of a listener who automatically monitors this phrase (*bottom*: **IEi (Ti)**: 600-564-654 ms). Finally, it is possible to claim that a production profile draws on the same attractor profile as a listener's involuntary expectancy profile. That is, both speaker and listener use the same, i.e., the nearest, local attractors where all *n:m* = 1:1; both reflect the impact of an underlying isochrony on both production and expectancy.

Involuntary and Voluntary Attending
The expectancy profile just described is not the whole story. This profile [notated as I Ei (Ti)]

assumes that a listener's corrective attending reactions to this quasi-isochronous phrase are entirely automatic (i.e., involuntary). However, this is not true. Not all of the corrections to expectancy violations are not voluntary. Listeners can also willfully correct an ongoing expectancy. That is, in addition to involuntary phase corrections, listeners can voluntarily correct ongoing expectancies. In this chapter, the distinction between an involuntary phase correction and a voluntary one is important [see VEi (Ti) in Figure 8.1]. It is important not only because it reflects results of accumulating research on attending, but also because most entrainment models typically assume that all adaptive phase corrections are automatic. Yet, mounting evidence suggests this is not so.

Accordingly, this chapter distinguishes involuntary expectancies, in which corrective responses of the manifest period of p′ are denoted by I∆p′, from voluntary corrections of p′, denoted as V∆p′. By definition, automatic changes are always present when a listener responds to fuzzy rhythms. Conversely, also by definition, voluntary corrections are optional. When present, a V∆p′

recognizes a listener's capacity to exert conscious control over phase corrections.

Involuntary Expectancy Profiles

Any expectancy profile typically incorporates some fundamental involuntary adjustments. In Figure 8.1, the involuntary expectancy profile spells out a listener's momentary expectancies about this phrase. This is formalized in Equation 8.1 as **I Ei** (Ti)) = (mi/ni) pi'+ ε (where ε is random error) (see Box 8.1). So, the momentary expectancy for Ti depends on a particular attractor plus the current manifest period, p'. Here notice that

p' = p + IΔpi. In other words, at any moment, the IΔpi represents a listener's involuntary correction in attending to an unexpected time span, Ti.

A detailed application of these constructs appears in Figure 8.1. For continuity with preceding chapters, the bottom panel summarizes entrainment terminology (e.g., phase shift [PS] and phase correct response [PCR]). Let us step through this example, beginning with assuming that a listener's latent oscillator period, given the first word of this phrase, is p = p' = T1 = 600 ms. This starts things off with an initial bias, i.e., an expectancy that T2, will continue with $m_2{:}n_2$

BOX 8.1
EXPECTANCY PROFILES AND PRODUCTION PROFILES

TWO TYPES OF EXPECTANCY PROFILES

An *expectancy profile* reflects a listener's internal expectancies based on a combination of an attractor profile and the period (latent or manifest) of an active oscillation. An *involuntary expectancy* about time spans depends on automatic phase corrections to unexpected timing variations. A *voluntary expectancy profile* about time spans includes automatic and voluntary phase adjustments combined additively.

An *involuntary expectancy profile* is:

$$\mathbf{IEi\big(Ti\big) = \big(mi\,/\,ni\big)p_i{}' + \varepsilon} \quad \text{where } \mathbf{p_i{}' = p + I\Delta p_i} \qquad \textbf{8.1}$$

This simplifies for prototypical (non-fuzzy) rhythms where pi' = p.
A *voluntary expectancy profile* is:

$$\mathbf{V\,Ei\big(Ti\big) = \big(mi\,/\,ni\big)pi' + \varepsilon} \qquad 8.2$$

where $\mathbf{pi' = p + }f\mathbf{(I\Delta pi + V\Delta pi)}$.

A voluntary expectancy profile reflects an additive combination of voluntary with involuntary corrections in the tempo curve. Together, the latter follows a (nonlinear) function, *f*.

PRODUCTION PROFILES

A production profile relies on an expectancy profile to produce a series of motor acts. It depends on changes in a tempo response curve, **rpi'** that parallels pi' but is *not identical* to pi'. Changes in **rpi** reflect both involuntary (**I**) and voluntary (**V**) influences on motor activity (i.e., **IrΔpi** and **VrΔpi**, respectively).

A *production profile* for surface time intervals (e.g., either T or Tg) is:

$$\mathbf{Pi\big(Ti\big) = \big(mi\,/\,ni\big)rpi' + \varepsilon} \qquad 8.3$$

where $\mathbf{rpi' = p + \Delta pi}$ and $\mathbf{\Delta pi = }f\mathbf{(Ir\Delta pi + Vr\Delta pi)}$.

Note: As $\mathbf{V\Delta p_i}$ *(in Equation 8.2) approaches* $\mathbf{Vr\Delta p_i}$ *(Equation 8.3), then* **Ei** (Ti) ~ **Pi** (Ti).

$(p_2') = 600$ ms. But, not uncommonly this expectancy, which is based on isochrony (i.e., mi:ni= 1:1), is violated by −60 ms with a T2 = 540 ms. Accordingly, an instant correction to this deviation shortens p′. This automatic correction delivers a momentary phase correction, a PCR of −36 ms; hence, IE_2 is 564 ms, which is closer to 540 (i.e., $p'_2 = p + I\Delta p_2 = 600 - 36$ ms). This is shown in a balloon outlined by dark gray line in Figure 8.1.

However, some listeners may go further, adding another correction that is consciously thought out, i.e., a voluntary correction. Figure 8.1 also illustrates this in the light gray balloon (as a change of -14 ms). Together, involuntary and voluntary corrections are shown to deliver an adjusted expectancy for the time span, T_2 of 550 ms (VE_2) (bottom row in Figure 8.1). In short, listeners who intentionally modify p′ will create a V∆pi. The result is $p' = p + f(I\Delta pi + V\Delta pi)$ (Equation 8.2).[3,4]

Arguably, the fuzzy surface structure of the phrases speakers produce, as in Figure 8.1, is rarely random. Instead, often such irregularities afford meaningful time changes produced by a speaker to highlight important words. For instance, both "Take" and "book" are longer than longer than "this." It is pertinent that automatic responses to surface changes preserve some informative surface features. This is accomplished with the manifest period, p′ (i.e., I∆pi′), which lead to the $I Ei$ (Ti) that retains some surface features.[5] Note that these automatic phase adjustments are typically *partial* corrections in that they reflect an incomplete "push" of the oscillator's period toward a deviant time span (e.g., here 540 and 660 ms).[6]

Finally, this example of involuntary and voluntary actions of an oscillation, while detailed, involves a relatively short and simple rhythm. Yet, concepts of involuntary and voluntary phase/period corrections are quite general, extending much beyond this tutorial example to more complex events in speech and music. The main goal in Figure 8.1 is to offer concrete illustrations of how people may generate dynamic expectancies that are continuously violated and corrected, involuntarily and, optionally, voluntarily. See also Box 8.1.[7]

Discussions of fuzzy rhythms are essential because most of the sound patterns we encounter in speech and musical domains *are* fuzzy rhythms; that is, they are not prototypical patterns. Instead, they are often interesting, meaningful, variations of a prototype. Therefore, it is important to recognize that we operate in acoustic environments filled with a variety of different fuzzy rhythms. For example, instead of the quasi-isochronous phrase of Figure 8.1, it is common to encounter a fuzzy version, i.e., a token, of a dactyl time pattern (e.g., 600, 290, 320 ms), which elicits expectancies based on the prototype of 600, 300, 300 ms.

More About Voluntary Expectancy Profiles

The preceding section used a speech example to illustrate the idea of fuzzy rhythms and our responses to them. These rhythms stimulate corrective inner responses in the form of either involuntary expectancies (**IEi** (Ti) or voluntary expectancies, **VEi**(Ti). This section focuses on voluntary expectancy profiles using an example from the musical domain. One aim is to highlight the communicative nature of certain irregularities. The term irregularity often suggests randomness or nose. But in the present framework, it can also reflect the presence of meaningful deviations from a prototype. This is evident in the fuzzy rhythms of music, where the distinction between involuntary expectancies and voluntary ones assumes a greater role.

A Music-Like Example

Bill has been fiddling with a new drum he received for his birthday. He playfully plans to tap out a string of grouped sounds. Figure 8.2 outlines a rhythm Bill produces that comprises groups of two, three, and four tones. Here, the louder sounds mark beginnings and ends of groups, suggesting two different time scales in this rhythm.

Let us focus on the slower time scale Bill produces. Here, the louder sounds define group time spans, Tgi. Thus, the top row of Figure 8.2 shows a series of seven rhythmic groups that constitute a musical production profile, **P**(Tgi). This stimulus rhythm is more complex than the speech rhythm of Figure 8.1. Not only is the produced surface structure longer and fuzzier than that of "Take this book," it does not hide an isochronous attractor profile. Instead, it hides a more complex series of hidden attractors, that are identified in this figure as *mi:ni* ratios (in black). If Bill's produced event is heard by friends, then one hypothetical listener would hear this by relying on an intrinsic oscillation with p ~600 ms. As such, this listener would sense a series of hidden attractors such as 1:2 and 3:2 and 1:1.

But the degree to which Bill communicates this to listeners depends on his musical skills. His production profile will be more or less successful in conveying such a hidden attractor profile to listeners. In this case, let us consider that a listener tracks this rhythm by relying on her voluntary

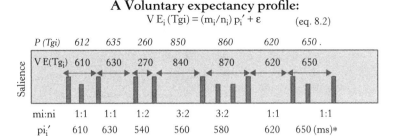

A Voluntary expectancy profile:

$$V E_i (Tgi) = (m_i/n_i)\, p_i' + \varepsilon \quad \text{(eq. 8.2)}$$

P (Tgi)	612	635	260	850	860	620	650 .
V E(Tg_i)	610	630	270	840	870	620	650

mi:ni	1:1	1:1	1:2	3:2	3:2	1:1	1:1
p_i'	610	630	540	560	580	620	650 (ms)*
pi'	610	620	560	590	590	610	620 (ms)

A fuzzy rhythm with two stimulus time scales:
Tg is higher level span; Ti is lower level span.

Intrinsic oscillation period for Tg time scale: p ~ 600 ms.
*p′ is a voluntary manifest period: $p_i' = p_i + f\,(I\Delta p_i + V\Delta p_i)$.
p′ is an involuntary manifest period: $p_i' = p_i + I\Delta p_i$

FIGURE 8.2 P(Tgi) is a production profile outlined for the slower time spans of a grouping pattern where successive time spans are marked by louder sounds. **V** Ei (Ti) is a voluntary expectancy profile which is based on an attractor profile (mi:/ni) and the voluntary period, p′ (asterisk; Equation 8.2). Note that a **V** Ei (Ti) based on this p′ is influenced by voluntary (V∆pi′) and involuntary phase corrections (I∆pi′).

expectancies, **V** Ei(Tgi). Figure 8.1 illustrated that such expectancies will include momentary adjustments to irregularities that are voluntary as well as involuntary corrections. Together, these adjustments allow listeners to more or less closely track Bill's performance (i.e., his production profile).

To be more precise, Equation 8.2 (Box 8.1) spells out a listener's attending as involving a voluntary expectancy profile, **VEi** (Tgi). This expectancy profile requires multiplying each *mi:ni* ratio in series of groups with a corresponding manifest attractor pi′. In turn, pi′ depends on *both* involuntary and voluntary corrections (i.e., I∆pi +V∆pi).[8] In this example, a listener then tracks Bill's production profile fairly well if **V** Ei(Tgi) ~ **P** (Tgi). In a sense, this illustrates an underlying parallelism between the voluntary expectancy of a listener and the voluntary production of a musical performer. It also suggests how listeners may achieve synchrony of attending with a musical performance.

Unpacking these ideas, we find that voluntary and involuntary factors contribute additively to the formation of the voluntary expectancy profiles of Bill's listeners. And these factors also figure in Bill's productions. Furthermore, while the automaticity of involuntary forces has been firmly established in research on produced and perceived phase-corrections, less is known about voluntary forces.[9,10] Nevertheless, voluntary factors may figure in listeners' fine-tuning of their phase corrections in response to certain deviations while listening to speech as well as musical events. By contrast, listeners have little control over responses

to other deviations that also violate expectancies. This refers to listeners' automatic phase correction to subtle changes in speech or musical production. For instance, detections of stimulus modulations that provoke ever-present automatic phase corrections cannot be suppressed by instructions to voluntarily ignore a particular modulation. For instance, people explicitly told to *ignore all timing deviations* in a produced sequence cannot do this! This is consistent with the theoretical assumption that manifest periods depend on default, automatic phase corrections that simply cannot be suppressed.[11]

The most important research on the topic of voluntary versus involuntary phase corrections is attributable to Bruno Repp.[12] For instance, Repp observed that during synchronous tapping people continuously refine their skills, shifting from automatic taps that lag sequenced sounds early in training to voluntary anticipations of sounds later in training. More generally, Box 8.2 summarizes Repp's prolific research on phase correction behaviors in responding to music-like sequences, research that has strongly influenced this discussion.

In light of discoveries of widespread adaptive behaviors, perhaps we underestimate the importance of commonplace activities on people's early brain "tuning." For instance, when infants play "paddy cake" with adults, they experience quite simple timing relationships that contribute to early refinements of their timing expectancies. Ultimately, these acquired expectancy profiles

---

BOX 8.2
Q AND A: EIGHT QUESTIONS POSED BY BRUNO REPP
(SEE TEXT FOR REFERENCES)

Here are extracted answers to a series of questions, all of which have been addressed at some point in the impressive research of Bruno Repp.

1. **Q:** Do listeners always *automatically* produce a phase correction response (a PCR) to a time change in rhythm?
   A: No. Sometimes the correction has a voluntary component.

2. **Q:** In a regular rhythm, if a PCR occurs to a time deviation (i.e., a phase shift [PS]), is this a rapid, immediate correction?
   A: Yes, theoretically. However, a motor manifestation of a PCR often appears later (e.g., with the next tone).

3. **Q:** In tapping tasks, is a corrective adjustment, a PCR, largely motor or perceptual?
   A: Perceptual.

4. **Q:** Do people only phase-correct to supraluminal (perceivable) time deviations?
   A: No. They phase-correct to both subliminal and supraluminal time deviations.

5. **Q:** Are subliminal phase corrections automatic?
   A: Yes.

6. **Q:** Is phase correction affected by marker salience?
   A: Yes. Perturbations by more intense sounds lead to greater adaptivity (larger PCRs) than those of less intense sounds.

7. **Q:** Is phase correction affected by the magnitude of a time deviation?
   A: Yes. The PCR increases linearly with magnitude of Δt up to a point that reflects a change of between 12% and 20% of the sequence rate (i.e., of the intrinsic p).

8. **Q:** Does the PCR always show complete (100%) correction; that is, is $|PCR| = |\Delta t|$?
   A: No. An automatic phase correction to a single phase shift typically covers about 60% of the PS (within entrainment limits); that is, PCR = .6PS. However, this may vary (e.g., see Repp references 9–12, 51–55, and 62–64).

---

come under voluntary control; that is, they serve as voluntary expectancy profiles. It turns out that voluntary expectancy profiles are more naturally embraced by listeners. By definition, they are more flexible because voluntary components are open to change. On the other hand, involuntary expectancies are less flexible; indeed, sequences based only on involuntary expectancies seem mechanical. In short, typically both inherent (involuntary) and acquired (voluntary) biases operate when listeners track attractor profiles (Box 8.2), but they are more aware of the voluntary influences.

Finally, this discussion invites a reflection on the practice of labeling certain variable rhythms as "fuzzy." In later sections, this term comes under scrutiny as various nonrandom deviations from attractors are shown to reflect meaningful crafted timing fluctuations.[13] In this vein, we cannot ignore the effectiveness of certain voluntary timing variations that result in gifted oratory in speech or in inspired interpretive musical performances of otherwise plain scores. Behind all the present notations/formulas surrounding this discussion of production and expectancy profiles is a simple truth: sound patterns in speech and music are filled with timing variations that are often cleverly shaped by skilled speakers and musicians to project specific, often hidden, meanings to a listener. This topic is revisited later in this chapter.

Alternative Views of Expectancies: Motor Productions

At this point, it is important to acknowledge alternative views of expectancies. Although the preceding account acknowledges a parallelism between production and expectancies, it focuses upon hypotheses about expectancies that putatively determine synchronized attending.

However, this view has been disputed. Prominent alternative explanations feature a major role for motor behaviors. These theories are motivated by motor tapping tasks which encourage people to synchronize motor gestures with rhythmically distributed sounds.

One shortcoming with motor explanation relates to findings that tappers often produce inexplicable anticipatory motor acts based on preceding time structures. People appear to effortlessly anticipate forthcoming sounds in some rhythms but not others. Although it is possible that a manifest (entrained) expectancy, p′, governs rhythmic responses in tapping experiments, most tapping theories focus strictly on motor activity and not on driving rhythms with the potential for entraining neural oscillations underlying attending/expectancies.[14,15]

Nevertheless, studies of synchronized motor tapping behaviors have illuminated much about phase corrections. However, explanations of motor models emphasize the temporal disparity between a sound's onset and a tap: $t_{tone\ onset} - t_{motor\ tap}$. By contrast, expectancy violations emphasize temporal disparity between a sound's actual and expected (pulse) onset time: $t_{tone\ onset} - t_{expected\ pulse}$. Also, motor models assume that the magnitude of a phase correction response is a linear function of the sound-to-tap time interval. Thus, whether a deviant time change is 10 ms or 100 ms, a corrective response is a fixed proportion of the resulting onset to tap interval.[16,17,18] Alternatively, with dynamical systems models, the sound-to-expected pulse interval has a nonlinear relation with phase correction (f in Box 8.1). Still other reasons to question a strictly motor account come from phase corrective behaviors that happen in the absence of overt taps, suggesting that people's responses depend on expectancies about sounds, not motor onsets.

Finally, linear models of corrective motor behaviors differ from a class of motor models originating from a dynamical systems approach, as described by Scott Kelso.[19,20,21,22] (See Large and Kolen[23] for an interesting discussion.) Generally, dynamical models hold that a driven oscillation determines a temporal expectancy based jointly on its period and phase, with expectancy violations leading to nonlinear corrections of phase and period.

SUMMARY OF EXPECTANCY PROFILES

Time patterns embedded in speech and music afford listeners a basis for transient mode-locking and attractor profiles. Attractor profiles form the core of expectancies for a listener when activated by an internal referent period, p, for an attractor profile (and manifest period of p′). The core of an expectancy profile is an attractor profile that realized in real time by a persisting referent tempo, p.

Expectancy profiles extend to fuzzy rhythms. These rhythms evoke phase corrections in response to deviations from attractor states in a (hidden) attractor profile. This section acknowledges that these phase corrections inevitably have an involuntary component, and they may also have voluntary contributions.

The major points in this section are:

- Listeners initially guide attending to an event using *involuntary expectancies* that depend on an attractor profile (*ni:mi*) combined with a latent (p) or manifest (p′) oscillator period (**I Ei** (Ti) = (*mi/ni*) pi′).
- Involuntary expectancies in fuzzy rhythms reflect manifest periods, pi′, influenced *only* by involuntary corrections (pi′ = p +**I**Δpi).
- Voluntary expectancies reflect manifest periods determined by *both* voluntary plus involuntary correction factors (**V**Δpi) = (*mi/ni*) pi′ where pi′ = p + f (**I**Δpi + **V**Δpi)).
- Motor models of synchronized tapping do not include temporal expectancies.

PRODUCTION PROFILES AND DRIVING RHYTHMS

The communicative events we routinely encounter in music and speech are acoustic rhythms packaged as *production profiles, P(Ti)*. This section pursues the idea that a production profile created by one person, induces a parallel profile, i.e., an expectancy profile, experienced by another. Ultimately, the rhythms within these two profiles form dyads that in ordinary environments lead to the loops of call-and-answer cycles between speaker and listener. In these exchanges, produced sound patterns created by one individual parallel expectancies of another individual. Effectively, speaker–listener interactions exhibit *parallelism*. Here parallelism simply means that a production profile and an expectancy profile share common core constructs. One shared construct is an *attractor profile*. Another is a *tempo curve*.

The tempo curve is a new concept. This idea builds on the primary rate of an external time pattern in a production profile. Simply put, this rate governs the onset times of successive local attractors in produced profiles. It expresses the tempo in which an attractor profile unfolds. Most interesting is the fact that in music and speech this tempo is typically modulated over the course of an attractor profile, creating a *tempo curve.* Modulations are conveyed by a speaker or performer who either unwittingly (involuntarily) or intentionally (voluntarily) speeds up or slows down his speaking rate during the production of an attractor profile. We have all experience that gifted speaker show slows her speech over certain phrases; similarly, who has not experienced the shifting tempo of musical patterns, designed to evoke tension in the listener.

Tempo curves of production profiles affect listeners' expectancies. Thus, in a listener's expectancy profile, these tempo modulations manifest as changes in the basic referent periodicity of a strong oscillation. In a listener's expectancy profile, the opening tempo of production, together with subsequent tempo modulations, lead to manifest changes in the periodicity of the ongoing referent oscillation as experienced by a listener. Listeners not only experience this oscillation's stable latent period, p, they also experience manifest periods, p′ which follow from their own involuntary and (optionally) voluntary corrective activities, sparked by modulations of the produced tempo. That is, a listener exposed to local event time changes created by a produced tempo curve will not only resonate to the latent tempo, but this listener will also attempt to adaptively track the produced period's ups and downs with momentary changes in her own internal periodicity (p′).

Creating a Production Profile: The Origin of Driving Rhythms

In the larger scheme of things, an entrainment scenario holds that production profiles still consist of driving rhythms. Speakers and musicians produce these profiles, which function as temporal skeletons of their communications. So, we must not forget elements that make constituent driving rhythm effective. Given the general attending hypothesis, it seems clear that effective driving rhythms must have important time marker properties, among them strength and regularity. This section reviews these properties.

Marking Time: Physical Determinants of Time Markers of Driving Rhythms

In theory, forceful driving rhythms that figure in a production profile must have salient time markers. That is, recurrent time spans stand out when outlined by certain physical changes, discontinuity, or acceleration along a dimension. For instance, a change in intensity (or frequency,

duration) effectively "marks" the onsets of time spans (e.g., louder sounds of Figure 8.2). The idea of physical change prompts the question: Change relative to what? The answer is that a physical change is calibrated relative to a preceding serial context. Candidate dimensions are the usual suspects: intensity, duration, frequency, and a few others.[24] Also, stress is a common time marker in fluent speech; stress may depend on increments either in intensity or duration (or both). But intensity changes often top the list of effective time markers in both music and speech.[25]

Is force all there is? Arguably, in sound sequences, intensity modulations are a major source of driving rhythm force, consistent with the general attending hypothesis. Although external force, loosely associated with stimulus intensity/amplitude, is an undeniable source of marker strength (e.g., K levels), physical change along other dimensions cannot be ruled out. For instance, in a time pattern, a lengthened ending sound, as in an iambic rhythm (short-long), typically captures attention, whereas heightened intensity beginning a sequence (loud-soft) often identifies a trochaic figure (long-short).[26] Debates surround the role of sound frequency as a source of time-marking.[27,28] Undoubtedly, co-variation of physical changes heighten marker salience (louder-plus-longer or longer-plus-higher frequency). Moreover, physical change is validated as a source of subjective salience by Kluender and colleagues who discovered that people exhibit enhanced perceptual sensitivity to physically changed sounds.[29,30]

Temporal Regularity of Objective Time Markers: Zeitgebers

An effective driving rhythm is not only forceful, it must also be temporally regular. Well—sort of. In the world of entrainment models, regularity is a relative matter. Curiously, timing of distinctive time markers is not *rigidly* regular. In fact, this laxness complicated the original discovery of "driving rhythms," deemed *zeitgebers*.[31] That is, one of several (admittedly circular) definitions of *zeitgeber* is "A time giver: Any external stimulus that will entrain or re-phase a biological rhythm."[22][p.366] Curiously, *rigid* regularity is not even mentioned in defining a *zeitgeber*! So the idea of "approximate" regularity lives on: a critical time marker must recur, but not with strict isochrony.

Since its relatively recent origin in biological sciences, the idea of time markers spread widely, culminating in the respected field of chronobiology.[32] Despite early debates over circadian rhythms, it is now broadly accepted that recurring physical changes, not only in light, but in many other salient physical changes, definitely entrain biological rhythms.[33,34]

How Much Irregularity?
There is a Goldilocks principle in play on this topic: no irregularity is dull, and too much irregularity in a sequence won't work. Effective driving rhythms must have "just enough" irregularity to keep a listener engaged but not so much that one becomes disengaged.

So, if temporal irregularity is admissible, what is "too much?" A psychophysics perspective on this topic claims that average deviations exceeding 5% of a hypothesized time marker period are intolerable. This converges with the Weber fractions discovered in time discrimination.[35] Yet numerous examples in this and preceding chapters exceed this limit.

Dynamic attending models dramatically loosen the Weber fraction constraint. Given entrainment principles, limits on driving rhythm variations are not fixed in stone. Instead, the disruptive potential of deviant time spans depends on many factors including the surrounding context of driving rhythms and driven rhythm strength (i.e., push–pull factors). Consequently, all-or-none psychophysical thresholds differ from those of entrainment region limits. Accordingly, in an entrainment framework, it is not uncommon to find tolerance for timing deviations exceeding 15% of a mean intermarker time interval in a surrounding context.

Time Scales of Time Markers
Theoretically, regularity applies universally to successive time intervals within any time scale, fast or slow. So, too, driven rhythms have varying biological time scales, from the very fast events supporting pitch perception (Chapter 6) to other, somewhat slower periodicities of EEG categories (beta, gamma) as well as the much slower neural oscillations (circadian, seasonal period). In principle, if these oscillations include limit cycle properties, then all may function as endogenous driving (or driven) rhythms. Driving rhythm regularity abides within different time scales.

Importantly, we can identify distinctive time markers of various time scales in light of an interesting correlation between marker strength and rhythmic time spans: stronger time markers are correlated with longer time intervals in a sequence. This correlation is confirmed by Tilsen and Johnson.[36] Using Fourier analysis to decompose filtered complex speech signals, they identified multiple overlapping quasi-isochronous component rhythms. The resulting *rhythm spectrum* ranged from fast driving rhythms (e.g., periods of 167 ms) to slower ones (e.g., 2 seconds) marked by stronger time markers. In short, rough regularity of overlapping rhythmic components, with different time scales (tempi), is real in speech.

These discoveries of Tilsen and Johnson are important. First, they show that beneath the surface timing of a composite speech signal lurk many candidates for driving rhythms of different rates. Second, they recovered time scales correlated with marker strength where slower rhythms are marked by correspondingly stronger time markers (i.e., higher amplitudes).[37,38] This echoes certain earlier approaches to speech timing.[39] Remarkably, they uncovered a strong rhythm with a period near 600 ms, commonly associated with P-centers (e.g., in nuclear vowels). Tilsen and Johnson conclude: "Our method finds that while some utterances in English do exhibit stress-based rhythm, others have a clear syllable-based rhythm, and still others exhibit more regular intervals on a phrasal time-scale, i.e., between pitch-accented syllables."[36]

In sum, along with the discovery of a rhythm spectrum, the role of marker strength reinforces a marker strength, **MS**, rule: *faster rhythms, marked by weaker time markers, nest within slower rhythms with periods outlined by stronger timemarkers.*[40] This idea is illustrated in Figure 8.2 for two time scales. Longer group time spans (Tgi) are outlined by time markers with correspondingly higher salient markers. The **MS** rule suggests an Alice in Wonderland shrinkage: as marker salience attenuates, their time intervals shrink.

Production Profiles: Parallels with Expectancy Profiles
Production profiles, unlike expectancy profiles, are observable. This is evident in Figures 8.1 and 8.2. In speech, production profiles appear in the phrases people utter, whereas in music they appear in the songs we sing. In both domains, a production profile is the temporal skeleton of driving rhythms. In speech, they feature phrases devoid of meaty semantics. In music, they trace out the abstract timing (e.g., meter, rhythm) of a musical event devoid of its melody.

In the Beginning . . . Are Expectancy Profiles

A premise in this framework maintains that while production profiles emerge early in life, within a maturing listener they are preceded by growing expectancy profiles. As evident in the preceding chapters on aging, early in life, infants tend to orient to certain sound patterns *before* they can produce them. This suggests a primacy for the development of expectancy profiles. Moreover, early expectancies are triggered by automatic responses of infants to ambient sounds produced by caregivers. In short, in a maturing infant, rudimentary expectancies—namely, involuntary expectancy profiles—begin to develop before corresponding motor activities that support an infant's own production profiles.

Infants' involuntary expectancies ride on culture-general attractor profiles. In the first year of life, these involuntary expectancy profiles begin to plant roots of primitive production profiles based largely on involuntary expectancy profiles.[41] And, eventually, with exposure, these initial expectancies grow into voluntary expectancies that reinforce certain culture-specific attractor profiles. Later in the first year of life, refined voluntary expectancies emerge (e.g., **Ei** (Ti)) which then facilitate the generation of parallel production profiles (e.g., **P**(Tgi)).

Attractor profiles, then, are naturally hidden in both expectancy and production profiles. This implies that attractors are the heart of parallelism. Expectancies of young infants draw on certain attractor profiles that lead to archetypical production profiles, evident in babbling and other common vocal gestures in infants. Nevertheless, initial "starter" expectancy profiles are incomplete. They provide infants with a production plan for a first pass at creating novel time patterns. In the arc of maturation, early expectancy profiles, acquired from listening to caretakers, set the stage for an infant's later mastery of more challenging production profiles. Expectancy profiles offer stepping stones to production profiles. And at the core of both profiles is the (often) hidden attractor profile.

Attractor Profiles

As defined, an attractor profile is the rhythmic core of an expectancy profile. And, as seen, they form a major source of the parallelism between expectancy profiles and production profiles. This is illustrated in Figure 8.2. Here, attractor profiles reflect the serial order of attractors as a series of seven special time ratios. Theoretically, these are stepping stones within a profile, from one *ni:mi* attractor to the next that are constrained by each attractor's entrainment region. Figure 8.3 shows an Arnold tongue regime suggesting this serial order of these attractors (i.e., common to Figures 8.2 and 8.4). In this figure, for a particular expectancy profile, solid circles reflect produced prototype attractor ratios, and *x*'s values reflect stimulus deviations from attractor ratios. Differences between *x* and prototype values, realize timing variations (for each attractor). Basically, these deviations represent contributions from both involuntary (I∆pi)

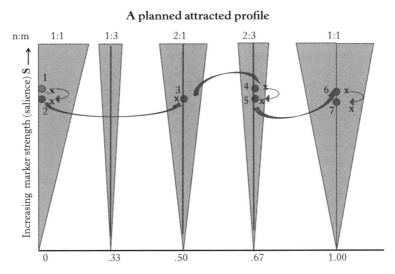

FIGURE 8.3 Arrows indicate planned serial order of attractors for the attractor profile featured in Figures 8.2 and 8.4. Numbers 1–7 correspond to serial order of attractors. The X values indicate locations of Tgi/p relative to prototype ratios (solid circles).

and voluntary (**V**Δpi) corrections originating from expectancy profiles that carry over to production profiles (see Equations 8.2 and 8.3).

The close connection between expectancies (**V E**i (Ti) and productions (**P**i (Ti)) means that, while producing an event attractor in real time, the underlying relationships of expectancies linger. In both speech and music, an inherent parallelism persists between the production and the perception of an event. Consistent with the centrality of hidden attractors in this parallelism are findings indicating that people who have produced a musical event tend to remember its abstract time relationships, not the specific gestures previously used to ornament its production profile.[42] In other words, musicians recall an abstract attractor profile more readily than particular tempo modulations involved in producing it.

Production Profiles, Response Tempo Curves, and Parallelism

The preceding discussion argues for the centrality of attractor profiles in defining both expectancy profiles and production profiles. However, the role of tempo in parallelism cannot be ignored, as this section illustrates.

The tempo of a pattern reflects the basic rate at which a string of attractors unfolds. Although tempo can be fixed over time, more often it varies. In fact, tempo variations raise a fascinating issue related to expressive timing. In production profiles, tempo variations are often expressive in bringing an attractor profile to "life". For a listener, the resulting expectancy profile carries variations in, the produced tempo that yield changes of a manifest period, pi', over time. Unlike the latent oscillator period, p, pi' changes as a listener responds to momentary timing variations in a produced time pattern. But, these tempo changes in a production profile must be distinguished from their counterpart, pi', in expectancy profiles. That is, a production profile controls motor modulations, hence its manifest tempo involves response as **r**pi' (compare Equations 8.2 and 8.3).

A production profile is a timed succession of motor responses based on a marriage of an

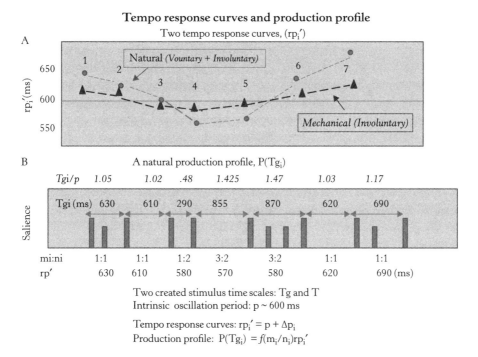

FIGURE 8.4 (**A**) Two different tempo response curves, **rp**'. One, a natural curve, combines voluntary within involuntary components (i.e., **V**Δpi' plus **I**Δpi') as in Equation 8.3. The other, a mechanical curve, depends only on automatic phase/period corrections (i.e., **I**Δpi').

(**B**) A natural production profile, P(Tgi) based on the natural tempo response curve here and the attractor profile (later). This tempo response curve is applied to group time spans, Tgi. Also shown are Tgi/p ratios that indicate X points in Figure 8.3.

attractor profile (*mi:ni*) with a *tempo response curve* (i.e., **rpi**′). This is precisely expressed in Equation 8.3. Parallelism refers to a resemblance between two components: A production profile (Equation 8.3) and an expectancy profile (Equation 8.2). In short, maximal parallelism occurs when both components (i.e., the attractor profile and pi′~ rpi′) are identical in expectancy and production profiles.

Parallelism is typically more pronounced in attractor profiles than in tempo curves. For instance, Figure 8.4A shows two examples of tempo response curves (**rpi**) producing the same attractor profile (Figure 8.4B). One curve labeled Natural (light short dashes) is noticeably more variable than the other, termed Mechanical (dark long dashes). Generally, tempo response curves in production profiles assume many forms.

In this context, we can now expand upon the topic of *expressive timing*. This refers to timing variations (i.e., deviations from an expected form) typically used by speakers or performers to instill emotion in listeners. Simply put, it involves a producer's "interpretation" of an attractor profile as expressed by a tempo response curve. In speech, for example, when talking to a friend, a speaker may momentarily vary his speaking rate by conforming to one tempo response curve, but, when speaking to a stranger he may be more constrained. That is, despite relying on the same attractor profile, in speaking to a stranger this speaker may cautiously enlist a slower, less variable, tempo response curve. Similarly in music, a sudden slowing in music, for instance, can forecast danger, thus motivating anxiety, whereas speeding up may convey gaiety. Alternatively, an isochronous rhythm, which produces a flat tempo response curve, usually conveys little emotion.

Generally, in music, tempo response curves are essential to expressive timing. They often reflect a musician's intentional plan. So, one musician may employ a plan that includes a tempo response curve designed to highlight special parts of an attractor profile, slowing at one point in time, then speeding up for other attractors. Another performer, however, may perform the same piece designed to express a very different tempo response curve, although retaining the same (scored) attractor profile.

These plans resemble consciously developed expectancy profiles. That is, what a speaker or performer produces has roots in expectancy profiles which function as action plans for production. In particular, the tempo response curve of a production

created by a speaker or performer contains tempo modulations based on plans for shaping a referent period. Such changes in a referent period, p, then refer to intended modulations of productions, pi′ (i.e., in **V**Δpi′ of Equation 8.2). Executing this plan, however, yields a production profile based on voluntary aspects of the produced response tempo curve (rpi; i.e., in **Vr**Δpi′ of Equation 8.3).

This suggests how speakers and performers can shape a listener's interpretation of a given attractor profile. It also implies that, depending on a creator's whim, two events with identical attractor profiles may be interpreted quite differently by virtue of how this creator executes the tempo response curve. It is the parallelism between voluntary expectancy profiles and production profiles that allows expectancy profiles to *implicate a course of action*.

Tempo Response Curves in Action

This theoretical approach implies that production profiles follow a course of planned action involving response tempo. This idea builds on the concept of *incremental planning* originally proposed by Caroline Palmer and Peter Pfordresher.[43] They argued that people (here, musicians) use a tacit plan to produce a series of rhythmic groups within a musical event. The plan operates incrementally on successive group time spans by heightening one's concentration on the time span of one rhythmic group (i.e., Tgi) at a time within a longer series of such groups.

In the present discussion, this concept is generalized to include a tempo response curve. This curve spells out an enlarged plan for developing produced time spans over an entire series of event time spans. As suggested, this plan draws on a voluntary expectancy profile by substituting motor responses, **rpi**′ (Equation 8.3) for expected manifest periods of pi′ (Equation 8.2). Thus, in this example, when applied to *i*th attractor, **rpi**′ generates an observable group time span, Tgi. In this fashion, a tempo response curve then maps onto a given attractor profile buried in an expectancy profile, thereby creating an expressive production of an attractor profile.

More generally, as a voluntary expectancy profile is translated into tempo response curves, resulting plans for producing an event open a range of different forms, each with different modulating patterns for **rpi**′. For instance, the voluntary expectancy profile of Figure 8.2 has the same attractor profile as the production profile shown in Figure 8.4B. But the latter profile is one among several possible profiles where p′ is replaced by different values of **rpi**. The impact of different tempo response curves becomes clear in Figure 8.4A. This panel of Figure 8.4 shows different tempo response curves for the same attractor profile, as in Figure 8.4B and Figure 8.2. In panel A of Figure 8.4, a voluntary modulation of tempo (light gray short dashed line) is shown along with a contrasting tempo curve created with involuntary modulations (dark gray dashes) by relying only on automatic $\mathbf{r}$pi changes (with the same attractors).

Clearly, Figure 8.4A illustrates that voluntary adjustments to the group time spans in this pattern are more pronounced and interesting than are the involuntary ones. Indeed, the voluntary curve is often deemed a Natural tempo response curve because it seems more expressive; by contrast, involuntary curves are dubbed Mechanical curves. More precisely, the Natural curve is produced from a production plan of Equation 8.3, wherein both voluntary and involuntary $\mathbf{r}\Delta$pi$'$ factors are present, whereas the Mechanical curve is produced by the same equation, but only the involuntary factor ($\mathbf{r}\Delta$pi$'$) is operative.

Tempo modulation is a major tool that speakers and musicians use to create different interpretations of the same attractor profile. Despite an equivalence of attractors, an artfully designed (i.e., natural) production profile rarely exactly matches its expectancy profile. In other words, attractor parallelism refers to an *abstract* similarity between constructs of expectancy and production profiles, one that transcends absolute rate. An expectancy profile may be abstractly similar to a production profile, but not identical to it.

Disparity between an expectancy profile and related production profiles is due mainly to differences between pi$'$ (of a voluntary expectancy profile) and the $\mathbf{r}$p$_\mathrm{i}'$ (of a production profile). Ultimately, tempo response curves are important for their potential in offering a wide variety of different production profiles with the same core rhythmic relations. In a nutshell, this approach formalizes a temporal aspect of theme and variation.

Voluntary and Involuntary Factors in Production Profiles

The tempo response curve is fundamental in theory-building. Specifically, this curve functions as a communicative vehicle that conveys to listeners both voluntary and involuntary information delivered in a production profile.

Theoretically, involuntary factors in a production impact the automaticity of a listener's entrainment because they are carried by critical driving rhythm properties, such as force and regularity. In theory, any tempo fluctuations carrying

these involuntary properties will determine the strength of momentary perturbations and resulting corrections as $\mathbf{I}\Delta\mathbf{r}p'$ (i.e., Equation 8.3 with $\mathbf{V}$rpi = 0). Consequently, a listener exposed to such a production will react with parallel automatic fluctuations in his expectancy profile, which shows up in the manifest period, p$'$, due to automatic corrections, $\mathbf{I}\Delta$pi (Equation 8.1). Voluntary factors, on the other hand, reflect a producer's creative imagination. Although more speculative, as a speaker finds ways to intentionally shape his tempo response curve (via $\mathbf{V}\Delta$rpi$'$), these voluntary aspects of a production profile are designed to affect a listener's conscious experience of the produced curve (via $\mathbf{V}\Delta$pi).[44]

A portrayal of two different types of tempo response curves appears in Figure 8.4A. The mechanical curve reflects a tempo response curve generated only by involuntary factors ($\mathbf{I}\Delta\mathbf{r}p'$). By contrast, the natural curve reflects joint effects of involuntary-plus-voluntary factors ($\mathbf{I}\Delta\mathbf{r}p'$ + $\mathbf{V}\Delta\mathbf{r}p'$). Panel B in this figure details the production profile, $\mathbf{P}$(Tgi) for the natural curve. Not surprisingly, listeners usually find natural production profiles more pleasing than mechanical ones. Apparently, we are more comfortable with timing variations that are intentionally generated by another human than when such variations are 'machine' made (i.e., automatically generated). Simply put, people prefer expressive modulations of tempo to unexpressive changes.

Ingenious Tempo Response Curves

A few popular tempo response curves appear in Figure 8.5. For explanatory clarity, panel A outlines the difference between an involuntary expectancy profile (dashed line) and its parallel natural production profile (solid line); that is, both share the same attractor profile. However, this expectancy profile reflects only involuntary changes in the manifest period, pi, whereas its counterpart production profile is expressively shaped by a natural motor response curve, $\mathbf{r}$pi$'$, based on both involuntary and voluntary factors.

Other panels offer a very small sample of different tempo response curves. All reflect the additive effects of involuntary and voluntary factors on $\mathbf{r}$pi. Their differences suggest the novelty of human expressions as conveyed by voluntary timing factors. These curves reflect significant, nonrandom timing configurations that can highlight certain attractors (by locally slowing) or obscure them (by locally speeding up). They also showcase a few ingenious interpretations conveyed

Examples of tempo response curves: $rp' = p + r\Delta p$

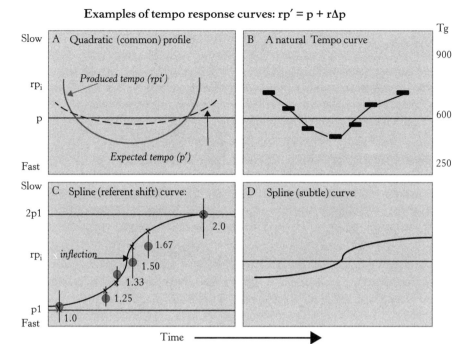

FIGURE 8.5 Examples of four different tempo response curves all reflecting **rp′** changes for a referent oscillator period of p. Most common in speech and music are variations on the quadratic curve (**A, B**). Also in music common are deep (**C**) and shallow (**D**) spline curves.

by tempo response curves mapped onto attractor profiles.

A natural U response tempo profile of slow-fast-slow appears in Figure 8.5B. This curve contrasts with the S shapes of a spline curve in Figure 8.5C,D. The spline curve is ingenious. It plays a special role in musical rhythms because it schedules paths between different time scales; that is, two referent tempi (p1 versus 2p1). In Figure 8.5C, the path of local response tempi (**rp**i′) is initially near a fast intrinsic period (e.g., p1), but over time it slows to a significantly slower intrinsic period (2 p1). Momentary values of **rp**i′ also wander intriguingly about the succession of hidden attractors (filled dots for attractors of 1.25, 1.33, etc.). These attractor states provide hidden stepping stones along a spline path to a slower rate. Also popular are subtle spline curves that capture the end-lengthening of a rhythmic group, as in Figure 8.5D. David Epstein[45] was fond of the spline curve, arguing for its effectiveness in shifting a listener's functional temporal referent.

Response tempo curves reveal the production origins of fuzzy rhythms. A tempo response curve carves out a calculated series of timing deviations that creates an *expressive* fuzzy rhythm. In music, this amounts to planned

time-warping. Either consciously or unwittingly by habit, people modulate the surface pattern of a hidden attractor profile simply by varying local tempo. This happens in speech as well as musical events. We all know someone who chatters at a fast local rate but slows down near phrase endings (following a spline curve). On the other hand, the popular U curve describes talkers who begin a phrase hesitantly then speed up as the phrase continues, finally slowing again near the end (a U curve). These and other speaking tendencies reflect an individual's unwitting use of a favorite tempo response curve shaped by overlearned habits.[46,47,48]

People use tempo response curves to advance their communicative goals. We all have a natural need to be understood, and, to achieve this goal, we unknowingly shape our production profiles, slowing down, even pausing, at an important time point then speeding up at other time points. These are often speaker-specific tendencies motivated by spontaneous emotions and/or habitual plans we use when producing a sound pattern, plans that find a way into motor response curves. Great orators have internalized creative plans along these lines. It is not merely simpler or more artful attractor profiles that help effective speakers or talented musicians achieve momentary performance goals: overall plans about a response tempo curve also further a performer's broader communicative goals. By contrast, there are also those plan-less speakers who, oblivious to connecting with their listeners, ramble on at a boring, almost fixed tempo. Ideally, effective speakers and musicians rely on implicit plans that feature compelling timing modulations designed to regulate a listener's attending by activating in listeners experience expectancy profiles that shape accessible hidden attractors.

Synchronizing Expectancy with Production Profiles

Finally, effective listening rests on synchronicity. This is what makes parallelism important. Synchrony requires a simultaneous matching of a listener's expectancy profile with the unfolding production profile of a speaker or musician. In this duet, two profiles operate concurrently: multiple neural oscillations of an expectancy profile of one person (a listener) must synchronize with parallel exogenous time spans in the production profile of another (e.g., a speaker). Of course, ultimately, acoustic production profiles spring from a creator's tunable brain where neural activity gravitates to a producer's motor/premotor cortex. Presumably, correlated neural oscillations of the listener, activated within expectancy profiles, originate in the auditory cortex along with closely related regions. This adds a twist to the old phrase "a meeting of minds." In speech, decomposing this joint activity means that production profiles in the brain of a speaker generate the basis of overt actions for coupling with covert expectancy profiles in the brain of a listener.

In light of some contemporary theories of attending, a scenario dedicated to oscillatory synchronicity between an attender and the creator of a sound pattern may seem far-fetched. However, recent neuroscience research eerily confirms this perspective. Stephens et al.[49] discovered parallelism in correlations between the brain activity of a speaker and neural recordings of a listener. Using functional magnetic resonance imaging (fMRI), they recorded activity in both parties during natural verbal communication and discovered neat couplings between speaker and listener neural activities when communication was successful. On these occasions, the neural expectancies of listeners could both slightly lag as well as clearly anticipate changes in the speaker's brain signal. Noteworthy, this brain-to-brain coupling is widespread across brain areas in speakers and listeners.[50]

Subsequent studies add further support for the synchrony of parallelism. For instance, Silbert and colleagues[51] found that brain activities in a listener correlated with those of a speaker during a 15-minute narrative. Examinations of brain activities in both listener and speaker showed that neural production activities (including motor brain regions) in a speaker's brain were correlated with a listener's comprehension neural activities (expectancies). Finally, not to be overlooked is the discovery that neural activity was not limited to one hemisphere. Rather, synchronies involved widespread, bilateral brain activity. Importantly, in this research, listeners' brain activity was coupled with parallel activity in the production (neural) profiles of speakers, supporting inherent parallelism.[52]

Summary of Production Profiles and Driving Rhythms

In sum, the dynamics of produced events can be described in terms of the same basic concepts used to portray expectancies. That is, in speech and music, it is hypothesized that both production and expectancy profiles embed attractor profiles and tempo curves. This parallelism facilitates entrainments of listeners' driven rhythms with speaker's driving rhythms. Emerging evidence, consistent with this framework suggests that this parallelism exists as it is revealed in neural synchronies.

Major points of this section are:

- Production profiles yield a series of event driving rhythms ($\mathbf{Pi}$ (Ti) = f ($mi{:}ni$) $\mathbf{r}pi'$ + ε)).[53]
- Production profiles parallel expectancy profiles ($\mathbf{Pi}$ (Ti) ~ $\mathbf{Ei}$ (Ti) = f ($mi{:}ni$) pi' + ε).
- Mismatches in coordinating a listener's $\mathbf{Ei}$ (Ti) with another's $\mathbf{Pi}$ (Ti) create expectancy violations.
- Synchronizing a listener's expectancy profile, $\mathbf{Ei}$ (Ti), with a production profile from another individual, $\mathbf{Pi}$ (Ti), creates in the listener a series of entrainment states, namely an attractor profile.
- Maximal parallelism of expectancies with productions rests on identical attractor profiles and on similarities of tempo curves where $\mathbf{I}\Delta pi$ ~ $\mathbf{Ir}\Delta pi$ for involuntary factors and $\mathbf{V}\Delta pi$ ~ $\mathbf{Vr}\Delta pi$ for voluntary factors.
- Parallelism emerges from dynamics of speaker–listener exchanges as synchronization of a listener's neural expectancy profiles with the neural production profiles of a speaker.

EXPERIMENTAL APPROACHES TO PRODUCTION AND PERCEPTION OF MUSICAL EVENTS

The final section of this chapter samples a few experimental forays into behavioral parallelism. To review, parallelism refers to the hypothesis that expectancy and production profiles depend on identical hidden attractor profiles. Moreover, it can be argued that parallelism is *maximized* when production and expectancy profiles not only share the same attractor profile but also operate with the same tempo curve. Thus, it is possible that maximal parallelism occurs when an involuntary expectancy profile reflects a listener's involuntary production profile. This might happen, for example, if a listener generates an involuntary expectancy that tracks a speaker's mechanical production profile, thus inducing the same attractor profile together with a tempo response tempo curve based only on automatic corrective responses.

However, this is unlikely to happen in real life. Typically we don't produce mechanically generated profiles. Our ordinary encounters with speech and musical productions created by others are far more likely to involve production and expectancy profiles than incorporate both voluntary and involuntary components. Basically, people don't like involuntarily generated production profiles. They sound dead. The latter claim is supported by the careful research of Bruno Repp.[54] Across a range of studies, Repp concluded that listeners not only automatically adjust to the timing variations of fuzzy rhythms, but they are also strongly inclined to voluntarily improve upon these involuntary corrections when these deviations increase to provocative magnitudes (Box 8.2).

Background: Isolating Voluntary and Involuntary Factors

In theory, maximal parallelism between expectancy and production profiles depends not only on shared attractor profiles, but also to an important degree they depend upon shared tempo curves, including voluntary as well as involuntary factors. To pursue this means teasing apart these factors.

Repp did just this.[55,56,57,58] Box 8.2 presents a condensed overview of Repp's major findings. In several studies, Repp asked people to synchronize taps to an isochronous rhythm containing one or several deviant time intervals. Thus, as a listener taps to such a rhythm, she automatically adapts her response to each deviation with the correction evident in her next tap. More to the point, however,

Repp discovered that involuntary corrections happen mainly for small timing changes. Relatively large deviations, by contrast, evoked voluntary corrections in addition to involuntary ones (cf. Equations 8.2, 8.3).

To clarify the issues at stake, consider a thought experiment for two extreme scenarios. In a *robot scenario*, a listener relies solely on involuntary expectancies, effectively running mechanically on automatic pilot. This listener will *always* track a production profile using an involuntary expectancy profile with automatic adaptions to time variations (i.e., $\mathbf{V}\Delta\mathrm{pi}' \sim 0$, for all i in Equation 8.2). The other extreme is a "control freak" scenario. In this case, *all* phase corrections, regardless of their magnitude, are voluntary (i.e., $\mathbf{I}\Delta\mathrm{pi}' \sim 0$, for all i in Equation 8.2).

Neither scenario is plausible. Wisely, Repp carves out a middle path in which voluntary and involuntary factors jointly constrain people's response to timing modulations in a production profile. Under the assumption that non-zero values of $\mathbf{I}\Delta\mathrm{p}'$ and $\mathbf{V}\Delta\mathrm{pi}'$ combine additively, Repp used a subtraction strategy to validate the contribution of each effect.

The subtraction strategy forces decomposition of a response tempo curve into involuntary and voluntary components. As described by Caroline Palmer,[59] the methodological trick is straightforward: an experimenter explicitly instructs expert musicians to produce a musical piece mechanically by suppressing all voluntary expressions (the robot scenario). In a contrasting condition, the musicians are told to expressively create a more natural production of the same piece (e.g., "perform musically"). The latter invites use of the voluntary factor (a control freak scenario).

The subtractive experimental strategy assumes a tempo response curve, $\mathbf{rp}_i'$, rests on an additive combination of involuntary ($\mathbf{I}$) plus voluntary ($\mathbf{V}$) factors across all profile attractors, $\mathbf{i}$ (Equation 8.3). Consequently, suppressing the voluntary factor ($\mathbf{Vr}\Delta\mathrm{pi}'$) eliminates it, hence isolating the involuntary factor ($\mathbf{Ir}\Delta\mathrm{pi}'$) in a mechanical production. By contrast, a production based on additive contributions of both voluntary and involuntary factors is arguably more natural. Subtracting $\mathbf{Ir}\Delta\mathrm{pi}$ of the mechanical performance from ($\mathbf{Ir}\Delta\mathrm{pi} + \mathbf{Vr}\Delta\mathrm{pi}'$) of a natural performance isolates estimates of voluntary phase corrections at various time points in a profile.

The remainder of this section considers validations of ideas associated with parallelism. Necessarily, this research exploits the subtraction strategy to assess voluntary factors. The first, a study by Bruno Repp, documents parallelism of expectancy and production profiles. Following in this vein is a study by Amandine Penel and Carolyn Drake. A third set of studies by Caroline Palmer and Edward Large expands on voluntary control of tempo responses curves in musical productions given an entrainment framework.

Voluntary Determinants of Expressive Timing: Studies of Bruno Repp

Expressive timing in music usually refers to artistic modulations of the surface timing in producing a musical piece. It reflects artful speeding or slowing at "just the right moments" in producing a piece. Given the DAT framework outlined in preceding sections, this entails a time-warping of the surface structure that hides an attractor profile. These surface distortions expressively deliver an artful fuzzy rhythm to a listener. Experimentally, the subtraction strategy allows an experimenter to gauge the effects of eliminating certain tempo changes. They permit an answer to the following question: "How much do listeners rely on automatic versus voluntary control of attending as they attempt to synchronize with a musical pattern?"

Expectancy Versus Production Profiles

According to attending dynamics, listeners naturally synchronize their own expectancy profiles to the expressively produced profile of a musician (or speaker). Nevertheless, certain modulations within a musical piece (or utterance) can result in a mismatch of these two profiles which creates expressive violations of listeners' expectancies.

To assess this, Repp[60] created a mechanical (computerized) version of a production profile based on a Chopin étude (Figure 8.6A). Using the subtraction strategy, he eliminated *both* involuntary ($I\Delta$rpi′) and artful voluntary ($V\Delta$rpi′) components of a produced response tempo curve; this essentially reduced the piece to a strictly isochronous sequence.[61] Listeners (musicians and nonmusicians) then were asked to synchronize taps with these isochronous sounds. The critical discovery was that listeners' resulting taps were distinctly *not* isochronous! This is evident in Figure 8.6B.

Most interesting, Repp found that people showed automatic timing adjustments in taps, producing longer time intervals at beginnings and ends of musical groups (e.g., revealing a U-shaped response tempo curve as in Figure 8.5A). Apparently, people cannot fully comply with synchrony instructions. Instead, they exhibit certain ever-present involuntary biases captured by basic forms of tempo response curves, curves that do not reflect strict isochrony.

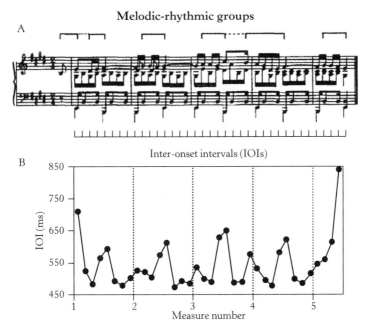

FIGURE 8.6 (**A**) Excerpt from computer generation of Chopin's Etude in E Major, op. 10 No. 3. Initial context set by first eighth note. Following measures show regularly marked note onsets with eight per measure (see grid).

Repp wondered if his tappers were aware of their biases. So he planted a few longer time intervals in otherwise isochronous productions and asked listeners to detect these changes. All listeners failed to detect those deviations at serial locations where they *expected* to find a longer time interval. In other words, *perceived time changes accompany only stimulus fluctuations that violate a listener's involuntary expectancy profile.* And—people are unaware of these biases.

Intuitively, this makes sense. Our most basic expectancies operate on automatic pilot. They allow effortless alignment with certain grouping features in the environment. Following up on this, Repp and colleagues[62,63] found that people also cannot suppress certain corrective reactions to deviant time changes. Especially with small timing irregularities, these corrective reactions just happen—because they are automatic (see Box 8.2).

Perceiving Time in Fuzzy Rhythms: A Study by Penel and Drake

Amandine Penel and Carolyn Drake also pursued parallelism in perception and production using musical events.[64] Building on Repp's findings[65,66,67] they aimed to disentangle the roles of voluntary from involuntary factors in expectancy (a perception task) and production profiles (a tapping task).

However, unlike Repp's design, in this perception task musicians were told to both detect a target deviation and to restore the patterns to isochrony. Presumably, they should fail at this if they cannot detect a deviation given an involuntary expectancy profile. And indeed, consistent with Repp's finding, these researchers also found that listeners detect and restore *only relatively large time deviations* (i.e., ones associated with voluntary factors). They also discovered, in a related production task, that musicians told to voluntarily produce an expressive sequence created a more variable time pattern than musicians told to produce a mechanical sequence. In particular, the former group modified tempo response curves in ways suggesting intentional blurring (hiding) of certain attractor relations, but not others.

In sum, both involuntary and voluntary factors influence listeners' temporal expectancies. Furthermore, listeners' dynamic expectancy profiles are correlated with their production profiles as they are shaped by a tempo response curve. This confirms the general nature of parallelism.

Tempo Response Curves: Research of Caroline Palmer and Edward Large

Parallelism of expectancy and production profiles applies across different time scales. This conclusion emerges from research of Caroline Palmer and Edward Large.[68] This study differs from preceding ones in its explicit reliance on entrainment explanations of people's ability to track different tempo response curves.

Large and Palmer developed a two-oscillator entrainment model of an ideal listener we shall term "Joe." In this simulation, Joe operates with two simultaneous entrainable oscillations, where each tracks a different time scale. (e.g., as in group vs. subgroup timing; i.e., related by 2:1). Joe had to synchronize with both mechanical and natural versions of a Bach polyphonic composition.[69]

In this simulation, Joe nicely followed entrainment principles, showing adapting expectancies to rather large temporal fluctuations of the natural driving rhythms of a Bach performance. Finally, Joe also distinguished among three different types of coordination between expectancy and production profiles. A produced sound can be *on-time*, *unexpectedly early*, or *unexpectedly late* relative to its parallel expectancy profile. In this piece, Joe correctly phase-adapted to all three timing types. This relatively simple entrainment model elegantly captures rhythmic themes as well as expressive, i.e., interpretive, variations of a natural musical pattern.

One fact seems clear: expectancy violations posed by natural, i.e., fuzzy, time patterns are *not* perceived as random noise. Rather, they are perceived as part of a tempo response curve shaped by both involuntary and voluntary factors. Such curves wind around a hidden attractor profile to create distinctively modulated time patterns. "Wind around" here implies that the creator of a production profile "knows" when to voluntarily slow down or speed up a motor tempo in order to highlight one or another aspect of an attractor profile (as in a spline curve).

More on Tempo Curves

Theoretically, a tempo response curve created by a musician schedules a pattern of local tempo modulations. Practically speaking, there is much we do not know about tempo curves and their role in synchronizing an expectancy profile with a production profile. However, entrainment models offer a reasonable launching pad for advancing our knowledge about these constructs.[45,70]

Loehr, Large, and Palmer[71] also used a two-oscillator entrainment model to describe a musician synchronizing overt responses to a musical rhythm as its tempo changes. In this task, musicians had to "keep pace" with a speeding or slowing production profile at two different time scales. They succeeded in this, faltering only with the fastest tempi (3% speeding).[72] Importantly, this entrainment model successfully portrayed adaptive rate tracking. Finally, it is likely that both involuntary and voluntary factors contributed to this performance, given task instructions.[73]

Fascinating Fractals

On a grander scale, the idea of tempo response curves opens a door to a range of different modulating tempo patterns. Effectively, higher order time patterns are those created by different local perturbations which implicate multiple, overlapping time scales. In turn, these lead to a rich, fascinating temporal texture induced by the unfolding shape of a tempo response curve.

Pushing boundaries, such configurations lead to the exciting discoveries of Ed Large and his colleagues. In probing the timing variability of natural musical productions of pianists, they discovered reliable serial autocorrelations among timing deviations of several coinciding production profiles.[74,75] For instance, larger time deviations in a tempo response curve tended to be consistently separated by longer time lags, whereas smaller time deviations were regularly separated by shorter time lags. These patterns indicated recurrent self-similarity across time scales symptomatic of fractal structure (i.e., $1/f^{\alpha}$ structure).[76] In short, multiple "tempo-like" response curves exist that are more complex and fascinating than those implied by Figure 8.5.

Summary of Production and Perception of Musical Events

In sum, the communicative signals we create and receive are acoustic patterns defined by their inner rhythms and rates. More specifically, the inner time structure of such productions carries attractor profiles accompanied by fluctuating tempo curves. As listeners, our first, and automatic, response to such patterns is a barely conscious one. But often this is followed by a more engaged response as our attending to them becomes intentionally shaped by naturally acquired habits.

Studies probing expectancy and production profiles reviewed in this section support the idea of parallelism and its extensions to include involuntary and voluntary components of tempo curves. Finally, it is clear that the variability of timing in these profiles during dyadic communications is not random. It may be chaotic sometimes, but it is not stochastically random.

Finally, the concept of parallelism invites comparisons with interpretations of *mirror neurons*. Rizzolatti and colleagues[77,78] proposed mirror neurons to account for findings of parallel neural activity in macaque monkeys who observed other monkeys producing certain motor gestures. The viewing monkeys showed neural activity in perceptual regions of their brains that corresponded to the active regions of the produced gestures. However, this chapter does not interpret parallelism to mean that perception/attention is *equated* with action. It merely highlights abstract structural similarities of expectancy (attention/perception) and production (action) profiles that advance, possibly fallible, entrainments. Moreover, others sound reasonable warnings of premature generalizations of mirror neuron research.[79] Nevertheless, the overriding concept of parallelism is worth pursuing.

The major points in this section are:

- Parallelism between the expectancy profiles of a listener and the production profiles of a speaker/performer is evident in correlations between these profiles reported across experimental studies.
- Attractor profiles are a core feature of parallelism between expectancy and production profiles. Contributing to parallelism are tempo curves (pi′ in expectancy profiles) and tempo response curves (**r**pi′ in production profiles).
- Tempo response curves may obscure or highlight different underlying attractors in an attractor profile. These curves rise from involuntary and voluntary factors.

CHAPTER SUMMARY

This chapter continues themes of synchrony. It broadens the portrayal of synchronous activity to include whole profiles of patterned event rhythms as production profiles that are created by speakers or musicians. In turn, production profiles can elicit expectancy profiles in listeners. Conversely, in other contexts, acquired expectancy profiles can supply plans for production profiles. In either case, the stage is set for synchrony between parallel expectancy and production profiles.

The chapter aimed to convey the gist of the synchronous interplay between expectancy profiles and parallel production profiles. Synchrony between these profiles depends on their shared constructs: attractor profiles and tempo curves. Maximum parallelism between profiles holds when production and expectancy profiles share attractor profiles and have identical tempo curves. The issue of parallelism is critical to ensuring synchrony between a listener and a speaker.

A second goal aimed to clarify involuntary and voluntary factors that shape tempo curves. A tempo response curve of a production profile (**rpi**) is the motor correlate of the tempo curve (pi′) of an expectancy profile over time (i). Particularly for tempo response curves, voluntary factors add expressive shape in creating these curves, which then become crafted fuzzy rhythms. Looping full circle in a hypothetical speaker–listener exchange, such crafted rhythmic productions of a speaker then inspire corresponding corrective changes in the expectancy profiles of a listener.

A third goal was to provide experimental support for distinguishing between expectancy and production profiles in the context of parallelisms. Several illustrative studies confirm the relevance of parallelism between expectancy and production profiles as well as clarify the respective roles of voluntary and involuntary factors in these profiles.

NOTES

1. Margaret Wilson and Thomas P. Wilson, "An Oscillator Model of the Timing of Turn-Taking," *Psychonomic Bulletin & Review* 12, no. 6 (December 2005): 957–68, doi:10.3758 /BF03206432.

2. For tutorial reasons, this assumes time spans at the word level; later chapters acknowledge syllable and phoneme rhythms.

3. Bruno H. Repp, "Phase Correction, Phase Resetting, and Phase Shifts after Subliminal Timing Perturbations in Sensorimotor Synchronization," *Journal of Experimental Psychology: Human Perception and Performance* 27, no. 3 (2001): 600–21, doi:10.1037/ 0096-1523.27.3.600.

4. Bruno H. Repp, "Processes Underlying Adaptation to Tempo Changes in Sensorimotor Synchronization," *Human Movement Science* 20, no. 3 (June 2001): 277–312, doi:10.1016/ S0167-9457(01)00049-5.

5. Note that, by definition, the latent period, p, does not change.

6. A full PCR to a phase shift (PS) would be −60 ms.

7. Equations are spelled out for the ith point in time to highlight the fact that these are in-the-moment expectancies.

8. Note: the red p′ of the voluntary expectancy is $p' = p + f(I\Delta pi + V\Delta p')$ which includes an involuntary component shown below as a black p′ in this figure.

9. Repp, "Processes Underlying Adaptation to Tempo Changes in Sensorimotor Synchronization."

10. Bruno H. Repp and Yi-Huang Su, "Sensorimotor Synchronization: A Review of Recent Research (2006–2012)," *Psychonomic Bulletin & Review* 20, no. 3 (February 9, 2013): 403–52, doi:10.3758/ s13423-012-0371-2.

11. Repp and Su, "Sensorimotor Synchronization."

12. B. H. Repp, "Sensorimotor Synchronization: A Review of the Tapping Literature," *Psychonomic Bulletin & Review* 12 no. 6 (December 2005): 969–92, accessed January 17, 2016, http://link.springer. com.proxy.library.ucsb.edu:2048/ article/ 10.3758/ BF03206433#page-1.

13. Marilyn G. Boltz, Rebecca L. Dyer, and Anna R. Miller, "Jo Are You Lying to Me? Temporal Cues for Deception," *Journal of Language and Social Psychology* 29, no. 4 (December 1, 2010): 458–66, doi:10.1177/ 0261927X10385976.

14. John Michon, "*Timing in Temporal Tracking*," (Netherlands: Van Gorcum, 1967).

15. Jiří Mates et al., "Temporal Integration in Sensorimotor Synchronization," *Journal of Cognitive Neuroscience* 6, no. 4 (July 1, 1994): 332–40, doi:10.1162/jocn.1994.6.4.332.

16. D. Hary and G. P. Moore, "Synchronizing Human Movement with an External Clock Source," *Biological Cybernetics* 56, no. 5–6 (July 1987): 305–11, doi:10.1007/BF00319511.

17. Dirk Vorberg and Hans-Henning Schulze, "Linear Phase-Correction in Synchronization: Predictions, Parameter Estimation, and Simulations," *Journal of Mathematical Psychology* 46, no. 1 (February 2002): 56–87, doi:10.1006/jmps.2001.1375.

18. Alan M. Wing and A. B. Kristofferson, "The Timing of Inter-response Intervals," *Perception & Psychophysics* 13, no. 3 (October 1973): 455–60, doi:10.3758/BF03205802.

19. Kelso has convincingly shown that principles of dynamics apply to motor coordinations.

20. R. G. Carson and J. A. S. Kelso, "Governing Coordination: Behavioural Principles and Neural Correlates," *Experimental Brain Research* 154, no. 3 (November 8, 2003): 267–74, doi:10.1007/ s00221-003-1726-8.

21. John J. Jeka and J. A. S. Kelso "Manipulating Symmetry in the Coordination Dynamics of Human Movement," *Journal of Experimental Psychology: Human Perception and Performance* 21, no. 2 (1995): 360–74, doi:10.1037/0096-1523.21.2.360.

22. E. W. Large, P. Fink, and J. A. S. Kelso, "Tracking Simple and Complex Sequences," *Psychological Research* 66 no. 1 (February 2002): 3–17, accessed January 17, 2016, http://link.springer. com.proxy.library.ucsb.edu:2048/ article/ 10.1007/ s004260100069#page-1.

23. Edward W. Large and John F. Kolen, "Resonance and the Perception of Musical Meter," *Connection Science* 6, no. 2–3 (1994): 177–208.

24. Duration tradeoff with intensity at fast rates. And, P-centers, defined largely by shifts from

dissonance to consonance, are accompanied by heightened energy.

25. Greg Kochanski and Christina Orphanidou, "What Marks the Beat of Speech?" *The Journal of the Acoustical Society of America* 123, no. 5 (May 1, 2008): 2780–91, doi:10.1121/1.2890742.

26. Jessica S. F. Hay and Randy L. Diehl, "Perception of Rhythmic Grouping: Testing the Iambic/Trochaic Law," *Perception & Psychophysics* 69, no. 1 (January 2007): 113–22, doi:10.3758/BF03194458.

27. Peter Q. Pfordresher, "The Role of Melodic and Rhythmic Accents in Musical Structure," *Music Perception: An Interdisciplinary Journal* 20, no. 4 (2003): 431–64, doi:10.1525/mp.2003.20.4.431.

28. Robert J. Ellis and Mari R. Jones, "The Role of Accent Salience and Joint Accent Structure in Meter Perception," *Journal of Experimental Psychology: Human Perception and Performance* 35, no. 1 (2009): 264–80, doi:10.1037/a0013482.

29. Keith R. Kluender, Jeffry A. Coady, and Michael Kiefte, "Sensitivity to Change in Perception of Speech," *Speech Communication* 41, no. 1 (August 2003): 59–69, doi:10.1016/S0167-6393(02)00093-6.

30. Explanations focus on suppression of a listener's neural response to a preceding context, thus releasing a heightened reaction to a physical change.

31. Colin S. Pittendrigh and Serge Daan, "A Functional Analysis of Circadian Pacemakers in Nocturnal Rodents," *Journal of Comparative Physiology* 106, no. 3 (October 1976): 333–55, doi:10.1007/BF01417860.

32. Early debates contesting biological entrainments questioned the validity of circadian rhythms in animals. Initially, these were treated, after the fact, as mechanical reactions to light–dark cycles unrelated to any internal, adaptive biological rhythm (with a period near 24 hours).

33. J. D. Palmer, *An Introduction to Biological Rhythms* (New York: Academic Press, 1976).

34. S. Daan et al., "Assembling a Clock for All Seasons: Are There M and E Oscillators in the Genes?" *Journal of Biological Rhythms* 16, no. 2 (April 1, 2001): 105–16, doi:10.1177/074873001129001809.

35. Ilse Lehiste, "Isochrony Reconsidered," *Journal of Phonetics* 5, no. 3 (1977): 253–63.

36. Sam Tilsen and Keith Johnson, "Low-Frequency Fourier Analysis of Speech Rhythm," *Journal of the Acoustical Society of America* 124, no. 2 (August 1, 2008): EL34–EL39, doi:10.1121/1.2947626.

37. Sam Tilsen and Amalia Arvaniti, "Speech Rhythm Analysis with Decomposition of the Amplitude Envelope: Characterizing Rhythmic Patterns within and across Languages," *Journal of the Acoustical Society of America* 134, no. 1 (July 1, 2013): 628–39, doi:10.1121/1.4807565.

38. James G. Martin, "Rhythmic (Hierarchical) Versus Serial Structure in Speech and Other Behavior," *Psychological Review* 79, no. 6 (1972): 487–509, doi:10.1037/h0033467.

39. Martin, "Rhythmic (Hierarchical) Versus Serial Structure in Speech and Other Behavior."

40. The MS rule is credited to James Martin and his hierarchical theory of speech timing.

41. See discussion of Trehub's research in Chapter 7.

42. Rosalee Meyer and Caroline Palmer, "Temporal and Motor Transfer in Music Performance," *Music Perception: An Interdisciplinary Journal* 21, no. 1 (2003): 81–104, doi:10.1525/mp.2003.21.1.81.

43. Caroline Palmer and Peter Q. Pfordresher, "Incremental Planning in Sequence Production," *Psychological Review* 110, no. 4 (2003): 683–712, doi:10.1037/0033-295X.110.4.683.

44. At least one study measuring this effect suggests that increased amplitude of neural oscillations during selective attending affects the phase coupling (Lakatos et al., 2008).

45. David Epstein, *Shaping Time* (New York: Schirmer, 1994).

46. Tempo curves in speech are likely based on syllable timing which varies within and between speakers, but Ghitza and colleagues have explored this topic, focusing upon a role for theta driven oscillations.

47. Oded Ghitza, "On the Role of Theta-Driven Syllabic Parsing in Decoding Speech: Intelligibility of Speech with a Manipulated Modulation Spectrum," *Frontiers in Psychology* 3 (2012), https://doi.org/10.3389/fpsyg.2012.00238.

48. Reinisch, Eva, Jesse, Alexandra, McQueen, James M. Speaking rate from proximal and distal contexts is used during word segmentation. Journal of Experimental Psychology: Human Perception and Performance, Vol 37(3), Jun 2011, 978–996

49. Greg J. Stephens, Lauren J. Silbert, and Uri Hasson, "Speaker–Listener Neural Coupling Underlies Successful Communication," *Proceedings of the National Academy of Sciences* 107, no. 32 (August 10, 2010): 14425–30, doi:10.1073/pnas.1008662107.

50. Arjen Stolk et al., "Neural Mechanisms of Communicative Innovation," *Proceedings of the National Academy of Sciences* 110, no. 36 (September 3, 2013): 14574–79, doi:10.1073/pnas.1303170110.

51. Lauren J. Silbert et al., "Coupled Neural Systems Underlie the Production and Comprehension of Naturalistic Narrative Speech," *Proceedings of the National Academy of Sciences* 111, no. 43 (October 28, 2014): E4687–96, doi:10.1073/pnas.1323812111.

52. Controls ruled out time warping distortions and explanations based on semantics and grammar in the contexts.

53. The symbol ε here refers to statistical error i.e., noise; i.e., it is not a phoneme.

54. Repp, "Sensorimotor Synchronization."

55. Bruno H. Repp, "Automaticity and Voluntary Control of Phase Correction Following Event Onset Shifts in Sensorimotor Synchronization," *Journal of Experimental Psychology: Human Perception and*

Performance 28, no. 2 (2002): 410–30, doi:10.1037/0096-1523.28.2.410.

56. Bruno H. Repp, "Phase Attraction in Sensorimotor Synchronization with Auditory Sequences: Effects of Single and Periodic Distractors on Synchronization Accuracy," *Journal of Experimental Psychology: Human Perception and Performance* 29, no. 2 (2003): 290–309, doi:10.1037/0096-1523.29.2.290.

57. Bruno H. Repp, "Detectability of Duration and Intensity Increments in Melody Tones: A Partial Connection between Music Perception and Performance," *Perception & Psychophysics* 57, no. 8 (November 1995): 1217–32, doi:10.3758/BF03208378.

58. Bruno H. Repp, "Detecting Deviations from Metronomic Timing in Music: Effects of Perceptual Structure on the Mental Timekeeper," *Perception & Psychophysics* 61, no. 3 (April 1999): 529–48, doi:10.3758/BF03211971.

59. Caroline Palmer, "Music Performance," *Annual Review of Psychology* 48, no. 1 (1997): 115–38, doi:10.1146/annurev.psych.48.1.115.

60. Repp, "Detecting Deviations from Metronomic Timing in Music."

61. All time spans were inter-onset-intervals (IOIs) of 500 ms; Ti = IOI in Figure 8.6A.

62. Repp, "Sensorimotor Synchronization."

63. Repp and Su, "Sensorimotor Synchronization."

64. Amandine Penel and Carolyn Drake, "Timing Variations in Music Performance: Musical Communication, Perceptual Compensation, and/or Motor Control?" *Perception & Psychophysics* 66, no. 4 (May 2004): 545–62, doi:10.3758/BF03194900.

65. Carolyn Drake, Amandine Penel, and Emmanuel Bigand, "Tapping in Time with Mechanically and Expressively Performed Music," *Music Perception: An Interdisciplinary Journal* 18, no. 1 (October 1, 2000): 1–23, doi:10.2307/40285899.

66. This is Bach's two and three part inventions.

67. Carolyn Drake, "Perceptual and Performed Accents in Musical Sequences," *Bulletin of the Psychonomic Society* 31, no. 2 (February 1993): 107–10, doi:10.3758/BF03334153.

68. Edward W. Large and Caroline Palmer, "Perceiving Temporal Regularity in Music," *Cognitive Science* 26, no. 1 (January 2002): 1–37, doi:10.1016/S0364-0213(01)00057-X.

69. Bach's two- and three-part inventions.

70. Edward W. Large and Mari Riess Jones, "The Dynamics of Attending: How People Track Time-Varying Events," *Psychological Review* 106, no. 1 (1999): 119–59, doi:10.1037/0033-295X.106.1.119.

71. Janeen D. Loehr, Edward W. Large, and Caroline Palmer, "Temporal Coordination and Adaptation to Rate Change in Music Performance," *Journal of Experimental Psychology: Human Perception and Performance* 37, no. 4 (2011): 1292–309, doi:10.1037/a0023102.

72. Tempo changes conformed to a constant 1% or 3% to an overall level of 15% change.

73. The manifest period, p′, here is modeled as a motor periodicity (thus, technically, it is rpi′). Tempo changes conformed to a constant 1% or 3% to an overall level of 15% change. In this two-oscillator model, one oscillation entrains to rhythmic time spans (Tgi = beat period ~pi′), other tracks the faster time level (beat subdivisions).

74. Summer K. Rankin, Edward W. Large, and Philip W. Fink, "Fractal Tempo Fluctuation and Pulse Prediction," *Music Perception* 26, no. 5 (June 2009): 401–13, doi:10.1525/mp.2009.26.5.401.

75. These involved recorded performances of scores by composers such as Bach, Chopin, and others.

76. To the extent that the production profile formula is correct, some self-similarity is not surprising as it springs from attractor multipliers.

77. Giacomo Rizzolatti and Laila Craighero, "The Mirror-Neuron System," *Annual Review of Neuroscience* 27, no. 1 (2004): 169–92, doi:10.1146/annurev.neuro.27.070203.144230.

78. Giacomo Rizzolatti, Leonardo Fogassi, and Vittorio Gallese, "Neurophysiological Mechanisms Underlying the Understanding and Imitation of Action," *Nature Reviews Neuroscience* 2, no. 9 (September 2001): 661–70, doi:10.1038/35090060.

79. Gregory Hickok, "Eight Problems for the Mirror Neuron Theory of Action Understanding in Monkeys and Humans," *Journal of Cognitive Neuroscience* 21, no. 7 (January 13, 2009): 1229–43, doi:10.1162/jocn.2009.21189.

PART II

Applications of Theoretic Constructs: Domains of Music and Speech

9

Meter and Rhythm

How We Hear Them

This opening chapter of Part II focuses on musical events. These are events conceived as slowly timed patterns which are effective in governing a listener's attending. Although the examples employed in this chapter are musical ones, the explanatory concepts involved are general ones introduced in Part I. In slightly disguised form, the concepts used in this chapter echo those of preceding chapters, and they recur as well in future chapters dressed in new garb. Also, basic premises concerning attending and its roots in universal principles remain. The Part 11 portion of the book applies the theoretical ideas of Part I to consider contemporary issues in music and speech.

The present chapter begins this endeavor by addressing meter and rhythm in music. In listening to a melody, we are often unaware of the many different layers of timing floating beneath its surface. Instead, we are drawn to melodic flourishes and surface patterns without realizing the fundamental, but subtle, influence that various time layers levy on our listening. Time structure, in its various forms, gently shapes our monitoring of musical events. This chapter is about certain musical time scales and the hierarchies they form, wherein fast time layers are embedded in slower ones. It also distinguishes hierarchical timing, typically equated with musical meter, from serial time patterns that form rhythmic groups. This distinction is a central topic in this chapter.

CHAPTER GOALS

Classic perspectives often differentiate meter, as a hierarchical time pattern, from rhythm, as a serial time pattern. One goal of this chapter is to provide a dynamic attending explanation for this distinction. A second goal centers on applying entrainment concepts to explain important features of musical meter and rhythm such as accents (time markers) and time periods (of driving and driven rhythms). For instance, in musical events, it is useful to distinguish the salience of *objective* time markers, as accents, from the salience of *subjective*

time markers, as internalized accents. Respectively, such accentuations correspond to time markers associated with external (driving) rhythms versus those associated with internal (driven) rhythms. Also returning in this chapter are two familiar entrainment concepts: oscillator clusters (as *metric oscillator clusters*) and internalized time patterns (as *rhythmic attractor profiles*). Respectively, these constructs pertain to the synchronous activities defined by traditional and transient mode-locking entrainment protocols. That is, metric clusters emphasize vertical (hierarchical) embedding of different time periods, whereas rhythmic attractor profiles feature horizontal (serial) arrangements of different time periods.

Finally, a unifying theme in this chapter addresses a central issue in studies of musical timing. This concerns the relationship between meter and rhythm perception: Do they rely on inherently different psychological processes, as some imply? Or, are meter- and rhythm-related constructs within a larger theoretical framework?

BACKGROUND

It is common to draw a strict dichotomy between meter and rhythmic grouping. And, often, this motivates psychological explanations based on different underlying perceptual mechanisms. But historically, the criteria supporting such a dichotomy have varied, ranging from descriptions of meter as a grid or a rigidly periodic clock contrasted with specific grouping rules for rhythm based on Gestalt principles, for instance. Also popular is the assumption that meter perception depends largely on acquired skills, whereas rhythm perception is explained by appeals to innate grouping tendencies. There is some truth in all of these descriptions. However, an a priori judgment that meter and rhythm are inherently different constructs discourages pursuit of important ways in which they are related.

By way of background, the current section describes three influential approaches to this topic.

One is a rule-based grid approach to meter and rhythm, a second focuses on rhythmic grouping using Gestalt principles, and the third is a coding model that differentiates metric coding from rhythmic grouping. In different ways, all support a meter–rhythm dichotomy.

METER PERCEPTION: GRIDS AND ABSTRACT RULES

Meter perception has come into its own as a topic of perceptual research in recent decades. Music theorists supply a rich body of literature on these topics that validates the complexity in metrical and rhythmic timing across cultures.[1,2] It would be folly to discount the wealth of these insights. In the past 30 years, the disciplines of music and psychology converged to jointly examine issues of meter (and rhythm). Admittedly, the current multidisciplinary orientation now removes musical listeners from concert halls, dance clubs, and honky-tonk bars to place them in less celebratory laboratory settings where people are simply invited to listen to subsets of monotonic, highly simplified sequences (which some rightfully claim as boring). Yet, careful manipulations of metric versus rhythmic timing in such sequences, born of this interdisciplinary effort, has advanced our understanding. The landmark book of Lerdahl and Jackendoff[3] can be justly credited for jump-starting this interdisciplinary adventure.

Generative Rules of Meter

According to Lerdahl and Jackendoff, meter follows distinct rules. In their remarkably detailed analyses of musical structures (metric, rhythmic, tonal), they laid forth a rule-based approach which entailed five *well-formedness rules* for describing meter. These rules were then combined into recipes for how listeners "hear" well-formed metric patterns using *preference rules*. Both kinds of rules are best understood in the context of a metric grid, as expressed by Liberman and Prince[4] and others. Figure 9.1A, for instance, interprets time spatially in a metric grid. Different vertical grid lines cross various (horizontal) time levels that range from fast (level 1) to slow (level 6) timing. Many musical and linguistic theories (past and present) endorse this spatial grid concept.[5]

The prominent metric grid of Lerdahl and Jackendoff is the focus of this section. Their theory formalized metric relations in communicative sound patterns using generative rules. For example, well-formedness rules specify the grid of Figure 9.1 using *multiple strings of concurrent beats* (vertical lines) at different time levels. Each level has fixed spacing (e.g., levels 1–6 in Figure 9.1). From these rules, a *tactus* level is identified as a well-formed referent string. Another well-formedness rule holds that beats in any hierarchical level must coincide with beats in all lower levels. Furthermore, beats within a level must be

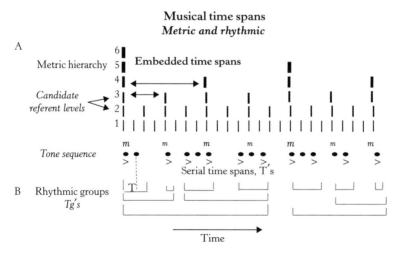

FIGURE 9.1 Musical time spans (metric layers, rhythmic groups). (**A**) Six hypothetical metric time levels with shorter time spans nested within longer ones; stronger metric accents (*M*, *m*, . . . etc.) that outline respectively longer metric times. A tone sequence (dots indicate onsets) outlines a series of inter-onset time (IOIs) spans, T (see dashed dark gray line). Rhythmic groups are marked by rhythmic accents, >. (**B**) Grouped time spans, Tg, are also nested.

Adapted from figure 1 in Mari Riess Jones, "Musical Time," in *Oxford Handbook of Music Psychology*, eds. Susan Hallam, Ian Cross, and Michael Thaut (Oxford: Oxford University Press, 2011).

separated by two or three time spans, gauged by the next lower level beat string. Aggregating over layers, stronger beats occur at points where beats of several different time layers coincide. These rules, then, specify an ideal, internalized configuration of time layers that putatively determines meter perception. Indeed, these well-formedness rules do circumscribe a range of acceptable metric patterns. They represent a built-in bias for "good" meters, namely those with 2:1 and 3:1 time ratios between beat-defined time spans of adjacent time levels. Finally, any rule violation weakens this percept of metricality.

However, well-formedness meter rules also lead to several different "good" metric forms for the same musical event. Here, rhythm enters the grid picture. Meter perception is disambiguated by a surface rhythm formed using preference rules; some groups are preferred over others (e.g., groups of two beats might be preferred over those of four beats). Preference rules, then, ultimately determine what is heard as the "the real meter" of a tone sequence. In this way, internalized metric generations depend on preference rules that link a surface rhythm to an internalized meter.

The dichotomy of meter and rhythm in this theory resides in distinctions between well-formed rules (meter) and preference rules (rhythm), where the latter are also sensitive to parallel placements of groups and so on. For instance, consider the tone sequence suggested in Figure 9.1 (black dots). Although all tone onsets coincide with beats of level 1, the duple meter structure of this hierarchy is reinforced if accents (e.g., phenomenal accents of louder and/or longer tones) coincide with beats at odd-numbered locations (gridlines 1, 5, 9, 17 of level 1). This highlights level 3 with a corresponding group of beats. In turn, this instills a preference for a duple meter.

This theory has been widely influential. It intuitively captures basic aspects of meter as conceived by composers and musicians, stimulating as well other rule-based approaches (reviewed by Temperley and Bartlett, 2002).[6] Most such theories are *beat-finding models* that focus on effective determinants of specific metrical levels, such as the tactus, in a complex pattern of successive sounds.[7] However, some approaches also introduce temporal quantization and connectionist principles.[8] Still others raise profound questions about a perceiver's reliance on static grids and abstract rules.[9,10]

One scholar raising such questions is Justin London.[11] He keenly observed that Lerdahl and Jackendoff's abstract well-formedness rules may be unnecessary for explaining the down-to-earth experiences of typical listeners when listening to time patterns. He argues: "Why not ask just ask what affects people's responses to various time patterns?" (p. 72). In other words, we don't need to extract well-formedness rules if some time patterns automatically dominate attending, thereby facilitating certain responses. Furthermore, London's hypothesis paves the way for a more dynamic approach to meter that incorporates inherently cyclic relationships implied by different metric time layers. His listener-oriented approach opens the door to modeling meter perception using internalized, overlapping cycles at different, but related, rates (periods).

In sum, scholarly thinking about meter perception has progressed from a tradition rooted in abstract rules to one that conceives of listeners as oriented to cycles (i.e., periodicities). Yet distinct differences remain between meter, with its hierarchical layers, interrelated by simple time relationships (1:2, 1:3, etc.), and rhythms consisting of serially patterned groups. Therefore, let us turn to approaches that consider rhythm perception.

PERCEIVING RHYTHMS AND GESTALT RULES

Psychology also has a long history of fascination with pattern formation, especially as bequeathed by Gestalt theory. Although Lerdahl and Jackendoff identified abstract rules for music and speech based on well-formedness and preference rules, their rules differ from the "good forms" of Gestalt rules, long popular in psychology. Gestalt rules are more general than generative grammar rules in that they apply to the perception of visual and auditory configurations in time and space.

Historically, Gestalt theory influenced Fraisse's explanations of people's rhythmic percepts of non-isochronous tone sequences. For instance, if a fuzzy dactyl rhythm (short-short-long, as 300-289-540 ms) occurs, according to Gestalt theory, people will tend to distort it toward a simpler form (e.g., 300-300-600 ms). Fraisse enlisted Gestalt rules of assimilation and simple "good form" to explain the attracting power of time ratios of 1:1 and 1:2. As discussed in Chapter 7, Fraisse was fascinated by what he described as the anchoring "pull" of certain simple time ratios.

However, others cast a broader net. These researchers explored the nature of group formation specified with Gestalt rules of principles of proximity, contiguity, similarity, and inclusiveness. Thus, rhythmic groups can form from temporal proximity (e.g., XXX...XXX) or pitch similarity (e.g., HHHLLL for high and low pitches), and so on. For instance, Gestalt principles guided Garner's influential *run-gap principle*.[12] He described listeners' tendencies to "reorganize" recycled monotone time patterns into "good forms" where perceptual organizations favored longer rhythmic groups (runs) at the beginning of a lengthy pattern and longer empty intervals (silent gaps) ending a rhythm. Also in this spirit, Stephen Handel's work confirms the power of various Gestalt rules using recycled rhythmic figures.[13,14]

This brief overview of approaches to rhythm identifies issues that continue to occupy contemporary scholars. Yet one thing seems clear: People can perceive rhythmic patterns quite apart from a metrical framework. So, does this mean that rhythm and meter perception are entirely different and independent constructs? One line of thought implies this is so. It holds that meter rests on recursive, learnable rules whereas rhythm is based on innate Gestalt grouping principles.

However, if two different constructs respectively underlie percepts of meter and rhythm, then why are biases favoring simpler time ratios evident in both cases? And why does learning benefit percepts of both meter and rhythm? And what if it can be shown that rhythm and meter somehow have an interacting effect on perception? What if rhythm primes a meter percept or vice versa? These questions bring us to a third approach to meter and rhythm suggested by Dirk Povel.

METER AND RHYTHMIC GROUPS: A CODING MODEL

Dirk Povel outlined a clear distinction between meter and rhythm wherein meter is represented internally by "ticks" of an internalized mechanical clock,[15] and a rhythmic time pattern creates grouping accents that may, or may not, align with these clock ticks. Importantly, these ideas were formulated in a testable coding model.

Povel's coding theory, proposed 1985, met with great success due to its elegant simplicity.[16,17] The model is limited to two different time levels: namely, a referent (clock) level of clock ticks and level of subdivisions conveyed by rhythmic grouping accents.

An Emergent Clock

Povel proposed that rhythm depends on a listener's emergent, internal clock. Interestingly, a particular metric clock is induced by contextual regularities in a tone sequence initially created by *grouping accents*, >. Once a "best" clock, based on regular grouping accents, emerges, it then operates as a fixed temporal grid (i.e., as a referent time level). For example, in Figure 9.1, if level 3 in this hierarchy produces a best clock, then it marks out meter-like clock ticks (i.e., **m . . . m . . . etc.**), each such tick is a *metric accent*. Next, all grouping accents (>) are assessed relative to the clock ticks; they are gauged as more or less deviant from metrical tick accents. Overall coding strength increases with fewer misalignments of rhythmic grouping accents with metric clock ticks. Example rhythms in Figure 9.2 show two different "clocks" (i.e., referent levels are marked by clock ticks, **o,** for 800 or 400 ms). In this case, a code of four deviations determines the weakest clock.[18]

Povel proposed an important and widely confirmed algorithm for identifying grouping accents, >, in sequences.[19] Specifically, salient grouping accents occur on (1) isolated tones, (2) the second tone in a two-tone group, and (3) initial and ending tones in groups of three or more sounds (see Figure 9.2).

This coding model suggests that meter and rhythm interact via alignments of metric (**o**) and rhythmic grouping (>) accents. Note that the example sequence of Figure 9.1 has many (70%) grouping accents, >, that coincide with **m** accents. Also, the examples of Figure 9.2 show different alignments of grouping with meter accents. Although both the number of grouping accents aligning with clock "ticks" and the number of misalignments are potentially important, the coding model emphasizes the latter as clock violations (stars). In Figure 9.1, the number of clock violations leads to codes indexing no violations (pattern 1) and to four violations (pattern 4), for good and bad clock fits, respectively.

Finally, from a psychological perspective, it is important to note that this is a memory model. Memory codes in Figure 9.2 reflect the number of clock violations (stars) collected over a completed sequence. Thus, at some later time, pattern 1 should be more accurately reproduced than patterns 3 or 4. Memory code predictions underscore the fact that the clock model does not describe real-time attending because such a code depends on a completed sequence.

Evidence for a Memory Code Model

Povel's model remains wildly successful. Originally, it received strong support in tasks requiring people to reproduce recycled metrical and non-metrical sequences.[20] And it continues to reap empirical success. For instance, recently, Patel et al.[21] induced a strong clock in listeners who tapped in synchrony to a pattern resembling pattern 1 in Figure 9.1. Next, these listeners successfully continued this tapping pattern to a different, metrically weaker, phase-shifted ambiguous rhythm. This is consistent with predictions of this memory model. Other support comes from perception tasks where metrically "good" clock patterns improve temporal acuity.[22,23,24,25]

Despite its success, some question assumptions of the clock model. Devin McAuley[26] noted that a clock emerges mainly from negative evidence (clock violations) denying a role for positive evidence when **m** and > accents coincide. For instance, patterns 1 and 2 (in Figure 9.2) not only offer little negative evidence (0 and 2 clock violations, respectively), but they also provide positive evidence (i.e., **m** and > coincide at 5 and 7 loci). McAuley and Semple[27] found that Povel's clock model worked for non-musicians but not for musicians who used both positive and negative evidence. In short, skilled listeners rely on the reinforcing effects of synchronous alignments of metric and grouping accents as well as the absence of misalignments, a process that makes intuitive sense.

Summary of Background Approaches

The three different approaches to meter and rhythm reviewed here all acknowledge a dichotomy between these two constructs. Moreover, these approaches also imply that meter and rhythm perception reflect inherently different internal mechanisms. For meter, this may involve abstract rules for the development of a static grid or an emergent clock. Conversely, popular Gestalt rules offer ways to describe temporal groups. Finally, all three approaches fail to address real-time attending activities of listeners as they respond in-the-moment to meter and rhythm. The remainder of this chapter explores the latter perspective.

The main points in this section are:

- Meter and rhythm are often assumed to reflect inherently different, dichotomous functions.
- Meter is popularly conceived as a fixed grid or mechanical clock.
- Contemporary thinking distinguishes meter from rhythm. One view stipulates abstract generative rules for a well-formed metric

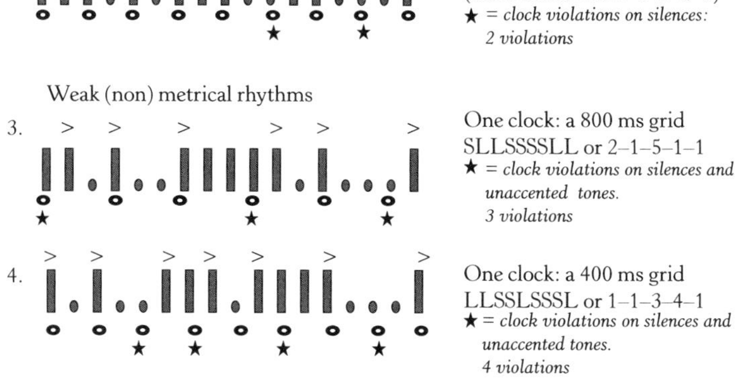

Examples of povel & essens' sequences

FIGURE 9.2 Four-tone sequences (gray bars) illustrating predictions of Povel's coding model for a mechanical clock given strong and weak metric rhythms. Clock "ticks" ⭘ mark out a grid (analogous to **m** in Figure 9.1). A violation ★ indicates a mismatch of a clock tick with a group accent, >. Two clocks are shown (for 800 and 400 ms grids) for patterns with few violations (strong metrical rhythms) and for ones with several violations (weak metrical rhythms).

grid and preferred rhythms. A second appeals to Gestalt laws of grouping/assimilation. A third view replaces a hierarchical grid with a mechanical clock. Rhythms supply grouping accents that may or may nor coordinate with this clock.

ENTRAINMENT APPROACHES: IDENTIFYING DRIVING AND DRIVEN RHYTHMS

The remainder of this chapter advances a real-time approach to attending as it applies to people's ability to track musical meter and rhythm. It applies (and extends) major hypotheses from Part I to explain dynamic attending to metrical and rhythmic aspects of music. As such, the present applications assume that "[t]he human system in general and the perceptual system in particular depends upon properties of endogenous rhythmic processes in the nervous system. These rhythms differ in frequency and may increase or decrease in amplitude within a given frequency."[28][p.328]

To preview, apparent dichotomies of meter and rhythm can be addressed using different applications of basic entrainment mechanisms that explain differences in listeners' attending to these aspects of events. To clarify this, it is necessary to first identify the nature of driving and driven rhythms involved in entrained attending of metrical and rhythmical events. The primary argument in this chapter holds that differences in external properties of meter and rhythm force basic entrainment mechanisms to operate with correspondingly different protocols. In brief, this chapter proposes that meter perception depends largely on the traditional mode-locking protocol, whereas rhythm perception relies on the transient mode-locking protocol (Chapter 7).

Distinctions between these two entrainment protocols were introduced in Part I. In this chapter, they return to explain constraints imposed by metrical versus rhythm time relationships. The traditional mode-locking protocol leads to the familiar construct of an oscillator cluster, here a *metric oscillation cluster*. Metric clusters are endogenous configurations of multiple, simultaneously active neural oscillations that together represent an internalized metric hierarchy. By contrast, the transient mode-locking protocol, also based on entrainment mechanisms, describes real-time attending to rhythmic patterns. However, in this case, the resulting internalization is an attractor profile, termed a *rhythmic attractor profile*. In brief,

we have a superficial dichotomy that is profoundly grounded in a common framework, an entrainment framework.

Reinterpreting the Metric Grid

Given the preceding distinctions, let us return to a metric grid, as sketched in Figure 9.1A. Although this is a useful sketch, within an entrainment frame, each level of a stimulus time hierarchy is now recast as a functional driving rhythm. In an originating stimulus sequence, each level represents an exogenous driving rhythm that is approximately regular, with a "roughly" constant rate. Furthermore, an internalization of each driving rhythm within such a hierarchy is represented in a listener as a correlated cortical oscillation, i.e., its driven rhythm, with a corresponding latent period. And, once listeners develop multiple active oscillations resonant to respectively different metric levels, they will have internalized a dynamic metric time hierarchy.

In this entrainment scenario, the simultaneous activity of multiple tunable oscillations leads to the endogenous entrainments described in Part I for the traditional mode-locking protocol. And the result is a malleable internalized hierarchy, termed a *metric oscillator cluster*. "Malleable" here means that these neural oscillations fluctuate (within limits); moreover, as limit cycle oscillations, members of a cluster operate adaptively vis-á-vis various driving rhythm changes. Evidence favoring neural entrainment to metric time levels comes from Nozaradan and colleagues.[29]

To illustrate this idea, consider the stimulus driving rhythm of level 3 in Figure 9.1; let its **m** markers recur every 1,200 sec. This slow periodicity, then, will engage a spontaneously fluctuating driven neural oscillation with an approximately similar resonant period. Next, assume that a different exogenous entrainment occurs at level 1 (where T = 300 ms is an inter-onset-interval [IOI]; i.e., here, a quarter note). The latter stimulus driving rhythm then induces activity in a faster neural oscillation. These two active oscillations then engage in endogenous entrainment following a 4:1 ratio. In turn, this allows a listener to sense a duple (4/4) meter. By contrast, imagine that a different level 1 oscillation happened to be activated, one with a period of 400 ms, creating a 3:1 ratio; in this case, this would elicit in a listener the sense of a triple meter. Such recursive embedding relationships look suspiciously like attractor ratios (e.g., 1:2, 1:4, etc.), a point to which we return.[30]

Next, this reinterpretation of a metric grid can be supplemented by inviting in rhythmic time patterns. So, let's focus on onsets of successive tones (black) depicted below in Figure 9.1B. These trace out a coherent but non-isochronous time pattern that exhibits different serially ordered driving rhythms. Individual time spans, T, as well as the group time spans, Tg, are shown in this figure; the latter are marked by rhythm grouping accents, >. Any succession of varied time spans is a candidate for transient mode-locking, as described in Chapter 7. With this entrainment protocol, we may assume that a persisting referent oscillation emerges based on some initial time span marked by grouping accents (>). For example, perhaps the first group time span, Tg (star), establishes a persisting internal referent period that listeners use to gauge future group time spans, large and small, throughout the remainder of this pattern. The result is a *rhythmic attractor profile*.

In short, the temporal distributions of metric and rhythm accents in musical events, so neatly identified by Povel, can be seen from a different perspective. Here they play an instigating role in awakening oscillators that figure in metric clusters, and they also figure in the development of rhythmic attractor profiles. Clearly, both time markers (accents) and the periods they outline are critical to a listener's final percept of an event's time structure. So, let's next unpack a theoretical account of accents.

Accents: Reinterpreting Time Markers of Driving and Driven Rhythms

In any acoustic sequence, certain points in time inevitably draw our attention. Often these are points marked by forceful external time markers. In this case, they serve as objective *accent points* which draw peaks of attending energy. While some accents are objectively marked in the surface structure of a time pattern, curiously, in other cases the salience of a time point resides only in the mind of a listener. Thus, let us distinguish *objective* from *subjective salience* of a time point.

Objective salience refers to the measureable strength of a physical time marker. For instance, a louder sound that marks a metric accent has objective salience wherein this salience is an objectively measureable physical property. However, if a weak time marker appears at a metrically prominent point in time (e.g., the tenth note in Figure 9.1), a skilled listener may nonetheless *sense* this as strong subjectively salient point in time. In this case, salience is subjective because it is associated with internal attending energy; it refers to a local peak of attending, in the form of either an *expectancy pulse* (i.e., attentional anticipation) or a *reactive energy burst* (i.e., attentional capture). In either case, what is critical is the occurrence of a *heightened burst of attending energy* which defines a functional accent at a particular point in time.

This psychological approach focuses on local boosts of attending neural energy. Four different categories of accent boosts are outlined in Table 9.1. Note that this approach to accenting differs from that of Lerdahl and Jackendoff,[31] who differentiated *phenomenal accents* (emphatic physical changes in a rhythm) from both *structural accents* (beginnings/ends of phrases) and *metrical accents* (strong metric beats). Instead, in the present breakdown, accents are either metric or rhythmic (columns in Table 9.1). And in both cases, accents can express either subjective (internal) or objective (external) salience, leading to the four accenting categories shown in Table 9.1. These distinctions are illustrated schematically in Figure 9.3.

More About Metric Accents: Subjective Versus Objective Salience

Metric accents in a musical event depend on the contextual regularity of physical time markers (**m** accents), as in Figure 9.1. *Objective salience of metric accents* is linked to an observable driving rhythm. It derives from a discretely heightened physical change (e.g., intensity) in an external rhythm. This might reflect a marker high in a produced metric hierarchy, for example. By contrast, *subjective salience of metric accents* is linked to

TABLE 9.1 SOURCE OF ACCENT TIMING

Source of Accent Salience	Meter	Rhythm
Objective (from driving rhythms)	Context regularity: moutlining metric time layers	Local changes: > Outlining group boundaries
Subjective (from driven rhythms)	Expectancy pulses: "Expectancy"	Reactive pulses: "Capture"

an internal, driven rhythm; it derives from a discretely heightened change in internal energy associated with a driven oscillation.

Expanding on this topic, subjective metric accents reflect the activity of a strong driven rhythm created by a regular metric context. Subjective salience derives from elicited expectancy pulses; strong pulses usually accompany strong driven oscillations. Subjective salience refers to a listener's "felt" strength of an entrained expectancy pulse.

Figure 9.3 illustrates reactions of strong and weak oscillations of a hypothetical listener who entrains to a sequence containing regularly recurring metrical accents. In the top row of this figure, tx is the expected time of contextually recurring metric accents. Here, a strong, phase-specific expectancy pulse conveys subjective salience at metrically expected times, tx. Such a pulse not only anticipates a physically strong time marker, at tn (e.g., see the physical change bar), but it also occurs at an expected time where *no physical marker occurs*. Importantly, this creates a *silent expectancy pulse*. Expectancy pulses slightly anticipate an expected stimulus onset.

The bottom row of Figure 9.3 features the activity of a weaker driven oscillation. Note that its phase-specific expectancy pulses are weaker than those in the top row. However, following a sudden encounter with a physical stimulus (blue bar), a relatively strong reactive pulse is evoked by this stimulus. As shown, reactive pulses happen automatically *after* surprising physical events for both strong and weak oscillations.

More About Rhythmic Accents: Subjective Versus Objective Salience

Rhythmic accents are linked to stimulus groups, as Povel proposed. Their objective salience is determined by Povel's algorithm. Importantly, these accents do not necessarily coincide with metric accents. For instance, the rhythmic groups in Figure 9.1 b (time spans of Tgs) do not always "fit" neatly into the contextual regularity of this duple meter: **m** and > accents. Nevertheless, in an entrainment scheme, the subjective salience of grouping accents (as reactive pulses) depends on the "surprise" value of an unexpected accent. Unexpected sounds automatically capture attending, as shown in attending energy profiles (AEPs; see Chapter 4).

In sum, musical sequences lay a foundation for the arousal of two types attending pulses that are linked, respectively, to expectancy and capture

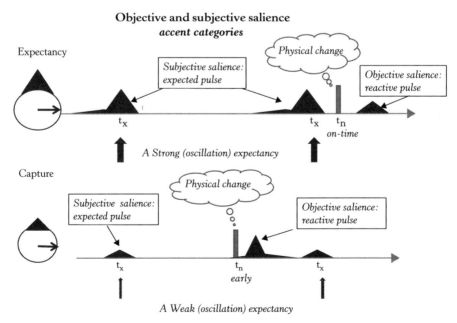

FIGURE 9.3 Two types of accents expressing expectancy and capture. Top row shows a strong entraining oscillation with strong expectancy pulses (hence, high subjective salience) at times, tx. Subjective accent salience depends on pulse energy. Expectancy pulses occur at anticipated time points regardless of stimulus (gray bar). Bottom row shows a weak entraining oscillation with weak expectancy pulse (hence, low subjective salience). In both rows, a physical change, whether expected or not, evokes a reactive pulse, which is correlated with objective salience.

profiles (in the phase response curves [PRCs] and AEPs of Chapter 4). As internal pulses they specify subjective salience of metric and rhythmic accents, respectively. Figure 9.3 suggests that both types of accents come in two flavors: namely, objective and subjective:

- *Objective metric accents* are distinguished by physical changes, usually in intensity. *Subjective metric accents* depend on the internal energy of an expectancy pulse.
- *Objective rhythmic accents* are physically distinguished as markers of a (local) driving rhythm. *Subjective rhythmic accents* depend on neural correlates, which are either expectancy pulses (for meter) or reactive pulses (for rhythm).

How Do Accents Work?

According to the Dynamic Attending Theory (DAT), accenting draws on theoretical distinctions between expectancy and capture. However, this entrainment account has been disputed by current research which suggests that accents are not time markers of driving and driven rhythms. Instead, an alternative position is that accents are motor-driven images.

The Dynamic View of Accenting

A DAT account, just previewed, proposes that the subjective salience of accents depends on entraining neural activities involving expectancy and reactive pulses, both of which are operative within an established context. In music, driving rhythms within an extended metric context deliver objective metric accents, while locally rhythmic groups supply objective rhythmic accents. Patterns of objective metric accents lead to expectancy pulses, whereas external stimulations by rhythmic groups tend to evoke reactive pulses, as depicted in Figure 9.3. Ultimately, the subjective salience of any accent is rooted in neural entrainments.

Empirical support for this view comes from Joel Snyder and Ed Large.[32] They presented non-musicians with an isochronous sequence of loud/soft duple-meter time markers and recorded magnetoencephalogram (MEG) activity in listeners' auditory cortex. Recorded bursts of neural activity, indicative of expectancy pulses, were found preceding expected tone onsets (i.e., at time tx). Also, silent expectancy pulses appeared during random silences. These expectancy bursts involved high gamma, γ, frequencies (28–40 Hz). By contrast, reactive attending pulses were beta pulses β (15–20 Hz) that followed tone onsets.[33]

A Motor Imagery View

This dynamic account of accenting has been questioned by John Iverson and colleagues.[34] Following studies suggesting that beta pulses reflect motor activities,[35] they proposed that accents are auditory images voluntarily produced by activating a listener's covert motor behavior. Clearly, this picture differs from that painted by DAT. It implies that gamma bursts do not reflect the subjective salience of expectancy pulses, but instead this gamma activity merely reflects reactive activities.[36] Consistent with this view, the beta frequencies reported by Large and Snyder have been interpreted as signs of motor-generated images governed by voluntary (instructions) and involuntary (stimulus) factors.

Support for a motor imagery view involves MEG recordings of musicians' selective responses to tones in rhythmic groups (beta bursts of 20–30 Hz). These responses of listeners supply evidence for their voluntary compliance with instructions to imagine certain accents in a triple meter sequence. Because beta is often linked to motor activity, these findings were interpreted as support for motor imagery: "the motor system may reciprocally affect the auditory system, possibly by setting up precisely timed beat-related expectancies or alternative subjective perception via subjective accentuation."[33]

Summary of Meter Perception

Currently, two different views of meter perception are in play. One holds that anticipatory neural energy signifies metrically entrained attending, evident in expectancy pulses. The other view maintains that reactive neural bursts reflect motor images, favoring a motor imagery explanation. Unfortunately, these disparate findings arise from experimental designs that differ in many variables, including rhythmic patterning, sequence rates, implied meters (duple vs. triple)m participants' musical skills, and criteria for beta versus gamma frequencies, to list a few. As a result, resolving theoretical differences on the basis of these studies is problematic. Nevertheless, it is apparent that neural correlates of accents exist, and future pursuit of these issues will no doubt be productive.

METER PERCEPTION AND OSCILLATOR CLUSTERS: AN ENTRAINMENT PERSPECTIVE

Musical meter is conventionally associated with hierarchical time structure. However, in a dynamic attending framework, this hierarchy is not a grid. Rather, it is a more malleable construct in which objective accents outline multiple, overlapping driving rhythms at different time scales (layers); furthermore, these driving rhythms are assumed to induce corresponding subjective accents. Moreover, as driving rhythms become internalized as resonant neural correlates, an even more structured internal brain configuration emerges in the form of an oscillator cluster. That is, sets of simultaneously active internal oscillations endogenously entrain with one another thereby leading to a metric oscillator cluster.

Formation of any oscillator cluster follows the traditional mode-locking profile. This protocol is reviewed in Figure 9.4. Here, a referent oscillation, with a fixed (latent) period p (top row, lighter gray triangles), aligns (below) with four external driving rhythms, each with a different fixed rate, T (larger, dark triangles). The stationarity of both the internal period, p, and that of each external driving rhythm period, T, yields four different traditional mode-locking protocols involving exogenous entrainment.

To preview the next section, imagine now that each of the external periods, T, depicted in Figure 9.4 also elicits a resonant internal periodicity. In this case, several different active oscillations also come into play. Consequently, endogenous dyads will also emerge based on endogenous entrainments among these oscillations.

Given traditional mode-locking, a variety of related oscillations can connect with one another thus forming an oscillator cluster.

The Tunable Brain on Music: Forming Metric Clusters

Meter perception ultimately depends on what is inside a listener's head. So, let's hypothesize that this "what" is a process which involves coordinated activities of many endogenous cortical oscillations activated by a metrical event. In a listener, the sense of meter begins to grow with exposure to external regularities of **m** accents, as shown in Figure 9.1.

To begin, we must acknowledge that metrical accents appear almost regularly. This regularity is evident, for instance, with accents at different metric levels in Figure 9.1. This means that metric accents outline a roughly constant driving rhythm which, via traditional mode-locking, should elicit distinct neural oscillations as driven rhythms. Given this time hierarchy, let's consider four different driving rhythms at respectively different hierarchical levels, with external periods between 200 and 1,600 ms. Once active, such oscillations endogenously entrain to one another following various traditional mode-locking protocols (e.g., n:m = 2:1, 1:1, 1:2, 1:3, etc.). This flurry of oscillations eventually settles into a metric oscillator cluster, which represents an internalized duple meter.

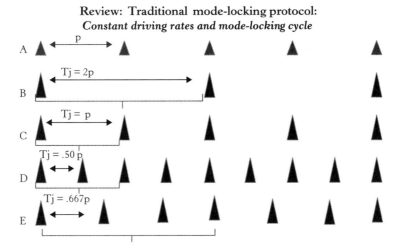

Review: Traditional mode-locking protocol:
Constant driving rates and mode-locking cycle

A   p

B   Tj = 2p

C   Tj = p

D   Tj = .50 p

E   Tj = .667p

FIGURE 9.4 Review of traditional mode-locking modes. (A) A referent oscillation with small periodically recurring pulses, pj, appears in the top row. Rows **B–E** show four driving rhythms with periodic time-markers, each with a different rate. Resulting entrainments between each driving rhythm, the referent rhythm, as a driven oscillation, are shown to follow traditional mode-locking protocols. Brackets indicate a mode-locking cycle.

Consider a situation in which a listener is exposed to the very simple *loud-soft-loud-soft* cadence of a marching band, where strong and weak **m** accents alternate. Such a 1:2 pattern is hard to ignore. Indeed, automatic entrainment to a duple meter is swift, evident in prompt head-nodding and/or foot-tapping in listeners. The compelling timing of alternating strong–weak sounds instills in most listeners a duple meter via exogenous entrainments. Moreover, this process may become so entrenched that it outlasts the presence of the originating stimulation.

Most music buffs testify to the internal reality of the "sense" of meter—even in the absence of a stimulus. For example, it is difficult to dispute musicians' claims that upon encountering a 6/8 musical score, they can "call up" a sense of six eighth notes recurrently clustered within longer (measure) time spans. Musically savvy people carry around in their heads a variety of meters. Granting that various exogenous entrainments occur between the impact of some external metric driving rhythms and what ends up in a musician's head, the next step requires contemplation of endogenous entrainments among driven neural rhythms activated in a listener. When two or more metrically related internal oscillations become active in a tunable brain, this leads to endogenous entrainments. And, following the traditional entrainment mode-locking protocol (Figure 9.4), multiple oscillations activated by these driving rhythms begin to interact.

The result of all this activity is that endogenous couplings end up forming a *metric oscillator cluster*. From a DAT perspective, then, what ends up in musicians' heads are entrenched metric oscillator clusters. In fact, this description of a metric oscillator cluster should be familiar to readers because, if it is speeded up, it will resemble a pitch oscillator cluster, which involves fast complex sounds (from Chapter 6). Metric oscillator clusters are simply much slower versions of the micro-timed pitch clusters elicited by partials of a complex harmonic sound. All such clusters, regardless of component rates, share a defining feature: they gravitate to time-honored relationships that are invariant throughout a metric event.

Metric clusters will include a referent periodicity. Whereas in pitch clusters the referent was the fundamental frequency, in meter this privileged time level is termed the tactus. Generally, a metric cluster expresses abstract harmonic relations among different neural oscillations which form a fluent *internalized metric frame* which includes neural representative of the tactus.

Evidence for Metric Oscillator Clusters

Despite its abstractness, the reality of an internalized metric frame is bolstered by several findings. A classic paper by Palmer and Krumhansl[37] provides strong validation of internalized metric timings. Musicians readily imagine multiple metric levels implied by fragments of an auditory event; even nonmusicians can induce a few metric levels from fragments of duple and triple meter sound patterns. Furthermore, duple meter stimulus patterns enhance performance in a time discrimination task, especially for musicians.[38] Finally, although tapping tasks typically encourage selective attending to a single metrical level, tapping performance is enhanced by the presence of surrounding metric levels.[39,40]

Converging evidence based on proof of existence is offered by Edward Large.[41] He presented a 2 Hz tactus (500 ms) to a "listener" simulated by a bank of endogenous oscillations (periods of 125 ms to 2 sec). In theory, metrical listening should occur only if those oscillations of metrical time levels congruent with the referent period become active (e.g., relative to p in Figure 9.4). Over a large range of stimulating driving rhythms, Large observed that selective phase-locking activity happened only for pairs of oscillations observing metric time ratios (1:2, 1:3, 2:3, etc.).

Unlike views of meter as a static grid, a dynamic approach incorporates a self-organizing potential. This is evident in the formation of metric oscillator clusters. Figure 9.5 suggests how an unfolding metric frame might activation neural oscillations at each of four different metric levels in a musical event. In such an example, cluster formation implies that a single strong endogenous oscillation (here $p_2 = p_R = 400$ ms) acts as an internal (referent) driving rhythm that then awakens other related (but resting) members of a metric oscillator cluster. Specifically, oscillator amplitudes are selectively heightened. Also an internal "domino effect" may occur, with active oscillations waking other related but resting oscillations. The operating "awaking" principle is typically resonance, but simple entraining ratios also play a role. Thus, skilled musicians might readily "call up" relevant mental metric frames by just viewing a musical score. And, once one internal oscillation gains strength, this flows to others with related periodicities. In such cases, one oscillation, Oi, excites another, Ok, and so on, looping back and forth, thereby promoting healthy metric persistence. Looping interactions are especially possible with coupled oscillations of equal strength (symmetric coupled). Finally, such self-organizing/spreading activations are keys to creativity.

In sum, meter perception begins with stimulus-driven activities that lead to multiple exogenous entrainments of related oscillations. And it continues, driven by the arousal of sets of strong, connected internal oscillations (with skill, a likely differentiating factor). In this section, the news centers on the construct of a metric oscillator cluster produced with traditional mode-locking. A metric oscillator cluster functions as an endogenous frame for meter. This process explains how activities of multiple, nested, endogenous oscillations can express the constraints of metric timing constraints on attending.

What's Inside a Metric Cluster?

This seems like a question already answered: clusters are filled with related (i.e., member) oscillations. But a more detailed answer fleshes out cluster features that promote how listeners perceive meter. Specifically, two properties of metric clusters are important. One concerns specific attractor relationships among oscillator members of a cluster as defined by a set of global attractors. The other concerns relative amplitudes of oscillations. Both factors figure in a familiar Arnold tongue regime, shown in Figure 9.6. In this figure, the abscissa identifies attractor ratios and the ordinate plots the amplitude (i.e., strength) of an oscillation that functions as a driving rhythm.

Global Attractors

Global attractors result from the traditional mode-locking protocol (Chapter 7). Particularly in describing meter, this entrainment protocol expresses constant, commensurate time relationships between two (or more) active oscillations. Figure 9.6, for instance, shows endogenous time relationships among three hierarchically overlapping oscillations from Figure 9.5 (e.g., periods of 200, 400, 800 ms; with p_R = 400 ms). In pair-wise interactions among periods, all adjacent oscillations realize a simple global attractor of 1:2, but different global attractors emerge to connect other oscillations e.g., *n:m* of 1:1 or 1:4. Generally, Western music showcases a range of relationships that figure in metric clusters.

Limits of Attractors and Entrainment

All entrainment models place limits on entrainment.[42] And such limits are closely connected to attractors, where constraints are expressed by an attractor's entrainment region (where region boundaries of tongues are bifurcation limits). Each global attractor in a cluster specifies an entrainment region, as suggested in Figure 9.6. Here, the amplitude of a particular driving oscillation is plotted on the ordinate (Aj).[43] Member oscillations of a cluster are internal rhythms that couple with other internal rhythms, forming endogenous dyads. Thus, for example, in this figure cluster members observe three fixed dyadic ratios (.50, 1.0, 2.0). Each is one of several global attractors for the metric pattern of Figure 9.5. From the aging hypothesis, such attractors are critical, life-long components in governing attending dynamics.

Figure 9.6 shows the three cluster members with periods of p_1 = 200 ms, p_2 = 400 ms, and p_3 = 800 ms. For instructive purposes, assume p_2 functions as a referent oscillation, $p_2 = p_R$. Referent periods are typically carried by a stable, persisting referent oscillation. Thus, hypothesized attractor ratios (p_R:pj ratios) each fall on vertical prototype line within a entrainment tongue, V, in Figure 9.6.

Four active oscillations: *A metric oscillator cluster*

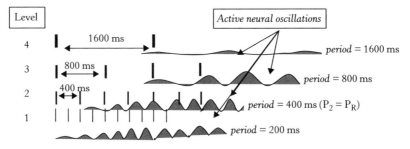

FIGURE 9.5 A metric cluster induced by external driving rhythms at four different time scales in a metrical rhythm. This figure depicts activation of hypothesized neural oscillations at different metric time scales. The formation of a metric oscillator cluster is the result of endogenous entrainments among these neural oscillations.

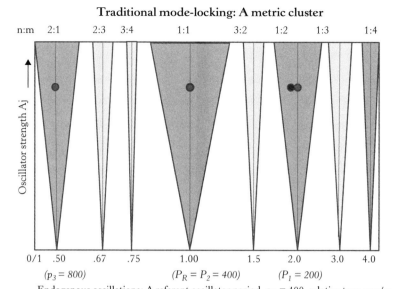

FIGURE 9.6 An Arnold tongue regime applied to oscillations in an oscillator cluster. Period ratios (on abscissa) reflect relationships between a referent oscillation's period (400 ms) and that of two different endogenous driving oscillations (800 ms, 200 ms) within a cluster resulting from a traditional mode-locking protocol. A set of three attractors (.50, 1.00, 2.0) reflects prototypical relations (light gray circles); a slightly deviant oscillation is also shown (darker gray circle). The ordinate reflects strength of a driving rhythm oscillation (not necessarily the referent).

These are operative attractors ratios of .50, 1.0, and 2.0 etc. (abscissa). Also shown is a slightly deviant version of one oscillation, with a period, $p_1 \sim 210$ ms (darker dot in the 2.0 entrainment region). This illustrates that some oscillator fluctuations are harmless, given a referent period, p_R, of 400 ms, in an adaptive brain system (i.e., its endogenous ratio is 1.91 instead of 2.00). Deviations are typical of brain oscillations which spontaneously fluctuate yet hover near their latent value. In this scenario, the functional global attractors function as keys to effective attending.

Amplitudes of Pulse and Oscillations: Selective Attending

In the present discussion of oscillator clusters, "selective attending" refers to the activity of one or several entraining oscillations in a cluster. Two aspects of selective attending to an external driving rhythm are pertinent. One concerns the impact of an external driving rhythm on phase entrainments of a driven oscillation within a cluster. The other concerns the role of a dominant oscillation on selective attending to one versus another metric time layer. These two aspects of selective attending (whether voluntary or involuntary) are termed, respectively, *phase-based focal attending* and *period-based focal attending*.

Phase-Based Focal Attending

Phase-based focal attending refers to situations in which a phase-specific expectancy pulse of a cluster oscillation targets peak attending energy at a particular phase point (previewed by AEPs of Chapter 4). Edward Large pursued this idea. He proposed that an internal expectancy pulse carried by a driven (entraining) oscillation is locally sharpened at a particular, expected phase point within the period of a driven oscillation (e.g., tx in Figure 9.3).[44,45] Effectively, this describes a hyper-sensitive (high energy) region within the orbit of an oscillation. In theory, this pulse may be influenced by the regularity of an external driving rhythm for a given oscillation with an oscillation cluster.

Figure 9.7 illustrates phase-based focal attending as a function of driving rhythm regularity. In panel A, an expectancy pulse appears at an expected phase point, tx (i.e., $\varphi = 0$), in the regular period of this oscillation (from times ti to ti + 1). This pulse is strongly peaked for a regular external driving rhythm (finely phase-tuned) but becomes diffuse for irregular driving rhythms (poor phase corrections), as shown in panel B. Within a metric cluster, this driven oscillation becomes "phase-tuned" to expected time points of an external driving rhythm (e.g., for **m** accents) depending on contextual regularity.

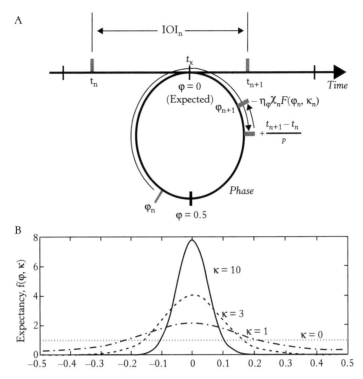

FIGURE 9.7 (A) Times of stimulus onsets, tn and tn + 1 (for a recurring inter-onset period, IOI), relative to contextually expected time, tx, are shown as phase points in an entraining oscillation where the expected phase is $\varphi = 0$. (B) An expectancy pulse centered at the anticipated phase point, tx, can be strongly focused or weakly focused as shown.

Reproduced from Large and Palmer, "Perceiving Temporal Regularity in Music," *Cognitive Science* 26, no. 1 (January 2002): 1–37, doi:10.1016/S0364-0213(01)00057-X.

The amplitude of an expectancy pulse increases as phase-tuning becomes more precise. In other words, a pulse strengthens with the enhanced recruitment of phase-aligned oscillatory activities. This pulse, then, represents the neural correlate of the momentary experience of subjective salience conveyed by a stimulus. Even in the absence of an objective accent, strong pulses persist as *silent expectancy pulses*. A number of studies confirm the validity of phase-based expectancy pulses using MEG/event-related potential (ERP) recordings.[46,47,48, 49 ,50, 51, 52]

Period-Based Focal Attending

Period-based focal attending refers to selectively heightening the overall amplitude of a single oscillation of a metric cluster. This revives the construct of a *dominant* oscillation, one based upon the relative heightening of amplitude (from Chapter 5). In music, a dominant oscillation determines period-oriented attending. For instance, in a metrical context, it describes a listener who momentarily focuses on the recurring period of one metrical

level over others in a time hierarchy. Moreover, in theory, such period-based allocations of attending energy can be brought under voluntary control. For instance, to follow a slow melodic theme within a musical event that contains multiple interleaved voices, one must consciously "pay attention" to sounds happening at this slow rate and ignore others. This entails voluntarily heightening the amplitude of a relevant oscillation, rendering it dominant.

Jones and Boltz[53] previewed this idea in differentiating *future-oriented attending*, which assigns greater attending energy to oscillator periods entraining to slower driving rhythms (higher metric layers), from *analytic attending*, which entails voluntary shifts of attending energy to faster driving rhythms. Both are tethered to a referent oscillation, the tactus, which reflects a basic beat period. Support for period-oriented attending comes from Carolyn Drake and colleagues.[54,55,56] They found evidence of voluntary attending to certain metric levels, relative to a referent level, in the synchronized tappings of musicians and non-musicians. Although musicians were better than non-musicians, all showed voluntary analytic attending (to faster metric levels) and voluntary future-oriented attending (to slower metric levels). Drake et al. summarized their results within a dynamic attending schematic, reproduced in Figure 9.8.[57]

Special Entrainment Models of Meter Perception: Perspectives from Edward Large

Preceding sections suggest that attending, especially selective attending, depends on the amplitudes of an entraining oscillation. A formalization of entraining oscillations in which amplitude appears in the pioneering modeling of Edward Large.[58,59,60] Initially, Large's models were based on classic sine-circle mappings describing phase-locking as a function of the frequency and strength of an external driving rhythm.[61,62] Subsequently, he outlined a more general entrainment model featuring a role for the amplitude of an internal (i.e., driven) rhythm that is based on an Andronov-Hopf bifurcation equation (Equation 9.1; Box 9.1).[63,64] This model not only predicts that phase coupling increases with driving rhythm strength, but it also features a role for supra-threshold amplitude variations in driven rhythms that express selective attending.[65]

Summary of Meter Perception from an Entrainment Perspective

Meter perception when considered from an entrainment perspective relies upon the coordinated activities of multiple, commensurately related oscillations in a listener's tunable brain. Such oscillations can be activated either by external driving rhythms or by other internal oscillations. Three aspects of meter perception are central in a listener's response to a metrical stimulus. First, sets of simultaneously activated oscillators form metric clusters via endogenous entrainments; these clusters function as flexible internalized frames for different musical meters. Second, within a metric cluster, a persisting referent-level oscillation emerges as common source of endogenous coupling. Third, the formation of metric clusters importantly depends on traditional mode-locking. In this view, once strong metric clusters become active, metric sensibility takes on a "life of its own."

The major points of this section are:

- Multiple, simultaneously active oscillations endogenously couple to form metric oscillator clusters.
- Oscillations in a cluster offer an internalized, stable referent period (p_R) for various p_R/pj oscillator relations within a traditional mode-locking protocol.
- Attractor relationships in a cluster capture metric relationships. They be mapped into an Arnold tongue regime where simpler ratios determine attractor regions of greater width (i.e., for e.g., $n{:}m$ = 1:1, 2:1, 3:1), hence greater stability.
- Entrainment models most promising for understanding selective attending feature a role for the varied amplitudes of driven oscillations within a metric cluster.

ENTRAINMENT APPROACHES TO RHYTHM PERCEPTION

Rhythm perception poses a challenge to established entrainment theories. The reason for this centers around the fact that conventional entrainment

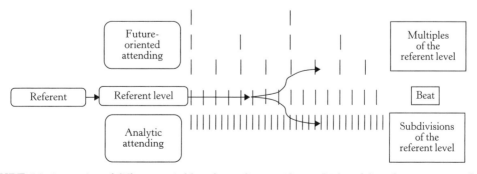

FIGURE 9.8 A mapping of different period-based attending to either multiples of the referent time period, as in *future–oriented attending,* or to subdivisions of the referent, as in *analytic attending.* This is summarized here.

Reprinted from figure 1 in Drake et al. "Tapping in Time with Mechanically and Expressively Performed Music," *Music Perception: An Interdisciplinary Journal* 18, no. 1 (2000): 1–23, doi:10.2307/40285899.

BOX 9.1
ENTRAINMENT MODEL EXAMPLES

Two examples of entrainment models following a traditional mode-locking protocol have been developed by Edward Large (see text for references). Both models predict Arnold tongue regimes.

THE SINE CIRCLE MAP

The simplest entrainment model addresses discrete changes of phase, φ, in a limit cycle (driven) oscillation and involve a sine circle map; that is, a mapping of one (e.g., oscillation) circle onto another. A phase at time n (φ_n) becomes a new phase location on a circle at time n + 1 (φ_{n+1}). A difference equation describes this, assuming the discrete periodic forces of a driving rhythm:

$$\varphi_{n+1} = \varphi_n + \Omega - K[\sin(2\pi\varphi_n)] / 2\pi \ (mod -.50, .50, 1) \qquad 9.1$$

This equation maps phase changes in a two-dimensional ($\Omega \times K$) mapping. It captures mode-locking and Arnold tongues; parameters define a plane with Ω on the abscissa and K plotted on the ordinate.

The parameter, Ω, is the manifest frequency of a driven rhythm. When $K = 0$, Ω is estimated using the average period of a driving rhythm, T, relative to a given intrinsic period, p_j: T:p_j. The Ω is typically plotted as a bare winding number on the abscissa of an Arnold tongue plot.

A CANONICAL ENTRAINMENT MODEL INCORPORATING AMPLITUDE

Edward Large (see text for references) also developed a generalized model of entrainment that includes amplitude modulations, **A** (absent in sine circle models). He adapts a canonical version of the Andronov-Hopf model, which applies to weakly connected sets of oscillations. The model predicts changes in amplitude and phase for an arbitrary oscillation with an intrinsic frequency, ω. It can explain listeners' sensitivities to a variety of metric properties in music where the acoustic stimuli vary over time, s(t). Two differential equations describe changes in amplitude, **A**, and phase, φ, respectively. Amplitude changes depend on a bifurcation control parameter, α, where $\alpha = 0$ denotes a threshold bifurcation point associated with the onset of a spontaneous oscillation; negative and positive α values (near $\alpha = 0$), respectively, describe declining versus increasing amplitudes. Persisting oscillator behavior is modeled for the case of removing a driving stimulus, s(t), if $\alpha > 0$. This allows for spontaneous oscillator activity. By contrast, negative α values dampen oscillations:

$$dA / dt = A(\alpha + \beta A^2) + cs(t)\cos\varphi + \text{h.o.t} \qquad 9.2$$

Other parameters affecting amplitude are beta, which controls an oscillation's amplitude asymptote, and c, which reflects the coupling strength between an endogenous oscillation and the stimulus time pattern.

Equation 9.3 describes phase changes as a function not only of ω, but also a weighted frequency detuning parameter, δ ($\delta = \omega i - \omega j$), for driving and driven periods (i,j). The coupling parameter, c, is qualified by the **A**, implying that the coupling connection with an external driving rhythm is attenuated with a strong driven oscillation (large **A**):

$$d\varphi / dt = \omega + \delta A^2 - \{cs(t)\sin\varphi\} / A + \text{h.o.t} \qquad 9.3$$

In general, when a driving rhythm is present (i.e., s(t) >0), entrainments with it are possible. Moreover, expanding higher order terms (h.o.t.) allow for multiple resonance relations between a single neural oscillation and a stimulus input. And, as **A** increases, so do nonlinearities in this system.

approaches require almost stationarity (i.e., quasi-isochrony) of both driving and driven rhythms. As discussed in Chapter 7, several quasi-isochronous driving rhythms contribute to traditional mode-locking protocols. The overlapping nature of several different driving rhythms in metric hierarchies meets this requirement, fitting neatly into a traditional protocol. However, this succession of different time spans is characteristic of truly patterned rhythms, but it does not neatly fit into the traditional mode-locking protocol.

Issues concerning non-isochronous, but coherent, rhythmic patterns were resolved in Chapter 7, with the introduction of the transient mode-locking protocol. Transient mode-locking explains how entrainment applies to coherent time patterns. This section continues that line of thought by applying it to rhythmic time patterns that unfold within a metrical context. This raises new and interesting issues.

Rhythm Perception and Rhythmic Attractor Profiles

This section revives core issues surrounding the dichotomy of meter and rhythm. It details both superficial differences between meter and rhythm as well as unescapable dependencies between meter and rhythm arising from aspects of attending dynamics.

To begin, rhythm perception depends on transient mode-locking. In this view, rhythm perception is explained by the activity of a single, persisting oscillation which serves a referent role for a listener who experiences a coherent non-isochronous stimulus rhythm. As discussed in Chapter 7, such rhythms comprise a series of time spans, each functioning as a fleeting driving rhythm. Consequently, transient mode-locking yields a corresponding series of local attractors that form a *rhythmic attractor profile*.

Such attractor profiles are not new. However, what is new in this chapter concerns the role of rhythmic attractor profiles in a metric context. In particular, rhythmic attractor profiles now emerge within a context that also elicits a metric oscillator cluster. In these circumstances, such a rhythm becomes a special time pattern, familiarly termed a *metrical rhythm*. Unlike the non-isochronous rhythms of Chapter 7, in this chapter, metrical rhythms invite listeners to rely on the joint activity of a metric cluster *and* a rhythmic attractor profile. For simplicity, in this discussion, imagine a metrical rhythm that elicits *both* a metric cluster and a rhythm attractor profile and that they *share the*

same *referent oscillation*. Thus, the same referent period functions in a cluster during traditional mode-locking functions and in transient mode-locking for the rhythmic pattern.

Entraining to a Metrical Rhythm: A Detailed Example

To flesh out these ideas, Figure 9.9 presents a breakdown of the metric and rhythmic components hypothesized to influence how a listener hears a metrical pattern. The stimulus sequence is a pattern of time spans (T's) marked by filled gray ovals at the bottom of this figure. The top portion of the figure shows a listener's hypothetical metrical engagement with this stimulus sequence. This top portion of the figure portrays traditional mode-locking. The rhythms involved are coded as driving (dark gray triangle markers) and driven (light gray markers) rhythms. The top three rows show a few members of a metric oscillator clusters, with a 400 ms referent period, p_R all of which co-occur, forming traditional mode-locking for a three oscillator cluster. This cluster comprises two internal driven rhythms and an internal driving rhythm (p_3 of 800 ms). Notice that the driving rhythm ($p_3 = 800$ ms) of this cluster covers two cycles of the referent period for the rhythmic pattern (e.g., $p_R = 400$ ms). The metric cluster in the top rows represents part of a listener's larger internal metric frame, as it is captured by various global attractors. Although this figure displays only three oscillations, it spells out the respective roles of referent periods and driving rhythms within such a cluster. An internal metric frame induced by this traditional mode-locking protocol is expressed by global attractors consistent with a duple meter (e.g., 1:2, 2:1, etc.).

Figure 9.9 also portrays a rhythmic attractor profile (cf. Chapter 7). This appears in the bottom portion of this figure. From Chapter 7, the attractor profile results from transient mode-locking to the series of brief, exogenous driving rhythms (i.e., single Ti time spans). A succession of such time spans can also include groups (Tg), here as fleeting exogenous driving rhythms (200, 400, 800 ms). Nevertheless, in this example, the sustaining referent oscillation that supports transient mode-locking is oscillation remains: $p_{2 = p_R =}$ 400 ms. This shows the development of a rhythmic attractor profile (via transient mode-locking) happening concurrently with the growth of a metric frame (via traditional mode-locking).

Finally, metric rhythms are typically characterized by rhythmic attractor profiles that share the same referent oscillation as the metric frame in

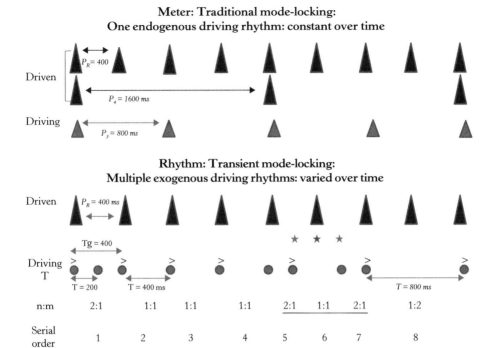

FIGURE 9.9 Joint activity of traditional mode-locking and transient mode-locking operating in a listener following a metrical tone sequence (bottom; light gray filled circles). Generally light gray codes driving rhythms and dark gray codes driven rhythms. *Top*: Metric oscillator cluster. Endogenous metric relationships appear in the top two rows, with two driven oscillations (dark gray triangles i.e., pulses) with periods of 400 and 1,600 ms. The third row shows an internal driving rhythm (light gray triangles, i.e., pulses) with a $p_3 = 800$ ms. Note: the referent oscillation is the same for both metric (top) and rhythm (bottom) Figs: $p_R = 400$ ms. This metric cluster has a global attractor of .50 (for duple meter). *Bottom*: Rhythmic attractor profile. Endogenous rhythm relationships appear in the two bottom rows. Row 4 shows the driven referent period (dark gray) $p_R = 400$ ms. Row 5 shows external driving rhythms (light gray) as a succession of different driving rhythms. Below is the rhythmic attractor profile.

Rows 3 and 4 show impacts of rhythmic time spans, T (a series of external driving rhythms). Here, the driving rhythms are external. However, the internal referent oscillation, p_R, remains 400 ms. In this example, this oscillation is a driven rhythm. Transient mode-locking leads to an attractor profile with n:m states shown in row 5. (Misalignments [stars, row 3] result from incomplete mode-locking cycles, creating local attractor ambiguity [row 5; see Note 62]).

which the rhythm operates, as illustrated in this example. Together, a listener experiences the following rhythmic attractor profile of 1:2-1:1-2:1 of local attractors (ratios of .50, 1.0, 2.0; see row 5 for n:m attractors) as these unfold within a global duple meter frame.[66]

Shared Constructs in Meter and Rhythm: Some Implications

At a more general level, it is possible to see that the time structure of meter and that of rhythm fit into the larger theoretical framework of dynamic attending. That is, both metric and rhythmic time structures tap into entrainment mechanisms. In fact, three theoretical commonalities link meter with rhythm in this chapter. One obvious shared

entrainment concept involves listeners' responses to both meter and rhythm as involving driving–driven dyads. A second commonality is that percepts of both meter and rhythm pattern begin with positing a reliance on exogenous entrainment. Initially, an external driving rhythm excites resonant activity in a listener that, in turn, leads to some form of endogenous entrainment involving internal oscillations. In this regard, meter and rhythm also share the common concept of referent oscillation. Finally, a third overarching shared construct between meter and rhythm that emerges from this discussion is that both rely on entrainment protocols that feature attractors. In meter, a metrical category is defined by a set of global attractors that remain unchanged over the course of a musical event. One prominent global attractor often speaks for the whole set of global attractors, as when a meter is identified by a single ratio for duple or triple meters. Attractors also define rhythmic time patterns, but here transient mode-locking delivers rhythmic attractor profiles.

Implications of Shared Constructs

Commonalities between meter and rhythm spark new theoretical explanations about the impact of interactions of meter with rhythm on listeners' percepts. Such interactions certainly raise tantalizing questions about attentional dependencies of rhythm on meter or of meter on rhythm. For instance, it implies that rhythm can prime a listener's percept of meter (and vice versa). This idea is based largely on shared (hidden) attractors, which occupy a common entrainment region. Conversely, meter can prime percepts of rhythmic figures, as Stephan Handel has shown.[67,68]

In the current framework, the basic idea is that when meter and rhythm share attractors they are inherently compatible. In turn, compatibility leads to enhanced performance in certain tasks. Unifying elements in these tasks are attractors and their respective entraining regions. To some extent, a global attractor in a metric cluster is likely to be mirrored in the local attractors of a rhythmic attractor profile in metrical rhythms. Metric and rhythmic attractors for a given sequence will tend to share the same attractor entrainment regions. This also suggests that a rhythmic sequence can

prime a listener to hear a certain metric frame. Such priming is illustrated in Figure 9.10 (a variant of the Figure 9.2 sequence). In this example, the metric cluster and the rhythmic attractor profile share the same referent oscillation (p_R = 400 ms). Moreover, the global attractors of the metric cluster (*left column*) share many local attractors in the rhythmic attractor profile (*bottom*). This figure illustrates compatibility that invites *temporal priming*.

Temporal priming happens when a relatively strong priming stimulation (meter or rhythm) shares attractor regions with a somewhat weaker, primed stimulus (rhythm or meter). In an entrainment framework, the entrainment region and its limits provide a gauge for assessing the presence of a common attractor. Thus, the Arnold tongue regime functions as a source of effective priming, where priming depends upon enhanced stability of a driving–driven dyad. For instance, local attractors activated by an external rhythmic pattern may match global attractors of the prevailing meter of this pattern. This means that momentarily activated local attractors of a rhythmic patteren will fall into an entrainment region established by a metrical context and its global attractors.

Summary of Rhythm Perception

A rhythmic pattern is a coherent series of time spans (Ti) as discussed in Chapter 7. This section introduces coherent time patterns that also happen to be metrical rhythms in that they also

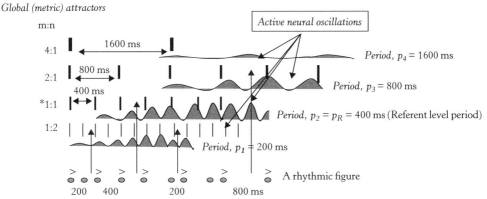

Rhythmic priming of a metric cluster

FIGURE 9.10 Temporal priming. From Figure 9.4, showing a metric cluster, this figure presents a rhythmic attractor profile priming the activity of metric cluster. Both assume a common internal referent period (p_R = 400 ms) which persists throughout this sequence. Thus, serial placements of external time spans (200, 400, 800 ms) in this rhythmic figure create local attractors that prime congruent metric cluster oscillators and related global attractors. Metric clusters and rhythmic attractor profiles share many of the same attractors

fit into a larger metric framework. Specifically, the layered time patterns of metrical rhythms allow compliance with a hierarchical embedding of slower time spans that jointly form a metric frame. Respectively, this leads to two different types of entrainment protocols, namely traditional mode-locking, which supports metrical relationships, and transient mode-locking, which supports rhythmic attractor profiles.

The major points in this section are:

- Meter and rhythm have been conventionally attributed to distinctly different underlying mechanisms: this section disputes this distinction.
- In a dynamic attending framework, meter and rhythm place respectively different constraints on a common set of underlying resonance and entrainment mechanisms.
- Meter capitalizes on a traditional mode-locking protocol in an entrainment framework, whereas rhythm is based on transient mode-locking,
- Traditional mode-locking leads to metric oscillator clusters, whereas transient mode-locking creates a rhythmic attractor profile.
- Priming of rhythm by meter or priming of meter by rhythm both depend upon shared attractors and entrainment regions of the underlying two constructs.

CHAPTER SUMMARY

This chapter describes new ways to think about metrical and rhythmic relationships. Against the backdrop of classic positions on meter and rhythmic grouping, principles of entrainment are introduced to explain attending/perception of meter and rhythm. Meter perception is hypothesized to depend on metric oscillator clusters, where a cluster emerges from endogenously entrained driven oscillations following a traditional mode-locking protocol. A metric cluster is summarized by internalized global attractors. These attractors reflect unchanging relative time relationships among metrically accented layers of a musical event.

Contrary to many conventions, this chapter describes rhythm perception using entrainment principles similar to those involved in meter perception. Specifically, these principles involve driving and driven rhythms, as well as attractors. However, rhythm perception is more stimulus-driven than is meter perception. This is evident in alignments of successive time spans for external grouping patterns that involve reliance upon successive exogenous driving rhythms. Each of these brief stimulus driving rhythms exogenously entrains with a persisting driven referent oscillation. In this way, a transient mode-locking protocol generates a series of local attractors that form a rhythmic attractor profile.

Similarities and differences between meter and rhythm perception raise several issues. These include their respective accents: metric versus rhythmic accents, both of which can convey subjective and/or objective salience. Also the role of driving rhythm differs when describing listeners' responses to meter versus rhythm. In metrical patterns, people rely on individual, metrically marked driving rhythms that are roughly constant throughout a musical pattern. By contrast, rhythm perception requires attending briefly to changing time spans, namely driving rhythms, as a pattern unfolds. These differences explain why metric oscillator clusters emerge with metrical patterns and rhythmic attractor profiles emerge with rhythms.

Finally, this entrainment narrative is about the ways that meter and rhythm differentially shape attending in real time. In this, the dichotomy of meter and rhythm reduces to differences in mode-locking protocols (traditional vs. transient) involving synchronies of attending. Nevertheless, both protocols incorporate predictions about attending dynamics that depend on momentary amplitudes of entraining oscillations. And, although these internalized portraits of meter and rhythm admit certain differences, their allegiance to entrainment principles means that they preserve important commonalities, such as a referent level and shared attractors, which lead to interesting predictions about temporal priming of rhythm versus meter.

NOTES

1. Grosvenor Cooper and Leonard B. Meyer, *The Rhythmic Structure of Music*, vol. 118 (Chicago: University of Chicago Press, 1963), https://books-google-com.proxy.library.ucsb.edu:9443/books?hl=en&lr=&id=V2yXrIWDTIQC&oi=fnd&pg=PA17&dq=Book:+++Cooper+and+Meyer+++music+&ots=QuX-MLXMWn&sig=sZxu99Nu42IonZ0V7pUj3uhNWw8.

2. Jonathan Kramer, *The Time of Music: New Meanings, New Temporalities, New Strategies* (New York: Schirmer Books, 1988).

3. Fred Lerdahl and Ray S. Jackendoff, *A Generative Theory of Tonal Music*, The MIT Press, Cambridge, Massachusetts, 1983. com.proxy.library.ucsb.edu:9443/books/about/A_Generative_Theory_of_Tonal_Music.html?id=6HGiEW33lucC.

4. Mark Liberman and Alan Prince, "On Stress and Linguistic Rhythm," *Linguistic Inquiry* 8, no. 2 (1977): 249–336.

5. As Robert Port notes (personal communication), such grids allow reversibility in space not available to dynamic portrayals of grids where time is not reversible.

6. David Temperley and Christopher Bartlette, "Parallelism as a Factor in Metrical Analysis," *Music Perception* 20, no. 2 (December 2002): 117–49, doi:10.1525/mp.2002.20.2.117.

7. H. Christopher Longuet-Higgins and Christopher S. Lee, "The Perception of Musical Rhythms," *Perception* 11, no. 2 (1982): 115–28, doi:10.1068/p110115.

8. Peter Desain and Henkjan Honing, "Time Functions Function Best as Functions of Multiple Times," *Computer Music Journal* 16, no. 2 (1992): 17–34, doi:10.2307/3680713.

9. Edward W. Large and John F. Kolen, "Resonance and the Perception of Musical Meter," *Connection Science* 6, no. 2–3 (1994): 177–208.

10. Justin London, *Hearing in Time: Psychological Aspects of Musical Meter* (New York: Oxford University Press, 2012), https://books-google-com.proxy.library.ucsb.edu:9443/books?hl=en&lr=&id=8vUJCAAAQBAJ&oi=fnd&pg=PP2&dq=London,+Justin++++Book++music,++time+&ots=HFpduOgCMz&sig=GUw88Sqc3DqABQfzCRJnYS51TbQ.

11. London, *Hearing in Time*.

12. Wendell R. Garner, *Uncertainty and Structure as Psychological Concepts*, vol. ix (Oxford, England: Wiley, 1962).

13. Stephen Handel, "The Differentiation of Rhythmic Structure," *Perception & Psychophysics* 52, no. 5 (September 1992): 497–507, doi:10.3758/BF03206711.

14. Stephen Handel, "The Interplay Between Metric and Figural Rhythmic Organization," *Journal of Experimental Psychology: Human Perception and Performance* 24, no. 5 (1998): 1546–61, doi:10.1037/0096-1523.24.5.1546.

15. This mechanical clock should not be confused with neural oscillations in entrainment theories, where the neural periodicity is an adaptive limit cycle oscillation.

16. Dirk-Jan Povel, "Internal Representation of Simple Temporal Patterns," *Journal of Experimental Psychology: Human Perception and Performance* 7, no. 1 (1981): 3–18, doi:10.1037/0096-1523.7.1.3.

17. Peter J. Essens and Drik-Jan Povel, "Metrical and Nonmetrical Representations of Temporal Patterns," *Perception & Psychophysics* 37, no. 1 (January 1985): 1–7, doi:10.3758/BF03207132.

18. The complex process of arriving at the "best" clock entails exhaustive matching of > and *m* accent timings.

19. Dirk-Jan Povel and Hans Okkerman, "Accents in Equitone Sequences," *Perception & Psychophysics* 30, no. 6 (November 1981): 565–72, doi:10.3758/BF03202011.

20. Dirk-Jan Povel and Peter Essens, "Perception of Temporal Patterns," *Music Perception: An Interdisciplinary Journal* 2, no. 4 (July 1, 1985): 411–40, doi:10.2307/40285311.

21. Aniruddh D. Patel et al., "The Influence of Metricality and Modality on Synchronization with a Beat," *Experimental Brain Research* 163, no. 2 (January 15, 2005): 226–38, doi:10.1007/s00221-004-2159-8.

22. Jaan Ross and Adrianus J. M. Houtsma, "Discrimination of Auditory Temporal Patterns," *Perception & Psychophysics* 56, no. 1 (January 1994): 19–26, doi:10.3758/BF03211687.

23. Mari Riess Jones and William Yee, "Sensitivity to Time Change: The Role of Context and Skill," *Journal of Experimental Psychology: Human Perception and Performance* 23, no. 3 (1997): 693–709, doi:10.1037/0096-1523.23.3.693.

24. Jessica A. Grahn and Matthew Brett, "Impairment of Beat-Based Rhythm Discrimination in Parkinson's Disease," *Cortex* 45, no. 1 (January 2009): 54–61, doi:10.1016/j.cortex.2008.01.005.

25. Handel, "The Differentiation of Rhythmic Structure."

26. J. Devin McAuley and Peter Semple, "The Effect of Tempo and Musical Experience on Perceived Beat," *Australian Journal of Psychology* 51, no. 3 (December 1, 1999): 176–87, doi:10.1080/00049539908255355.

27. McAuley and Semple, "The Effect of Tempo and Musical Experience on Perceived Beat."

28. Mari R. Jones, "Time, Our Lost Dimension: Toward a New Theory of Perception, Attention, and Memory," *Psychological Review* 83, no. 5 (1976): 323.

29. Sylvie Nozaradan et al., "Tagging the Neuronal Entrainment to Beat and Meter," *Journal of Neuroscience* 31, no. 28 (July 13, 2011): 10234–40, https://doi.org/10.1523/JNEUROSCI.0411-11.2011.

30. The term "beat" is defined as a recurrent time unit by the *Harvard Dictionary of Music*. However, sometimes "beat" is used to implicate only the time marker, suggesting that a beat is an accent. To avoid confusion, terms such as "time spans," "accents," or "time markers" are usually used in this chapter.

31. Lerdahl and Jackendoff, *A Generative Theory of Tonal Music*.

32. Edward W. Large and Joel S. Snyder, "Pulse and Meter as Neural Resonance," *Annals of the New York Academy of Sciences* 1169, no. 1 (July 1, 2009): 46–57, doi:10.1111/j.1749-6632.2009.04550.x.

33. Takako Fujioka et al., "Beta and Gamma Rhythms in Human Auditory Cortex During Musical Beat Processing," *Annals of the New York Academy of Sciences* 1169, no. 1 (July 1, 2009): 89–92, doi:10.1111/j.1749-6632.2009.04779.x. This research confirmed that both beta and gamma excitations happened in the auditory cortex.

34. John R. Iversen, Bruno H. Repp, and Aniruddh D. Patel, "Top-Down Control of Rhythm Perception

Modulates Early Auditory Responses," *Annals of the New York Academy of Sciences* 1169, no. 1 (July 2009): 58–73, doi:10.1111/j.1749-6632.2009.04579.x.

35. C. Pantev et al., "Human Auditory Evoked Gamma-Band Magnetic Fields.," *Proceedings of the National Academy of Sciences* 88, no. 20 (October 15, 1991): 8996–9000, doi:10.1073/pnas.88.20.8996.

36. This is in spite of the fact that expectancy pulses were recorded as anticipatory.

37. Caroline Palmer and Carol L. Krumhansl, "Mental Representations for Musical Meter," *Journal of Experimental Psychology: Human Perception and Performance* 16, no. 4 (1990): 728–41, doi:10.1037/0096-1523.16.4.728.

38. William Yee, Susan Holleran, and Mari Riess Jones, "Sensitivity to Event Timing in Regular and Irregular Sequences: Influences of Musical Skill," *Perception & Psychophysics* 56, no. 4 (1994): 461–71.

39. Bruno H. Repp, "Metrical Subdivision Results in Subjective Slowing of the Beat," *Music Perception* 26, no. 1 (September 2008): 19–39, doi:10.1525/mp.2008.26.1.19.

40. Edward W. Large, Philip Fink, and Scott J. Kelso, "Tracking Simple and Complex Sequences," *Psychological Research* 66, no. 1 (February 2002): 3–17, doi:10.1007/s004260100069.

41. Edward W. Large, "Neurodynamics of Music," in *Music Perception*, eds. Mari Riess Jones, Richard R. Fay, and Arthur N. Popper, Springer Handbook of Auditory Research 36 (New York: Springer, 2010), 201–31, doi:10.1007/978-1-4419-6114-3_7.

42. Large and Kolen, "Resonance and the Perception of Musical Meter."

43. A referent oscillation is not necessarily the dominant oscillation of a cluster.

44. Edward W. Large and Mari Riess Jones, "The Dynamics of Attending: How People Track Time-Varying Events," *Psychological Review* 106, no. 1 (1999): 119–59, doi:10.1037/0033-295X.106.1.119.

45. Edward W. Large and Caroline Palmer, "Perceiving Temporal Regularity in Music," *Cognitive Science* 26, no. 1 (January 2002): 1–37, doi:10.1016/S0364-0213(01)00057-X.

46. Joel S. Snyder and Edward W. Large, "Gamma-Band Activity Reflects the Metric Structure of Rhythmic Tone Sequences," *Cognitive Brain Research* 24, no. 1 (June 2005): 117–26, doi:10.1016/j.cogbrainres.2004.12.014.

47. Theodore P. Zanto, Joel S. Snyder, and Edward W. Large, "Neural Correlates of Rhythmic Expectancy," *Advances in Cognitive Psychology* 2, no. 2–3 (2006): 221–31.

48. Fujioka et al., "Beta and Gamma Rhythms in Human Auditory Cortex During Musical Beat Processing."

49. Donna Abecasis et al., "Differential Brain Response to Metrical Accents in Isochronous Auditory Sequences," *Music Perception: An Interdisciplinary Journal* 22, no. 3 (March 1, 2005): 549–62, doi:10.1525/mp.2005.22.3.549.

50. Renaud Brochard et al., "The 'Ticktock' of Our Internal Clock: Direct Brain Evidence of Subjective Accents in Isochronous Sequences," *Psychological Science* 14, no. 4 (July 1, 2003): 362–6, doi:10.1111/1467-9280.24441.

51. Douglas D. Potter et al., "Perceiving Rhythm Where None Exists: Event-Related Potential (ERP) Correlates of Subjective Accenting," *Cortex* 45, no. 1 (January 2009): 103–09, doi:10.1016/j.cortex.2008.01.004.

52. Mari R. Jones and Marilyn Boltz, "Dynamic Attending and Responses to Time," *Psychological Review* 96, no. 3 (1989): 459–91, doi:10.1037/0033-295X.96.3.459.

53. Jones and Boltz, "Dynamic Attending and Responses to Time."

54. Carolyn Drake, Mari Riess Jones, and Clarisse Baruch, "The Development of Rhythmic Attending in Auditory Sequences: Attunement, Referent Period, Focal Attending," *Cognition* 77, no. 3 (December 15, 2000): 251–88, doi:10.1016/S0010-0277(00)00106-2.

55. Carolyn Drake, "Psychological Processes Involved in the Temporal Organization of Complex Auditory Sequences: Universal and Acquired Processes," *Music Perception: An Interdisciplinary Journal* 16, no. 1 (1998): 11–26, doi:10.2307/40285774.

56. Carolyn Drake, Amandine Penel, and Emmanuel Bigand, "Tapping in Time with Mechanically and Expressively Performed Music," *Music Perception: An Interdisciplinary Journal* 18, no. 1 (2000): 1–23, doi:10.2307/40285899.

57. Drake, Penel, and Bigand, "Tapping in Time with Mechanically and Expressively Performed Music."

58. Karl D. Lerud et al., "Mode-Locking Neurodynamics Predict Human Auditory Brainstem Responses to Musical Intervals," *Hearing Research* 308 (February 2014): 41–49, doi:10.1016/j.heares.2013.09.010.

59. Edward W. Large and Felix V. Almonte, "Neurodynamics, Tonality, and the Auditory Brainstem Response," *Annals of the New York Academy of Sciences* 1252, no. 1 (April 1, 2012): E1–7, doi:10.1111/j.1749-6632.2012.06594.x.

60. Large, "Neurodynamics of Music."

61. Large and Kolen, "Resonance and the Perception of Musical Meter."

62. Large and Jones, "The Dynamics of Attending."

63. Frank Hoppensteadt and Eugene Izhikevich, "Canonical Neural Models," 2001, http://www.izhikevich.org/publications/arbib.pdf.

64. Frank C. Hoppensteadt and Eugene M. Izhikevich, "Synaptic Organizations and Dynamical Properties of Weakly Connected Neural Oscillators,"

Biological Cybernetics 75, no. 2 (August 1996): 117–27, doi:10.1007/s004220050279.

65. Review issues of neural amplitude in Chapter 4.

66. Perceptual errors may occur in a sequence at points where a local attractor predicts a mode-locking cycle that is not completed in the sequence. In Figure 9.9, stars reflect points where such errors (underlined) are likely, as Povel has observed. Here the series 2:1-1:1-2:1 implicates missed accents and/or incomplete cycles.

67. Handel, "The Interplay Between Metric and Figural Rhythmic Organization."

68. Handel, "The Differentiation of Rhythmic Structure."

10

Learning Time Patterns

Attending and learning are two different yet intimately related activities. Consider, for instance, the morning walk of a listener who briefly observes a butterfly hovering over a flower, then arrives at traffic light to cross the street, where she greets a neighbor also out on a walk. At each moment on this walk, our subject is attending to different things (butterflies, traffic lights, the neighbor, etc.). These are episodes of attending that change effortlessly to accommodate each new event, with the preceding event fading quickly from consciousness. Later in the day, little of this journey may be recalled. Yet, if our subject repeated this journey in exactly the same fashion for a series of morning (as in the movie *Groundhog Day*), then learning sets in and recall improves.

Attending and learning serve different functions. Attending is a flexible, in-the-moment, activity essential to survival for its ready responses to momentary changes in an environment. But it comes and goes. Learning, on the other hand, reflects a lasting predisposition to react in certain ways due to past experiences. Both are necessary to survive. This chapter proposes relevant differences between attending, rooted in entrainment principles, and learning, based on binding principles. Despite these differences, it can be argued that learning grows out of attending.

In this chapter, attending and learning are examined in the context of musical patterns. These are acoustic events with time patterns that carry constraints associated with rhythm and meter, as well as tempo. In music, metrical events are typically distinguished from nonmetrical ones. In terms of attending dynamics, this means we continue to entertain different entrainment protocols for metric versus rhythmic events. Specifically, as outlined in Chapter 9, metrical time constraints appeal to a traditional mode-locking protocol whereas rhythmic constraints call for transient mode-locking. This chapter pursues this distinction to examine the general implications of both processes for perceptual learning of time patterns.

The approach to learning in this chapter qualifies certain beliefs about learning. That is, it is generally accepted that exposure frequency of to-be-recalled events determines learning. While exposure frequency is undeniably essential to learning, it is also true that some things are more complex than others and they seem intrinsically harder to learn. To address this, the argument developed in this chapter assumes that learning rides on entrained attending. Furthermore, it also suggests that such learning is often implicit. This means that implicit learning is *implicit* because it occurs during episodes of involuntary entrainment. And it also implies that certain complex musical events will be harder to learn than simpler ones.

Preceding chapters have established that the complexity of musical time patterns can be linked to the time structure of underlying attractors. In particular, more complex attractors are less stable with narrower entrainment regions than simpler ones. The present view maintains that although people can learn complex time patterns, they require more exposures to these events. This chapter explores how entrainments affects this learning process.

A related topic pertinent to speech as well as music concerns cultural differences in time patterns. Different cultures feature different time patterns, evident in favored metric relationships and culture-specific rhythmic figures. Across the globe, musical meters differ, with some cultures favoring complex time ratios (e.g., 4:3) and others favoring simpler ratios (2:1). And the fact that even complex meters are eventually learned is clear evidence that exposure frequencies are important.[1] But, finally, the automaticity we feel in listening to a culturally familiar musical piece is based not only on the strength of familiar relationships acquired from learning, but also on our immediate engagement with the inherent nature of certain time relationships.

This chapter maintains that certain temporal biases function as unacknowledged launching pads for learning novel time patterns. The rationale for this holds that a listener must be attending at the "right" moments in time to grasp a particular relationship, a view that applies to learning of both metrical relationships and rhythmic patterns.

CHAPTER GOALS

Classic learning questions concern the "what" that is acquired and "how" it is acquired. One goal of this chapter is to set the stage for answering these questions when the skill in question is perceptual mastery of time patterns. The first section provides a background that briefly reviews skill acquisition capacities in listeners of different ages. This illustrates that perception of time patterns is strengthened by implicit learning; namely, involuntary learning that occurs in the absence of explicit instructions.

A second goal involves identifying "what" is learned in metric and rhythmic time patterns. Following the distinctions between meter and rhythm explored in Chapter 9, the "what" that is learned about metrical patterns involves embedded (hierarchical) time relationships and related categories (from metric oscillator clusters). On the other hand, the "what" that is acquired with rhythmical patterns involves serial time patterns (from rhythmic attractor profiles).

A third goal involves identifying "how" learning of meter and rhythm occurs. The general working framework posits that attending to the time structure of any event must be differentiated from learning this time structure. Preceding chapters have emphasized that attending depends on the synchronous phase couplings of active oscillations. This chapter makes the case that these synchronous alignments of attending, then, afford learning opportunities that reinforce bindings among periods of the involved entraining rhythms. The end product—namely, meter learning—is summarized by a *metric binding hypothesis* that extends meter learning to the learning of meter categories.

BACKGROUND: SKILLS AND MUSICAL TIMING

That a musical skill gap exists, no one disputes. Musicians simply have superior listening skills not only for metric relationships but also for timing patterns in general.[23,4,5,6,7,8] "Musician" here will refer to an individual who reports substantial formal musical training, usually beginning at an early age. In reviewing this literature, Laurel Trainor[9] convincingly documents the superiority

of musicians' listening skills relative to those of non-musicians in performing tasks of identification/detection of rhythmic and metric properties in musical patterns. Typically, the skill gap is a matter of degree: a musician's ear (or brain) is simply more "finely tuned" than that of a non-musician. This section provides a backdrop on perceptual learning of time relations by describing proclivities and skill differences of learners at different ages as they respond to various time patterns.

Origins of Metric Skills in Young Listeners

Learning begins at birth or before; biases in listening are found even in young infants. Thus, in addition to questions about the "what" and "how" of learning, we must also take note of "who" can learn. Infants do not enter the world as empty vessels. Following Jusczyk's[10] view that early learning is *innately guided,* we may anticipate certain findings that reveal infants' early ability to respond to simpler time relationships; arguably, given the aging hypothesis corollary, these simpler relationships offer ready-made "hooks" that guide attending toward "what" to learn. An infant who is naturally "prepared" for certain time ratios will readily "tune in" to patterns with simpler attractors. For such infants, attending biases open a path for acquiring lasting internalizations of these time relations.

These ideas about early attending predispositions and guided learning converge with revised thinking about critical learning periods. Historically, a *critical learning period* was identified as a single "critical" developmental stage where exposure to an event putatively had maximum impact in promoting language and/or musical learning. However, newer approaches propose that several age-dependent sensitive periods exist, where each successive stage grants a maturing child greater readiness to learn specific aspects of language and music.[11,12] Thus, in acquiring proficiency in speech, infants move from sensitivities to fast sound patterns (e.g., phonemic patterns) to a readiness to learn slower regularities of syllables and words at respectively older ages.

Very Young Listeners and Meter Learning

Perhaps very young infants can selectively learn meter-like time patterns with sufficient exposures. And, if this learning is hastened by early entraining proclivities, then even very young infants should be capable of mastering fast but structurally simple time patterns. A caveat is that unskilled listeners rely mainly on simpler time regularities that are clearly outlined (i.e., by distinctively marked time spans). This is consistent with findings in infant-directed speech. In other words, certain prominent physical changes (e.g., in intensity, frequency, duration) grab the attending of novices. Thus, newborns should be more likely to react to recurrent musical periodicities when these time spans are distinctively outlined by salient markers. Not only does this seem to be the case, but marker salience appears to apply to even prominent physical changes in tactile forces, such as rhythmical bouncing.[13,14,15,16] Moreover, such early exposures testify to early implicit learning of metric relations which has a lasting impact on listening proficiency later in life.[17,18]

Although infants' early learning capacities are dazzling, very young infants can hardly be considered skilled musical listeners. Rather, they come equipped with a general ability to focus on the core timing properties common in the domains of music and speech. In theory, their ability to permanently internalize (i.e., learn) certain sets of time patterns begins with wobbly attending due to poor phase-locking and biased endogenous attending resulting from predispositions for simple resonance ratios.[19] However, infants also come equipped with relatively weak cortical oscillations which operate as relatively responsive driven rhythms.[20] This means that, despite the weakness of their phase-locking, infants' reliance on weak driven oscillations means they are also ripe for engaging in stimulus-driven attending.

Given such inborn constraints, it is reasonable to ask: Can young listeners learn to differentiate complex (and simple) metric patterns with repeated exposures if the relevant time spans are distinctively marked? Hannon and colleagues provided an affirmative answer. They found naïve young listeners can do this, within limits.[21] Five- and seven-month-old infants as well as adults heard metric patterns of differing complexity (meters of 2:1, 3:2, and 7:4 metric ratios). The youngest infants were indeed challenged by ratio complexity, failing to react to meter ratios of 3:2 and 7:4; however, older infants and adults showed positive responses to certain complex ratios based on prior exposures (e.g., 2:1 or 3:2), but not 7:4. Finally, 12-month-old infants mastered the more complex time metric ratios.[22,23] Thus, exposure due to an infant's musical/linguistic environment shapes attending even in the first year of life, suggesting that babies enter the world prepared to exploit implicit learning opportunities, beginning with simple commensurate time ratios.

In sum, infants are born with a greater capacity than we may credit them. Although they require distinct time markers of time patterns, young infants appear to respond effortlessly to the simpler time ratios characteristic of duple meter, with their potential for learning more complex time ratios increasing rapidly with exposures during the first year of life.

The Musical Skill Gap in Older Children: Age and Experience

As children age, their exposure to the music and language of their culture naturally increases. A perennial dilemma in assessing the relative contributions of maturation and exposure frequency (training) concerns the natural co-variation of these factors.

Carolyn Drake and colleagues addressed this dilemma in a study that controlled exposure frequency using children ranging in age from 4 to 10 years.[24] Focusing directly on meter learning, participants had to synchronize taps to multilayered duple (2:1) metric rhythms of different rates. The marker distinctiveness of rhythmic time spans was also varied.[25]

Both age and exposure training affected performance. Importantly, across age groups, trained listeners synchronized better than those with no musical training (except for 4-year-olds with weak motor skills). Older children with more training performed best, showing sensitivity to higher metric time levels. Finally, this acquired skill gap was most apparent in tapping to impoverished music that contained no distinctive time markers.

In sum, metrical expectancies strengthen with both maturation and exposure/training. Also, older, more skilled children appear more likely than others to target their attending over multiple (slower) metric time levels. By contrast, both the younger and the less skilled listeners rely disproportionately on distinctive time markers than do others (as did less skilled young adults).[26] It appears that, regardless of age, listeners without explicit training are less effective in internalizing metric relationships than are musicians.

The Musical Skill Gap in Adults: Consequences of Meter Learning

The listening superiority of musicians over nonmusicians is quite prominent in adult populations. Relative to nonmusicians, adult musicians have access to more metric time levels, are better at detecting small timing deviations, and show a greater ability to segment metric levels outlined by subtle (or missing) metrical accents.[27,28,29]

Basically, musicians appear to have internalized metric time relationships. Arguably, this is responsible for their heightened sensitivity to metric layers even in the absence of salient objective time markers. It suggests that musicians operate with refined temporal expectancies that supply them with their own (internal) time markers. That is, musicians rely on their own subjectively salient metric accents.

Further support for this interpretation comes from a study that disentangled the impact of *subjective metric* accents from that of *subjective grouping* accents (see Chapter 9). Kung and colleagues orthogonally varied placements of these two types of subjective accents with the aim of assessing the metric segmenting skills of adult musicians and nonmusicians.[30] Using the classic click location task, they gauged the strength of listeners' internalized segmentations in the *absence of objective time markers*.[31,32] Musicians were dramatically more accurate in identifying metric segmentations than were nonmusicians, particularly with events lacking objective metric accents (e.g. when an implicated, i.e., subjective, **m** accent is centered in a group). This is strong support for the claim that musicians operate with internalized metric time frames.

Of course, if sensitivity to metric timing is reserved only for people with extensive musical training, then music would not be the widely popular art form that it is. Accordingly, for broad appeal, composers frequently "help out" untutored ears by strategically placing several strong (i.e., objectively salient/ interesting) markers throughout a musical piece. This type of "guidance" may range from subtle indications of a complex pattern, such as the drum introduction to Dave Brubeck's *Take Five* or Bruce Springsteen yelling a simple "one, two, three, four!" during the break in *Born to Run*. Presumably, this enables unskilled listeners to tune in to critical metrical time layers (other clever composition aids for untutored ears are given by Temperley and Bartlette[33]).

Learning Simple and Complex Meters

Clearly, infants as well as adults can learn individual metric patterns, whether simple or complex. But do they learn simple and complex patterns with equal ease? Evidence that implicit learning is slower for a complex metric pattern than a simple one is provided by Barbara Tillman

and colleagues.[34] They presented adults with the same number of repetitions of a simple meter (duple, 2:1) and a complex (3:2) metric pattern. Predictably, the complex meter was harder to learn (see also Brandon et al. 2012).[35] Generalizing, given the frequency of exposure over a life span, it is quite likely that adult musicians have acquired a stronger internalized sense of complex meters than have nonmusicians. Nevertheless, in related studies Barbara Tillmann and her colleagues confirm that adults with little musical training are quite capable of implicitly learning metrical relationships.[36,37,38] For instance, in one task, participants learned metrical relationships among groups of syllables even when these metrical relationships were weakly instigated.

This section suggests that people perceptually learn time patterns, especially metrical ones, based largely on exposure frequencies. At the same time, several factors qualify this learning. In addition to exposure frequency, both time marker (objective) salience and time ratio complexity affect this learning curve.

One explanation of findings discussed in this section maintains that more exposures to distinctively marked external rhythms invite involuntary entrainment of oscillations, which, in turn, eventually leads to a more lasting "internalization" of these external driving rhythms. In this internalization process, subjectively salient accents (as internalized expectancy pulses) may come to substitute for objectively salient ones. And with more stimulus exposures, internalizations of relevant event time periods become stronger. In addition, internalized time relations, such as metric ratios, persist in a listener's memory even when the original stimulus pattern vanishes. In short, with exposure to metrical events, "what" listeners acquire is a heightened internalized sensitivity to time relations that belie a metric attractor.

Summary of Musical Skill Gap

The accumulating research on the acquisition of metrical skills suggests that maturation, exposure frequency, and metric complexity are all factors in skill acquisition. To understand how these factors converge to influence meter learning, it will be important to also pursue how they affect a learner's ability to dynamically attend to individual metrical patterns unfolding in real time. Perceptual learning of relevant time relationships is often implicit. And, in this view, implicit learning begins with involuntary entrainment of attending which leads to mastering an ability to track relationships that define a metric category. Ultimately, with more exposure (hence more entrainment opportunities) this culminates in a more permanent internalization of relevant attractor relationships.

To preview later discussions, a full understanding of meter learning must also recognize that "what" is learned likely extends beyond internalization of the time relationships of an individual metric pattern. Finally, to learn meter will entail mastering a *category* of time relationships that share certain metric relations. In other words, meter learning becomes category learning. For instance, people come to recognize a duple meter across a range of different rhythmic patterns (and melodies). In this expansion of learning, "what" is learned becomes abstract metrical knowledge that is eventually summarized in a metric binding hypothesis.

Major points in this section are:

- Early in life, children show sensitivity to metric relationships. Both age and experience affect this sensitivity.
- A musical skill gap is pronounced in adults. Relative to nonmusicians, musicians show greater sensitivity to (1) metric time layers (without objective/prominent markers), (2) multiple metric time levels, and (3) complex meters.
- Meter learning begins with involuntary attending to individual metric patterns. Frequent exposure to such patterns leads to implicit learning and internalization of relevant periodicities of a metrical stimulus.

FUNDAMENTAL PRINCIPLES IN LEARNING TIME PATTERNS

Historically, learning is defined as the acquisition of a more or less permanent change in behavior resulting from practice. With implicit or passive perceptual learning, "practice" is best described as repeated exposures to a stimulus. Note that confining this discussion to implicit learning means excluding formal aspects of musical training where practice includes explicit instructions about scales, chords, and the like accompanied by refinements of motor activities. Instead, here the focus is on involuntary aspects of implicit learning due primarily to exposures to metrical and nonmetrical rhythmic sequences.[39,40]

A common observation about music points to the creative repetitiveness embedded in the music of all cultures. Themes and similar rhythmic patterns recur, with artistic changes, throughout a musical episode, and certain invariant metric relationships make measures and hypermeasures repetitive. Stylistically, a culture's music highlights certain groups of sounds and particular meters through culture-specific repetitiveness of certain time patterns. Not to be overlooked is the obvious fact that repetition is conductive to both entrainment and learning. Let an *entrainment episode* connote the total duration of several (repeated) exposures of certain external sets of driving rhythms. At the same time, lengthy and/or repeated episodes also offer multiple learning opportunities.

This section describes a role for entrainment in promoting learning. It proposes that learning is distinct from entrainment but that these are co-occurring, indeed intertwined, activities. Entrainment is important because it guarantees attending "at the right time" for learning to happen. Both entrainment and learning depend on synchrony, but with entrainment synchrony refers to fleeting mode-locking states, whereas with learning synchrony delivers reinforcements that accumulate to bind oscillations together.

Entrained Attending and Learning

We learn about things to which we attend. This happens even if attending energy is modest and/or involuntary, as in implicit learning. Entrained attending, at some level, is a precondition for perceptual learning. However, entrainment only temporarily phase-connects an attending periodicity to an environmental driving rhythm. All else equal, *when a phase-coupling parameter linked with the driving rhythm is reduced or disappears, so does driving-driven entrainment.* Learning, by contrast, is a phenomenon that builds a lasting internal binding between a driven rhythm and driving rhythm based on the exposure frequency of stable dyad coupling during an entrainment episode. Importantly, entrainment is a gate-way to learning, but once established learning then survives the disappearance of an driving rhythm whereas entrainment does not.

To understand how entrainment and learning work together, it is useful to review two types of entrainment described in preceding chapters: exogenous and endogenous entrainments, shown in Figure 10.1A,B. Exogenous entrainment, depicted in panel A, has been defined as involving an external (stimulus) driving rhythm. Endogenous entrainment, shown in panel B, involves dyads where both driving and driven rhythms are internal periodicities.

Exogenous entrainment, as featured in this figure, shows a tone sequence (light gray ovals)

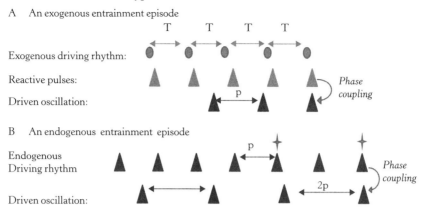

FIGURE 10.1 Schematic examples of exogenous and endogenous entrainments. (**A**) An isochronous series of tone onsets (light gray ovals) has a fixed inter-onset period, T. Each tone instantly evokes a reactive pulse which initially "internalizes" this external driving rhythm. An exogenous dyad forms based on phase coupling with an emerging driven oscillation (dark gray pulse) of period, p (p~T). (**B**) A fast driven oscillation, with period, p, forms an endogenous dyad with a slower, driving oscillation (period of 2p) following a traditional mode-locking order of n:m of 1:2.

with roughly identical stimulus time spans, T, outlined by time markers that evoke an isochronous series of reactive pulses (light gray pulses in panel A). This sequence of *reactive pulses* is series of evoked pulses that respond to each tone onset in this stimulus sequence. By contrast, a true endogenous driven rhythm (dark gray pulses) phase locks with the driving rhythm. This driven rhythm carries emerging (recurring) *expectancy pulses* that recur with period, p (~T). With phase-coupling between driving and driven rhythms, expectancy pulses grow and begin to align, then even to anticipate the automatically evoked, reactive pulses. This figure depicts one example of traditional mode-locking between two isochronous rhythms. This entrainment protocol should be familiar as it reflects the simplest of global attractors (n:m = 1:1 for elementary event tracking).

The entrainment portrayed in Figure 10.1B shows a coupling of two different rhythms, one automatically evoked and fleeting indicative of world events, the other induced and self-sustaining representing neural activity. Note that here the period (2p) of the slower stimulus rhythm is twice than of the oscillation's period (p). Nevertheless, panel B shows the possibility of phase-coupling between two rhythms due to a 2:1 ratio of their periods. This ratio serves as a global metric attractor; it may express the beginning of a metric oscillator cluster if additional neural oscillations emerge. In the present chapter, endogenous entraining concepts discussed in Chapter 9, such as metric clusters (with global attractors) and

rhythmic attractor profiles (with local attractors), return to play important roles in promoting the learning of meter and rhythm, respectively.

Coupling Versus Binding Parameters

Learning differs from entrainment in several respects. Most importantly, entrainment depends on *phase-coupling parameters*, whereas learning depends on *period-binding parameters*. Coupling parameters of entrainment regulate temporary phase connections between driving and driven rhythms, whereas the binding parameter of learning calibrates longer lasting connections among the periods of different rhythms.

That this distinction is warranted is illustrated by unpacking a simple formulation of entrainment given by the *sine circle map* (Box 9.1). This elementary model used a difference equation to map a phase change of a driven oscillation at time i as a function of its phase on i – 1. Mathematically, this expression does what most entrainment models do: it specifies a *coupling parameter* that quantifies phase changes in a driven rhythm as a function of the force applied to its driving rhythm[41] (e.g., the coupling parameter, **k**, where $0 \leq \mathbf{k} \leq 1.0$). So, does this mean that the coupling parameter functions also as a learning parameter? Probably not. Coupling parameters reflect the momentary force of a prevailing driving rhythm. However, this force immediately vanishes when a driving rhythm is withdrawn: *If the force of driving rhythm "dies," coupling strength also dies* (**k** → *0*). And, of course, removal of a coupling force means that entrainment vanishes. And this allows attending to drift into asynchronies between the driving and driven rhythm. Synchrony is lost. Finally, and most critically, if a coupling parameter is used as a learning parameter, then, due to this dual role, any "learning" accumulated during an entrainment episode must vanish as the coupling parameter now drops to zero.

This is bad news. If learning is based on phase-coupling, then the function of a coupling parameter, which is temporary, conflicts with learning. It denys the building of lasting associative connections among various driving and driven rhythms. In short, phase connections between oscillations are temporary; they depend on a momentary coupling force. Consequently, phase coupling parameters are good for installing synchrony between rhythms, where they explain flexible shifts of attending. But coupling parameters are not good for learning because they cannot ensure that this "togetherness" will last once a driving rhythm loses its force.

Introducing . . . a Binding Parameter

A solution to this problem is to add another parameter, one for learning. Ideally, this new parameter depends on exposure frequency; it cannot be linked directly to the external driving rhythm force. A *binding parameter* comes into action during an entrainment episode at points in this process where the pulses of two rhythms coincide (i.e., are synchronous), as in Figure 10.1B.

Even a momentary experience of synchrony is reinforcing. An instant of synchrony strengthens a binding link between periods of coordinating oscillations. Importantly, unlike a phase coupling parameter, a binding parameter applies to internalized time periods, *regardless of driving rhythm force*. A binding parameter depends only on alignments of internalized periods of driving and driven rhythms. Alignment, not force, determines binding reinforcement of a driving-driven dyad. Whereas coupling parameters are determined by force factors that function in the moment, binding parameters are determined by period alignment factors that deliver reinforcements based on synchrony and which serve a lasting function. Proposed details of reinforcements and their schedules for binding are outlined in Box 10.1.

The *principle of synchrony*[42] affects both entrainment and learning parameters but in very different ways. During endogenous entrainment among active oscillations, the force of an internal coupling parameter moves the peak pulse of a driven oscillation toward a momentary alignment with a corresponding peak phase of its driving oscillation. It accomplishes this by phase shifts that reduce phase differences in order to align pulses of a driving and a driven rhythm. Asymptotically, the entrainment goal is complete phase synchrony ($\Delta\varphi = 0$).

Learning, by contrast, depends on the degree of phase synchrony (pulse alignments) established

---

BOX 10.1
REINFORCEMENT SCHEDULES: INDIVIDUAL
AND CATEGORICAL TIME PATTERNS

1. *Phase alignments of internal pulses (reactive with expected) increase binding strength.*
   a. *Individual instances*: Precise phase alignments of expectancy with reactive pulses in a sequence strengthen bindings among all active oscillations and a stimulus.
   b. *Individual instances*: Phase alignments of expectancy with reactive pulses that only approximate synchrony (fuzzy rhythms) provide correspondingly weaker binding strength.
   c. *Category prototypes*: The number of precise pulse alignments affects prototype strength.
2. *Frequency of reinforcements increase binding strength.*
   a. *Individual instances*: Instance repetition increases overall binding reinforcement, with binding strength increasing with more/longer entrainment episodes.
   b. *Individual instances*: Relative frequency of reinforcement in an instance depends on mode-locking constraints.
   c. *Individual instances*: Frequency of reinforcement depends on attractor simplicity.
   d. *Category prototypes*: Reinforcement frequency is highest for one global attractor of a metric cluster.

during the span of an entrainment episode. However, asymptotically, coinciding pulses *reinforce* the binding strength between the periods of driving and driven rhythms. Figure 10.2 provides two examples of binding based on entrainment where pulses (reactive, expectancy) effectively internalize periods of a stimulus driving sequence during phase entrainment with an internal driven rhythm. Each moment of pulse synchrony between a driving-driven pair during this entrainment episode provides an opportunity for strengthening bindings between periods of the two rhythms, via reinforcement. Reinforcements (stars) are hypothesized to arise from the impact of synchrony on release of a rewarding neurochemical, such as dopamine.[43,44,45] In turn, with more pulse synchronies, increased reinforcements selectively strengthen the mode-locking relationship among these synchronized rhythms i.e., binding strength increaes. Thus, in Figure 10.2A, an external sequence (driving referent period) spells out its internalized stimulus rhythm (S_R) via resonance or a series of reactive pulses during an exogenous entrainment episode. In this example, the stimulus rhythm yields seven reinforcement moments (stars) for binding with an isochronous driven rhythm.

Accordingly, a binding parameter is *not dependent on the force of the stimulus driving rhythm.* Rather, binding strength lasts regardless of coupling strength. In fact, in this scenario, a removal of the external stimulus driving rhythm leaves only a faint skeleton of it, but this does not weaken the acquired binding strength, which lives on. That is, any reappearance of this external stimulus rhythm in the future will immediately restore the impact of past exposures. Effectively, the established bonds facilitate "recognition" of that stimulus rhythm.

Figure 10.2B illustrates another exogenous entrainment situation, one that leads to weak binding due to fewer reinforcements. This happens when a stimulus driving rhythm (referent in light gray) is slower than a driven rhythm. As shown in this figure, this paradigm offers relatively few binding opportunities. Moreover, here silent pulses of an entraining oscillation do not receive reinforcements. Nevertheless, even this experience is a prelude—a weak prelude—to meter learning. In part, this is because each exogenous entrainment episode also offers opportunities for strengthening of bonds between simultaneously occurring oscillations in, for example, a metric cluster.

Meter Learning: Examples
Basically, whether a metrical pattern is simple or complex, it can elicit a metric cluster (from Chapter 9). To briefly review, let us consider a

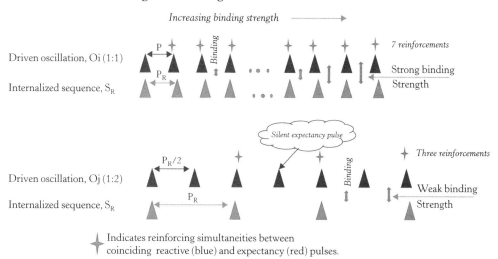

Exogenous bindings and reinforcements

Increasing binding strength ⟶

Driven oscillation, Oi (1:1)

Internalized sequence, S_R

7 reinforcements

Strong binding Strength

Driven oscillation, Oj (1:2)

Internalized sequence, S_R

Silent expectancy pulse

Three reinforcements

Weak binding Strength

Indicates reinforcing simultaneities between coinciding reactive (blue) and expectancy (red) pulses.

FIGURE 10.2 Examples of bindings between an internalized stimulus sequence as referent (light gray S_R) and a resonant internal (dark gray) driven oscillation. *Top dyad*: Each of seven alignments of reactive with expectancy peaks strengthens, via synchronous reinforcement, a binding of the two rhythms. Over time, this leads to stronger bindings (light gray arrow). *Bottom dyad*: Fewer reinforcements from a synchronized pulse occur when a slow referent, p_R (light gray pulses) aligns with alternate peaks of a faster driven oscillation. A total of three alignments leads to weaker binding than in top dyad.

few stimulus examples of a simple meter, the duple meter. In this case, a single metrical pattern embeds at least two different (hierarchical) metric layers, each of which can function as an external driving rhythm for a neural correlate. Four such metrical tone sequences appear in Figure 10.3. In theory, these sequences (light gray filled circles) stimulate resonant activity in several different oscillations that coalesce, via traditional mode-locking, into a metric cluster; this cluster is controlled here by global duple meter attractors. Simplifying matters, this figure focuses only on two oscillator members of such a cluster with neural correlates, O1 and O2 (dark gray), with respective oscillation periods of 1 and 2 seconds.

Figure 10.3 outlines some features of meter learning. Learning is assumed to strengthened as a function of increasing numbers of driving/driven binding opportunities. These involve coincidences of reactive and expectancy pulses hypothesized to reinforce bindings. Consequently, different reinforcement frequencies happen with different metrical sequences (M1 and M2 and their fuzzy counterparts). Note that in this figure, each stimulus sequence offers different reinforcement opportunities. This is evident in the number

of aligned pulses (stars) which differs across sequences. For instance, the top row of this figure shows five alignments of expectancy pulses with reactive pulses for the O1 oscillation, three of which involve coinciding expectancy pulses of O2 (large stars). But, in the second row, a fuzzy version of the M1 metric sequence is shown. Here, fuzziness leads to pulse misalignments, hence fewer strong reinforcements (i.e., fewer large stars). Overall, these examples suggest that learning should be stronger for a duple meter relation in M1 and M2 than for their fuzzy versions because the latter offer fewer strong reinforcements.

Finally, Figure 10.3 does not show another aspect of learning during entrainment. In each of these four patterns, it is also possible for activated oscillations to endogenously entrain with each other. This is because they are governed by a 2:1 metric attractor. In fact, this global metric attractor holds for all four of the example sequences depicted in Figure 10.3, including the fuzzy rhythms, which are "good enough" approximations to this global attractor. Furthermore, given endogenous entrainments, the same principles of binding described for exogenous entrainments with metrical stimulus rhythms applies to endogenous entrainments

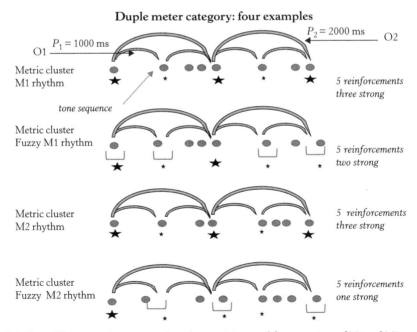

FIGURE 10.3 Four different metric sequences based on prototype and fuzzy versions of M1 and M2 sequences (light gray ovals). M1 and M2 are sequences of Figure 10.4 with two oscillator members of a cluster (O1, O2); each shows five reinforcements (stars) of members of metric clusters with sequences. Fuzzy versions of M1 and M2 have some weaker reinforcements due to asynchronies (brackets).

among oscillations of a metric cluster. As the number of coincidences between two entraining oscillations within a metric cluster increases so does strength their bindings. Overall, this means that more encounters with metrical events will strengthen future percepts of metric relationships.

Determinants of Binding: Reinforcements

Learning is essentially an internal process. Binding occurs with synchrony between pulses of internalized rhythms. As previous examples suggest, pulses arise from stimulus-driven sequences (reactive pulses) as well as from oscillations (expectancy pulses). Binding strength grows over time, with increasing opportunities for pulse synchrony. Major factors that affect reinforced binding fall into two categories: phase alignment and exposure frequency.

Phase alignments. Approximation to phase synchrony affects the strength of a reinforcement. Generally, misalignments (e.g., fuzzy rhythms) and silent expectancy pulses weaken underlying time relationships, thereby reducing opportunities for learning through binding.

Frequency of

phase   alignments. Exposure frequency increases opportunities for reinforcement of bindings among active oscillations. One factor that affects the exposure frequency of aligned pulses (hence reinforcements) is attractor complexity.

In general, complex attractors lead to fewer alignments between hypothesized oscillations than simple attractors. All else equal, this account predicts that simple attractors are learned more quickly than complex ones. Generally, reinforcement rate declines as attractor complexity increases. Although unsurprising, the underlying rationale places constraints on popular claims that event exposure alone is sufficient to explain learning. Instead, inherent structural properties of a stimulus rhythm mean that exposure to a time pattern is a necessary but not a sufficient condition for learning.

Stages of Meter Learning

All learning begins with a listener confronting a single novel instance. This truism applies to meter learning. Thus, one morning, a listener suddenly hears a new song on the radio with an unfamiliar time pattern; yet it happens to be a novel instance of a larger metric category. Even if this listener is notoriously unmusical, some implicit learning happens simply from her prior listening experiences. Tacit learning begins during an initial listening experience that supplies an entrainment episode. During this episode, attending to some embedded time relationships might instill a more lasting impression even for a naïve listener. A few opening elements of the song will "stick in her head" to facilitate later recognition. For instance, later in the day, this listener may find herself inadvertently humming a crude approximation of its rhythm (perhaps mangling its melody). The fundamental principles responsible for such behavior, outlined in preceding sections, are related to constraints on entrained attending (coupling) and on learning (binding).

A unique feature of the Dynamic Attending Theory (DAT) is the proposal that learning, even of a single metrical sequence, originates in entrained attending activities. Upon repetition of a metrical pattern, related resonant oscillations are activated that increase in number, expanding the reach of attending activities.

Stages of meter learning `represent uncharted territory. It is possible that the initial stages of meter learning simply involve learning of individual metric patterns. This means learning begins with the encounter of a novel metric pattern that invites exogenous entrainment. Thus, Stage 1 of meter learning would involve bindings arising from a single driving/driven dyad. Stage 2 then, might involve entrainments in whole sets of driving–driven rhythms with a variety of individual metric patterns. In each case, bindings follow suit. In Stage 3, the driving rhythms of many metric patterns (e.g., of a metric category) can be become internalized, leading to endogenous entrainments and the formation of metric oscillator clusters. With binding comes the discovery of different metric clusters that share common attractors. Finally, in this third stage, learning facilitates discovery of general (i.e., abstract) knowledge of time relationships through experiences with a number of different metric sequences having shared global attractors. Knowledge of metric categories emerges. For instance, in this stage, people learn that a common attractor (2:1) fits all duple meter clusters, whereas a different attractor (3:1) fits all triple meter clusters. This effectively unites a variety of different metric patterns with similar metric clusters.[46]

Summary of Learning Time Patterns

In sum, the three stages of Table 10.1 suggest a provisional progression for meter learning. Much of this is implicit learning, based on binding opportunities supplied by involuntary

TABLE 10.1 STAGES OF METER LEARNING				
Stage Progression	**From exogenous entrainment to endogenous bindings**			
Driving rhythm	**Driven rhythm**	**Entrainment**	**Binding**	
1. Novel metric time pattern: One driving rhythm	One driven oscillator.	Exogenous entrainment: A driving/driven dyad	Binding during entrainment. Synchrony of expectancy with reactive pulses	
2. Several different metrical patterns offer different sets o driving rhythms.	Several sets of driven internal oscillators are active.	Each pattern has exogenous entrainments for sets driving/driven dyads.	Each pattern grows bindings following entrainments of sets of driving/driven dyads.	
3. Multiple metric patterns offer sets of internalized rhythms.	All driven rhythms for each pattern are oscillations.	Driving and driven rhythms for each pattern endogenously entrain to form metric cluster.	Strong bindings in clusters among entraining oscillations. Clusters of different relate to common global attractor.	

entrainments.[47,48] As an initially novel time pattern repeats, we unwittingly grow accustomed to its rich inner structure. Learning, as described here, begins with a single instance, then develops through stages that include exposures to this and similar metric instances. Ultimately, a growing number of bindings in different dyads lead to discoveries of metric categories. Meter learning is ultimately category learning. With sufficient exposure to a range of metrical patterns, spontaneous cortical oscillations begin to align, with endogenous couplings leading to opportunities for long-lasting learning of metric clusters and their global attractors. And while metric oscillator clusters, introduced in Chapter 9, are not new, their role in learning discussed in this chapter is new.

The major points of this section are:

• Entrained attending is a platform for learning. Entrainment relies on phase coupling parameters, leading to driving–driven synchrony which, when achieved, results in reinforced binding among periods of active oscillations.
• An individual metric pattern offers several metric time layers, each functioning as a different external driving rhythm. Thus, it affords several exogenous entrainments leading to multiple oscillations that couple endogenously to form temporary metric clusters.
• Learning of a metrical pattern through binding improves with (1) good phase

alignment, (2) a high frequency of reinforced bindings, and (3) simpler (vs. complex) attractors associated with a to-be-learned stimulus rhythm.
• Stages of metrical learning begin with exogenous entrainment, then binding, with rhythms in a novel metrical pattern. Learning culminates with endogenous entrainments in multiple similar metrical patterns, followed by bindings in metric oscillator clusters and the discovery of metrical attractors that define a metric category.

CATEGORY LEARNING AND THE METRIC BINDING HYPOTHESIS

The preceding description suggests that, finally, the mastery of meter learning goes beyond the learning of one metrical pattern or even several such sequences. Meter learning actually operates on a grander scale than is suggested by enhanced familiarity with a single, recurring time pattern. It is useful to distinguish the learning of an individual metrical pattern from learning the abstract properties that define a whole metric category. For instance, M1 and M2 of Figure 10.3 belong to the same duple meter category. Does learning one of these patterns help in learning the other?

In fact it does. This is due to category learning. Ultimately, category learning springs from one's

Metric and non-metric stimulus rhythms

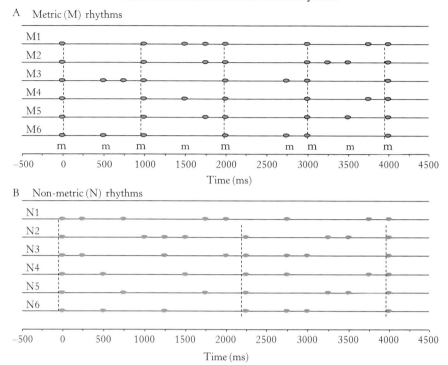

FIGURE 10.4 Six metrical, M, and six nonmetrical, N, tone sequences.

Reprint of figure 2 in Robert J. Ellis and Mari Riess Jones, "Rhythmic Context Modulates Foreperiod Effects," *Attention, Perception, & Psychophysics* 72, no. 8 (November 2010): 2274–88, doi:10.3758/BF03196701.

ability to differentiate whole sets of different time patterns that belong to one meter category from a different set of time patterns that do not belong to that category. This fleshes out the learning summarized stages 2 and 3 of Table 10.1. In these stages, a single pattern has several embedded (hierarchical) time layers wherein each layer functions as a driving rhythm that exhibits relationships to other time layers; these are metric relationships that will recur in other metrical patterns within the same metric category. This section pursues category learning of meter in more detail.

Let's begin with two different metrical sequences of the same duple meter category: M1 and M2. In fact, they are part of a set of six different instances (tokens) of the duple meter category shown in Figure 10.4. As a set, these token metrical, M, sequences differ from matched counterparts (same time spans) in a set of nonmetrical sequences, N, also shown in Figure 10.4. Notice that although the M patterns differ from each other, they seem to share some features (see vertical dashed lines) that are missing in the "matched" set of N patterns.

It turns out that musicians and nonmusicians alike hear this difference. Furthermore, individual exposures to different M tokens enhance a listener's sense that they belong to a common category; by contrast, little such awareness happens with N patterns.[49]

The Path of Category Learning

Category learning begins with acquiring familiarity with individual category instances (Table 10.1). Thus, simply repeating a single pattern, such as the M1 pattern, allows listeners to exogenously entrain, then bind, several endogenously coupled oscillations which then form metric oscillator clusters (see M1 of Figure 10.3). Similarly, exposures to different M tokens lead to the development of another related metric cluster of overlapping oscillations. And so it goes for exposures to all six M patterns. In stage 3, similar cluster relationships of all six M patterns facilitate listeners' reliance on traditional mode-locking relationships. Consequently, the metric clusters and global attractors of all M patterns in Figure 10.3 are quite similar.

Major properties relevant to M category learning are outlined in Figure 10.5. As an example, the top portion of this figure outlines traditional mode-locking/binding for the M1 tone sequence (light gray ovals). Hence, what is most relevant are global attractors and cluster reinforcements. The M1 sequence marks out accents that invite cluster formations of oscillations with periods of 500, 1,000, and 2,000 ms. Although other oscillations may contribute to this oscillator cluster, these are the primary ones. Let a referent oscillation be $p_R = 500$ ms.[50] Then, two slower oscillations, $p_1 = 1,000$ ms and $p_2 = 2,000$ ms, yield expectancy pulses spaced in time that reflect the periods of two higher metric time levels. Upon the presentation of an M1 stimulus token, salient markers are shown by vertical bars (of increasing thickness.). In this example, five reactive pulses from the tone sequence *align* with expectancy pulses for the referent period of 500 ms. In other words, exogenous entrainment bindings are reinforced (medium-sized stars). This strengthens links between these oscillations and the surface time of this sequence.

The preceding discussion suggests how learning via binding may begin. Taking this proposal a step further, in Figure 10.5 consider the tone sequence alignments of marked metric layers in the tone sequence (driving rhythms). As driving rhythms, these layers offer opportunities for entrainment and binding. For instance, the marked time layer with a time span of 2 seconds, will entrain a neural oscillation (period, $p_1 \sim 2$ seconds) to this metric layer; binding follows suit based on three reinforcements (large stars). Similarly, an oscillation with a 1 second period, p_2, for a lower level layer will garner five reinforcements (stars). Figure 10.5 documents these binding strengths for the M1 pattern. Finally, we can expect these activated oscillations to interact with one another to form an endogenous cluster. In this final stage, traditional mode-locking among oscillations within such a cluster will deliver three global (metric) attractors (e.g., 1:1, 2:1, and 4:1).

This returns us to category learning. Although Figure 10.5 focuses only on one metric pattern, M1, consider what happens if a different duple meter sequence from the set of tokens (M1–M6 in Figure 10.4) is examined. Most duple meter tokens will show very similar alignments among their slower driving rhythms, hence among the entraining oscillations. In fact all token metric sequences of Figure 10.5 embed slower driving rhythms that implicate the same duple meter global attractor of 2:1. Figure 10.5 shows that the strongest metric cluster

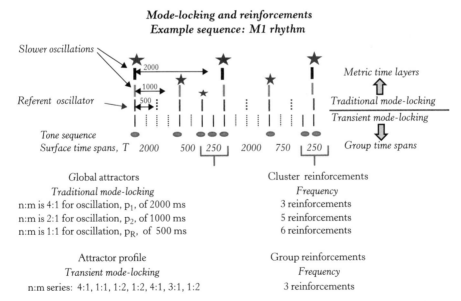

FIGURE 10.5 An example of entrainment, as mode-locking, and learning, as reinforcement frequency, for a tone sequence (M1). Layers of oscillator periods within a cluster are marked by vertical lines. Alignment strength of coinciding pulses (including reactive pulses to tones) are gauged by size of stars (number of coinciding, i.e., vertical, pulses). Detailed relationships between global attractors of this metric cluster, given traditional mode-locking, and related attractor reinforcement frequencies, are described in text. Concurrent transient mode-locking to the rhythmic figure also reaps some entrainments.

has global attractors of 1:1 and 2:1. Similarly, this global attractor is the one that is most reinforced across the set of metri patterns in Figure 10.4. Not surprisingly, this binding is strongest for the duple meter category.

This description has not emphasized the impact of simple repetition of a category token (or tokens) which also will reinforce metric relationships. That is, the mere repetition of a duple meter token will add reinforcements to a duple meter relationship, while also strengthening a listener's learning of that particular metrical pattern. For instance, in Figure 10.5, the strongest metric cluster for this particular token has global attractors with *n:m* relations of 1:1 and 2:1. Generally, tokens of a category exhibit the global attractors that are most reinforced within a musical culture.

Finally, "what" is learned by members of a given musical culture is an invariant subset of global attractors that applies to all tokens of metric category. In this case, it is the 2:1 abstract time relationships of a duple meter category. But the same reasoning applies to other metric categories. Binding parameters strengthen these attractors due to two main factors: metric complexity and exposure frequency.

The Metric Binding Hypothesis

The claim that people acquire keen meter perception with extended exposures to certain metrical stimuli is not especially controversial. What is important is understanding how we accumulate categorical knowledge about meter. This is abstract knowledge about time relationships in which internalized time relationships dominate.

An important aspect in mastering meter categories relates to this abstract property of invariant time relations. Although individual metric tokens differ, all retain an invariant relationship between at least two time levels in a metric hierarchy. In a Gibsonian fashion, a particular *n:m* relation between time levels reveals a defining invariance—a global attractor—that touches a variety of different tokens. Furthermore, this invariance translates into selective reinforcements of those oscillator dyads based on such an attractor. Category learning rests on the development of strong bindings within a metric cluster that outweigh other bindings, including local bindings within rhythmic groups of attractor profiles. Although exposure frequency alone plays a role in reinforcing driving/driven bindings of entraining dyads, the simplicity of attractor time relationships (e.g., 2:1, 3:1) also contributes to the popularity of a particular meter. Moreover, these simpler time ratios also beget more opportunities of binding through reinforcement. Consequently, in Western music, the duple meter exhibits both attractor simplicity and high exposure frequency.

The musical skill gap between musicians and nonmusicians is a stark reminder that exposure enables skilled listeners to effortlessly identify and classify different but novel musical patterns into distinct metric categories (e.g., duple vs. triple meters). The meter category of an unfamiliar march (duple meter) or waltz (triple meter) is easily recognized by an expert. Any card-carrying musician does this automatically, even without the presence of objective metric accents. Indeed, merely asking musicians if they can do this risks insulting them. Musicians provide powerful evidence for long-term perceptual and categorical learning of metrical relationships.

The metric binding hypothesis summarizes how training and exposure strengthens bindings among pertinent oscillators during endogenous entrainment. In our society, exposures to a range of different musical instances (tokens) of a particular category inescapably lead to heightened reinforcements of a lean version of a metric cluster; this refers to the strongest global attractor in a metric oscillator cluster. This global attractor defines a metric category.

A *metric category prototype* is a stimulus pattern that "stands" for an internalized category. In music, a prototype is a distillation of a particular attractor relationship defining a category. It reflects knowledge about the abstract time relations of novel but metrical rhythms.

Category Members and Their Rhythms

This account of meter learning leaves an unanswered question: What differentiates one individual metrical sequence from another in a metric category? A quick glance at the six M patterns in Figure 10.4 provides a short answer: rhythmic grouping patterns. For instance, both M1 and M2 tokens have duple meter patterns, but they differ in rhythmic groupings. A richer answer speaks to the nature of differentiation. Basically, M1 and M2 have different *rhythmic attractor profiles*. This brings us to the bottom portion of Figure 10.5. It features attractor profiles and group reinforcements of M1 which flow from the transient mode-locking entrainment designed to explain attending to rhythmic patterns.

Most sequence members of a metric category are decorated with rhythmic grouping patterns.

In contrast to truly nonmetrical patterns (N), a metrical pattern contains rhythmic groups that "fit" into a given meter. Both metrical and nonmetrical patterns have rhythms that invite transient mode-locking; consequently both deliver rhythmic attractor profiles. For example, the M1 sequence has a series of groups of one, two, and three tones (Figures 10.4 and 10.5). The three-tone group is formalized in an attractor profile (bottom of Figure 10.5) as n:m of 1:2-1:2 (bracket), and a two-tone group in M1 subdivides the referent period (n > m) as 1:2 (bracket, for final T of 250 ms). By contrast, in the N1 control sequence (of Figure 10.4), the surface rhythm, with alternating groups of one and two tones, has fewer compatible local attractors (e.g., 1:2).

Finally, although much research has focused on the mastery of individual sequences, our ordinary encounters with music expose us to a wide variety of different rhythmic sound patterns that may all belong to the same metric category. Indeed, a signature of the mastery of meter learning rests with an individual's ability to identify the meter of an entirely novel sequence. Category learning emerges when a listener has internalized an invariant (global) time relation that applies to a wide range of different rhythmic patterns. In short, "what" is learned is an abstract metric invariant: a global attractor.

Does Rhythm Learning Really Exist?

Category learning of meter does not mean that the learning of individual patterns is necessarily superior for metrical sequences compared to nonmetrical ones.[51] Nevertheless, theoretically, there is a tendency to treat rhythmic groups as perceptual primitives, essentially ruling out rhythm learning. But rhythmic patterns and related attractor profiles are indeed learnable. For instance, a nonmetric sequence may exhibit a compelling attractor profile that leads to faster learning than a metric counterpart that is governed by a complex global attractor.

Yet skepticism regarding rhythm learning remains. One reason for this skepticism arises from our subjective experience with rhythmic time patterns. Intuitively, grouping of items, adjacent in space and/or pitch sounds, just "seems" natural and immediate. This naturalness is often expressed in the nativism of Gestalt principles that specify perceptual "grouping" principles such as proximity or continuity and so on.

While granting the immediacy of percepts of rhythm groups, it remains possible that rhythm learning exists without denying its roots in innate relationships. This reasoning is predicated on an assumption that people rely on similar learning principles when mastering meter and rhythm. Both involve strengthening of oscillator connections that mirror innate attractors. With rhythm learning, it is possible that reinforcements of local attractors occur during transient mode-locking as an ongoing referent period briefly aligns with reactive pulses sparked by the salient tone onsets of successively changing driving rhythms. This learning through binding may produce a strong attractor profile.

Certainly, less is known about rhythm learning than meter learning. Nevertheless, evidence countering skepticism about the existence of rhythm learning comes from Stephen Handel.[52] He discovered that listeners who show poor sensitivity to time relationships after one presentation of a rhythmic pattern (metrical or nonmetrical), improve with exposures to grouping patterns.[53] In this vein, the presence of metrical properties also appears to facilitate this learning.[54]

According to Handel, grouping percepts depend on Gestalt principles, and learning consists of refining codes of group size. Alternatively, according to DAT, rhythm learning is directed toward strengthening connections associated with the local attractors of rhythmic attractor profile. In this respect, rhythm learning resembles meter learning by emphasizing a role for internalized attractor relationships that are reinforced during learning.

Evidence for a Metric Binding Hypothesis

The metric binding hypothesis offers predictions about listeners' acquisition of metric sensitivity. Support for these predictions comes from studies of musical skill reviewed earlier in this chapter which are briefly recapitulated here.

Exposure Frequency Versus Frequency of Reinforcements

The metric binding hypothesis implies that metric invariants (e.g., as global attractors) define a category. Their internalized representations are predicted to gain strength from exposure frequency (number of entrainment episodes), a prediction supported by a number of studies.[55,56,57,58]

Metric Markers and the Skill Gap

The metric binding hypothesis correctly predicts that musicians, with strong internalized metric clusters, rely heavily on relevant expectancy pulses that serve as subjectively salient accents. These expert listeners depend on salient *silent* expectancy pulses that allow them to "hear out" metrical markers even in sequences that contain no objective metrical accents. Nonmusicians cannot do this. Instead, average listeners rely on the stimulus-driven reactive pulses of external metric time markers. This is also confirmed.[59,60]

Multiple Metric Levels

The metric binding hypothesis also correctly predicts that musicians, who have permanently internalized metric clusters, will exhibit greater sensitivity to metric time layers than will nonmusicians.[61]

Metric Complexity

Complex meters are correctly predicted to be harder to learn as categories than are simpler meters.[62,63] Theoretically, this is because, relative to simple attractors, complex attractors lead to lower reinforcement rates.

Summary of Category Learning and the Metric Binding Hypothesis

In sum, the metric binding hypothesis builds on distinctions between entrainment (based on coupling parameters) and learning (based on binding parameters) to explain how people implicitly learn metric categories. In the end, meter learning is category learning; it draws on factors that explain attending to and learning of invariant time relationships common to different individual (i.e., token) rhythmic sequences. Finally, this learning rests on the acquisition, through binding, of a metric concept defined by a strong global attractor in a metric cluster. In sum, meter learning rephrases the familiar Hebbian rule: *oscillations that fire together bind together*.

Major features in this section are:

- Category learning of meter, described by a metric binding hypothesis, depends on selective strengthening of certain global attractors in a metric cluster due to bindings from reinforcement frequency.
- A metric category prototype is a stimulus pattern exhibiting strong global attractors of a metric category.
- Rhythmic structures of sequences distinguish metric instances (tokens) within a category. Concurrent with learning global attractors, rhythm learning rests on reinforcement opportunities for learning the profile of successive local attractors.

- Predictions of metric binding correctly identify factors such as phase alignment, exposure frequency, and attractor complexity as influencing category learning.

MODELING METER LEARNING

The metric binding hypothesis describes properties of meter learning that happen during entrainment episodes. As outlined, this hypothesis does not represent a rigorous binding model; mathematically, it may be expressed in various ways. Others have formulated rigorous models that address meter learning in different ways; two are mentioned here.

SONOR

One meter learning model created by Michael Gasser with colleagues Douglas Eck and Robert Port[64] extends earlier entrainment models.[65] Their model, Self-Organizing Network of Oscillators for Rhythm (SONOR), is inspiring. SONOR relies on a network of coupled oscillations that learns to both perceive and produce metrical sequences. It adapts a Hopfield attractor neural network to include oscillations connected by coupling weights that change following a Hebbian learning algorithm.[66] Gasser and colleagues were first to address issues of meter learning. Accordingly, this model inspired the current metric binding hypothesis.

Two general features of SONOR are worth noting. First, SONOR allows an oscillation in a coupled dyad to function interchangeably as either a driving or a driven rhythm. Second, in SONOR, a driving rhythm can be either endogenous (a neural oscillation) or exogenous (a stimulus cycle).

SONOR is an impressively broad model of meter learning, addressing both perceptual learning and motor production (Box 10.2). In this model, meter learning depends on weight changes of a phase coupling parameter that connects a pair oscillations. Coupling weights increase with the sum of weights of numerous simultaneously active oscillations, providing stronger coupling weights to improve oscillator phase alignments. Critically, this means that oscillator connections (i.e., their entrainments) become stronger due to increased coupling weights. In short, learning depends on phase parameters. Furthermore, attractor complexity affects weighting of coupling parameters. SONOR directly addresses learning by assuming that both activation levels of oscillations and their

BOX 10.2
TWO HEBBIAN MODELS OF RHYTHM LEARNING

SELF-ORGANIZING NETWORK OF OSCILLATORS
FOR RHYTHM (SONOR)

SONOR is a neural network of individual oscillations with fixed periods (biological primitives). Meter learning depends on strengthening coupling connections (W_{ij}) between two oscillations (O_i, O_j). An important architectural difference between SONOR and earlier entrainment models is its incorporation of momentary intensity variations of driving rhythms.

Formally, perception is given by the input, I, to an oscillator, $I_i(t)$, at time t. An oscillator, activated by these inputs, has output, O_i. The sum of all connective weights on other oscillations (j to n) affects the momentary output of a receiving oscillation (O_i). In turn, this determines the input:

$$I_i(t) = O_i(t)\sum_{j=0}^{n}[O_j(t)W_{ij}] \qquad\qquad 10.1$$

The output of an oscillation at time t, $O_i(t)$, determines production of a metrical sequences as a series of timed pulses, each with an amplitude level, $A_i(t)$. Peak activity level of oscillator i is determined by matching the activity levels of synchronous incoming pulses from other oscillations. Although pulse peaks differ, pulses occur regularly at a fixed phase (zero phase points/oscillation) for the period of each oscillation. In a series of unfolding phases, φ_i, with pulse amplitudes, $A_i(t)$, changes in the oscillator output at moment t are:

$$O_i(t) = A_i(t)[0.5\cos(\varphi_i(t)) + 0.5]^{\gamma_i(t)} \qquad\qquad 10.2$$

This function determines momentary activation height (via gain, $\gamma_i(t)$), including peak pulse heights. Activation levels change in response to pulses from other oscillations and external time markers. In addition, Hebbian changes in weights (ΔW_{ij}) depend on joint activation levels of coinciding pulses from two different oscillations (or an oscillation and an external salient marker). Coupling weight changes then accumulate over time as strengthened connections.

Finally, magnitude of a phase change in oscillator i, $\Delta\varphi_i$, depends on the relative phase of a pulse from an impacting oscillation (e.g., oscillation j) together with current weights of coupling oscillations (i and j). Generally, as W_{ij} increases, this model predicts that connection between two oscillations (i, j) benefits from joint exposure regardless of their commensurate periods. Effectively, coupling weights "pull" the pulse peak of a driving rhythm closer to the pulse peak of a driven rhythm. Finally, special relative period ratios (e.g., attractors) are not explicitly featured in this model.

SELIGER'S HEBBIAN LEARNING MODEL

A Hebbian model involving network oscillations is offered by Seliger and colleagues (see text reference). In this model, all connections are expressed by phase coupling coefficients (K_{ij}) that operate directly on phase differences between oscillations. It also incorporates slow dynamical changes in these coupling parameters (coefficients). Importantly, coupling parameters are supplemented by a "learning" parameter, e. Considering just two oscillations, O_i and O_j, differential equations express adaptive strength changes of a coupling force coefficient, K_{ij}, between oscillations (Equation 10.3). Phase change, φ_i (e.g., for oscillation i), is specified in Equation

10.4. These changes reflect oscillator couplings for a cluster of N oscillations (i.e., a cluster of $N = 2$ is a dyad).

$$\mathbf{d\,K_{ij}} / \mathbf{dt} = \mathbf{e}[-\cos(\varphi i - \varphi j) - \mathbf{K_{ij}}] \qquad 10.3$$

$$\mathbf{d\,\varphi i} / \mathbf{dt} = \omega i - 1 / N \sum_{j=0}^{N} \mathbf{Kij} \sin(\varphi i - \varphi j) \qquad 10.4$$

Equation 10.3 is a differential equation reflecting continuous changes in coupling strength between oscillation, **Kij** (note that **Kij** is **K** with symmetric coupling). Small values of **e** in this equation (i.e., close to a Hopf bifurcation) reflect dynamic changes that express learning as slow incremental changes in coupling strength due to phase differences. Assuming the parameter **α** is positive, fixed **α** values strengthen **Kij** over time with small phase differences (ideally zero). Thus, phase-coupling depends on internal driving rhythm force, although its final value also depends on acquired phase changes of a phase-aligned stimulus rhythm. Changes in **e** modulate the impact of alignments of two oscillations from **α** cos (φi – φj) and **Kij** (Equation 10.3). Note that some phase differences prohibit learning, whereas others promote it. Thus, if (φi – φj) is 90 degrees, then **cos** (φi – φj) = **0**, meaning no **Kij** increments. By contrast, if two oscillations are perfectly phase-aligned (a 0 degree difference) then **cos** (φi – φj) = **1.0,** indicating significant incrementing from phase-aligned couplings.

Equation 10.4 describes changes in phase over time. On one hand, these depend on parameter values (e.g., **Kij**) which can reduce phase differences (i.e., phase correction) between two oscillations; alternatively, resulting phase alignments feed back into Equation 10.3 to promote learning by strengthening the coupling coefficient **Kij**. This loop leads to strengthening of connections between simultaneous (aligned) oscillations within a larger oscillation cluster. Network learning appears in a persistence of an acquired phase configuration, given the withdrawal of an external driving stimulation.

This model does not single out couplings with commensurate integer ratios among oscillator periods. Instead of time ratios, the magnitude of a frequency difference, **Δω,** figures into this model as a detuning variable. Strengthened phase connections, due to a simple frequency ratio (**ωi:ωj**), depend on the degree to which their rotation number yields a **α** cos (φi – φj) > 0, creating a stronger **Kij**. Other implications related to frequency (period) locking are not specifically addressed.

In sum, acquisition of a connectivity configuration depends on the degree and number of phase alignments between oscillations of a cluster. It results from strengthening of coupling coefficients. Finally, as with SONOR, what is learned in this model is a configuration of relative phases associated with synchronized states of oscillations within a cluster.

coupling weights increase with exposure to simple metric sequences (e.g., duple meter sequences) but not for nonmetrical ones. In this way, behaviors in a driving–driven network depend on momentary coupling weights among active oscillations and the presence of simple attractor ratios; moreover, they are influenced by exposure frequency.

Finally, support for SONOR is found in successful simulations of meter learning. A three-oscillator network was exposed to a duple meter tone pattern in which the metrical pattern was outlined by intensity accents. Simulated SONOR network responses showed that increased coupling weights affected the network's preference for a 2:1 period relationship of the exposed duple meter over a nonexposed 3:1 (triple meter) pattern.

SONOR and the Metric Binding Hypothesis

SONOR assumes that meter learning is a function of both exposure frequency and attractor relationships, assumptions shared with the Metric Binding hypothesis of DAT. However, an important theoretical difference centers on the interpretation of coupling parameters. SONOR interprets changes in coupling weights as a source of learning. That is, coupling parameters do "double duty"; they operate as both coupling parameters (during entrainment) and as binding parameters (during learning). By contrast, the metric binding hypothesis distinguishes coupling parameters, which affect entrainment and depend largely on driving rhythm force, from binding parameters, which affect learning and depend on exposure frequency.

The distinction between entrainment and learning embedded in the metric binding hypothesis allows it to address momentary attending, short-term memory, and various temporal changes in a listener's sensitivity to a driving rhythm while preserving learning as a more permanent process based on binding parameters, which persist even when the force of a driving rhythm is removed.

Seliger's Learning Model

Another formalization of learning within an entrainment context is offered by Seliger and colleagues.[67] This model (Box 10.2) offers a more general approach to learning time relationships than either SONOR or the metric binding hypothesis. In fact, it does not explicitly address meter learning. Rather, it addresses learning predicated on entrainment. It shares with SONOR the assumption that learning depends on coupling parameter strength following a Hebbian algorithm. But it differs in adding a separate learning parameter (e) that is specifically sensitive to exposure frequency. In brief, this model incorporates a learning parameter that is solely linked to the exposure frequency of oscillator phase alignments.

Summary of Modeling Meter Learning

The two mathematical models described in this section provide important foundations for understanding entrainment and the learning of metric relations. However, as the origin of learning, both appeal to traditional mode-locking associated with a fixed global attractor. Consequently,

applied to musical time patterns, these models may be expanded to address learning of metric categories (e.g., metric oscillator clusters) but they do not address concurrent learning of categorical instances of metrical versus non-metrical patterns (e.g., attractor profiles).

The major points of this section are:

- Two formal entrainment models describe learning of time patterns given a traditional mode-locking protocol.
- SONOR explicitly addresses meter learning, assuming that exposure during entrainment leads to weighted coupling parameters that affect meter learning.
- A different entrainment model assumes that learning time patterns depends on both coupling (force-based) and learning (exposure-driven) parameters.

CHAPTER SUMMARY

This chapter outlines a general framework for understanding the "what" and "how" of learning time patterns that happens during an entraining episode. It articulates an intimate relationship between the phase-coupling activities that are deemed temporary and flexible and bindings among oscillator periodicities that lead to long-lasting learning. This framework underscores differences between attending based on entrainment and learning based on bindings. Although both are universal processes, in this scheme, attending and learning serve different functions. Attending is a flexible, force-driven activity that enables in-the-moment reactions to external events, whereas learning does not depend on driving rhythm force, drawing instead on strengthened bindings that yield more deliberative responses based on past experience. These two activities operate in tandem during an entrainment episode, with entrainment (and coupling) providing a platform for learning (hence binding). This chapter outlines factors that distinguish these two processes as they apply to skill acquisition with regard to musical meters.

Entrainment is shown to depend largely on the force associated with a relatively regular driving rhythm. In the development of metric categories, listeners must form metric clusters based on multiple driving rhythms of metric hierarchies that offer opportunities for endogenous entrainments among multiple resonant oscillations. The result is a metric oscillator cluster, governed by force-based coupling parameters and global attractors.

Learning is proposed to build on oscillator clusters. At various hypothesized learning stages, learning is strengthened by bindings between entraining oscillations. Unlike entrainment, which depends on driving rhythm force, learning depends on growing binding strengths among oscillator periods due to exposure frequency of aligned (synchronized) pulses.

A metric binding hypothesis describes the learning of metrical properties in individual sequences as well as learning of categories defined by invariant time relationships which specify different metric relationships. Extended experience with metrical time patterns (i.e., category tokens) promotes learning through binding, leading in turn to development of expert skills. Musicians benefit from selective strengthening from binding via exposure to the defining global attractors of meters. The "what" that is learned about meter is categorical knowledge captured by global attractors of a reinforced metric oscillator cluster. This abstract metric knowledge is long-lasting, arising from repeated exposures to metric instances of a category.

Finally, the broad theoretical perspective developed in this chapter suggests a complex picture of learning. Learning is based on both innate tendencies and exposure frequency. This story departs from some widely accepted views of learning as dependent largely on exposure frequency. It also contrasts with approaches to time patterns that endorse a dichotomy between meter perception as an acquired skill due to exposure frequency and rhythm perception that is innate and based on Gestalt grouping principles. The approach presented in this chapter suggests that innate (attractor) and acquired (binding) constructs are both involved, in different ways, in people's percepts of meter and rhythm.

NOTES

1. Erin E. Hannon and Sandra E. Trehub, "Metrical Categories in Infancy and Adulthood," *Psychological Science* 16, no. 1 (January 1, 2005): 48–55, doi:10.1111/j.0956-7976.2005.00779.x.

2. Sylvain Moreno and Mireille Besson, "Musical Training and Language-Related Brain Electrical Activity in Children," *Psychophysiology* 43, no. 3 (May 1, 2006): 287–91, doi:10.1111/j.1469-8986.2006.00401.x.

3. Manuela M. Marin, "Effects of Early Musical Training on Musical and Linguistic Syntactic Abilities," *Annals of the New York Academy of Sciences* 1169, no. 1 (July 1, 2009): 187–90, doi:10.1111/j.1749-6632.2009.04777.x.

4. Gabriella Musacchia et al., "Musicians Have Enhanced Subcortical Auditory and Audiovisual Processing of Speech and Music," *Proceedings of the National Academy of Sciences* 104, no. 40 (October 2, 2007): 15894–98, doi:10.1073/pnas.0701498104.

5. Nina Kraus and Bharath Chandrasekaran, "Music Training for the Development of Auditory Skills," *Nature Reviews Neuroscience* 11, no. 8 (August 2010): 599–605, doi:10.1038/nrn2882.

6. Gabriella Musacchia, Dana Strait, and Nina Kraus, "Relationships Between Behavior, Brainstem and Cortical Encoding of Seen and Heard Speech in Musicians and Non-Musicians," *Hearing Research* 241, no. 1–2 (July 2008): 34–42, doi:10.1016/j.heares.2008.04.013.

7. Mari Riess Jones and William Yee, "Sensitivity to Time Change: The Role of Context and Skill," *Journal of Experimental Psychology: Human Perception and Performance* 23, no. 3 (1997): 693.

8. Mari Riess Jones et al., "Tests of Attentional Flexibility in Listening to Polyrhythmic Patterns," *Journal of Experimental Psychology: Human Perception and Performance* 21, no. 2 (1995): 293–307, doi:10.1037/0096-1523.21.2.293.

9. Laurel J. Trainor and Kathleen A. Corrigall, "Music Acquisition and Effects of Musical Experience," in *Music Perception*, ed. Mari Riess Jones, Richard R. Fay, and Arthur N. Popper, vol. 36 (New York: Springer New York, 2010), 89–127, http://link.springer.com/10.1007/978-1-4419-6114-3_4.

10. P. W. Jusczyk, *Language, Speech, and Communication. The Discovery of Spoken Language* (Cambridge, MA: MIT Press, 1997).

11. Janet F. Werker and Richard C. Tees, "Speech Perception as a Window for Understanding Plasticity and Commitment in Language Systems of the Brain," *Developmental Psychobiology* 46, no. 3 (April 1, 2005): 233–51, doi:10.1002/dev.20060.

12. Laurel J. Trainor, "Are There Critical Periods for Musical Development?" *Developmental Psychobiology* 46, no. 3 (April 1, 2005): 262–78, doi:10.1002/dev.20059.

13. István Winkler et al., "Newborn Infants Detect the Beat in Music," *Proceedings of the National Academy of Sciences* 106, no. 7 (February 17, 2009): 2468–71, doi:10.1073/pnas.0809035106.

14. Henkjan Honing et al., "Is Beat Induction Innate or Learned?" *Annals of the New York Academy of Sciences* 1169, no. 1 (July 1, 2009): 93–96, doi:10.1111/j.1749-6632.2009.04761.x.

15. Eveline Geiser et al., "Refinement of Metre Perception – Training Increases Hierarchical Metre Processing," *European Journal of Neuroscience* 32, no. 11 (December 1, 2010): 1979–85, doi:10.1111/j.1460-9568.2010.07462.x.

16. Jessica Phillips-Silver and Laurel J. Trainor, "Vestibular Influence on Auditory Metrical Interpretation," *Brain and Cognition* 67, no. 1 (June 2008): 94–102, doi:10.1016/j.bandc.2007.11.007.

17. Gottfried Schlaug et al., "Increased Corpus Callosum Size in Musicians," *Neuropsychologia*, Neuropsychological And Developmental Studies Of The Corpus Callosum, 33, no. 8 (August 1995): 1047–55, doi:10.1016/0028-3932(95)00045-5.

18. Daniela Perani et al., "Functional Specializations for Music Processing in the Human Newborn Brain," *Proceedings of the National Academy of Sciences* 107, no. 10 (March 9, 2010): 4758–63, doi:10.1073/pnas.0909074107.

19. Erin E. Hannon and Laurel J. Trainor, "Music Acquisition: Effects of Enculturation and Formal Training on Development," *Trends in Cognitive Sciences* 11, no. 11 (November 2007): 466–72, doi:10.1016/j.tics.2007.08.008.

20. Recall that the width of an entrainment region is greater for weak than for strong latent oscillations. This should be distinguished from the other factor, effective coupling strength (e.g., K), which also affects entrainment region width.

21. Erin E. Hannon, Gaye Soley, and Rachel S. Levine, "Constraints on Infants' Musical Rhythm Perception: Effects of Interval Ratio Complexity and Enculturation," *Developmental Science* 14, no. 4 (July 1, 2011): 865–72, doi:10.1111/j.1467-7687.2011.01036.x.

22. Hannon and Trehub, "Metrical Categories in Infancy and Adulthood."

23. E. E. Hannon and S. E. Trehub, "Tuning in to Musical Rhythms: Infants Learn More Readily than Adults," *Proceedings of the National Academy of Sciences* 102, no. 35 (August 30, 2005): 12639–43, doi:10.1073/pnas.0504254102.

24. Carolyn Drake, Mari Riess Jones, and Clarisse Baruch, "The Development of Rhythmic Attending in Auditory Sequences: Attunement, Referent Period, Focal Attending," *Cognition* 77, no. 3 (December 15, 2000): 251–88, doi:10.1016/S0010-0277(00)00106-2.

25. Three marker properties were (1) distinctive metric markers conveyed by Ravel's *Bolero*, (2) moderately noticeable markers were intensity increments in an isochronous rhythm, and (3) weakly distinctive metric accents involved time spans implied only by a rhythmic pattern with no physical changes.

26. Robert J. Ellis and Mari R. Jones, "The Role of Accent Salience and Joint Accent Structure in Meter Perception," *Journal of Experimental Psychology: Human Perception and Performance* 35, no. 1 (2009): 264–80, doi:10.1037/a0013482.

27. Caroline Palmer and Carol L. Krumhansl, "Mental Representations for Musical Meter," *Journal of Experimental Psychology: Human Perception and Performance* 16, no. 4 (1990): 728–41, doi:10.1037/0096-1523.16.4.728.

28. Shu-Jen Kung et al., "Dynamic Allocation of Attention to Metrical and Grouping Accents in Rhythmic Sequences," *Experimental Brain Research* 210, no. 2 (March 26, 2011): 269–82, doi:10.1007/s00221-011-2630-2.

29. Mari Tervaniemi, "Musicians—Same or Different?" *Annals of the New York Academy of Sciences* 1169, no. 1 (July 1, 2009): 151–56, doi:10.1111/j.1749-6632.2009.04591.x.

30. Kung et al., "Dynamic Allocation of Attention to Metrical and Grouping Accents in Rhythmic Sequences."

31. J. A. Sloboda and A. H. Gregory, "The Psychological Reality of Musical Segments," *Canadian Journal of Psychology/Revue Canadienne de Psychologie* 34, no. 3 (1980): 274–80, doi:10.1037/h0081052.

32. J. A. Fodor and T. G. Bever, "The Psychological Reality of Linguistic Segments," *Journal of Verbal Learning and Verbal Behavior* 4, no. 5 (October 1, 1965): 414–20, doi:10.1016/S0022-5371(65)80081-0.

33. David Temperley and Christopher Bartlette, "Parallelism as a Factor in Metrical Analysis," *Music Perception: An Interdisciplinary Journal* 20, no. 2 (December 1, 2002): 117–49, doi:10.1525/mp.2002.20.2.117.

34. Barbara Tillmann, Catherine Stevens, and Peter E. Keller, "Learning of Timing Patterns and the Development of Temporal Expectations," *Psychological Research* 75, no. 3 (August 4, 2010): 243–58, doi:10.1007/s00426-010-0302-7.

35. Melissa Brandon et al., "Incidental Learning of Temporal Structures Conforming to a Metrical Framework," *Frontiers in Psychology* volume 3 (August 23, 2012): 1–10 , doi:10.3389/fpsyg.2012.00294.

36. Benjamin G. Schultz et al., "The Implicit Learning of Metrical and Nonmetrical Temporal Patterns," *The Quarterly Journal of Experimental Psychology* 66, no. 2 (February 2013): 360–80, doi:10.1080/17470218.2012.712146.

37. J. Terry et al., "Implicit Learning of Between-Group Intervals in Auditory Temporal Structures," *Attention, Perception, & Psychophysics* 78, no. 6 (August 2016): 1728–43, doi:10.3758/s13414-016-1148-x.

38. Tillmann, Stevens, and Keller, "Learning of Timing Patterns and the Development of Temporal Expectations."

39. M. Boltz, "The Incidental Learning and Remembering of Event Durations," in *Time, Action and Cognition*, eds. Françoise Macar, Viviane Pouthas, and William J. Friedman, NATO ASI Series 66 (Netherlands: Springer, 1992), 153–63, doi:10.1007/978-94-017-3536-0_17.

40. Joanna Salidis, "Nonconscious Temporal Cognition: Learning Rhythms Implicitly," *Memory & Cognition* 29, no. 8 (December 2001): 1111–19, doi:10.3758/BF03206380.

41. Continuous versions of this model have similar parameters in differential equations.

42. Mari R. Jones, "Time, Our Lost Dimension: Toward a New Theory of Perception, Attention, and Memory.," *Psychological Review* 83, no. 5 (1976): 323.

43. Shaowen Bao, Vincent T. Chan, and Michael M. Merzenich, "Cortical Remodelling Induced by Activity of Ventral Tegmental Dopamine Neurons," *Nature* 412, no. 6842 (July 5, 2001): 79–83, doi:10.1038/35083586.

5

67

44. Paul W. Glimcher, "Understanding Dopamine and Reinforcement Learning: The Dopamine Reward Prediction Error Hypothesis," *Proceedings of the National Academy of Sciences* 108, no. Supplement 3 (September 13, 2011): 15647–54, doi:10.1073/pnas.1014269108.

45. G. S. Medvedev et al., "Dendritic Synchrony and Transient Dynamics in a Coupled Oscillator Model of the Dopaminergic Neuron," *Journal of Computational Neuroscience* 15, no. 1 (July 2003): 53–69, doi:10.1023/A:1024422802673.

46. In stage 3, subjective salience of reactive pulses is hypothesized to wane as they are replaced by strengthened expectancy pulses during internalization.

47. Salidis, "Nonconscious Temporal Cognition."

48. Brandon et al., "Incidental Learning of Temporal Structures Conforming to a Metrical Framework."

49. Robert J. Ellis and Mari Riess Jones, "Rhythmic Context Modulates Foreperiod Effects," *Attention, Perception, & Psychophysics* 72, no. 8 (November 2010): 2274–88, doi:10.3758/BF03196701.

50. The referent could be any of these oscillations.

51. Benjamin G. Schultz et al., "The Implicit Learning of Metrical and Nonmetrical Temporal Patterns."

52. John R. Iversen, Aniruddh D. Patel, and Kengo Ohgushi, "Perception of Rhythmic Grouping Depends on Auditory Experiences," *The Journal of the Acoustical Society of America* 124, no. 4 (October 1, 2008): 2263–71, doi:10.1121/1.2973189.

53. Stephen Handel, "The Differentiation of Rhythmic Structure," *Perception & Psychophysics* 52, no. 5 (September 1992): 497–507, doi:10.3758/BF03206711.

54. Stephen Handel, "The Interplay Between Metric and Figural Rhythmic Organization," *Journal of Experimental Psychology: Human Perception and Performance* 24, no. 5 (1998): 1546–61, doi:10.1037/0096-1523.24.5.1546.

55. Hannon and Trehub, "Metrical Categories in Infancy and Adulthood."

56. Hannon and Trainor, "Music Acquisition."

57. Benjamin G. Schultz et al., "The Implicit Learning of Metrical and Nonmetrical Temporal Patterns," *The Quarterly Journal of Experimental Psychology* 66, no. 2 (February 1, 2013): 360–80, doi:10.1080/17470218.2012.712146.

58. Brandon et al., "Incidental Learning of Temporal Structures Conforming to a Metrical Framework."

59. Kung et al., "Dynamic Allocation of Attention to Metrical and Grouping Accents in Rhythmic Sequences."

60. Drake, Riess Jones, and Baruch, "The Development of Rhythmic Attending in Auditory Sequences: Attunement, Referent Period, Focal Attending."

61. Palmer and Krumhansl, "Mental Representations for Musical Meter."

62. Carolyn Drake, "Reproduction of Musical Rhythms by Children, Adult Musicians, and Adult Nonmusicians," *Perception & Psychophysics* 53, no. 1 (January 1993): 25–33, doi:10.3758/BF03211712.

63. Hannon and Trehub, "Metrical Categories in Infancy and Adulthood."

64. Michael Gasser, Douglas Eck, and Robert Port, "Meter as Mechanism: A Neural Network Model that Learns Metrical Patterns," *Connection Science* 11, no. 2 (June 1, 1999): 187–216, doi:10.1080/095400999116331.

65. Edward W. Large and John F. Kolen, "Resonance and the Perception of Musical Meter," *Connection Science* 6, no. 2–3 (January 1, 1994): 177–208, doi:10.1080/09540099408915723.

66. J. J. Hopfield, "Neural Networks and Physical Systems with Emergent Collective Computational Abilities," *Proceedings of the National Academy of Sciences* 79, no. 8 (April 1, 1982): 2554–8.

67. P. Seliger, S. C. Young, and L. S. Tsimring. Plasticity and Learning in a Network of Coupled Phase Oscillators. *Physical Review E* 65, no. 4 (2002): 041906.

11

Musical Melodies

Melody is arguably the queen of song. So it seems strange to find a well-known music dictionary defining melody with the mundane phrase: "A melody is a succession of musical tones."[1] Yet this definition has the merit of casting a wide net. Moreover, most of us have an idea of what constitutes a melody from tunes spontaneously hummed by friends to the more crafted sound patterns produced by musicians at concerts. This chapter aims to describe how we, as listeners, attend to melodies as they unfold in real time.

To begin, it is useful to recognize certain constraints on melodic structure that can affect the one's attending. One broad constraint, of course, concerns the individual tones that form a melodic pattern. Theoretically, these tones resemble the 'fast events' discussed in Chapter 6. Chapter 6 where complex sounds afford micro-driving rhythms that support pitch perception. However, musical tones belong to the special sets of complex sounds are culture-sensitive musical scales. A second constraint concerns the overall "shape" of a melody. Although a melody is a configuration of specially scaled pitch steps (i.e., pitch intervals), these pitches also contribute to a melodic contour that transcends their component pitch intervals. This chapter applies familiar concepts of dynamic attending to explain our responses to these and related aspects of musical melodies.

CHAPTER GOALS

This chapter explores entrainment concepts as they apply to people's response to events created by musical melodies. Although the time scales of melodic tones now shrink to the micro-rhythms of pitch, the basic entrainment concepts are familiar ones. Not only do certain recognizable concepts permit explanations of attending to melodies of music, they also foreshadow concepts relevant to speech melodies considered in later chapters. However, at first glance, any discussion of music raises issues seemingly unique to this domain, in part because music involves seemingly rarefied

topics such as tonality and implied harmony as well as characteristic melodic contours.

This chapter has three major sections. The first section introduces musical scales together with their psychological implications. This includes an overview of basic concepts such as musical key, tonality, and relative stability.

The second major section describes tonality in melodies from the perspective of dynamic attending. This builds on earlier discussions of pitch perception (Chapter 6), where tones are conceived as providing micro-driving rhythms that elicit resonant oscillations as fast driven rhythms. Other familiar concepts relate to endogenous entrainments among melodically activated oscillations. These include oscillator clusters and attractor profiles which support explanations about how we attend to chords and melodies, respectively.

The third major section addresses melody contour. This illustrates how elementary entrainment concepts apply to listeners' pitch tracking of the surface structure of melodic groups, manifest as contours. This introduces a new concept of *pitch tracking*, which involves modulating exogenous entrainments. That is, people virtually track rising and falling pitch contours of unfolding tone sequences.

BACKGROUND: MUSICAL SCALES AND TONALITY

Melodies are special because they rely on precisely scaled tones. Although musical melodies can express grand frequency excursions not found in speech, even these sweeping pitch shifts abide by the constraints of musical scales. Musical scales stipulate specific tone differences (i.e., *pitch intervals*) which are actually are frequency ratios. For readers unfamiliar with Western musical scales, Box 11.1 summarizes a few central properties. Typically, musical tones are rich, complex sounds with pitches determined by fundamental frequencies. Chapter 6 provides an important backdrop for the present chapter in that

---

BOX 11.1
TONALITY: WESTERN MUSICAL SCALES AND CHORDS

Western musical scales comprise sets of tones related by frequency ratios. The most stable relationships in Western scales involve tone pairs with frequency (time) ratios of 1:1 (unison) and 2:1 (octave). Conventionally, the octave is subdivided into smaller sets (i.e., musical scale sets). The nature of subdivisions has a long history dating to Pythagorean scales designed to maximize harmonic "pureness." The popular equal temperament (ET) tuning system is a compromise scale; the ET chromatic scale has 12 equal subdivisions of an octave (12 semitones) based on an irrational frequency ratio (1.0594). This scale preserves circular symmetries at the cost of reducing the "pureness" of frequency ratios. ET ratios only *approximate* simple time ratios.

This chromatic scale has 12 pitch classes per octave: C, C$^\#$, D, D$^\#$, E, F, F$^\#$, G, G$^\#$, A, A$^\#$, B. Thus, all tones with frequencies that are integer (n) multiples of 16.3 Hz (32.7 Hz . . . 261.63 Hz . . . 1,046.5 Hz . . .) belong to the C pitch class (middle C is 261.63 Hz). Other scales are subsets of the chromatic scale. Western diatonic scales have seven distinct *pitch classes*. Table 11.1 displays a familiar diatonic major scale, the C major scale (C, D, E, F, G, A, B, C′) with ET tuning. Major diatonic scales reflect an invariant sequence scale steps of: 2-2-1-2-2-2-1 (in semitones); minor scales have a different pattern. Each diatonic scale begins on specific keynote in 12 pitch classes of an octave.

Chords are simultaneous subsets of scale tones. A chord stacks one or more scale tones on a *root* tone with a scale frequency. Important roots are the first (tonic), fourth (subdominant), and fifth (dominant) tones in a scale (Table 11.1). These are C, F, and G in the C major scale. Prominent chords form the category of *major chords*: tonic, **I** (e.g., CEG); dominant, **V** (GBD); and subdominant, **IV** (FAC). These chord types have invariant frequency relationships among component scale tones, differing only in their roots.

Musical scales and chords reflect abstract patterns of frequency relationships among scale tones that transcend individual frequencies. Among important abstractions are *tonal relationships*. These involve invariant frequency relationships of a scale's keynote (i.e., the tonic) and other scale tones. For instance, in the C major scale, a perfect fifth between the tonic, C, and dominant tone, G, reflects a powerful tonal relation with a frequency ratio, 1.4981, that approximates 1.5 (3:2). This reflects a large skip in scale steps (seven semitones), but it remains a stable relationship because this ratio approximates a simple attractor ratios of 3:2.

---

both chapters acknowledge that individual complex tones typically consist of many, very rapid micro-driving rhythms.

Musical Scales: Calibrated Micro-Rhythms

Musical scales differ with culture.[2,3] Although cultural differences are central to the flourishing field of ethnomusicology, they are beyond the scope of this chapter, which concentrates on European musical scales. A working assumption is that, with some modifications, basic concepts underlying these scales generalize to scales in other cultures.

A Western musical scale is a set of tones with special interrelationships (Boxes 11.1 and 11.2). Each scale tone is a complex sound with its pitch based on the fundamental frequency (F0; or repetition frequency). In this ideal form, the pitch of a tone does not change over time.[4] A musical scale expresses tonal information arranged in an increasing order of scale tone pitches. An example of a Western tonal scale, the C major scale, is outlined in Table 11.1 for a single octave. These tones are a subset of a larger scale with 12 tones, the *chromatic scale* (assuming equal temperament [ET] tuning). The C major scale is one of many diatonic scales, each identified by an important referent tone, termed the *tonic*, or *keynote*. In this table, the tonic is C (e.g., C$_3$, C$_4$; C$_4$ is middle C). Critically, all tones in a scale are related to the tonic by defining frequency (F) ratios (Fi/Fj) or conversely period ratios; see column 3 in this table).[5] Notice that the simplest ratios are unison (C_3:C_3 with frequency ratios of 1:1)) and octave (C_3:C_4 with frequency ratios of 1:2)), which respectively capture identity and strong self-similarity of two tones. All tones related by an octave belong to the same *pitch class* (e.g., C_1, C_2, C_3, C_4, etc.). Finally, an abstract C major scale simply spells out successive scale steps as *pitch classes* (C, D, E . . . B, C′). Scale properties of Table 11.1 hold for other diatonic major scales (i.e., with tonics of $C^\#$, D, or E, etc.). For all such scales, adjacent tones in an ascending order differ in small intervals (one or two semitones, where a semitone ratio is 1.059). Relationships in Table 11.1 are collectively termed *tonal relationships* because all scale tones are referenced to the same tonic.[6]

Tonal Relations and Dynamic Terminology: A Preview

Musical scales, as such, do not explain tonality. However, it is difficult to grasp the dynamics of melodies without understanding tonal relationships. Not surprisingly, melodic dynamics rely on changing tone frequencies, which translate into dynamic tonal relationships.[7,8] From a dynamical perspective, the stimulus frequency, Fi, of each tone functions as an external micro-driving rhythm, with angular velocity, $\omega_i = 2\pi Fi$. And, the fast neural correlate of ω_i is notated as ω_{oi}. (For simplicity, throughout this chapter, scale tones are treated as pure tones, with external frequencies notated as *Fi*; when discussing complex harmonic tones, F0 continues to represent the fundamental frequency of a complex, as defined in Chapter 6.) More generally, external frequency relations among scale tones are reflected by ratio relations, ω_i : ω_j, where each tone is referenced to a particular frequency (ω_j). For example, in Table 11.1, the C_3, identifies the C major scale (Table 11.1). As tonal relationships, other frequency ratios in column 3 implicate different degrees of stability, shown in column 8.[9,10]

Theoretically, the external frequencies, often expressed as angular velocities, ω_j, describe micro-driving rhythms in a dynamic attending framework. Furthermore, a driving–driven relationship involving the neural correlate of ω_j, expresses an exogenous driving:driven entrainment relation as: ω_i:ω_{oi} (e.g., as in the generic *n:m* = 1:1). Table 11.1 shows frequencies of various external micro-driving rhythms and their scalar relationships. All the scale tones listed in column 2 have correlated frequency relationships with C_3 ratios in column 3; each ratio reflects the division of the tone's frequency (column 4) by the frequency of the scale tone, C_3. This allows an interpretation of column 6 in this table where entries reflect the nearest attractor ratios estimated by the observed stimulus ratios of column 3. Finally, stability distinctions (column 8) capture the complexity of hidden attractors, which inevitably finds its way into the experience of tonal aesthetics.[11]

BOX 11.2
FREQUENCY RELATIONSHIPS AND ANGULAR VELOCITIES OF MICRO-DRIVING RHYTHMS

As a frequency gradient, a linear scale of sound frequencies increases monotonically as cycles/second (Hz). Expressed as angular velocities, ωi (= $2\pi f_i$), a set of micro-driving rhythms, ωi, for different stimuli, i, is active for a given tonal scale. By contrast, with a curvilinear gradient, angular velocities, ω_j, are points along a, for example, logarithmic pitch spiral. This curvilinear gradient has two parameters: a dilation parameter, C_t, which is a basic ratio of two sinusoids, and unit rotation (polar angle) generator, $m\theta$, where *m* is an integer. Using the formula for a logarithmic spiral: $r_j = r_0 C t^\theta$ (with Ct = 1.1166 for one radian), where r_j is a radius spiral; it is possible to express all musical frequency relationships as relative distances along a spiral path. Converting ωi to frequencies (Hertz) means that the arc length (in tone frequencies) between any two points on the spiral path fj + m and fj, which are $m\theta$ steps apart is: $f_{j+m} = Ct^{(m+j)\theta j} f_j$. For instance, the frequency of the C and octave above middle C is C5 = $1.1166^{6.2831}$ (261.09) which is 523.09 Hz. In this description, high self-similarities emerge among remote frequencies, such as those in different octaves with the same polar angle (e.g., pitch classes).

TABLE 11.1 STABILITY TABLE FOR C MAJOR (DIATONIC) SCALE

Equal Temperament (ET) Tuning Ratios

1	2	3	4	5	6	7	8
Scale Degree	Diatonic Note	F_i/F_j for $F_j = C_3$	ET Frequency $Fi = 2\pi\omega i$	Micro-period, p(ms)	Hidden Attractors n:m	DeviationΔ (Hz)	Stability Rank
1	C_3	1.00	130.81	7.645	1:1	0	1
2	D_3	1.122..	146.83	7.215	9:8	0.33*	7
3	E_3	1.260	164.81	6.068	5:4	1.29	5
4	F_3	1.335..	174.61	5.727	4:3	0.197	4
5	G_3	1.498..	196.0	5.102	3:2	0.22	3
6	A_3	1.682..	220.00	4.545	5:3	1.98*	6
7	B_3	1.888..	246.94	4.049	15:8	1.67*	8
8	C_4 (middle)	2.00	261.63	3.823	2:1	0.01	2

Among the more stable and compelling tonal relations in musical melodies is the octave ratio of 2:1. Indeed, along with the unison (i.e., two identical tones), the octave has the highest stability rank in column 8. The least stable ratio, 15:8, reflects the relationship between the tonic and the seventh scale tone (i.e., between C and B).[12] Although less powerful than the octave, other pitch intervals are sufficiently stable to levy a real attractor pull. For instance, a perfect fourth (five semitones), with a tonal relation, $C_3:F_3$, approximates a fairly compelling attractor ratio of 4:3 (columns 3 and 6 for row 4). (By definition, ET tones always slightly "hide" attractors with deviations in Hertz under 1%.) The main point is that musical scales, translated into a dynamic system, provide a range of attractor-generated stabilities. In sum, tonal scales supply dynamic building blocks for interesting musical melodies.[13]

Frequency Gradients: Linear and Curvilinear

This chapter considers how the musical sounds of a melody contribute to listeners' perception of tonality and tonal melodies. To accomplish this, it is useful to examine the origin of scale tones as a subset of frequencies in an expansive frequency gradient.

Initially, musical tones are fast, complex sounds. In theory, a musical tone tone may feed into an internal frequency gradient, described in psychoacoustics as a peripheral bank of filters. Typically, such a filter bank functions as a unidimensional frequency gradient. For instance, critical bands, defined along the basilar membrane, are cast as spatially adjacent filters that process incoming sounds based on near-neighbor proximities of frequencies.[14] Along auditory pathways to cortical activity, some tonotopy is found in subcortical structures.[15] However, at the cortical level, reviews indicate a more complex picture, with some research reporting many as six different tonotopic pitch gradients.[16] For instance, Langers and Kijk report functional magnetic resonance imaging (fMRI) activity involving two prominent, overlapping, curvilinear frequency gradients near the Heschl's gyrus.[17] Such spatial gradients reflect neural activity implicating distinctive near-neighbor proximity frequency relations.[18,19]

Naturally, the search for neural correlates of scale-generated tonality is more challenging. One puzzle involves the fact that unidimensionality of any neural gradient renders problematic certain near-neighbor proximity perceptions. For instance, if percepts of tone similarity are based on a "nearest neighbor rule," the relevant gradient would predict that tones separated in frequency by a semitone will be judged to be far more similar than tones an octave apart. Such a finding would shock many musicians. Indeed, as famously demonstrated by Roger Shepard, this prediction is not borne out.[20,21]

One solution to this puzzle assumes that listeners use a unidimensional subjective (i.e., neural) gradient that functions merely as a primitive filtering bank for a more elaborate and overriding up-line neural network.[22] In such a network, different tonal relationships (octaves, fifths, etc.) are expressed by proposed connections among network nodes, perhaps strengthened by exposure frequency. That is, in the absence of innate gradient constraints, certain tonal relationships gain strength from learning in a connectionist network. Thus, the acquisition of tonal skills that facilitate identifying pitch classes and tonal relationships (e.g., tonics, etc.) depends on Hebbian learning.[23] An excellent review of implicit learning of tonality involving a self-organizing network is found in Tillmann et al.[24] Self-organizing neural networks are trained-up by exposing them to chords and tonal melodies;[25] this is also nicely illustrated in Bharucha's model, MUSACT.[26]

A variant of this approach, offered by Large,[27] incorporates other constraints that explain listener's inherent sensitivity to certain pitch classes and tonal relationships. In addition, this model is unique in treating upline network nodes as nonlinear limit cycle oscillations.[28] In this, a hypothetical 'starter' frequency gradient grounds a more elaborate, subsequent, neural network.[29]

Nonlinear Frequency Gradients: Spatial, Temporal, or Both?

Network models succeed in capturing tonal relationships. Nevertheless, their grounding in linear gradients can overlook special frequency ratios among remote tonal frequencies. For example, the explanatory burden of explaining heightened tonal sensitivity to more stable ratios (e.g., octaves) places heavy reliance on exposure frequency, hence learning. This denies the possibility that we are naturally sensitive to certain gradient relationships.

Roger Shepard raised the possibility of favored relationships with the proposal that people are inherently sensitive to two different frequency gradients. Expressing a listeners' proclivities in mental geometry, he proposed two subjective spatial dimensions: a pitch height dimension (low to high frequencies) and a circular dimension (chromatic frequencies within an octave). Using crafted complex tones, he demonstrated that listeners are not only sensitive to low/high differences along a linear gradient, but also to pitch differences expressed along a curvilinear gradient defined by an octave circle. Consequently, he proposed that musical pitch rests not only on *pitch height dimension*, reflecting pitch linearity along a low/high dimension, but also on a *chroma dimension,* reflecting pitch circularity within octave. Later, this mental geometry was expanded into a double helix wound around a torus to express pitch classes, scales, and the circle of fifths.[30] At the time, this proposal of internal geometry was stunning.

Shepard raised the startling possibility that, subjectively, a frequency continuum can contain at least one rotational component.

Finally, Shepard's mental geometry put in play issues that persist today. First, his rejection of a singular reliance on unidimensional gradients for musical events called attention to multidimensional subjective configurations of tonal relations in music. Second, mental geometry suggested that subjective dimensions may be inherently spatial, not acquired by learning.

Spatio-Temporal Portrait of Frequency Gradients

Mental geometry, in spite of its beauty, leaves unanswered questions. One is topological; it concerns how spatialized frequency relationships arise from vibrating sounds. It is possible to imagine a curvilinear tonotopy shaped by time relationships. For instance, instead of strictly linear gradients, a *logarithmic spiral* gradient (in two spatial dimensions) appears, as in Figure 11.1.[31] In this case, a tone's frequency, as angular velocity, ω_i $(= 2\pi f_i)$, is determined by two factors: a linear component governed by one parameter (Ct for tone height) and a rotational parameter (θj for chroma) described in Box 14.2. The tone height parameter, Ct, reflects a dilation expansion with a ratio of spiral arc lengths. The chroma parameter, θj, is a polar angle reflecting a difference (i.e., a pitch interval) between two tones. For example, θj, is 210 degrees and 360 degrees, respectively, for intervals of a perfect fifth and an octave. The idea is that people hear relations among melodic sounds as "dynamic distances" reflected by these parameters. This curvilinear portrait of tone frequencies realizes the special status of octaves.[32,33] Validation of distinct chroma and pitch height dimensions as natural primitives is supported by findings that 3-month-old infants differentiate these dimensions.[34,35]

Spiral Rhythms: Observations

As a growth curve, the spiral captures rhythms of life, regardless of time scale. At the fast time scales of pitch, it highlights two major aspects of pitch relations. One aspect is relevant in describing tonality; it is specified by points along the circular, chromatic scale where tones differ with θj. For this scale, Ct = 1 and θj is 30 degrees (a semitone). The second aspect is relevant in describing pitch height and melodic contour; it is specified by a constant a polar angle (at 360 degrees) while varying Ct.

Other relevant features involve gradient coarseness and its invariant time properties.

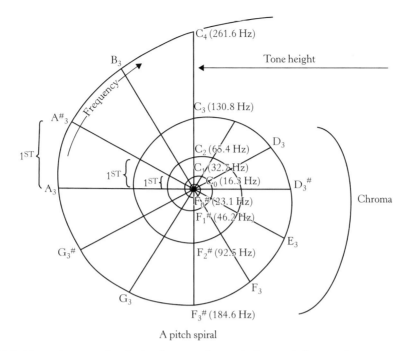

A pitch spiral

FIGURE 11.1 A logarithmic spiral applied to the micro-driving rhythms underlying pitch. Frequency is shown as arc length. Tone chroma relates to a circular dimension of pitch, and tone height relates to linearly expanding radii.

Adapted from June Hahn and Mari Riess Jones, "Invariants in Auditory Frequency Relations," *Scandinavian Journal of Psychology* 22, no. 1 (September 1, 1981): 129–44, doi:10.1111/j.1467-9450.1981.tb00388.x.

Coarseness depends on multiples versus subdivisions of different polar angles: Very fine-grained subdivisions involve small pitch intervals (e.g., in glides $\theta j < 10$ degrees) others are moderate (e.g., in the chromatic scale $\theta j = 30$ degrees) or coarse (e.g., for perfect fifths $\theta j = 210$ degrees).

Finally, spiral parameters, Ct and θj, are not confined to time scales of pitch. Rather, they can capture compelling attractor time relationships at the slower time scales discussed in preceding chapters. That is, invariant time relations glimpsed in the slice of a spiral in Figure 11.2 focus on the time relationships of fast micro-rhythms of pitch. However, this spiral extends to include slower macro-rhythms of meter and beyond. For example, an n:m (2:1) octave relationship reflects a compelling attractor at the slower time scales of meter and rhythm, where the attractor now defines a duple meter category (see Box 11.2).

Summary of Musical Scales and Tonality
The major points of this section are:

- Frequency gradients allow identification of special subsets of tones, as in chromatic and tonal scales.

- Tonal relationships are conventionally expressed as frequency ratios that translate into ratios of micro-driving rhythms.
- A set of frequency ratios defines a tonal scale. Ratios of scale tones differ, but all approximate hidden attractor ratios.
- Frequency gradients lead to neural correlates that may form linear or curvilinear configurations.
- One nonlinear gradient, a spiral, decomposes micro-driving rhythms into two components: a chroma (and tonal) component and a pitch height (contour) component.

CHROMA AND TONALITY
Contemporary research on melody has focused largely on perception of tonal melodies. In this context, tonality refers to the "keyness" of melody. One scale tone, the *tonic*, typically functions as a reference point from which other tones are perceived. This is suggested in Table 11.1 (column 3), where the common referent frequency for each scale frequency is the tonic frequency. Theoretically, such tonal relationships contribute to pitch chroma. Central issues motivating thinking about such

melodies concern how people sense (i.e., "pick up") special tonal relations, including the tonic.

Tonal Hierarchies: The Theory of Carol Krumhansl

Psychological explorations of melody center on the critical role of tonality. Psychological inquiries into this topic began with Carol Krumhansl's ground-breaking research and continues today as a thriving area of study.[36,37,38] Krumhansl studied tonality perceptions by asking listeners to judge how well a single chromatic tone (a probe) "fits" into a preceding tonal melody (or chord). A multidimensional analysis of listeners' judgments produced the cone-shaped pattern of Figure 11.2 (for a C major context). Clearly, good fits were found for probe tones C, E, and G as members of a *tonic triad*. These and related findings have been widely replicated, rendering Krumhansl's theory influential even today.[39,40]

Recently, Krumshansl and Cuddy[41] summarized tonality research using two principles. One assumes that listeners rely on a cognitive referent, such as a tonic, to judge individual tones (e.g., Rosch[42]). Second, listeners implicitly learn statistical regularities in melodies that summarize contingencies among a tonic tone and closely related (i.e., stable triad) tones (in Western music). Together, these principles build on the idea that a tone's relative stability is acquired through a listener's exposure to the statistical regularities of such tones within the musical corpus, an idea shared by the prominent music theorist David Huron.[43,44]

A Neurodynamic Approach to Tonality: Research of Edward Large

Dynamic approaches to tonality have also blossomed recently. Edward Large tackled percepts of tonal melodies using entrainment principles.[45,46] This approach dovetails with Krumhansl's theory, but it places greater emphasis on the role of entrainment and attractors in establishing differential stability of tonal relations. An internalized frequency gradient is proposed that casts gradient (scale) units as limit cycle oscillations. As such, these oscillations live along a linear gradient where they can adaptively "tune in" to corresponding micro-time driving rhythms of a tone's frequencies.[47] Figure 11.3A,B shows predictions and stability ratings for a range of chromatic scale tones. Also shown are entrainment region

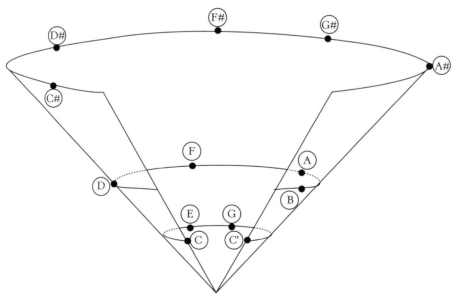

The idealized three-dimensional conical configuration.

FIGURE 11.2 An idealized three-dimensional conical configuration of musical pitch expressed by multidimensional scaling. It shows the psychological "strength" of different tonal relationships embedded with a chromatic scale, here for the scale of C major. Given a tonal context of C major, test tones of C, C′, E, and G are judged most relevant to that context.

Reprint of figure 3 in Carol L. Krumhansl, "The Psychological Representation of Musical Pitch in a Tonal Context," *Cognitive Psychology* 11, no. 3 (July 1979): 346–74, doi:10.1016/0010-0285(79)90016-1.

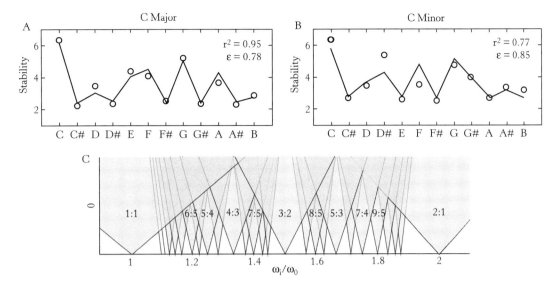

FIGURE 11.3 Panels **A** and **B** reflect stability judgments about test tones judged in either a C major context (**A**) or C minor context. Panel **C** shows an Arnold tongue bifurcation diagram developed from an entrainment model of Edward Large. Note that overlapping entrainment regions imply that less stable ratios will be psychologically "pulled" to a nearby more stable ones.

Reprinted from figure 7.7 in E. Large, "Neurodynamics of Music," in *Music Perception: Springer Handbook of Auditory Research*, eds. Mari Riess Jones, Richard R. Fay, and Arthur N. Popper, vol. 36 (New York: Springer, 2010).

constraints based on attractor ratio complexities (C). More stable scale tones (re: the tonic) correspond to wider, overlapping entrainment regions of attractors (Arnold tongue regimes). Large notes that the wider entrainment regions (for simpler attractors) imply more stable tonal relationships than do narrower entrainment regions (complex attractors). In this scenario, a hypothesized network of oscillations allows for adjustments of oscillator periods and/or amplitudes during entrainment (exogenous or endogenous).

Finally, in this dynamic approach, we find a wedding of entrainment and learning in considering time scales of micro-rhythms. That is, given attractor-governed entrainments, this network also learns from exposure frequency. Large's model acknowledges listeners' inherent tendencies to treat certain scale tones as special driving rhythms while also allowing for learning to strengthen unit connections evident in culture-specific musical scales.

Tonal Dynamics: Tonal Attractor Profiles and Tonal Oscillator Clusters

This section pursues a dynamic attending perspective on melody perception. It builds upon previous ideas of curvilinear gradients, to focus tonal dynamics at work in listening to melodies.

In tonal music, it is common to distinguish a melodic line, as a horizontal structure, from a vertical component of harmony, supplied by chords. From a dynamic attending perspective this distinction adapts familiar concepts in the form of a *tonal attractor profile,* which expresses horizontal structure as an internalized melodic line, and a *tonal oscillator cluster,* which reflects the vertical component of an internalized chord. The focus is largely upon people's ability to follow a melody as a function of the melody's particular referent oscillation that embodies the tonic frequency. However, it is also important to acknowledge the role of chords, which evoke oscillatory tonal clusters that facilitate listeners' ability to track a melodic line.

It is generally acknowledged that tonal melodies are "tonal" because in a series of tones, all of the member tones are 'tethered' to a common referent sound, the keynote. By this definition, the scale pattern of Table 11.1 becomes a tonal melody, albeit a boring one. It is fair to say that we prefer hearing *Twinkle Twinkle Little Star* to any unadorned musical scale. "Good" melodies display creative serial arrangements of scale tones, ones that cleverly juxtapose less stable versus more stable tones. Among other things, inspired composers instill suspense, tension, and resolution based on changing levels of stability at strategic points in a melody (cf. Chapter 8 on parallelism). For instance, a common ploy that commands a sense of tension, then resolution, occurs when the scale tone B (low stability) leads to the tonic C (high stability) in C major in a melodic line. Another composing device that teases listeners entails opening a melodic line with tones that are tonally ambiguous.

So, what does tonal ambiguity mean? Generally, it implies that a few tones of a melody jointly implicate more than one tonic. This raises a more basic question, one that has preoccupied scholars for years: namely, "How do listeners identify the tonic?" Or put another way: "Given tones within a melodic line, which one is heard as the referent (i.e., the tonic)?" Different answers have been advanced, all with some merit. A popular one maintains that the favored tonic candidate is the most frequently occurring tone (i.e., the mode).[48,49] This view gains support from research establishing the importance of a tone's exposure frequency in various cultures.[50,51] Also, people appear to learn novel scalar regularities, for example, those conveyed by artificial grammars, based simply on exposure frequency. Such findings suggest that Hebbian learning, based on exposure frequency, contributes to tonic identification, hence to melody learning.[52]

Yet closer scrutiny of this idea raises questions. Strengthening a tone's status by increasing its exposure within a melody implies that the serial order of tones in a melody doesn't matter. However, serial order *does* appear to matter in key identification. For instance, Matsunaga and Abe found that the opening portions of a melodic line levy a persisting influence, which they termed *perceptual inertia*, on a listener's choice of a tonic for both musicians and nonmusicians.[53,54] Also, David Butler and colleagues offer a related view, reviving an old serial recall favorite of psychologists, namely, the *primacy effect*.[55,56,57] Butler proposed an *intervallic rivalry hypothesis,* which maintains that the first one or two tones in a melody have *primacy priority* for serving as a referent—and this preference lasts until a better (i.e., a rival) tonic tone arrives. Butler maintained that key identification also relies on a cuing function by a rare scale interval, the tritone, which is uniquely correlated with a melody's key (in Table 11.1, it is the interval from notes F to B). Thus, when a melody contains tones F-then-B, this tritone (with another tone) invites the activity of the tonic referent of C.[58]

In sum, although exposure frequency is critical in establishing tonal sensitivity (i.e., a tonal referent), it is not the only factor involved. Returning

to an entrainment orientation, the primacy of beginnings is also important. Effectively, one of several opening tones in melody is also likely to serve as a referent oscillation as listeners involuntarily unpack a melodic attractor profile.

Melodic Lines: Tonal Attractor Profiles

Melodies are prime candidates for arousing attractor profiles in listeners. An internal attractor profile for a melody describes a listener's momentary expectancies based on transient mode-locking.[59] Here, a listener's momentary expectancies change while listening to an unfolding melody as each successive tone functions as an exogenous micro-driving rhythm. That is, with transient mode-locking, a listeners' fleeting adaptations to successive tones means that the micro-driving rhythm of each tone briefly "locks" with a sustaining referent oscillation established early in the melody. In this portrait, the stable referent oscillation reflects the periodicity of the tonic. In short, listeners follow such a tonal melody in real time as they realize a special attractor profile: a *tonal attractor profile.*

Although dressed in new clothes, this attractor profile is not a new concept. As with the slower rhythmic attractor profiles of Chapter 10, tonal attractor profiles emerge in reaction to a progression of varied (here micro-) driving rhythms. To illustrate, consider again the simplest, most mundane melody, namely the scalar melody of Table 11.1. It begins with C_3 and ends with C_4. Following the intervallic rivalry hypothesis, a primacy bias grants a provisional tonic of C_3 with a frequency of 130.81 Hz (i.e., for the referent period that persists as successive tones pass by; e.g. perceptual inertia). The emerging profile of local attractors begins with n:m = 1:1 (for C_3), then 9:8 (for D_3), then 5:4, and so on. Essentially, the profile of this scalar melody appears in column 6 of this table. Each new tone is a fleeting micro-driving rhythm gauged by a sustained referent period. Consequently, column 6 presents a series of hidden attractors, elicited by successive (fuzzy) frequency ratios. Of course, most melodies are far more interesting than scalar melodies. Nevertheless, with an entraining listener, all translate into profiles of hidden attractors.

Normally, attractors of tonal profiles differ in stability. The most stable, by definition, are tones equivalent to the tonic ($n{:}m = 1{:}1$). In fact, the tonic affords salience. Often it functions as an accent that marks out the longer time spans of slower macro-rhythms. As with metrical accents, tonal accents gain subjective salience from their internalized attractors. Simple, stronger internalized attractors "pull" attending toward local tonal accents. This is evident in the research of Marilyn Boltz[60] and in the melodic anchoring effect of Jamshed Bharucha.[61] Accents are discussed in more detail in later chapters.

Finally, let's return to prototypes, here melodic prototypes. In a musical context, melodic prototypes are stimulus patterns that correspond to specific tonal attractor profiles. The scalar melody of Table 11.1, for example, is a most elementary prototype. As a prototype, this attractor profile (column 6) is invariant across a range of scalar melodies with different pitch heights and different key notes.

Chords: Tonal Oscillator Clusters

Often in music a melodic line is accompanied by chords that add harmony. A chord has been defined as a co-occurrence of at least two tones. Chords in tonal music are interesting because they directly awaken in a listener corresponding *tonal oscillator clusters*. The latter are endogenous clusters that comprise phase-locked, often binded, micro-driven oscillations that resemble the pitch oscillator clusters described earlier for complex harmonious sounds (Chapter 6). Thus, tonal clusters reflect endogenous entrainments among several active oscillations; as such, they also foreshadow certain fast oscillator clusters to be discussed in speech. In music, tonal oscillator clusters of chords accompany a melodic line; hence, they extend in time along with the chordal driving rhythms. In fact, often chords persist over significant stretches of a melody that exceed durations of several individual tones in the melody.

The preceding discussion implies that means that strategically placed chords in a melody can induce in listeners tonal clusters that affect their perception of a melodic line. In fact, the joint occurrence of chords and melody parallels the joint occurrence of meter with a slow rhythm (Chapter 10; cf. Figure 10.5). In the present context, chords contribute *explicit harmony,* which induces tonal oscillator clusters, whereas melodic lines can induce *implicit harmonies* realized by tonal attractor profiles.

A tonal oscillator cluster is illustrated in Figure 11.4. In this example, it is elicited by a prominent C major chord (e.g., C_3EGC_4). This cluster is akin to an internalized chord, but these neural oscillations can add energy to other, related oscillations belonging to melodic tones. In this fashion, chords can actually prime certain oscillations that "fit" forthcoming melodic tones. More precisely, a chord explicitly supplies the global attractors that define a tonal oscillator cluster; in turn, this heightens listeners' anticipations (rightly or wrongly) of future compatible local (melodic) attractors. Various forms of priming are possible: Chord-to-chord, chord-to-melodic line, and melodic line-to-chord, and so on.[62,63,64,65] Often such effects are successfully described using the spreading activity of neural networks. However, this section suggests an alternative way of thinking about such spreading activity. A dynamic attending view suggests a form of priming in which explicit harmony is expressed as *a chord that induces a preliminary heightening of amplitudes of resonant oscillations that then are further strengthened by future melodic tones.*

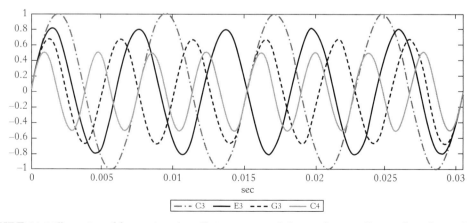

FIGURE 11.4 Illustration of four activated oscillations in a tonal cluster where oscillations (here depicted as sine wavers) correspond to frequencies of C3, E3, G3, and C4. In the tonal context of C major, these form an internalized **I** chord.

Tonal Melodic Lines: Implied Harmony

Some melodies, unaccompanied by chords, form powerful tonal attractor profiles that can prime a tonal oscillator cluster. This leads to *implied harmony*. For instance, theoretically, a melodic fragment, such as C_3-E_3-G_3, can induce a brief tonal attractor profile in listeners wherein the persisting tonal referent is elicited by the C_3 micro-driving rhythm. In this case, a different form of priming can happen: *A tonal attractor profile heightens the activity of a few, co-occurring oscillations that then automatically (endogenously) activate other, closely related harmonics. The result is that an implied harmony is realized by a primed oscillator cluster.*

Consistent with this idea, there is evidence that a melodic line alone can instill implicit harmony.[66] For instance, in one task, listeners had to detect in-key changes in a test region surrounded by either a melodic line or chords that were either harmonically related to the target key or not. Both nonmusicians and musicians found an in-key change implied by the context harder to detect than ones not implied by the context. Interestingly, the contextual melodic line was as effective in conveying implied harmony as the chord progression.

Musical Skill and Tonality

All of us have acquired some tacit knowledge of our culture's music.[67] Melodies of Western music creatively express a variety of tonal harmonies either explicitly, from series of chords, or implicitly, from a well-designed melodic line. Chord successions, termed *progressions*, are part of our tacit knowledge due to their prevalence in Western music.[68,69,70] Tonal clusters function as internalized chords. As such, they figure into our sensitivity to implied chord progressions in melodies that happen to lack explicit chords. Thus, implied harmony happens in tonal clusters that implicate

chords based on individual tones within a melodic line. Of course, musicians are especially alert to implied chord patterns as these listeners have acquired strongly reinforced bindings among members of tonal clusters.[61]

Nevertheless, most listeners have acquired some sensitivity to certain common chord progressions within culturally familiar context. In other words, with exposure bindings among oscillations in common chords and in chord progressions transpire. Common chord progressions often feature chords involving simple attractors (e.g., **I, IV,** and **V** or **V⁷**; see Box 11.1). This is true, for example, of the highly popular chord progression, **I-IV-V-IV** (famously known as *Louie Louie*). It is also pertinent that the more popular chords in Western music engage simple attractors.[71]

Dirk Povel and Erik Jansen asked "What makes a 'good' melody?"[72,73] Musicians heard melodies implied by different progressions as **I-a-V-I** where **a** was a target fragment for different implied chords: **I, II, III, IV, V,** or **VI,** as shown in Figure 11.5. Overall, melodic lines with implied chord progressions based on **I, V,** or **IV** received the best ratings. This prompted the conclusion that judgments reflect the familiarity of certain chord progressions (e.g., **I-IV-V-I**).

These findings underscore culture-specific preferences for certain melodic lines. However, these progressions also engage powerful tonal attractors (i.e., **I, V,** and **IV** chords represent attractors of 1:1, 3:2, and 4:3, respectively).[74] Finally, it is plausible that listeners were influenced not only by chord familiarity but also by attractor simplicity. Moreover, other research indicates pronounced effects of more extended tonal contexts on chord percepts.[75] Also, Tillmann et al. discovered that contextually induced temporal expectancies as well as tonal expectancies affected listeners' judgments about the "when" as well as the "what" of future chords in progressions.[76]

Sample chord progressions for implied harmony

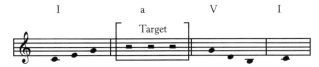

FIGURE 11.5 Four measures (see bar lines) in which three supply a musical context of implied chords in an **I a V I,** where the **a** bar contains a target chord. Bar lines indicate an induced triple meter. Implied chords are shown above each set of tones.

Adapted from Jansen and Povel, "The Processing of Chords in Tonal Melodic Sequences," *Journal of New Music Research* 33, no. 1 (March 1, 2004): 31–48, doi:10.1076/jnmr.33.1.31.35396.

Finally, the relative impact of learning in these paradigms remains an unsettled issue. Also, the roles of culture-specific exposure to certain entrainment properties as well as attractor simplicity all await future research. Nevertheless, current knowledge is generally consistent with the idea that listeners engage in dynamic attending as they track unfolding musical contexts.

Summary of Chroma and Tonality

Entrainment concepts offer a new perspective on tonal melody and harmony. Dynamic attending concepts applied to chroma relationships result in tonal attractor profiles (for melodies) and tonal oscillator clusters (for chords). At micro-time scales, these concepts feature entrainment, as endogenous oscillator couplings, and learning, as bindings among coupled oscillations. In this regard, they mirror distinctions at slower time scales which involve the entrainment and learning of meter and rhythm. Specifically, tonal oscillator clusters of chords resemble metric oscillator clusters, and melodic attractor profiles resemble rhythmic attractor profiles (cf. Chapter 10). The main difference involves time scale.

A full understanding of tonality and implied harmonies requires the acknowledgment of a basic, but perplexing, truth about musical scales and chord progressions. The most effective melodies, chords, and progressions are not only those commonly encountered, they are also ones with simpler attractor states. In other words, it is the simpler tonal attractors that are likely to be overlearned. This touches on a larger issue that haunts research in music cognition. It involves the seemingly unavoidable confounding of simplicity of time relations (e.g., of attractors) with their frequency of occurrence in a culture's musical corpus. The correlation of simplicity with commonality is responsible for distracting debates about which factor is "the" causative factor. Undoubtedly, both are important. Heavy exposure to the simpler micro-time ratios of 1:1, 2:1, and 3:2 in music inevitably contributes to perceptual overlearning of these tonal attractors and implied harmonies, especially for skilled listeners. Sandra Trehub neatly summarizes this issue, suggesting that people may innately favor simplicity and harmony over complexity and dissonance.[77]

Major points in this section are:

- Frequency gradients can be expressed as curvilinear configurations of micro-driving rhythms that embed dimensions of both chroma and pitch height.

- Hierarchies of tonal relationships reflect chroma differences in attractor complexity and/or exposure frequency of tonal attractor relationships.
- Real-time attending at micro-time levels of melodic tones is explained using three Dynamic Attending Theory (DAT) concepts: internalized tonal referent (for the tonic), tonal attractor profiles (for melodies), and tonal oscillator clusters (for chords).
- Both innate (tonal attractors) and acquired (learning) factors figure into tonality perception.

MELODIC CONTOURS: DYNAMICS OF PITCH UPS AND DOWNS

Melodic contours add a grand sense of undulating motion to music, creating drops in pitch from soaring heights to low valleys and vice versa. These shapes reflect shifts of the fundamental frequency of a musical instrument or the human vocal tract. The preceding section shows that melodies invite endogenous tonal attractor profiles in chroma. This final section shifts to the pitch height dimension to discuss exogenous pitch changes of tones and listeners' ability to track pitch contour (i.e., the *ups* and *downs* of these changes).[78] Dowling presciently observed that pitch contour alone exerts a strong influence on a listener's percept of a melody,[79] a point echoed by Mark Schmuckler in a review of this topic.[80]

Background: What's Melodic Contour?

The import of melodic contour in music was highlighted in Dowling's classic essay.[81] He showed that musicians and nonmusicians alike confuse melodies that share a common melodic contour even when differing in tonality (i.e., different attractor profiles). Conversely, average listeners do not confuse transposed melodies (i.e., in different keys) when they are correlated with differences in pitch contour. By contrast, if two different tonal melodies have identical pitch contours, only musicians reliably differentiate them.[82] On first exposure, most listeners "get" the ups and downs of a novel melody, but they tend to err in reporting the precise frequency relations (i.e., intervals between tones), an error that rarely happens with familiar melodies. As Dowling observes, our memory is quite good for tunes like *Twinkle, Twinkle Little Star*.

Clearly, pitch contour is critical in music perception. However, understanding "what" contour is must begin with a workable definition of it. First, pitch contour is shaped by serial changes in frequency of many successive tones.[83] In this respect, it departs from the pitch perception issues of Chapter 6, which centered on listeners' responses to single complex tones comprising unchanging frequencies. Instead, here, we examine how pitch percepts change over time as tones shift up and down in frequency (i.e., along the pitch height dimension).

Consider, for example, the tonal melody in the key of C, shown in Figure 11.6. It features a tone sequence based on a series of attractors (i.e., an attractor profile). This profile includes hidden attractors, locked to a tonal referent. Therefore, as preceding discussions imply, this melody should elicit tonality percepts due to refined endogenous entrainments of oscillations related to these hidden attractors.

Yet the melody of Figure 11.6 tells us more than an attractor profile. It also projects another pitch structure that grabs listeners' attention. This refers to the dazzling up and down sweeps in surface pitch (tone frequency, in light gray). Psychologists have toyed with different ways to formally define such melodic contours. One approach relies on pivot points, others appeal to Gestalt principles. As background, these views are briefly discussed; however, a primary aim in this section is to outline a DAT position on pitch contour.

Pivot Point Problems

A popular description of melodic contour relies on pivot points, which code successive changes in pitch ordinally as "up" (+) or "down" (−). For instance, a pivot point code for the melody of Figure 11.6 lists pitch changes as: < − + − = + − + >. Although parsimonious, pivot codes reduce pitch height modulations to ordinal directional changes. This ignores the height of a pitch rise or the depth of a pitch fall. Yet both adults[84] and children[85] are quite sensitive to these properties. Also, pivot codes ignore underlying transformations responsible for contours.[86,87] For instance, this melody shows two types of pitch height symmetry transformations (mirror image, pitch transpose). Finally, all pivot points are deemed equal; yet, perceptually, troughs (−) differ from pitch peaks (+).[88,89,90]

Despite upgrades, pivot point codes fail as satisfactory launching pads for modeling pitch contour. For example, Heather Johnston showed that listeners tend to extrapolate attending to anticipate the 'when' of future 'ups' and 'downs' of an ongoing pitch contour on the basis of a preceding context.[91] This suggests that a more complicated response to contour patterns is underfoot. In this spirit, Mark Schmuckler rightly argues for more promising approaches, ones that include Fourier analysis which speak to relative timings of contours 'ups' and 'downs.'[92,93]

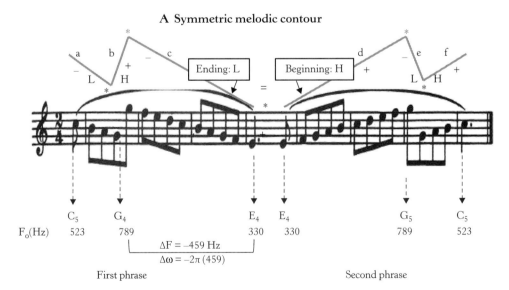

A Symmetric melodic contour

FIGURE 11.6 A schematic of a symmetric melodic contour in a duple meter. Blue lines follow pitch trajectories of noted notes; they express glides (technically faux glides) showing peaks (light gray *) and valleys or troughs (darker gray *) of melodic contour. Two kinds of pitch accents are previewed: beginning (H) and ending (L) accents (relevant to the on/off hypothesis of pitch tracking).

Classic Gestalt Principles

Other, more promising, candidates for formalizing contour appeal to Gestalt grouping principles applied to pitch (frequency) changes, especially *proximity* and *continuity*. Both principles figure in pitch glides, for instance. Thus, in Figure 11.6, high (H) and low (L) pitches together create ascending (/; i.e., LH) or descending (\; i.e., HL) glides that determine perceptual groups. That is, within each glide group, adjacent tones are proximal in frequency and pitch intervals are organized to exhibit continuity (i.e., as all semitones).[94] Additionally, even the popularity of the "hat pattern," formed by two glides (/\), can be explained as expressing pitch proximities of tones across adjacent glides. Undeniably, Gestalt principles offer apt descriptions of prominent melodic shapes. Nevertheless, after almost a century of success, we still don't know *why* Gestalt principles work.

The Implication-Realization (I-R) Theory

The I-R Theory of Eugene Narmour[95] rests on basic (archetypal) contour patterns, which presumably guide a listener's musical pitch expectancies. Consequently, this approach offers a richer description of melodic contours than previous accounts. At the risk of oversimplifying, this section briefly summarizes pertinent aspects of the I-R Theory.

The path toward describing a proverbial "good" melodic shape, trod by Narmour, was initially paved by the influential theorist Leonard Meyer[96] who identified archetypical contours of melodies. Perhaps the most famous, a "*gap-fill*" shape, features a large ascending pitch interval (the "gap") followed by a descending series of shorter intervals (the "fill"). Figure 11.6 illustrates this with the ascending octave leap (i.e., a gap between G tones) at the fourth tone, followed by a descending series of smaller (proximal) pitch intervals.

Narmour's theory widens the range of archetypal patterns using grouping principles. A basic melodic group of three tones has two pitch intervals: an initial *implication interval (I)* which instills an expectancy about the following *realization interval (R)*. Although originally Narmour posited five I-R expectancy principles,[97] Schellenberg[98] reduced these to three. A *registral direction,* in which a large implication pitch interval (over six semitones) leads to an expectancy for a large realization pitch interval of reversed direction (e.g., / →\ or \ →/). *Registral return* embodies an expectation based on the *continuation principle,* wherein the realized interval is one

that ends with a tone close to the first tone (within two semitones) of the implication interval. Finally, the third principle retains the general fondness for the Gestalt principle of *proximity*. Thus, in this principle Narmour describes an expectancy for the realized interval that ends with a tone close to the immediately preceding tone (i.e., 0, 1, or 2 semitones). Importantly, Schellenberg discovered that the proximity principle dominated people's pitch judgments about three tone groups.

Finally, Narmour's theory has more depth than other approaches to melodic contour. It pinpoints archetypal relationships that shape people's musical expectancies. Moreover, it is noteworthy that Gestalt principles remain prominent in I-R Theory. In this respect, Narmour's theory converges with another influential Gestalt picture of auditory perception painted by Al Bregman.[99]

A Dynamic Approach to Contour

This final section develops a contrasting view of melodic contour. This approach rests on principles of dynamic attending as they apply to surface contour groupings. In this view, contour groups depend on two prominent surface (stimulus) features: one involves group boundaries, which are based on segmenting *accents*. The other feature involves *pitch relationships*, which glue together tones in a group.[100] In particular, pitch (expressed by frequency relations) perceptually connects grouped tones based on adherence to stimulus proximity and continuation. A dynamic interpretation of such grouping appeals to stimulus-driven attending, i.e., the driving rhythm is an external periodicity. Specifically, this involves exogenous entrainment, described as *pitch tracking*.[101]

Pitch Accents: What's an Accent?

Pitch accents happen at change points in a melodic contour, such as the peaks and troughs of frequency undulations. Although pitch accents gain objective salience at these change points, they should not be confused with pivot points.

So what exactly *is* an accent? Lerdahl and Jackendoff[102] broadly defined *phenomenal* accents as surface changes in frequency or duration, distinguishing them from *structural* and *metric accents* (respectively, for tonality and meter). Although valid, these labels do not fully explain why accents work. To be fair, this is not an easy task. In fact, Cooper and Meyer[103] remarked on its impossibility, lamenting that "we cannot precisely stipulate what makes a tone seem accented" (p. 7). Their solution defined an accent as a stimulus (in a series) that is "marked for consciousness in some way." For decades, this justified the common credo of psychologists: "An accent is anything that grabs a listener's attention."

Yet, this, too, suffers from circular logic. Perhaps it is more manageable to consider an accent as a *stimulus, ωi, that locally phase-locks (briefly grabs/pulls) attending from a locally prevailing resting state, ωoi*. Alas, an air of circularity remains. However, this circularity weakens if determinants of attending can be specified. So, it is worth considering certain contextual influences on accentuation. Pitch accents segment groups because they physically "stand out" relative to local surrounds. For instance, consider group boundary accents.

Group Boundaries: A Fast/Slow Rule

The melodic contour in Figure 11.6 (gray lines) projects ups and downs in pitch that segment it into several groups (and subgroups) based on boundary accents. For instance, the sudden high-frequency change of the fifth tone in this melody gains objective salience as a pitch accent due to its stark difference from the preceding context of four falling tones. This sudden frequency increase (after G_4) means the next tone (G_5) has a much faster micro-driving rhythm, hence is attention-getting (i.e., $\omega_5 >> \omega_4$). Accordingly, as shown, the slower G_4 becomes an ending boundary accent, whereas the faster G_5 is a beginning boundary accent for the next group. Generally, group segmentation is determined by placements of low (L) and high (H) boundary accents (*). Finally, in addition to beginning and ending boundary accents, there are pitch peak accents. Pitch peak accents depend on the *fastest* local micro-driving rhythms (peak asterisks in Figure 11.6); such accents can also signal the beginning accents of subgroups (e.g., G_5 in this figure).[104]

Importantly, people hear L and H pitch accents as qualitatively different. Beginning H accents *seem* stronger than ending L accents. Theoretically, this is because accents with contextually higher frequencies (H) have correspondingly faster micro-rhythms as external driving rhythms. This automatically strengthens local exogenous entrainment activity that signifies the beginning of external driving rhythm. Conversely, accented tones defined by slower micro-rhythms (L) automatically weaken local entraining activities, indicating a 'dying' micro-driving rhythm within a melodic sequence. This idea is captured in a Fast/Slow rule.

The *Fast/Slow rule* holds that H accents are perceived to begin groups because they reflect a speeding up of entrainment (i.e. a starting) due to increased micro-rhythm rate.[105] These kinds of salient changes naturally convey a "beginning." By contrast, L accents are perceived as weaker because the sound signal is slowing in its entrainment cycles, hence implicating an ending. Such distinctions explain why listeners more readily notice rising (vs. falling ones) and are better at differentiating frequencies within rising than within falling glides.[106] Demany and colleagues refer to this as a *peak/trough perceptual effect*.[107,108,109]

Finally, although this discussion of melodic contour focuses on pitch accents, other stimulus properties (intensity, duration) also contribute to accent salience. For instance, the higher tone frequency of a beginning accent gains salience from temporal lengthening because the additional micro-driving rhythm cycles strengthen local entrainment between the latent oscillation, ω_{oi}, and its external driving rhythm, ω_i (for the *i*th tone). In this regard, duration variations among melodic tones created by a tempo response curve can also contribute to accent strength (cf. Chapter 8 for a review of tempo response curves).

Pitch Tracking Inside a Group: What Is It?

Next, let us consider why tones between beginning and end accents are perceived as a united group. A dynamic attending explanation continues to draws on pitch tracking activity. However, unlike the pitch perception paradigms described in Chapter 6, which focused on a listener's pitch percepts of single stationary tones, pitch tracking applies to common settings in music and speech where people involuntarily engage in adaptive exogenous entrainments that enable real time tracking of changing tone frequencies. In other words, we effortlessly follow the changing pitches within a melodic contour. But, the pitch tracking of musical contours contrasts with other entrainment constructs used to describe listeners sensitivity to tonality, namely tonal clusters and tonal attractor profiles. The latter depend on endogenous entrainments among different neural oscillations, whereas pitch tracking is based upon exogenous entrainment wherein the micro-driving rhythm reflects a continuously changing external tone frequency.

Here differentiating notation helps. So, consider that in pitch tracking, each tone within a group affords a brief external micro-driving rhythm, ω_i, that automatically engages a resonant neural correlate, ω_{oi}, where $\omega_{oi} \sim \omega_i$. Next, let external the micro-driving rhythms of successive tones in a group express stimulus frequency changes over time. For instance, in Figure 11.6, the initial downward glide of frequencies from C_5 to G_4 forms a group containing four different micro-driving rhythms that continuously slow down, beginning with C_5. People involuntarily adapt to the glide created by these changing stimulus-driving rhythms. It entails a series of brief exogenous entrainments involving successive activation of four different (adaptive) oscillations, each locking briefly to a new micro-driving rhythm (i.e., n:m = 1:1 in each case). Importantly, pitch tracking rides on stimulus-driven attending; absent are endogenous entrainments of clusters and attractor profiles. Instead, *pitch tracking is stimulus-bound, involving a series of exogenous entrainments.*

This dynamic portrait of melodic pitch tracking assumes that neural responses automatically follow successive discrete tone frequencies.[110] Neural evidence for such frequency following responses (FFR) has been found in brainstem recordings of oscillators tracking to sound sequences; these reveal different manifest frequencies (Ω) of responsive oscillations.[111,112] (Recall that Ω is a fleeting observable change of an adaptive oscillation's manifest, not latent, frequency during entrainment.)

Dynamic Proximity

The preceding paragraphs offer ways to explain how percepts of melodic contour groups are influenced by accents that segment groups and by pitch tracking that unites tones that "hang together" within an accented group. Nevertheless, Gestalt theory is right in highlighting two grouping principles: proximity and continuity. However, this section describes these principles from a new angle, one involving entrainment concepts. This section addresses proximity.

The melody of Figure 11.6 illustrates various segments filled with tones related by relatively small pitch intervals. Unquestionably, these small pitch intervals invite perceptual grouping, apparently validating the proximity principle. Yet vexing riddles remain about "*why*" this principle works. What does proximity mean, exactly? Why are melodic tones, separated by one or two semitones, judged as proximal when they also express *discernibly different* pitches? This universally acknowledged sense of proximity remains ephemeral. Where does it come from? Why does it disappear if tones differ by more than, say, two semitones, or if tones are

separated noticeably in time? Proximity is a powerful force, yet upgrading the term "proximity" to a Gestalt principle does not fully explain its power.

Dynamic proximity in music focuses on adjacencies of tones in pitch and time. Consider a melodic line in which two successive tones (at times of t_1, t_2) are close in frequency. Specifically, they have perceptible different, yet similar, micro-driving rhythms. Let these driving rhythms have angular velocities (ω_i, ω_j) mirrored by their neural correlates (ω_{oi}, ω_{oj}), where the latter are near neighbors along an internal frequency gradient. A crude analogy may clarify this: let a series of taps on adjacent piano keys provide an external gradient. As each successive key is depressed it briefly strikes a piano string and the string's external vibration (ω_i) is instantly matched, via resonance, with a neural correlate (ω_{oi}) in a listener. The latter correlates are driven micro-rhythms (adapting oscillations) situated along a neural frequency gradient.

A Dynamic Proximity Hypothesis: Entrainment Region Overlap (ERO)

Simply put, the innate sense of connectedness we experience as 'proximity' when tones are close in frequency (e.g., $[F_1 - F_2] < 3$ semitones) derives from overlapping entrainment regions of active near-neighbor oscillations (i.e., ω_{o1}, ω_{o2}). Micro-driving rhythms of neighboring tones successively activate corresponding driven rhythms along a neural gradient (i.e., at times t_1, t_2, t_3 ... etc.). Moveover, each driven oscillation carries a momentary entrainment region which can overlap with that of its activated neighbor. This is consistent with fMRI findings that activities of neighboring neural substrates in cortical gradients of the auditory cortex are highly correlated.[113,114]

In pursuing this idea, the external timing of tone onsets is also critical. This is because overlaps of entrainment regions are most potent when the relevant tones are close in both frequency and time. Vibrating activity in a phase space fades with the removal of any external driving rhythm. Thus, with two tones let the onset time of the first tone's driving rhythm be t_1 and that of the second be t_2. Even if near neighbors are close in frequency,[115] tones remote in time do not yield overlapping entrainment regions. As $[t_2 - t_1]$ increases, the entrainment region overlap (from tone 1) experienced at time t_2 with the second tone disappears due to fading of the earlier entrainment region.

Finally, a dynamic proximity hypothesis proposes that a listener's sense of proximity depends on the nature of this momentary overlap of two entrainment regions; the latter is termed the *entrainment region overlap* or ERO.

An ERO proximity hypothesis leads to two grouping predictions. First, dynamic proximity increases as ERO increases due to reduced frequency differences between the two tones. Second dynamic proximity also increases with the reduction of time differences between tones.

An Example of Dynamic Proximity

Figure 11.7 illustrates the ERO proximity hypothesis. Here, a melodic group consists of three neighboring tones (a few semitones apart). For instance, this may represent adjacent tones within any melodic group of Figure 11.6. Each tone has a distinct micro-driving rhythm (i.e., ω_1, ω_2, ω_3, at respective times: t_1, t_2, t_3).[116]

A listener engaging in pitch tracking such a melody will exogenously entrain briefly to successive micro-driving rhythms of melodic tones where each tone delivers an external ω_i and a resonant neural correlate (ω_{oi}). Given the gradient of Figure 11.7, the first tone (at t_1) activates its driven rhythm, ω_{o1}, with a fairly wide entrainment region (i.e., the n:m = 1:1). Phase-locking also

automatically generates a manifest frequency of ω_{o1} (i.e., Ω_1). Next, the second tone (ω_2) happens at time t_2^* with its resonant oscillation, ω_{o2}. At this point in time (*), the entrainment regions of these two latent oscillations briefly overlap. However, the region of ω_{o1} begins to fade as this stimulus is removed. Let t_2^* denote this point as the listener's moment of perception. At this instant, the stronger (darker) entrainment region dominates this listener's perception (i.e., ω_3 of the third tone has not yet occurred). Only entrainment regions elicited by ω_1 and ω_2 are currently active. (For completeness, shared manifest frequencies, Ω_1 and Ω_2 ~ ω_{o2} are also shown.) At this moment, the greater strength of ω_2, "pulls" the ambiguous manifest period Ω_1 toward it: $\Omega_1 \rightarrow \omega_2$. This n:m = 1:1 attractor pull on Ω_1 is strong enough to instill a palpable, but fleeting, sense of connection (i.e., *proximity*) between these two tones. In this fashion, the ERO hypothesis describes dynamic proximity.[117,118]

Auditory Streaming

This approach to proximity has broader implications. For instance, it sheds light on the famous phenomenon of *auditory pattern streaming*, introduced by Miller and Heise.[119] They presented melodic trills of alternating high (H) and low (L) frequencies to listeners who reported hearing

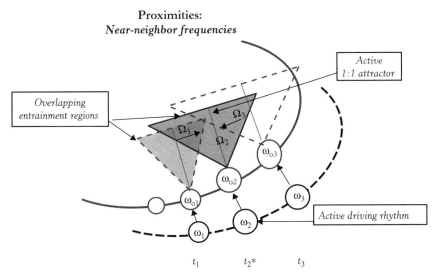

Proximities:
Near-neighbor frequencies

Active 1:1 attractor

Overlapping entrainment regions

Active driving rhythm

t_1 t_2^* t_3

Three successive driving rhythms separated by three semitones

FIGURE 11.7 A schematic of overlapping entrainment regions associated with near-neighbor neural oscillations in a circular gradient. Shifting driving rhythms (ω_i) at times t_1, t_2, t_3 (where the current, test time one is *) are shown progressively resonating (activating) their neural correlates (ω_{oi}). At time t^*, the strongest "pulling" force to ω_2: ω_{o2} is this dyad (n:m = 1:1) with darker region. Overlaps with adjacent oscillations mean that their manifest rhythms, Ω_i will gravitate to the currently active attractor, establishing a sense of proximity.

trills only when high and low tones were close (proximal) in frequency. Tones far apart in pitch (e.g., 8–14 semitones) caused listeners to hear two concurrent *streams*: L . . . L. . . L . . . and . . . H . . . H . . . H, and so forth. Such findings are typically cited as support for a Gestalt law of proximity.

The Gestalt proximity principle is central to the influential theory of *auditory scene analysis*[120] of Al Bregman, whose observations on streaming remain valid today.[121] For instance, in a classic paper, Bregman and Campbell[122] alternated low (L1, L2, L3) and high (H1, H2, H3) tones, notably at fast rates (i.e., small $t_{i+1} - t_i$ differences). They discovered that listeners reported hearing a high stream and a low stream concurrently. In this regard, the ERO hypothesis makes similar predictions because it incorporates differences in both time (Δt) and frequency (Δf) of adjacent tones.

Finally, this section has addressed percepts of melodic contour groups as these are influenced by local, within-group variations in tone frequency and timing. It illustrates how exogenous entrainments involving pitch tracking promote percepts of proximity among group tones. This approach confirms Gestalt emphasis on proximity while reinterpreting the power of proximity in an entrainment hypothesis. The idea of dynamic proximity underscores the inescapable fact that we experience melodic contours . . . in time.

A Dynamic Continuity Hypothesis

Continuity refers to persistence over time. This Gestalt rule holds that people group successive tones that express a recurrent (i.e., continuing) relationship. For example, the successive tones within a glide may be uniformly separated by three semitones (i.e., a constant scaled frequency difference). However, continuity also extends to true motions where discrete frequency and time separations between successive tones merge into continuous acoustic motions with an invariant velocity. In music, the power of continuity suggests a perceptual bias for invariance in implied (or real) motion. Moreover, as Narmour maintains, such frequency glides in melodies even invite anticipation of future continuation.

Dynamic Continuity as Implied Motion

In a dynamic attending framework, the sense of continuity rests on a listener's tendency to extract and use invariant relationships. This tendency is most successful in sequences with tones separated by the same, recurring pitch interval. Thus, in Figure 11.6, the descending glide of tones from the G_5 tone in constant (pitch interval) steps to E_4

(see bracket) provokes a sense of continuity. And this impression continues over time gaps, thereby *implying* constant motion. That is, although *technically* discontinuous (i.e., it is a faux glide), this faux glide segment nevertheless effectively implies a slow, continuously falling motion.

Historically, interest has centered on the implied motion of faux glides following theoretical lines established in classic Gestalt studies of apparent visual motion. Korte's third law posits that groups of discrete visual elements are perceived, within limits, as motions due to relative timing of onsets of spatially separated lights (visual phi phenomena).[123] In fact, it is widely accepted that, within limits, implied velocities instill in viewers motion-like visual percepts.

Visual motion percepts are linked to a continuity bias for constant motion. Diagnostic percepts, such as *tau* and *kappa* effects, support this bias. For instance, a visual tau happens when a single lengthened (shortened) time interval, T, in a sequence causes a viewer to report a correlated percept of spatial lengthening (or shortening) with this time interval. A temporal illusion, kappa, reflects an opposite effect. Given a constant context of spatial changes, this effect occurs when a single spatial change causes a correlated temporal illusion.[124,125,126] These illusions reflect listeners' involuntary biases to restore the constant velocity motion of a prior context.[127]

Auditory analogs of visual tau and kappa generalize to implied pitch motions.[128,129] Molly Henry and Devin McAuley found support for auditory illusions of both tau and kappa.[130,131] In both cases, listeners reported melodic illusions that preserved a pattern's continuation at a constant velocity (semitones/time). These intriguing phenomena are not merely laboratory curiosities. Similarly, Marilyn Boltz also showed that kappa illusions emerge in musical listening.[132]

In sum, dynamic continuity characterizes certain biases in people that influence their sense of a musical contour. Listeners favor illusory constant motions that perceptually "connect" tones within a melodic group. Finally, the "continuity as motion" bias draws on an implied velocity established by a prior context which has a sustaining quality. Thus, dynamic continuations may "continue" (i.e., persist in real time), leading listeners to generate an *extrapolated expectancy*.[133]

Illusions of Extrapolated Continuity

The idea that listeners extrapolate motion-like expectancies captures the sense of anticipation that often precedes a future happening. An underlying assumption holds that people rely on a recurring pitch–time relationship to anticipate similar future changes. This idea returns in recent research on the *continuity illusion.*

Melodic contours that support continuity expectancies are *true glides.* True glides present continuously ascending or descending frequencies; these rapidly excite overlapping entrainment regions of near neighbors. Faux glides, by contrast, comprise tones with similar frequencies separated by brief silences. Although listeners are better at detecting pitch changes in true than in faux glides, they efficiently track both in real time.[134,135] Importantly, there is general agreement that *continuity illusions* move listeners to literally "hear" a glide continue in time (i.e., through a sudden silent gap or one filled with soft noise).[136,137,138,139,140,141,142]   Explanations of these effects differ.[143,144,145,146,147,148,149]

A popular explanation of continuity illusions maintains that they are memory-driven, based on a listener's after-the-fact interpolation that retroactively "fills" the silent gap.[150,151] However, Polly Crum and Irv Hafter convincing ruled out an interpolation explanation in favor of an extrapolation hypothesis.[152] That is, they discovered that people engage in pitch tracking which can then be extrapolated in real time based upon the prior contextual velocity afforded by frequency glides.[153]

Summary of Melodic Contours

In sum, melodic contour offers patterns of tone frequencies to which listeners exogenously entrain, typically as pitch tracking. With these exogenous entrainments, listeners' grouping percepts reveal strong stimulus-driven influences based upon relationships among successive tone frequencies. One hypothesis features a role for overlapping entrainment regions elicited by micro-driving rhythms of proximal tones. A second hypothesis, addresses continuity percepts involving melodic groups of glides. Glides allow dynamic attending explanations involving the velocity of pitch tracking. In these ways, melodic contours, commonly explained by Gestalt proximity and continuation principles, may be addressed within a dynamic framework.

Major points about melodic contours are:

- Percepts of melodic contour are explained using stimulus-driven entrainment (i.e., variations of pitch tracking based on exogenous entrainments).
- Groups of tones, bounded by beginning and end accents, are carved out in melodic contour.
- Frequencies of accented tones, as micro-driving rhythms, conform to a Fast/Slow

rule which posits that stronger entrainments hold for frequencies serving as beginning (speed up) than for ending (slowing down) accents.
- Percepts of melodic contour groups based on proximities invite an ERO hypothesis involving pitch tracking and overlapping entrainment regions of near-neighbor oscillations.
- Percepts of melodic groups based on continuity are explained by pitch tracking based on dynamic continuities involving constant motion trajectories.

CHAPTER SUMMARY

Inspired by the original distinctions of Jay Dowling (1978), two major sections of this chapter concern, respectively, tonality and melodic contour in musical events An overarching aim was to illustrate how DAT approaches both topics.

Following a background section, the first major section considers the potential that entrainment theory holds for describing percepts of melodic tonality. Familiar entrainment concepts are enlisted to address perception of a musical keynote, as well as percepts of tonal melodies and chords. These entrainment concepts are internalized tonal structures, such as a tonal referent oscillation (key), tonal oscillator clusters (chords), and tonal attractor profiles (melodic lines). All concepts draw on common principles of resonance and entrainment. And all emphasize the refinement of endogenous entrainments which pave the way for learning harmony and melody.

The final section of the chapter concentrates on people's immediate responses to the surface of melodic contours. Unlike tonal aspects of music, which elicit culture-specific endogenous entrainment constructs (e.g., attractor profiles, oscillator clusters), melodic contour rests more on exogenous entrainments (e.g., pitch tracking). Three topics are relevant to contour perception. One involves pitch accents, which highlight contour boundaries. A second concerns dynamic proximity, which addresses near-neighbor grouping percepts. The third topic involves dynamic continuity, which explains musical glides as supporting velocity extrapolation. Although about melody, the aim of this chapter has emphasized time. As such, it resonates with a quote attributed to Debussy: "*Music is the silence between notes.*"

NOTES

1. Don Michael Randel, *The Harvard Dictionary of Music*, vol. 16 (Cambridge, MA: Harvard University Press, 2003), https://books-google-com.proxy.library.

ucsb.edu:9443/books?hl=enandlr=andid=02rFSecP hEsCandoi=fndandpg=PR5anddq=Harvard+Dicti onary+of+Music+andots=Ul8_OJ_hNPandsig=k_ 3bHszVZZWv-BtwF9aJ4Q_cvw4.

2. Rie Matsunaga, Koichi Yokosawa, and Jun-ichi Abe, "Magnetoencephalography Evidence for Different Brain Subregions Serving Two Musical Cultures," *Neuropsychologia* 50, no. 14 (December 2012): 3218–27, doi:10.1016/j.neuropsycholo gia.2012.10.002.

3. Psyche Loui, David L. Wessel, and Carla L. Hudson Kam, "Humans Rapidly Learn Grammatical Structure in a New Musical Scale," *Music Perception: An Interdisciplinary Journal* 27, no. 5 (June 1, 2010): 377–88, doi:10.1525/mp.2010.27.5.377.

4. In reality, for artistic reasons, slight (vibrato) modulations of an otherwise static sound are common.

5. Frequency, *f*, here refers to the F0 of a complex tone (or the frequency of a pure tone).

6. Tempered (ET) scales approximate ratios of "ideal" ratios of, e.g., a Just tuning scheme. Theoretically, tolerable ET approximations hide relevant attractor ratios.

7. Julyan H. E. Cartwright, Diego L. González, and Oreste Piro, "Nonlinear Dynamics of the Perceived Pitch of Complex Sounds," *Physical Review Letters* 82, no. 26 (June 28, 1999): 5389–92, doi:10.1103/ PhysRevLett.82.5389.

8. Julyan H. E. Cartwright et al., "Aesthetics, Dynamics, and Musical Scales: A Golden Connection," *Journal of New Music Research* 31, no. 1 (March 1, 2002): 51–58, doi:10.1076/jnmr.31.1.51.8099.

9. Recall that stability of such a ratio is the inverse of an attractor's complexity in DAT.

10. Also recall that Arnold tongue regimes specify stability differences. Attractor ratios resemble rate ratios of Chapter 6.

11. Cartwright et al., "Aesthetics, Dynamics, and Musical Scales."

12. The B tone (in C major scale) is often referred to as a "leading tone," since its low stability allows it to be "pulled" toward the tonic C.

13. Stability rankings correlate with the simplicity indices of Chapter 6; both can be linked to stability rankings of the devil's staircase.

14. Georg Von Békésy and Ernest Glen Wever, *Experiments in Hearing*, vol. 8 (New York: McGraw-Hill, 1960), http://www.abdi-ecommerce10.com/asa/ images/product/medium/0-88318-6306.pdf.

15. Federico De Martino et al., "Spatial Organization of Frequency Preference and Selectivity in the Human Inferior Colliculus," *Nature Communications* 4 (January 22, 2013): 1386, doi:10.1038/ncomms2379.

16. Dave R. M. Langers and Pim van Dijk, "Mapping the Tonotopic Organization in Human Auditory Cortex with Minimally Salient Acoustic Stimulation," *Cerebral Cortex* 22, no. 9 (September 1, 2012): 2024–38, doi:10.1093/cercor/bhr282.

17. Typically, measurements of these cortical activities do not involve recordings of different cortical layers (i.e., lamina).

18. S. Da Costa et al., "Human Primary Auditory Cortex Follows the Shape of Heschl's Gyrus," *Journal of Neuroscience* 31, no. 40 (October 5, 2011): 14067–75, doi:10.1523/JNEUROSCI.2000-11.2011.

19. Langers and Dijk, "Mapping the Tonotopic Organization in Human Auditory Cortex with Minimally Salient Acoustic Stimulation."

20. Roger N. Shepard, "Circularity in Judgments of Relative Pitch," *The Journal of the Acoustical Society of America* 36, no. 12 (December 1, 1964): 2346–53, doi:10.1121/1.1919362.

21. Roger N. Shepard, "Geometrical Approximations to the Structure of Musical Pitch," *Psychological Review* 89, no. 4 (1982): 305–33, doi:10.1037/0033-295X.89.4.305.

22. Diana Deutsch and John Feroe, "The Internal Representation of Pitch Sequences in Tonal Music," *Psychological Review* 88, no. 6 (1981): 503–22, doi:10.1037/0033-295X.88.6.503.

23. Jamshed J. Bharucha, "From Frequency to Pitch, and from Pitch Class to Musical Key: Shared Principles of Learning and Perception," *Connection Science* 21, no. 2–3 (September 1, 2009): 177–92, doi:10.1080/09540090902733822.

24. Barbara Tillmann, Jamshed J. Bharucha, and Emmanuel Bigand, "Implicit Learning of Tonality: A Self-Organizing Approach," *Psychological Review* 107, no. 4 (2000): 885–913, doi:10.1037/ 0033-295X.107.4.885.

25. Bharucha, "From Frequency to Pitch, and from Pitch Class to Musical Key."

26. Jamshed J. Bharucha, "Music Cognition and Perceptual Facilitation: A Connectionist Framework," *Music Perception: An Interdisciplinary Journal* 5, no. 1 (October 1, 1987): 1–30, doi:10.2307/40285384.

27. Edward W. Large, "A Dynamical Systems Approach to Musical Tonality," in *Nonlinear Dynamics in Human Behavior*, eds. Raoul Huys and Viktor K. Jirsa, vol. 328 (Berlin, Heidelberg: Springer, 2010), 193–211, http://link.springer.com/10.1007/978-3-642-16262-6_9.

28. Edward W. Large, Felix V. Almonte, and Marc J. Velasco, "A Canonical Model for Gradient Frequency Neural Networks," *Physica D: Nonlinear Phenomena* 239, no. 12 (June 15, 2010): 905–11, doi:10.1016/ j.physd.2009.11.015.

29. H. R. Wilson and J. D. Cowan, "A Mathematical Theory of the Functional Dynamics of Cortical and Thalamic Nervous Tissue," *Kybernetik* 13, no. 2 (September 1973): 55–80, doi:10.1007/BF00288786.

30. Shepard, R. N. (1982). Geometrical approximations to the structure of musical pitch. *Psychological Review*, 89(4), 305–33. http://dx.doi.org/ 10.1037/0033-295X.89.4.305

31. June Hahn and Mari Riess Jones, "Invariants in Auditory Frequency Relations," *Scandinavian Journal of Psychology* 22, no. 1 (September 1, 1981): 129–44, doi:10.1111/j.1467-9450.1981.tb00388.x.

32. Diana Deutsch, "Octave Generalization of Specific Interference Effects in Memory for Tonal

Pitch," *Perception & Psychophysics* 13, no. 2 (June 1973): 271–5, doi:10.3758/BF03214138.

33. Diana Deutsch and Richard C. Boulanger, "Octave Equivalence and the Immediate Recall of Pitch Sequences," *Music Perception: An Interdisciplinary Journal* 2, no. 1 (October 1, 1984): 40–51, doi:10.2307/40285281.

34. Laurent Demany, "The Perceptual Reality of Tone Chroma in Early Infancy," *The Journal of the Acoustical Society of America* 76, no. 1 (1984): 57, doi:10.1121/1.391006.

35. ET tuning leads to the chromatic scale with semitones, each with $\theta j = 30$ degrees.

36. Carol L. Krumhansl and Roger N. Shepard, "Quantification of the Hierarchy of Tonal Functions Within a Diatonic Context," *Journal of Experimental Psychology: Human Perception and Performance* 5, no. 4 (1979): 579–94, doi:10.1037/0096-1523.5.4.579.

37. Carol L. Krumhansl, *Cognitive Foundations of Musical Pitch* (New York: Oxford University Press, 2001), https://books-google-com.proxy.library.ucsb.edu:9443/books?hl=enandlr=andid=J4dJCAAAQBAJandoi=fndandpg=PT11anddq=+Krumhansl,+1990++Cognitve+foundations+of+music++andots=PEa3VF6_Goandsig=NdbOw1WawRIByvqt8esdZV089VE.

38. Carol L. Krumhansl and Lola L. Cuddy, "A Theory of Tonal Hierarchies in Music," in *Music Perception*, eds. Mari Riess Jones, Richard R. Fay, and Arthur N. Popper, Springer Handbook of Auditory Research 36 (New York: Springer, 2010), 51–87, doi:10.1007/978-1-4419-6114-3_3.

39. Krumhansl, *Cognitive Foundations of Musical Pitch.*

40. Carol L. Krumhansl and Edward J. Kessler, "Tracing the Dynamic Changes in Perceived Tonal Organization in a Spatial Representation of Musical Keys," *Psychological Review* 89, no. 4 (1982): 334–68, doi:10.1037/0033-295X.89.4.334.

41. Krumhansl and Cuddy, "A Theory of Tonal Hierarchies in Music."

42. Eleanor Rosch, "Cognitive Reference Points," *Cognitive Psychology* 7, no. 4 (October 1975): 532–47, doi:10.1016/0010-0285(75)90021-3.

43. David Brian Huron, *Sweet Anticipation: Music and the Psychology of Expectation* (Cambridge, MA: MIT Press, 2006), https://books-google-com.proxy.library.ucsb.edu:9443/books?hl=enandlr=andid=uyI_Cb8olkMCandoi=fndandpg=PR5anddq=David+Huron+Sweet+Anticipation++++++++++++++andots=ih7seC67sCandsig=ACCAI_IYRzxn5349_yvmlkDA2rg.

44. Huron, *Sweet Anticipation.*

45. Edward W. Large and Felix V. Almonte, "Neurodynamics, Tonality, and the Auditory Brainstem Response," *Annals of the New York Academy of Sciences* 1252, no. 1 (April 1, 2012): E1–7, doi:10.1111/j.1749-6632.2012.06594.x.

46. Large, Almonte, and Velasco, "A Canonical Model for Gradient Frequency Neural Networks."

47. Large, Almonte, and Velasco, "A Canonical Model for Gradient Frequency Neural Networks."

48. Krumhansl, *Cognitive Foundations of Musical Pitch.*

49. Laurel J. Trainor and Kathleen A. Corrigall, "Music Acquisition and Effects of Musical Experience," in *Music Perception*, eds. Mari Riess Jones, Richard R. Fay, and Arthur N. Popper, vol. 36 (New York: Springer, 2010), 89–127, http://link.springer.com/10.1007/978-1-4419-6114-3_4.

50. Krumhansl and Cuddy, *A Theory of Tonal Hierarchies in Music* (New York: Springer, 2010), http://link.springer.com.proxy.library.ucsb.edu:2048/chapter/10.1007/978-1-4419-6114-3_3.

51. Laurel J. Trainor and Kathleen A. Corrigall, *Music Acquisition and Effects of Musical Experience* (New York: Springer, 2010), http://link.springer.com.proxy.library.ucsb.edu:2048/chapter/10.1007/978-1-4419-6114-3_4.

52. Loui, Wessel, and Kam, "Humans Rapidly Learn Grammatical Structure in a New Musical Scale."

53. Rie Matsunaga and Jun-Ichi Abe, "Cues for Key Perception of a Melody," *Music Perception: An Interdisciplinary Journal* 23, no. 2 (December 1, 2005): 153–64, doi:10.1525/mp.2005.23.2.153.

54. Rie Matsunaga and Jun-ichi Abe, "Incremental Process of Musical Key Identification," *Proceedings of the 29th Annual Cognitive Science Society. Austin, TX: Cognitive Science Society*, 2007, 1277–82.

55. Helen Brown, "The Interplay of Set Content and Temporal Context in a Functional Theory of Tonality Perception," *Music Perception: An Interdisciplinary Journal* 5, no. 3 (April 1, 1988): 219–49, doi:10.2307/40285398.

56. Helen Brown, David Butler, and Mari Riess Jones, "Musical and Temporal Influences on Key Discovery," *Music Perception: An Interdisciplinary Journal* 11, no. 4 (July 1, 1994): 371–407, doi:10.2307/40285632.

57. David Butler and Helen Brown, "Tonal Structure Versus Function: Studies of the Recognition of Harmonic Motion," *Music Perception: An Interdisciplinary Journal* 2, no. 1 (October 1, 1984): 6–24, doi:10.2307/40285279.

58. The notation here for the musical scale note, F, should not be confused with same symbol, F, which conventionally refers to an acoustic frequency. Usually context clarifies the scalar note from the broader use of a sound's frequency.

59. Mary Farbood Morwaread, Gary Marcus, and David Poeppel, "Temporal Dynamics and the Identification of Musical Key," *Journal of Experimental Psychology: Human Perception and Performance* 39, no. 4 (2013): 911–8, doi:10.1037/a0031087.

60. Marilyn Boltz, "Perceiving the End: Effects of Tonal Relationships on Melodic Completion," *Journal of Experimental Psychology: Human Perception and Performance* 15, no. 4 (1989): 749–61, doi:10.1037/0096-1523.15.4.749.

61. Jamshed J. Bharucha, "Melodic Anchoring," *Music Perception: An Interdisciplinary Journal* 13, no. 3 (April 1, 1996): 383–400, doi:10.2307/40286176.

62. Jamshed J. Bharucha and Keiko Stoeckig, "Priming of Chords: Spreading Activation or Overlapping Frequency Spectra?," *Perception & Psychophysics* 41, no. 6 (November 1987): 519–24, doi:10.3758/BF03210486.

63. Barbara Tillmann et al., "Tonal Centers and Expectancy: Facilitation or Inhibition of Chords at the Top of the Harmonic Hierarchy?" *Journal of Experimental Psychology: Human Perception and Performance* 34, no. 4 (2008): 1031–43, doi:10.1037/0096-1523.34.4.1031.

64. Hasan Gürkan Tekman and Jamshed J. Bharucha, "Time Course of Chord Priming," *Perception & Psychophysics* 51, no. 1 (January 1992): 33–9, doi:10.3758/BF03205071.

65. Frédéric Marmel and Barbara Tillmann, "Tonal Priming Beyond Tonics," *Music Perception: An Interdisciplinary Journal* 26, no. 3 (February 1, 2009): 211–21, doi:10.1525/mp.2009.26.3.211.

66. Susan Holleran, Mari Riess Jones, and David Butler, "Perceiving Implied Harmony: The Influence of Melodic and Harmonic Context," *Journal of Experimental Psychology: Learning, Memory, and Cognition* 21, no. 3 (1995): 737–53, doi:10.1037/0278-7393.21.3.737.

67. This knowledge is acquired through tacit learning during entrainment at micro-time scales, following learning principles of Chapter 10.

68. Tillmann, Bharucha, and Bigand, "Implicit Learning of Tonality."

69. Emmanuel Bigand, "The Influence of Implicit Harmony, Rhythm and Musical Training on the Abstraction of 'Tension-Relaxation Schemas' in Tonal Musical Phrases," *Contemporary Music Review* 9, no. 1–2 (January 1, 1993): 123–37, doi:10.1080/07494469300640391.

70. Emmanuel Bigand et al., "Effect of Global Structure and Temporal Organization on Chord Processing," *Journal of Experimental Psychology: Human Perception and Performance* 25, no. 1 (1999): 184.

71. Walter Piston and Mark Devoto, *Harmony* (5th ed.) (New York: Norton, 1987).

72. Erik Jansen and Dirk-Jan Povel, "The Processing of Chords in Tonal Melodic Sequences," *Journal of New Music Research* 33, no. 1 (March 1, 2004): 31–48, doi:10.1076/jnmr.33.1.31.35396.

73. Erik Jansen and Dirk-Jan Povel, "Perception of Arpeggiated Chord Progressions," *Musicae Scientiae* 8, no. 1 (March 1, 2004): 7–52, doi:10.1177/102986490400800102.

74. Also I and V chord repetitions in this protocol may have affected ratings.

75. Bigand et al., "Effect of Global Structure and Temporal Organization on Chord Processing."

76. Barbara Tillmann and Géraldine Lebrun-Guillaud, "Influence of Tonal and Temporal Expectations on Chord Processing and on Completion Judgments of Chord Sequences," *Psychological Research Psychologische Forschung* 70, no. 5 (September 2006): 345–58, doi:10.1007/s00426-005-0222-0.

77. Sandra E. Trehub, "Musical Predispositions in Infancy," *Annals of the New York Academy of Sciences* 930, no. 1 (June 1, 2001): 1–16, doi:10.1111/j.1749-6632.2001.tb05721.x.

78. Jansen and Povel, "Perception of Arpeggiated Chord Progressions."

79. W. Jay Dowling, "Scale and Contour: Two Components of a Theory of Memory for Melodies.," *Psychological Review* 85, no. 4 (1978): 341–54, doi:10.1037/0033-295X.85.4.341.

80. Mark. A. Schmuckler, "Melodic Contour Similarity Using Folk Melodies," *Music Perception* 28, no. 2 (December 2010): 169–94, doi:10.1525/mp.2010.28.2.169.

81. Dowling, "Scale and Contour."

82. Walter J. Dowling and D. S. Fujitani, "Contour, Interval, and Pitch Recognition in Memory for Melodies.," *Journal of the Acoustical Society of America* 49, no. 2 (February 1, 1971): 524–31, https://utdallas.influuent.utsystem.edu/en/publications/contour-interval-and-pitch-recognition-in-memory-for-melodies(18de963b-3217-4b45-b530-e328e4739635).html.

83. The frequency of a pure tone or the fundamental of a complex tone.

84. Mari Riess Jones, Heather Moynihan Johnston, and Jennifer Puente, "Effects of Auditory Pattern Structure on Anticipatory and Reactive Attending," *Cognitive Psychology* 53, no. 1 (August 2006): 59–96, doi:10.1016/j.cogpsych.2006.01.003.

85. Stephanie M. Stalinski, E. Glenn Schellenberg, and Sandra E. Trehub, "Developmental Changes in the Perception of Pitch Contour: Distinguishing up from Down," *The Journal of the Acoustical Society of America* 124, no. 3 (2008): 1759, doi:10.1121/1.2956470.

86. Marilyn Boltz and Mari Riess Jones, "Does Rule Recursion Make Melodies Easier to Reproduce? If Not, What Does?" *Cognitive Psychology* 18, no. 4 (October 1986): 389–431, doi:10.1016/0010-0285(86)90005-8.

87. Mari Riess Jones, "A Tutorial on Some Issues and Methods in Serial Pattern Research," *Perception & Psychophysics* 30, no. 5 (September 1981): 492–504, doi:10.3758/BF03204846.

88. Laurent Demany and Sylvain Clément, "The Perception of Frequency Peaks and Troughs in Wide Frequency Modulations. II. Effects of Frequency Register, Stimulus Uncertainty, and Intensity," *The Journal of the Acoustical Society of America* 97, no. 4 (April 1, 1995): 2454–9, doi:10.1121/1.411966.

89. Laurent Demany and Sylvain Clément, "The Perception of Frequency Peaks and Troughs in Wide Frequency Modulations. III. Complex Carriers," *The Journal of the Acoustical Society of America* 98, no. 5 (November 1, 1995): 2515–23, doi:10.1121/1.413217.

90. Laurent Demany and Kenneth I. McAnally, "The Perception of Frequency Peaks and Troughs in Wide Frequency Modulations," *The Journal of the Acoustical Society of America* 96, no. 2 (August 1, 1994): 706–15, doi:10.1121/1.410309.

91. Johnston, H. M., & Jones, M. R. (2006). Higher order pattern structure influences auditory representational momentum. *Journal of Experimental*

Psychology: Human Perception and Performance, 32(1), 2–17. http://dx.doi.org/10.1037/0096-1523.32.1.2

92. Mark A. Schmuckler, "Testing Models of Melodic Contour Similarity," *Music Perception: An Interdisciplinary Journal* 16, no. 3 (April 1999): 295–326, doi:10.2307/40285795.

93. Schmuckler, "Melodic Contour Similarity Using Folk Melodies."

94. Recall that *pitch interval* refers to a scalar difference in tone frequencies, (fi–fj) where the unit semitone is (fi–fj)/fi = .0578.

95. Eugene Narmour, *The Analysis and Cognition of Melodic Complexity: The Implication-Realization Model* (Chicago: University of Chicago Press, 1992), https://books-google-com.proxy.library.ucsb.edu:9443/books?hl=enandlr=andid=vfbwkoJFxQUCandoi=fndandpg=PR9anddq=Eugene+Narmour+++book+andots=iVItyBmJ_wandsig=PIJFq51FoeUk5T3R3ofcZnJhAik.

96. Leonard B. Meyer, *Emotion and Meaning in Music* (Chicago: University of Chicago Press, 2008), https://books-google-com.proxy.library.ucsb.edu:9443/books?hl=enandlr=andid=lp07ZMAczT8Candoi=fndandpg=PR11anddq=Leonard+Meyer+++book+on+musicandots=QwYWdJz74gandsig=X1Ex09f5SZNZFIPpX8c9dYMqiz4.

97. The five principles are registral direction, intervallic difference, registral return, proximity, closure.

98. E. Glenn Schellenberg, "Simplifying the Implication-Realization Model of Melodic Expectancy," *Music Perception: An Interdisciplinary Journal* 14, no. 3 (April 1, 1997): 295–318, doi:10.2307/40285723.

99. Albert S. Bregman, *Auditory Scene Analysis: The Perceptual Organization of Sound* (Cambridge, MA: MIT Press, 1994), https://books-google-com.proxy.library.ucsb.edu:9443/books?hl=enandlr=andid=jI8muSpAC5ACandoi=fndandpg=PR11anddq=Bregman,+A.++Auditory+Scene+analysisandots=SFq_D6BIwEandsig=wCOGtOtK1wh7yXN0eOQnc8X1pGA.

100. Pitch is used to refer to frequency in this section for simplicity; this assumes a direct relation between the frequency of a pure tone and its percept as pitch.

101. This is also termed frequency following.

102. Fred Lerdahl and Ray Jackendoff, "A Generative Theory of Tonal Music," *Journal of Aesthetics and Art Criticism* 46, no. 1 (1987): 94–8.

103. Grosvenor Cooper and Leonard B. Meyer, *The Rhythmic Structure of Music*, vol. 118 (Chicago: University of Chicago Press, 1963), https://books-google-com.proxy.library.ucsb.edu:9443/books?hl=enandlr=andid=V2yXrIWDTIQCandoi=fndandpg=PA17anddq=Book:+++Cooper+and+Meyer+++music+andots=QuX-MLXMWnandsig=sZxu99Nu42IonZ0V7pUj3uhNWw8.

104. This discussion of accenting is confined to pitch (i.e. frequency) accenting properties. Clearly, if sound intensity is considered, then the issue of dominant frequencies enters the discussion because louder sounds also contribute to accentuation.

105. This relates to the number of cycles per unit of absolute time (e.g., a T:p ratio; see Chapter 6).

106. Demany and Clément, "The Perception of Frequency Peaks and Troughs in Wide Frequency Modulations. III. Complex Carriers."

107. Demany and Clément, "The Perception of Frequency Peaks and Troughs in Wide Frequency Modulations. II. Effects of Frequency Register, Stimulus Uncertainty, and Intensity."

108. Demany and McAnally, "The Perception of Frequency Peaks and Troughs in Wide Frequency Modulations."

109. Nina Kraus and Bharath Chandrasekaran, "Music Training for the Development of Auditory Skills," *Nature Reviews Neuroscience* 11, no. 8 (August 2010): 599–605, https://doi.org/10.1038/nrn2882.

110. Laurent Demany and Christophe Ramos, "On the Binding of Successive Sounds: Perceiving Shifts in Nonperceived Pitches," *The Journal of the Acoustical Society of America* 117, no. 2 (February 1, 2005): 833–41, doi:10.1121/1.1850209.

111. Gavin M. Bidelman, Jackson T. Gandour, and Ananthanarayan Krishnan, "Cross-Domain Effects of Music and Language Experience on the Representation of Pitch in the Human Auditory Brainstem," *Journal of Cognitive Neuroscience* 23, no. 2 (November 19, 2009): 425–34, doi:10.1162/jocn.2009.21362.

112. Nina Kraus and Bharath Chandrasekaran, "Music Training for the Development of Auditory Skills," *Nature Reviews Neuroscience* 11, no. 8 (August 2010): 599–605, doi:10.1038/nrn2882.

113. Christoph E. Schreiner and Jeffery A. Winer, "Auditory Cortex Mapmaking: Principles, Projections, and Plasticity," *Neuron* 56, no. 2 (October 2007): 356–65, doi:10.1016/j.neuron.2007.10.013.

114. Heather L. Read, Jeffery A. Winer, and Christoph E. Schreiner, "Functional Architecture of Auditory Cortex," *Current Opinion in Neurobiology* 12, no. 4 (August 1, 2002): 433–40, doi:10.1016/S0959-4388(02)00342-2.

115. Note that proximity in frequency within a curvi-linear frequency gradient is gauged along two dimensions: pitch height and chroma. That is, two sounds separated by an octave express greater proximity than two sounds separated by tritone interval.

116. Driving rhythm separations can *exceed* discrimination thresholds.

117. With tonal attractors along a neural gradient, a variation of this analysis describes stability differences of strong versus weak scale tones in melodic anchoring.

118. Bharucha, "Melodic Anchoring."

119. George A. Miller and George A. Heise, "The Trill Threshold," *The Journal of the Acoustical Society of America* 22, no. 5 (September 1, 1950): 637–38, doi:10.1121/1.1906663.

120. Bregman, *Auditory Scene Analysis.*

121. Bregman, *Auditory Scene Analysis.*

122. Albert S. Bregman and Jeffrey Campbell, "Primary Auditory Stream Segregation and Perception

of Order in Rapid Sequences of Tones," *Journal of Experimental Psychology* 89, no. 2 (1971): 244–9, doi:10.1037/h0031163.

123. Harry R. DeSilva, "An Experimental Investigation of the Determinants of Apparent Visual Movement," *The American Journal of Psychology* 37, no. 4 (1926): 469–501, doi:10.2307/1414909.

124. John Cohen, Ian Christensen, and Akio Ono, "Influence of Temporal Intervals on Comparative Judgements of Pitch: A Study of Subjective Relativity," *Tohoku Psychologica Folia* 33, no. 1–4 (1974): 76–87.

125. Bill Jones and Yih Lehr Huang, "Space-Time Dependencies in Psychophysical Judgment of Extent and Duration: Algebraic Models of the Tau and Kappa Effects," *Psychological Bulletin* 91, no. 1 (1982): 128–42, doi:10.1037/0033-2909.91.1.128.

126. H. Helson and S. M. King, "The Tau Effect: An Example of Psychological Relativity," *Journal of Experimental Psychology* 14, no. 3 (1931): 202–17, doi:10.1037/h0071164.

127. Jones and Lehr Huang, "Space-Time Dependencies in Psychophysical Judgment of Extent and Duration."

128. John Cohen, C. E. M. Hansel, and J. D. Sylvester, "Interdependence of Temporal and Auditory Judgments," *Nature* 174 (October 1, 1954): 642–4, doi:10.1038/174642a0.

129. Sumi Shigeno, "The Auditory Tau and Kappa Effects for Speech and Nonspeech Stimuli," *Perception & Psychophysics* 40, no. 1 (January 1986): 9–19, doi:10.3758/BF03207588.

130. Molly J. Henry and J. Devin, "Evaluation of an Imputed Pitch Velocity Model of the Auditory Kappa Effect," *Journal of Experimental Psychology: Human Perception and Performance* 35, no. 2 (2009): 551–64, doi:10.1037/0096-1523.35.2.551.

131. Molly J. Henry, J. Devin McAuley, and Marta Zaleha, "Evaluation of an Imputed Pitch Velocity Model of the Auditory Tau Effect," *Attention, Perception, & Psychophysics* 71, no. 6 (August 2009): 1399–413, doi:10.3758/APP.71.6.1399.

132. Marilyn G. Boltz, "Tempo Discrimination of Musical Patterns: Effects Due to Pitch and Rhythmic Structure," *Perception & Psychophysics* 60, no. 8 (November 1998): 1357–73, doi:10.3758/BF03207998.

133. Mari R. Jones, "Time, Our Lost Dimension: Toward a New Theory of Perception, Attention, and Memory," *Psychological Review* 83, no. 5 (1976): 323.

134. Aleksander Sek and Brian C. J. Moore, "Discrimination of Frequency Steps Linked by Glides of Various Durations," *The Journal of the Acoustical Society of America* 106, no. 1 (1999): 351, doi:10.1121/1.427061.

135. J. Lyzenga, R. P. Carlyon, and B. C. J. Moore, "The Effects of Real and Illusory Glides on Pure-Tone Frequency Discrimination," *The Journal of the Acoustical Society of America* 116, no. 1 (2004): 491, doi:10.1121/1.1756616.

136. Lyzenga, Carlyon, and Moore, "The Effects of Real and Illusory Glides on Pure-Tone Frequency Discrimination."

137. J. Lyzenga, R. P. Carlyon, and B. C. J. Moore, "Dynamic Aspects of the Continuity Illusion: Perception of Level and of the Depth, Rate, and Phase of Modulation," *Hearing Research* 210, no. 1–2 (December 2005): 30–41, doi:10.1016/j.heares.2005.07.002.

138. Lyzenga, Carlyon, and Moore, "Dynamic Aspects of the Continuity Illusion."

139. Valter Ciocca and Albert S. Bregman, "Perceived Continuity of Gliding and Steady-State Tones Through Interrupting Noise," *Perception & Psychophysics* 42, no. 5 (September 1987): 476–84, doi:10.3758/BF03209755.

140. Keith R. Kluender, Jeffry A. Coady, and Michael Kiefte, "Sensitivity to Change in Perception of Speech," *Speech Communication* 41, no. 1 (August 2003): 59–69, doi:10.1016/S0167-6393(02)00093-6.

141. Richard M. Warren et al., "Auditory Induction: Reciprocal Changes in Alternating Sounds," *Perception & Psychophysics* 55, no. 3 (May 1994): 313–22, doi:10.3758/BF03207602.

142. Poppy A. C. Crum and Ervin R. Hafter, "Predicting the Path of a Changing Sound: Velocity Tracking and Auditory Continuity," *The Journal of the Acoustical Society of America* 124, no. 2 (2008): 1116, doi:10.1121/1.2945117.

143. Laurent Demany, Daniel Pressnitzer, and Catherine Semal, "Tuning Properties of the Auditory Frequency-Shift Detectors," *The Journal of the Acoustical Society of America* 126, no. 3 (2009): 1342, doi:10.1121/1.3179675.

144. Laurent Demany, Robert P. Carlyon, and Catherine Semal, "Continuous Versus Discrete Frequency Changes: Different Detection Mechanisms?" *The Journal of the Acoustical Society of America* 125, no. 2 (2009): 1082, doi:10.1121/1.3050271.

145. Lyzenga, Carlyon, and Moore, "Dynamic Aspects of the Continuity Illusion."

146. Ciocca and Bregman, "Perceived Continuity of Gliding and Steady-State Tones through Interrupting Noise."

147. Kluender, Coady, and Kiefte, "Sensitivity to Change in Perception of Speech."

148. Warren et al., "Auditory Induction."

149. Crum and Hafter, "Predicting the Path of a Changing Sound."

150. Ciocca and Bregman, "Perceived Continuity of Gliding and Steady-State Tones through Interrupting Noise."

151. Kluender, Coady, and Kiefte, "Sensitivity to Change in Perception of Speech."

152. Poppy A. C. Crum and Ervin R. Hafter, "Predicting the Path of a Changing Sound: Velocity Tracking and Auditory Continuity," *The Journal of the Acoustical Society of America* 124, no. 2 (August 1, 2008): 1116–29, doi:10.1121/1.2945117.

153. Velocities were 3 Hz/ms; gaps were filled with noise.

12

Speech Timing

Speech timing has inspired many thoughtful theories; some emphasize how speakers produce coherently timed utterances, whereas others focus on listeners' percepts of speech timing. In the latter, a persistent puzzle concerns how people manage to hear discrete words in fluent (i.e., continuous acoustic speech signals). Still other theories grapple with cultural variety in speech timing, aiming to explain apparent rhythmic differences among three classical linguistic categories: stress-based (e.g., Dutch, English), syllable-timed (e.g., Spanish, French), and mora-timed (e.g., Japanese).[1]

One unifying idea centers on the role of a somewhat elusive regularity in speech timing, one that borders on isochrony. Applied to the preceding "big three" linguistic categories, temporal regularity is granted to interstress durations in *stress-based languages*, to syllable durations in *syllable-timed languages,* and to *morae* in other languages. Yet even these categorizations are disputed. As early as 1983, Dauer[2] questioned their usefulness. More recently, the preceding linguistic categories have been dismissed as overly simplistic.[3,4,5] In line with this criticism, statistical metrics of speech timing do not confirm the existence of such rigid category boundaries, favoring instead a continuum of timing differences between culturally different languages. Other scholars, arguing against a strict statistical metric, favor a more fruitful path to explaining speech timing, one that focuses on respective roles of rate and relative timing in speech of different cultures.

This chapter follows the latter path. It pursues applications of dynamic attending concepts to the rate and rhythm of sequences of syllables and words in phrases. In this, it does not address linguistic phonologies, but instead focuses on how people use speech (i.e., what governs productions and perceptions of speakers and listeners). Moreover, this approach concentrates on pre-lexical (i.e., prosodic) aspects of speech utterances with the aim of understanding how speech prosody affords driving rhythms that figure in entrainment

by a listener's tunable brain. Because this aim implicates novel ideas, it is important to unpack these concepts against the background of conventional descriptions of speech timing behaviors that embrace lexical and/or statistical approaches to speech timing.

CHAPTER GOALS

The first section of this chapter outlines the origins of thinking about speech timing. We find that early views centered on speech isochrony. The downfall of these approaches is sketched as they are challenged by other perspectives on speech timing that feature segmented durations instead of isochronous rhythms. Following this overview, a second section revives rhythmic features of speech prosody, including time hierarchies. This endeavor recognizes multiple rhythms that are hypothesized to serve as driving rhythms in an entrainment framework.

A third section unpacks this framework. It proposes that some meter-like properties abide in speech production, as expressed by (hidden) attractor ratios. This is followed by a section reviving entrainment constructs such as oscillator clusters, based on traditional mode-locking, and attractor profiles, based on transient mode-locking. Together, both concepts are among a set of entrainment tools that apply to spontaneous speech. A final section returns to the challenging issues surrounding the parsing speech to highlight the "right" attractors. Accordingly, a new way of describing prosodic grouping extends entrainment rules, outlined in the preceding chapter, to introduce additional grouping rules in speech.

BACKGROUND: SPEECH RHYTHMS

Prosody typically expresses the surface timing of speech created by a flow of syllables and words. And, somehow, prosodic timing allows us to perceptually pluck out, from this flow, groupings that we term syllables and words. But what marks these groups? What holds them together? And how does timing enter this picture? To address these and related questions, let us begin with simply identifying some prosodic timing features that arguably exist in different forms, across linguistic categories.

Speech Rate

The rate of speaking, roughly indexed by syllables per second, is a fundamental feature of all languages, although it differs with dialect, age, and other factors.[6,7,8] Syllable- and mora-based languages have faster speaking rates than stress-based languages. Nevertheless talking rate is a fairly basic property.

Temporal Distribution of Stressed Sounds

In stress-based languages, some syllables are more prominent, via *stress* (**S**), than others.[9] In syllable-timed languages, such as Spanish (mostly consonant-vowel-consonant [CVC], CV syllables), stress is distributed evenly over all syllables, whereas in stress-based languages, such as English (which adds CVCC and CCVCs to CVC, CV syllables), stress markers are more likely to land on CVCs than on CVs.

Marker Density

Syllable-timed (and mora-timed) languages typically feature a single prominent timing level based on strings of similar syllables (with few stress markers). By contrast, in so-called stress-based languages there exist putative identifiable time markers of different timing levels (e.g., syllables or morae, words, phrases).

Group Size

Lengths of prosodic groups (i.e., syllables, words) vary with linguistic culture. In stress-based languages, groups of syllables rarely exceed four or five syllables, whereas groups in the faster, syllable-based languages contain up to six or seven syllables (or more).

Together, these four properties offer touchstones for distinguishing among world languages. They summarize general constraints that must be considered by any universal theory of speech timing. A successful theory must include mechanisms that flexibly accommodate these properties.

Isochrony Theories

An early theory of speech timing embraced a strict conception of isochrony. Moreover, the first isochrony hypothesis addressed speech production, maintaining that isochrony holds across all spoken languages based on different, culture-specific prosodic units of fixed duration (e.g., interstress interval, syllable, or mora).

Many reviews document the checkered history of this early isochrony hypothesis.[10,11,12] Original attempts to explain speech timing appealed to temporal regularities of stressed syllables.[13] This idea stipulates that a universal temporal invariant exists, evident in the produced speech of any language. This invariant is a *tendency toward producing isochrony*.

These theories assumed that time markers are specific to a given linguistic culture, differing, respectively, in categories of stress-based, syllable-timed, and mora-timed. As a linguistic time marker, stress is variously realized as a lengthened duration and/or heightened intensity. In stress-based languages, such as English, objective time markers putatively outline *almost* equal interstress time spans (e.g., a metric foot, as in a *strong–weak* trochee). By contrast, in syllable-timed languages, such as French, time markers correspond to syllable onsets; hence, all syllable durations show a tendency to be equal. Mora-timed languages follow suit, with morae functioning much as syllables, hence determining an almost constant speech rate. Thus, the original isochrony hypothesis assumed speakers in any linguistic culture regulated their vocal productions *in the direction of* isochrony.[14]

Finally, early isochrony theories included the important constraint that meaningful speech timing derives from, at most, *two* stimulus time scales. Thus, in syllable-timed languages, such as French, a single time level of syllables is proposed. However, English was allowed two time levels where stress points outlined group time spans and intervening (briefer) syllables supplied the second time scale.

Historically, isochrony theories faced justifying the role of temporal regularity of pertinent time markers in a given language. Thus, in English, a constant interstress interval is a given; this should constrain the productions of intervening syllables, which must be shortened or lengthened to preserve the isochrony of stressed sounds. Naturally, this invites the following question:

How Isochronous Are Produced Speech Rhythms?

A strong prediction of early isochrony theories maintained that strict isochrony applies to produced interstress intervals in English. Hence, intervening syllable durations of stress-based languages must expand or shrink to accommodate stress isochrony. Support for this prediction appeared in Allen's original demonstrations that people regularly tap, with low variability, to a perceived beat in a spoken utterance.[15,16,17] Other research, also based on tapping to spoken passages, confirms the regularity of tapping to heightened intensity (stress) points.[18,19] These studies clearly reveal the influence of "something" in a speech signal that approximates isochrony.

Such findings were compelling. But they did not firmly nail down isochrony. In fact, subsequently troublesome statistical evidence revealed significant temporal variability of stress time markers across cultures. Although no guidelines stipulate what is "too much" marker variability, later research[20] indicates remarkable variability in both syllables and interstress intervals across different languages. For instance, instead of finding fixed interstress intervals, measured time intervals in English typically increase distinctly with the number of intervening unstressed syllables.[21,22,23,24,25,26] A telling road-block came with the following finding concerning direct assessments of produced time spans between stressed markers: Each increase in the number of intervening unstressed syllables (i.e., in an interstressed interval) added 110 ms to the speaker's interstress interval in English.[27] Similar problems occur with syllable- or mora-timed speech.[28,29,30] Such findings make it implausible that a simple isochrony hypothesis explains all classes of world rhythms.

In sum, surface time patterns reveal sizeable statistical variability in culture-specific time markers (stress, syllables, morae). Although the use of conventional statistical tools in assessing timing can be questioned, these findings remain problematic for any isochrony hypothesis.

Isochrony Theory Reconsidered

The challenge to early isochrony hypotheses posed by statistical variations in speech timing added urgency to questions about speech time markers and their regularity. Originally, isochrony hypotheses held that people who produce speech exhibit *motor biases* favoring the production of regular time markers. Yet it remains possible that, instead, listeners are actually *perceptually predisposed to isochrony*. In other words, people tend to *perceive* speech as isochronous by simply ignoring various timing deviations. This was the reasoning of Ilse Lehiste, who reformulated the original isochrony theory to posit that *listeners have a bias for hearing isochrony* even in speech

with distinctively varied timing. In other words, rhythmic regularity is in the head of a perceiver.

Consistent with this view, very young infants show orienting predispositions to isochrony.[31,32,33,34] This suggests that newborns who cannot produce rhythmic utterances remain somehow perceptually wired to isochrony. Also, classic findings of Demany and colleagues[35] confirm that 2-month-old infants distinguish isochronous from non-isochronous rhythms in nonspeech acoustic patterns.

In 1977, Ilse Lehiste tackled this puzzle in a now famous article, titled "Isochrony Reconsidered."[36] She eloquently argued for *a perceptual bias toward isochrony* while squarely confronting accumulated evidence of objective temporal variability in motor-generated stress-based time markers. Acknowledging produced motor biases, she nevertheless maintained that listeners tend to *perceive* speech as isochronous, given irregularly produced utterances. To this point, Lehiste provided data from a time judgment task where listeners had to identify the single "different" time in a sequence of four intervals (speech or nonspeech). Listeners' poor performance supported her conclusion that people simply *do not perceive spoken deviations from isochrony*.[37]

In sum, the sense of rhythmicity we experience is real according to Lehiste. She maintained that isochrony is in the head of a perceiver, not in an acoustic signal, a position shared by the Gestalt psychologist Stephen Handel.[38] This view differs drastically from the original isochrony theory rooted in motor production.

More Theories: Time Hierarchies

Another perspective entered the picture around this time with James Martin's claim that many more than two time layers of speech rhythms are operative.[39] He advanced the idea of speech time hierarchies in which fast isochronous rhythms are recursively embedded in slower ones, an idea found also in early entrainment theories.[40,41] Furthermore, Martin's marker salience (MS) rule holds that stronger (more salient) markers tend to outline relatively longer time spans in a hierarchy of different time spans, as suggested in Figure 12.1.

Recently, the idea of speech time hierarchy has been strengthened. A creative adaptation of Fourier decompositions of ordinary speech utterances revealed a wide range of different quasi-isochronous speech periodicities. Keith Johnson and Sam Tilsen termed this discovery a *rhythm spectrum*.[42] This concept is further enriched by other research

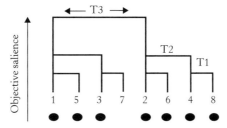

A rhythmic time hierarchy
Adapted from James Martin (1972)

Marker strength: Highest for markers 1 and 2; lowest for markers 7 and 8.

FIGURE 12.1 A rhythmic time hierarchy for speech proposed by James Martin. Three different stimulus time levels (T1, T2, T3) reflect component periodicities marked by accents of respectively different strengths.

Adapted from James G. Martin, "Rhythmic (Hierarchical) Versus Serial Structure in Speech and Other Behavior," *Psychological Review* 79, no. 6 (1972): 487–509, doi:10.1037/h0033467.

that decomposes surface timing of complex speech waveforms using filtered speech techniques which isolate different periodicities ranging from 12 ms to more than 2 seconds embedded in acoustic speech signals.[43,44,45,46] A sampling of this research, summarized in Table 12.1, shows stimulus periods modulated by fluctuations of different time markers, notably frequency modulations (FM) and/or amplitude modulations (AM), correlated with various speech time levels (e.g., phonemes, syllables, etc.).

Time Hierarchies

The concept of time hierarchies in produced speech moves the theoretical discussion into an entirely different theater. Instead of one or two semi-regular speech rhythms, this concept implicates a wide range of rhythmic components, each with a distinct (average) rate. Certainly, limiting candidate levels of temporal regularity to two or fewer is no longer feasible given the range of rates summarized in Table 12.1.

But not all time hierarchies are alike. Time hierarchies have been conceived in different ways. One approach advances the idea that these newly discovered speech rhythms serve as potential driving rhythms within an entrainment framework. However, it is also possible that the array of different time spans in Table 12.1 simply reflect different, important prosodic segments.

Mehler and colleagues[47] have advanced the latter view. That is, each time scale in such a hierarchy reflects a discrete duration of a particular prosodic segment (phoneme, syllable) with edges defined by distinctive markers. In other words, time hierarchies are built on discrete

speech segments and not on recurring rhythmic periods.[48,49] For instance, with English vowel intonations, specific edges distinguish verb from noun segments. This is not an uncommon view of timing in that it focuses upon individual speech segments, extracted from their surrounding context. These segments are shown to be variously outlined by distinctive prosodic features which then "bootstrap" listeners' percepts of speech timing early in life.

Bootstrapping ideas, formalized by Ramus and colleagues, explain newborns' reactions to sentences of different linguistic rhythms.[50] They formulated the *Proportional Vowel Time* (PVT) model that statistically differentiates codes of short consonants from those of longer vowel segments. Specifically, in a sentence, the proportion of total vowel durations is gauged relative to the variance of consonant durations. The resulting PVT metric successfully predicts infants' differentiation of linguistic categories. And, because various PVT scores fall along a continuum, such models also support claims that speech timing is not adequately described by three strictly defined linguistic categories (e.g., stress-timed, syllable-timed, mora-timed).

But . . . Where's the Rhythm?

Reponses to such PVT models raise questions about statistical coding which fails to capture rhythmic structure and/or rhythm perception. Rhythmic structure, whether isochronic, trochaic, iambic, or otherwise plays only an indirect role in the PVT metric.[51,52,53] In fact, Arvaniti[54] has questioned the PVT metric of the prosodic bootstrapping approach (i.e., as well as similar

TABLE 12.1 MULTIPLE TIME SCALES: A SELECTIVE SAMPLING OF CANDIDATE DRIVING RHYTHMS IN SPEECH

Filtered Rhythms: Rates and Time Markers

Hierarchical level	Rate	Time marker	
Speech correlate	Time scale	Intensity Amplitude Modulation	Frequency Frequency modulation
Phonemes (consonants)	12–20 ms (gamma)	50–80 Hz*	60–80 Hz
Phonemes (vowels/formant transitions)	20–60 ms (beta)	17–50 Hz*	25–40 Hz[X]
Short syllables	60–125 ms (alpha)	8–17 Hz[*X]	8–15 Hz
Long syllables	125–200 ms (theta)	5–8 Hz[*X]	5–8 Hz
Rhymes	200–500 ms (theta)	2–5 Hz[*X·]	2–5 Hz*
Words	500–2000 ms (delta)	.5–2 Hz[*X·]	.5–2 Hz*

• Elliot and Theunissen,[162] Ding and Simon,[163]
• Drullman, Festen and Plomb[164,165]

metrics, such as nPVI and rPVI of Grabe and Low[55]) for failing to express important rhythmic differences among languages (e.g., Bulgarian, English, vs. German).

Finally, the allure of isochrony may live on—but in different forms. Clearly, a simple version of the isochrony hypothesis is insufficient. Perhaps new perspectives, inspired by filtered speech findings, can explain the function of various speech rhythms. Such an approach to time hierarchies is considered in the next section.

Summary of Speech Rhythms

Major points of this section are:

- Classic categories of linguistic rhythms suggest differences in culture-specific speaking rates and metric-like time layers in speech timing, but category boundaries may overlap.
- Shortcomings appear both in early theories of isochrony and in those contemporary theories that eschew rhythmic patterns in favor of statistical codes.
- Some approaches assume that prosodic features outline discrete segments in speech timing.

PROSODIC TIME RELATIONS AND ENTRAINMENT

The remainder of this chapter unwraps a dynamic attending approach to speech timing. In this, time hierarchies are recognized as expressing many different speech-driving rhythms. Accordingly, the theoretical emphasis shifts to focus to the potential that prosodic rhythms may have for entraining related neural rhythms in listeners' tunable brains.

This dynamic attending approach shares an important assumption with prosodic bootstrapping hypotheses. Both assume that running speech is shaped, in part, by prosodic contours (i.e., *prelexical*) features. However, in Dynamic Attending Theory (DAT), these features are not edges; instead, they involve the time markers of periods of exogenous driving rhythms. This theory assumes that multiple driving rhythms of various rates and degrees of fuzziness abide in speech as real functional rhythms. Together, these rhythms deliver comprehensible utterances aimed at maximizing communication. The goal of communication invites parallelism between speaker and listener. As discussed in Chapter 8, parallelism refers to the shared tendencies of speakers and listeners who rely on similar prosodic constraints for producing and attending to speech signals. Moreover, parallelism between a speaker's production profile and a listener's expectancy profile implies that a *person who is speaking can voluntarily influence (i.e., shape) a listener's entrainment to the speaker's produced rhythms.*

More About Time Markers

Time hierarchies reveal multiple speech rhythms, as the prolific research of David Poeppel has convincingly established.[56,57,58] And, if we assume that these speech rhythms function as exogenous driving rhythms across different time scales in an entrainment framework, then it is useful to identify potential time markers of relevant stimulus periods. Although admittedly tricky, clues to such time markers appear in Table 12.1, which features prominent roles for modulations of amplitude (AM) and frequency (FM). Both modulations mark out onsets of salient markers of driving rhythms at time scales ranging from 12 ms (phonemes) to 2 sec (words). Criteria suggested by the general attending hypothesis merely stipulate that these stimuli carry effective driving rhythms (as *zeitgebers*) when objectively salient (forceful) and roughly regular in time (Chapter 8). Other caveats may involve species-specific and domain-specific features for certain rhythms.[59]

The many fast and slow rhythms summarized in speech hierarchies are components filtered out of a more complex acoustic signal of an utterance. Decomposing this envelope leads to individual driving rhythms, which differ in overall rate and in the nature of fluctuating time markers. Arguably, identifying these distinct levels of driving rhythms in speech is only part of an entrainment story. Driving rhythms, as part of dyadic entrainment, implicate driven rhythms as oscillations specific to different hierarchical levels. Emerging research on cortical speech rhythms, although mostly in theta and delta ranges, nonetheless confirms that specific entrainments of cortical oscillations transpire over time scales ranging from phonemic, syllabic, and word levels within overall speech envelopes.[60,61,62]

Syllables and Speaking Rate

Of special interest is one component rhythm in the speech signal, specifically that involving syllable rate. Among other component rhythms of a speech envelope is the rhythm of syllables that determines a speaker's talking rate. Speaking rate not only varies with speaker, it changes throughout a speaker's utterance, slowing or speeding up to shape a communicative tempo response curve, as described in Chapter 8. Nevertheless, despite such variability, average syllable rate (i.e., articulation rate) is around 200 ms (i.e., in the theta range; Table 12.1).[63]

Especially pertinent is the role that strings of syllables play for a listener. Articulation rate has long been recognized for its normalizing role in speech.[64] In this spirit, we might assume that this driving rhythm offers a referent period against which other concurrent driving rhythms are gauged (whether faster and slower). In a rough analogy with music, speaking tempo functions as a tactus for listeners. However, unlike music, the range and diversity of speaking rate of fuzzy speech rhythms is less crafted; speech is more spontaneous than music. And, extending this hypothesis implies that each of us carries our own, speaker-specific

talking rhythm. In this respect, syllable rate serves an important normalizing function. At the same time, to the extent that talking rate supplies a referent periodicity, its modest fluctuations (within the theta band) will be adaptively tracked by listeners. This idea is buttressed by recent magnetoencephalography (MEG) studies revealing the entrainment of neural oscillations to speech segments in frequency-following, with phase patterns of theta band neural oscillations.[65,66,67]

Problems with P-Centers

One complicating issue in this story arises in calibrating syllable timing (i.e., articulation rate). At first glance, it might seem that intensity changes at the onset of an initial consonant (when present) in a syllable functions as a time marker. But much evidence suggests that actually the initial vowel in a syllable levies a strong impact on the functional time marker. For instance, in a laboratory utterance of syllables such as *mad-glad-mad-glad*, listeners often do not "hear" syllable onsets beginning with onsets of consonants. Instead, the effective time markers of successive CVC or CCVC syllables are often marked by distinctive frequencies of the vowel; such markers have been termed perceptual-centers or *P-centers*. Originally discovered by Morton and colleagues,[68] research on P-centers suggests that onsets of nuclear vowels often function as syllable time markers. Experimental protocols have verified the salience of such vowel onsets in adults tapping to alternating monosyllables.[69] People, and even pre-babbling infants, successfully produce isochrony based on estimated P-centers.[70,71,72,73,74,75,76]

Finally, the import of P-center markers is underscored in a study that used listeners' phase-correction responses to index P-centers: "without knowledge of P-centers, the rhythm of spoken language cannot be measured accurately, and thus questions about the perceived timing of individual languages can be answered only on the basis of flawed or indirect data at best."[77[p.1615]]

It is difficult to disagree with this humbling dictum. Yet uncertainty remains regarding the objective (physical) correlates of subjectively salient P-centers.[78,79] In fact, a single phonemic feature (e.g., fundamental frequency, spectral harmonies, intensity) is unlikely to define P-centers. Nevertheless, following Cummins and Port,[80] let us assume that the best estimate of a syllable time marker is the onset of the first vowel (specifically a local spot of maximal energy of low frequencies). Adding to this, Doelling et al. found that a marker's "sharpness" (i.e., this objective salience is indexed by relatively large and rapid changes in an amplitude envelope) facilitates the entrainment of a related oscillation with this stimulus periodicity in the acoustic signal.[81]

Stress Beats

Stress beats mark out a different component speech rhythm in acoustic signals. These are time markers with greater salience conveyed by heightened energy. Following the MS rule, stress beats outline slower driving rhythms than syllables.[82] They differ physically from syllable markers as they are based largely on timed intensity modulations; hence, they project heightened loudness of certain syllables, as demonstrated by Kochanski and colleagues.[83]

Kochanksi and Orphanidou[84] asked people to repeat brief phrases (1,240 ms), such as "we always do", while aligning their vocal beats with metronome ticks (a 710 ms period). This created the waveform of Figure 12.2. Fluctuations of vocal intensity within this amplitude envelope translate into a series of *local loudness contrasts* (via a psychophysical function).[85] For instance, a local region of maximal loudness appears for "al" (in *always*), in Figure 12.2. This clearly demonstrates that local loudness changes are subjectively salient correlates of objectively salient stress markers. They confirm findings that the interstress time

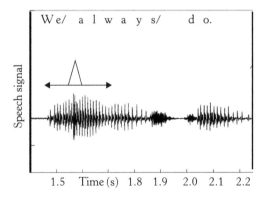

FIGURE 12.2 An example of the speech signal (audio waveform) for an experimental phrase "We always do" extracted from Kochanksi and Orphanidou (2008). Unlike the original figure, this figure omits certain features (e.g., spectral information). Here, a pulse outline is added to convey the gist of authors' complex loudness contrast algorithm.

Adapted from figure 10 in Greg Kochanski and Christina Orphanidou, "What Marks the Beat of Speech?," *The Journal of the Acoustical Society of America* 123, no. 5 (May 1, 2008): 2780–91, doi:10.1121/1.2890742.

scales which outline groups of syllables, are indeed longer than embedded time scales of syllables that carry an articulation rate (i.e., in the delta range).[86]

Finally, syllable and stress beat rhythms are two of many speech rhythms implicated in Table 12.1. To preview later discussions in this chapter, it is useful to remember that, as driving rhythms, all these rhythms are ideally outlined by objective time markers (identified in Table 12.1); hence, they automatically evoke in listeners reactive pulses. Yet, from a dynamic attending perspective, a 'fuzzy regularity' of time markers also invite entrainments. Driven rhythms emerge to support expectancies that tolerate occasional missing time markers, as silent expectancy pulses. That is, a dynamic attending account distinguishes stimulus-driven reactive pulses from internally driven expectancy pulses carried by an entraining driven rhythm.

Multiple Driving Rhythms: Dependent or Independent?

Taken together, syllable/vowel onsets and stress beats mark out two different speaker-specific time scales within a larger speech time hierarchy. Such acoustic markers may not always be prominent in ordinary speech, yet they remain critical to initial entrainment/learning. Especially useful in an utterance are the initial time markers of successive syllables as they highlight an important, referent driving rhythm. Let syllable time spans that specify a recurring referent time span be denoted by T_R (i.e. an external rhythm). By contrast, stress beats, which appear on *nonadjacent syllables*, carve out longer, recurring stimulus time spans, such as phrases, which are denoted by T_{RM}. Both these external quasi-periodicities meet criteria for salient time markers as *zeitgebers*. In short, both these speech rhythms qualify as critical, exogenous, driving rhythms in an entrainment framework.

Next, let us describe the production profile of a speaker (from Chapter 8). It entails two or more produced driving rhythms. It is important to note that these rhythms are not only speaker-specific, but they are typically fuzzy rhythms due to natural fluctuations vulnerable to modulations based on both involuntary and voluntary factors. Nevertheless, the DAT claim is that such fuzzy rhythms can nonetheless *implicate* coherent timing relations. For instance, the stress rhythm with a period of T_{RM} typically only *approximates* some multiple of T_R where T_R represents speaking rate.

To flesh out the function of speaking rate as a referent supplied by a speaker, let us assume that this stimulus periodicity elicits/entrains a driven rhythm in a listener. Here, for a listener such a speech context sets in motion a driven rhythm as a cortical oscillation with a latent period, $p_R \sim T_R$. In this scenario, a listener's p_R carries syllable-timed expectancy pulses. Support for such tracking behaviors at the speaking rate level by neural oscillations is found in the research of Lou and Poeppel who recorded MEG patterns of auditory cortical responses of a listener responding to a fluctuating syllable rhythm (theta band) within a spoken sentence.[61] Related behavioral support for this view shows that a speaker's articulation rate activates timed neural expectancies in listeners.[87,88,89,90,91]

In theory, similar entrainments apply to rhythms other than a speaker's referent rhythm. For example, in addition to automatically entraining a listener to his talking rate, a speaker producing a sentence naturally also creates slower rhythms, such as one with the recurring longer time spans of T_{RM}, marked by a stressed syllables. Together with talking rate, the T_{RM} rhythm also automatically entrains a listener by exogenously phase-locking with resonant slower oscillations. Indeed, from a dynamic attending perspective at both time scales, the fluctuations of external rhythms in a speaker's productions are automatically accommodated by a listener's corresponding neural driven rhythms, given entrainment limits.

This scenario offers an interesting validation of the phenomenon known as *speaker accommodation*. Speaker accommodation refers to a curious parallelism often observed between speaker and listener wherein one speaker unintentionally gravitates to *match* the speaking rate of another. This phenomenon is a clear and simple illustration of entrainment at work.[92,93]

Summary of Prosodic Time Relations and Entrainment

In sum, two prominent exogenous time scales with different prosodic time markers (syllable markers, stressed beats) have been enlisted to illustrate, respectively, driving rhythms of speaking rate and stress intervals. In theory, speaker-produced periodicities guide a listener's attending to future time markers in a speaker's speech. Ultimately, this story becomes more complicated, and interesting, with the discovery of still more exogenous driving rhythms.

Major points in this section are:

- Time hierarchies raise the possibility of multiple, quasi-isochronous, exogenous driving rhythms in ordinary speech.

- A dynamic attending approach assumes at least two exogenous driving rhythms figure in real speech, one based on the articulation rate of a speaker and the other based on the timing of stress beats.

PRODUCTION PROFILES AND METRICAL SPEECH: RESEARCH OF ROBERT PORT

In ordinary speech, phrases such as "Butter cream freezes well," figure into real conversational exchanges.[94] Somehow, the complex timing of this production profile allows listeners to track such speaker productions. The current section begins to address the "nuts and bolts" of this process. It concentrates on a basic element in speech production profiles: the relative timing of attractors.

Yes. Fuzzy speech rhythms indeed do hide attractors. Robert Port describes his discovery of this. He noticed that whenever a speaker continuously repeats a short fuzzy phrase (e.g., "Buy your friend a sandwich"), the initial fuzziness begins to slip away as the speaker's utterance falls into one of several patterns with highly simplified time relationships.[95] Basically, Port suspected that metric attractors hide beneath fuzzy speech. So he and his colleagues developed a *recycling task* wherein speakers repeated speech phrases such as "Big for a duck."[86]

Although this task simplifies speech productions, Port rightly observed that, in science, the simplest cases are portals to fundamental mechanisms. He argued that mechanisms underlying speakers' production profiles are best revealed when people recite memorized phrases as in "Hail, Mary full of grace," which fall into a duple meter frame. Or, when people read aloud word lists or speak to children. Port argued that generally repetitive speech encourages a reliance on universal (but hidden) speaking mechanisms.[96,97] Thus, recycling a phrase pushes a speaker to rely on vital regularities that ground produced speech.

Speech Production Profiles and Traditional Mode-Locking Protocols

A recycling task invented by Cummins and Port aimed to capture people's attraction to attractors. In ordinary speech, the "pure" harmonic ratios of meter are sporadic, largely due to a lack of repetition. However, in a recycled phrase, such as "big for a duck," the emergence of a simple time ratio, based on n:m = 1:2, emerges from repetitions as a speaker regularizes the timing of strong–weak

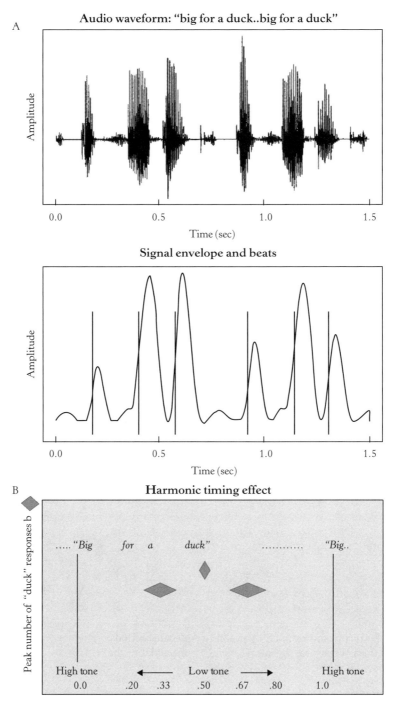

FIGURE 12.3 **(A)** Auditory waveform (top) and signal envelop with beats (bottom) for "Big for a duck" phrase reprinted from a study by Cummins and Port. **(B)** An adaptation of speech production paradigm/results designed to study the harmonic timing effect (see text for details).

Adapted from figure 1 in Fred Cummins and Robert Port, "Rhythmic Constraints on Stress Timing in English," *Journal of Phonetics* 26, no. 2 (April 1998): 145–71, doi:10.1006/jpho.1998.0070.

stresses. The resulting production profile contains two stimulus-driving rhythms (T_R, T_{RM}) that, together, create a duple meter. Waveforms from this phrase (and its smoothed amplitude envelope) appear in Figure 12.3A. In ordinary (i.e., fuzzy) speech, relevant attractors are typically hidden by the shape of a tempo response curve as well as by spontaneous fluctuations in speaking rate. By contrast, the task Port and Cummins devised minimizes (and controls), but does not eliminate such sources of fuzziness Figure 12.3.

Speakers repeatedly produced phrases similar to "Big for a duck." Both articulation rate and the slower cycle time period appear in a simplified format in Figure 12.3B. The acoustic waveform in panel A reflects this four-syllable phrase; it comprises components of two different time scales, one for speaking rate (T_R), the other for cycle time (T_{RM}) (i.e., a recurring stressed syllable group). Theoretically, a salient frame happens when $T_{RM} \sim nT_R$ (n is a small integer). Group time spans (T_{RM}), initially marked by high (H) tones, varied randomly over trials (1.0–2.33 sec) whereas articulation rate, T_R, initially marked by low tones (L), assumed one of two fixed values (T_R = 700 ms or 450 ms). Speakers began by synchronizing their utterance with "Big" (high tones) and "duck" (low tones), then continued speaking without tones. Cycle spans for relative phases (.20–.80 of cycle span) are determined for a given referent (articulation) rate.

As shown in Figure 12.3, people's produced speech gravitated to simple time ratios between cycle span (T_{RM}) and speaking rate (T_R) with phase alignments of "Big" relative to "duck." Most interesting is the strong tendency to produce "duck" halfway through a cycle period (i.e., phase of .50), thus highlighting a dependence on *simple duple meter attractors* of 1:2 (.50). Although clear tendencies toward the 1:3 attractor (.33, .67) are evident in Figure 12.3B (flatten darker gray rectangles, normalized to cycle span), the duple meter attractor (1:2) appears dominant. Variability (rectangle width) was lowest for the simplest (1:2) metric attractor. Cummins and Port termed this production profile the *harmonic timing effect*.

Port's discovery of these neat production profiles has broad implications. It shows that tendencies for specific dependencies among driving rhythms are based on synchronous relationships. Generalizing, this suggests that listeners in speaker–listener dyads are biased in favor of certain time ratios produced when a talker's stress rhythm cycle is one, two, or three times the articulation period of this speaker. Attractors are also evident in other motor productions, as famously modeled by Haken, Kelso, and Bunz (HKB).[98,99] Kelso's dynamical approach features a model of relative phase biases for bimanual gestures (two fingers), where attractor ratios (0, .50) describe favored finger configurations.

Multiple Driving Rhythms of Production Profiles

Port's seminal work reinforces the idea that at least two exogenous speech rhythms are at play in speech (i.e., syllable-based and stress-based driving rhythms). Yet a reliance on recycling techniques prompts concerns about the degree to which such tasks capture "real" (i.e., spontaneous) speech. After a few repetitions of the monosyllables "What's up doc?" even Bugs Bunny loses his charm. Arguably, more realistic time patterns side-step recycling in favor of stringing together various monosyllables with disyllables and trisyllables.

In pursuing this topic, Samuel Tilsen and colleagues used ordinary, noncycled, speech phrases in search of uncovering multiple driving rhythms.[100,101,102] For example, Tilsen and Arvaniti[103] used sophisticated filtering techniques to decompose complex but natural speech utterances into several component driving rhythms (e.g., sentences such as "ever went to the electric chair that they . . . "). These produced phrases expressed greater variability than the simpler, cycled ones used by Cummins and Port. Nevertheless, they could be decomposed into multiple layers of component rhythms hidden beneath the surface envelope.

Tilsen and Arvaniti recovered a number of potential driving rhythms despite nonstationary (fluctuating) components. Of special interest are two different time levels indicating, respectively, the production of a syllable-paced rhythm, T_R, and a slower production delivering a stress-timed rhythm, T_{RM}. Finally, they also isolated stretches of meter-like timing (n:m) relationships involving different driving periods.[104] These discoveries are important in validating the presence of multiple rhythmic time scales (and their interactions) hidden in the surface structure of normal speech. They converge with claims of a hierarchy of speech time scales.[105]

Finally, it is useful to remember that time hierarchies in speech, at least with respect to speech productions, imply that multiple individual rhythmic components are interdependent (i.e., they comply with relative timing constraints). This is most evident in the recycling tasks of Cummins and Port, among others. These discoveries support hypotheses about compelling, but hidden, time relationships among speech-driving rhythms, relationships that serve as guiding time constraints although obscured by normal speaking fluctuations. Of course, these constraints are rather abstract (i.e., they are attractors). In sum, speech production profiles are based on two major factors: attractor configurations and referent articulation rates.

Summary of Production Profiles and Metrical Speech

In sum, these studies illustrate that produced driving rhythms in a speaker–listener dyad have the potential to induce parallel driven rhythms in the tunable brain of a listener. Listeners exposed to such speech tend to align different oscillations with corresponding exogenous driving rhythms at respectively different time scales. Furthermore, we can assume that eventually the various, simultaneously active driven oscillations all endogenously lock to a, persisting referent oscillation.

From the perspective of an attender, it is fair to conclude that the speech patterns produced in the study of Cummins and Port invite in listeners a reliance on traditional mode-locking, which leads to the formation of *metrical speech clusters*. Applying this idea to explain listeners' attending to truly spontaneous speech remains a future challenge. But, as Port notes, "My hunch is that these attractors remain relevant in all speech although their effects are most clearly seen in simple repetitive speech."[106] Port's hunch may be correct.

The major points in this section are:

- Speech production profiles comprise multiple exogenous driving rhythms embedded in amplitude envelopes; two such rhythms are marked, respectively, by vowel onsets and stressed beats.
- Controlled speaking productions exhibit metric relationships between different produced driving rhythms; namely, between a fast articulatory driving rhythm and a slower, stress-based driving rhythm.
- Endogenous entrainments among multiple neural correlates, activated by different metric time scales, lead to *metrical speech clusters*.

PERCEIVING SPEECH TIMING: A CONTINUUM FROM METER TO RHYTHM

If ordinary speech is filled with many different time scales, as preceding sections imply, then we may expect to find a range of different driving rhythms embedded in casual conversations. A pertinent line of inquiry pursues questions about attending to natural, or spontaneous, speech. That is, to this point, the laboratory speech phrases outlined have been reasonably constrained to uncover hidden, meter-like relationships, as in the harmonic tuning effect. These phrases arise from production constraints that create simple metric time relationships with a tempo curve of fixed rate (i.e., a constant referent period). Consequently, listeners encountering such phrases tend to rely on metric clusters with fixed global attractors and stable referent oscillations.

By contrast, tackling the mysteries of ordinary speech perception is daunting. Not only is everyday speech normally filled with fuzzy rhythms, it is often rhythmically complex, involving coherent, but non-isochronous rhythmic patterns, as described in Chapters 7 and 8. Moreover, spontaneous speech not only reflects complex production profiles in which external referent rhythms—hence hypothesized—change over time, but these natural production profiles also ride on variations in speaking rate. That is, speech tempo curves of referent periods are not flat (i.e., speaking rate is not constant). On the other hand, the attractor relationships highlighted in the paradigm of Cummins and Port are essentially metrical ones. While metric attractors are sure to be found in patches of speech, it is also likely that between sporadic bursts of metrical timing are stretches of speech in which local attractors change and/or articulation rates varies. All this introduces subtle uncertainties in listeners about forthcoming driving rhythms in a speaker's utterance.

Imagine a speaker who utters a single, simple phrase. Such a phrase might be crafted to implicate a metrically constant (global) attractor together with a stable response tempo (unchanging referent period). In short, such a phrase is music-like in its metric properties. Consequently, this phrase occupies one end of a speech timing continuum that ranges from highly metrical to highly nonmetrical timing. Highly metrical phrases are ones that elicit a single metric cluster and perhaps one or two (possibly simple) global attractors depending upon the number of hierarchical levels involved. By contrast, highly nonmetrical speech passages elicit attractor profiles with a serial mixture of a number of different (possibly complex) local attractors. For instance, in the latter kind of speech passage, we might find a variety of different, intermingled syllable groups, including monosyllables, as disyllables and trisyllables of variable durations. In other words, the time structure of the former resembles a musical meter whereas that of the latter resembles timing characteristic of musical rhythms.

Two familiar properties figure into this continuum. First, at one end, simple meter-like configurations invite traditional mode-locking (i.e., with invariant driving rhythms), while at the opposite end of the continuum, complex time patterns maximize reliance on transient mode-locking (i.e., with variable driving rhythms). Second, the referent driving rhythm of production profile also figures in, creating both metric clusters (from traditional mode-locking) and attractor profiles (from transient mode-locking). However, this rhythm, too, is likely to vary, creating a tempo response curve with correlated expressive fuzziness (see Chapter 8).

Perceiving Meter in Speech

At the extreme metrical end of this hypothetical continuum are phrases with only meter-like attractor properties and constant tempo. These involve simpler phrases that supply examples of stress hierarchies or grids of speech prosody that are popular in linguistic theorizing.[107,108,109,110,111] However, linguistic hierarchies are distinguishable from the time hierarchies implied in Table 12.1 because they rely on abstract rules or syntactic constraints. For instance, Selkirk[112] carefully identifies multiple hierarchical levels ranging from syllables to phrases to sentences based on alignment rules (e.g., of pitch accents), but neither rhythm nor relative timing among hierarchical levels is accommodated. Although such linguistic approaches overlap in some ways with musical meters, they do not directly address metric timing and related synchronies.

Returning to speech continuum issues, let us situate true time hierarchies with simple timing relationships at the metrical end of this continuum, where it putatively describes the strongly metrical phrases/sentences that naturally happen in ordinary speech. This includes examples Cummins and Port have supplied. This continuum also describes meter-like relationships in ordinary speech reported by Lidji and colleagues.[113] They used Allen's classic tapping task[114] to study tapping to French and English sentences (articulation rates of T_R = 236 ms).[115] An example English sentence, "*Rats* and *mice* are *in* the *grass*, but *some* run *through* the *house*" shows stressed syllables (italicized). Quantifying listeners' production profiles revealed the impact of both syllabic rhythms, T_R, and stress-timed rhythms, T_{RM}, in English participants. English utterances are perceived as metrical with 1:2 and 1:4 attractors.

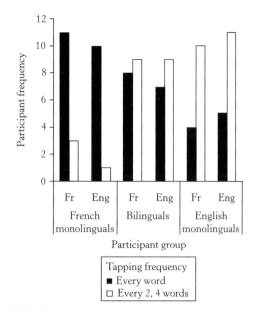

FIGURE 12.4. Results of tapping to French and English phrases by three groups of participants with different linguistic backgrounds.

Reproduced from Pascale Lidji et al., "Listeners Feel the Beat: Entrainment to English and French Speech Rhythms," *Psychonomic Bulletin & Review* 18, no. 6 (December 2011): 1035–41, doi:10.3758/s13423-011-0163-0.

However, French participants mainly tapped to the faster syllable-timed rhythms of French sentences, as shown in Figure 12.4 (implying n:m = 1:1 attractors). Generalizing, it is possible that languages differ not only in articulation (referent) rate, but also in preferred metric attractors. In sum, linguistic categories are defined, in part, by prevalent attractors.

From Meter to Rhythm in Speech

In a particular linguistic culture, a spoken phrase may fall somewhere along this imaginary continuum of temporal coherence, ranging from highly metrical to highly nonmetrical. Certainly classical poetry is likely to align with meter-like phrases. Poetic lines feature repeating rhythmic patterns, as evident in a famous bit of poetry children learn early in school that alternates weak and strong (**ws**) iambic syllables:

w S w S w S ... S w w .. S w   12.2
To be or not to be, that is the question

Spoken poetry inspires artistic license leading to interesting fuzzy rhythms that nonetheless hide a chosen metric frame (cf. Chapter 8). Creative pauses, usually between phrases, contribute to expressive tempo response curves that embellish attractors but do not banish them.

However, moving along this continuum, we encounter more complex phrases. For example, the phrase: "Big for a duck dressed elegantly in a tuxedo" exhibits a string of changing stimulus-driving rhythms created by a combination of monosyllables, disyllables, and trisyllables. As a result, this phrase is no longer precisely metrical. Nevertheless, such phrases schedule a series of different core time patterns: anapest, iambic, dactyl, and the like. These are the coherent but non-isochronous time patterns discussed at length in Chapter 7. They return us to contemplating coherent nonmetrical time patterns. Considering all such patterns allows us to pursue the idea that nonmetrical speech phrases are comprehensible whenever a series of changing driving rhythms approximates a coherent time pattern. This is because these rhythms invite transient mode-locking. Depending on a speaker's (admittedly flexible) assignment of stress to successive syllables, the transient mode locking protocol will deliver attractor profiles in speech that comprise various patterns of hidden local attractors (e.g.,

1:1, 1:2, 1:3, etc.). This assumes that the speaker's articulation rate realizes a driven periodicity that functions as a steady referent rhythm.

Transient mode-locking occurs with culture-specific, non-isochronous time patterns. Figure 12.5 illustrates two such patterns as anapest and dactyl rhythms (underlined). The anapest time pattern (short, short, long) is a non-isochronous time pattern, whereas the dactyl pattern, expressed as a strong-weak-weak stress sequence, is also non-isochronous, given the assumption that stress is expressed by temporal lengthening (e.g., long, short, short). In speech, just as a referent articulation rate (i.e., T_R) is critical to instilling metric clusters, so, too, such a referent facilitates the development of speech attractor profiles. That is, a listener tracking coherent time patterns in speech depends on attractor profiles of 1:2:1-1:1-1:1 (for the anapest rhythm) and 1:1-1:1-1:2 (for the dactyl rhythm). Again, this assumes that a roughly constant speaking rate, T_R, functions as a stable referent period for these serially changing driving rhythms. Of course, speaking rate differs with speakers; –some folks are naturally fast talkers, whereas others "take their time." Thus, stress-based time spans of produced phrases, when gauged

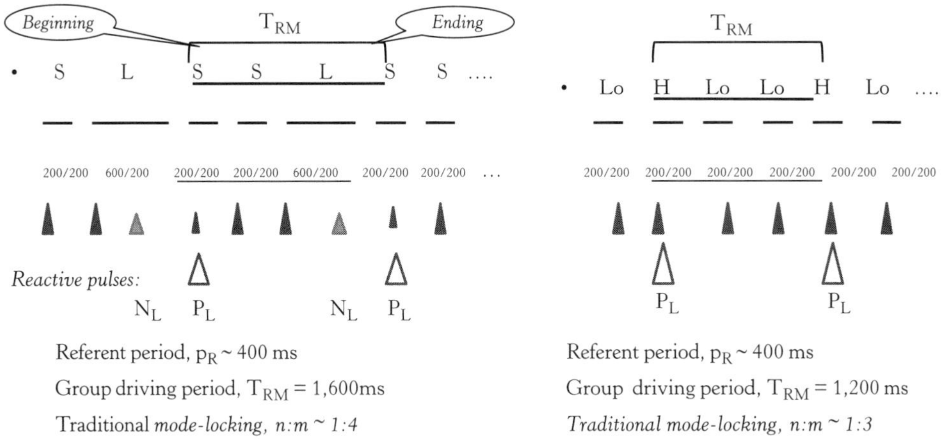

Rhythmic entrainment groups

FIGURE 12.5 Top rows shows the two *recurring* time patterns, each comprising three time spans, that are differently grouped (unbroken underline). The anapest rhythm is typically heard as ending with the lengthened time interval, L (due to linguistic stress). A recurring dactyl patter is isochronous, but it is typically heard as beginning with the stressed sound (higher intensity or frequency).

relative to a particular talking rate, lead to a series of simple attractors, given relatively simple stimulus time patterns. But, speaking rate can also fluctuate within a speaker (e.g., as a tempo response curve), a point to which we return.

To the extent that a culture's vocabulary is stocked with words comprising few syllables, a predominance of attractors involving the simple $nT_{RM}:mT_R$ relationship are likely wherein changes involve the driving rhythms, T_{RM}. For instance, a series of different driving rhythms may encourage listeners' reliance on transient mode-locking. Thus, a sentence like "This iron is horrible" comprises two monosyllabic words, one disyllable, and a trisyllable, thus implicating an attractor profile of 1:1 - 1:2 - 1:1 -1:3. This assumes a roughly constant speaking rate (T_R) based on syllable durations. Thus, the longer words (disyllable, trisyllable) have T_{RM} spans that hide attractors of 1:2 and 1:3 as they briefly grab a listener's attending during transient mode-locking. This results from entrainment tracking where T_R is expressed as an internal driven rhythm (with period $p_R \sim T_R$) that persists to briefly lock on to these successive external driving rhythms. Although this is a simple example, transient mode-locking extends to more complex attractor profiles with more complex attractors. All of this depends on the time pattern and hidden attractors. Still other, more interesting, complications interesting, complication when considering idiosyncrasies of speakers' tempo response curves.

Speech Structure: An Example

Recently, Ding and colleagues manipulated speech timing in a manner that touches on the distinction of metrical versus rhythmic patterning of timing in speech.[116] In one study, listeners heard sentences based on isochronous syllables in groups formed by repetitions of one, two, or four syllables presented in their own language and in a foreign language. All listeners showed cortical tracking (MEG) of talking rate (based on single syllables), implicating a referent oscillation with $p_R \sim T_R$. But only listeners familiar with the language showed additional neural tracking of sentences with higher (meter-like) levels of two- or four-syllable time spans. According to DAT, the latter finding provides evidence of a tacit reliance on traditional mode-locking, hence on meter-like oscillator clusters that are hierarchically linked, endogenously, with driving-to-driven ratios of 1:1, 1:2, and 1:4 of global attractors; these n:m estimates assume that the internalized periodicity

of the speaking rate (here, 4 Hz or 250 ms) serves as an internalized driven referent periodicity.

Ding and colleagues subsequently assessed listeners' responses to sentences containing words of variable durations (4–8 syllables, creating word durations of 250, 500, 1,000 ms). In this case, with continuous sentences, such as "Over the street is a museum," we expect to find evidence for transient mode-locking. Recorded listeners' responsive cortical activity (using electrocorticography [ECoG]) showed prominent neural activity in gamma and lower frequency activities (around the superior temporal gyrus). More relevant were lower frequencies distilled from a Fourier analysis of neural tracking of certain rhythms. Again, cortical activity emerged at the speaking rate level of 4 Hz. In addition, slower, related oscillatory frequencies of 2 and 1 Hz emerged.[117]

These findings also raise issues of intelligibility. They suggest that certain attractor patterns emerge when a listener is familiar with certain culture-specific time relationships, due to prior learning, with certain culture-specific time relationships. Of particular relevance is the fact that knowledge of a culture's grammar instills in a listener a predisposition to parse neutral (e.g., isochronous) sequences in certain culture-specific ways. This makes sense. Exposure frequency and binding cannot be ignored. Moreover, as these authors point out, linguistic predispositions are only loosely tied to acoustic cues or specific fluctuating frequencies. Instead, they are abstract. Indeed, following a DAT view, such acquired biases reflect states of synchrony described by attractors.

Summary of Speech Timing

In sum, a listener who confronts a speaker talking at an average rate will automatically track the acoustic signal based on the degree to which successive syllables or words elicit in this listener metric oscillator clusters (for speech meter) and/ or attractor profiles (for speech rhythm). This approach implies that we automatically greet successive time intervals with fleeting attending activities given basic entrainment constraints. This is not an unreasonable assumption considering that a listener's instant comprehension of a speaker's words, phrases, and sentences in conversations happens in the moment. Such an analysis also implies that a listener's attending relies on both traditional and transient mode-locking protocols as these weave into a listener's manner of entraining to various speech phrases.

The main point of this section holds that the production and perception of speech events rest on familiar entrainment concepts, which bend into action depending on the structural constraints of particular sound patterns.

Finally, there remains a hitch in this depiction of mode-locking associated with syllable groups (either in meter-like or rhythmic configurations). For instance, in previous examples, words, as groups of syllables, are expressed by *n:m* attractors. For instance, a two-syllable word is expressed as a 1:2 relationship, but these syllable pairs run together with surrounding syllables within fluent speech. That is, it remains unclear how this entraining system parses local attractors of successive syllables such that it highlights the "right" syllable groups. How does one know a repeating syllable *is* a repeating syllable? For instance, how does an entraining system "know" when a monosyllabic word (e.g., "this") ends and a new word "iron" begins or that "museum" is one word. Uncertainties about beginnings and endings of attractor groups invite an examination of the role of tempo response curves, a topic considered in the next section.

Major points in this section are:

- A continuum of speech timing relationships is based on the nature of relative timing, which ranges from highly metrical in music-like phrases to highly nonmetrical (patterned rhythms) in spontaneously spoken phrases.
- Meter-like constraints on speech lead to traditional mode-locking, with internal metric clusters and global attractors.
- Nonmetrical constraints arise from non-isochronous time patterns of spontaneous speech; these patterns invite transient mode-locking and attractor profiles.

PROSODIC GROUPS AND TEMPO RESPONSE CURVES

This final section returns to a prominent topic in speech timing, namely, *prosodic grouping*. Group perception was touched on in the preceding chapter in discussing the ups and downs of musical contour groups. This chapter (and the next) expand on this topic by considering ways in which superficial prosodic features in speech (e.g., intensity, timing) promote parsing of produced attractor profiles.

This section also revives the topic of tempo response curves. A speaker who cleverly speeds and slows his tempo response curve often creates

interesting, and systematic, variability among successive time spans (cf. Chapter 8). As in music, in speech, tempo response curves influence listeners' ability to group local attractors that figure in attractor profiles. For instance, in a typical speech production profile we may find words that implicate one, two, or three different local attractors, but lacking superficial changes in produced intensity and timing, it is not clear how a listener will parse a series of local attractors to correctly perceive the appropriate syllable groups for different words. How does a listener know one word ends and the next starts, given an attractor profile? People need cues to highlight beginnings and endings of successive attractor sets.

A dynamic attending approach to this problem appeals to surface features of speech, features that signal beginnings and endings of groups (of certain hidden attractors). The idea is simple: a speaker involuntarily (or sometimes voluntarily) signals a forthcoming beginning or ending of group by subtly modulating properties of stimulus-driving rhythms, including articulation rate. In theory, these modulations arise from superficial fluctuations either in the speech envelop or in the articulation rate or both. From a listener's perspective, this means that perceived prosodic groups will depend on certain properties of exogenous driving rhythms. Here we illustrate this idea using articulation rate. Finally, although it likely that certain patterns of tempo response curves are acquired or are culture-specific, we keep this discussion simple by focusing on a few illustrative examples.

Historically speech prosody and group segmentation have not been explained using entrainment principles. Instead, popular explanations of grouping percepts in speech dwell on segmentations based on lexical properties that are proposed to determine discrete speech units such as syllables and words. Therefore, a brief overview provides some necessary background.

A Segmentation Hypothesis: A Lexical View

Anne Cutler and Dennis Norris[118] argued that a lexical process accounts for perceptual speech segmentations. They proposed that strong (stressed) syllables in words trigger a listener's access to a mental lexicon. And, because accessing the lexicon takes time, a segmenting pause emerges. Furthermore, stressed syllables in English motivate this lexical segmenting heuristic: "Insert a word boundary before a strong syllable and assume what follows is a word." Thus, in a word recognition task that requires detection of real words, a word such as *mint* is shown within a connected string of nonsense syllables, as in *mintayve*. A listener typically experiences a pause that segments this disyllable word into two strong syllables (*min* and *tayve*).[119] However, such segmenting is absent in the word *mintesh* because only the initial syllable (*mint*) is strongly stressed.[120] A flood of related hypotheses ensued attributing such felt pauses to the segmenting effects of semantic cues, linguistic knowledge, and lexical competitions.[121,122,123] In fact, some have pitted lexical primes of embedded words against prosodic primes to support a lexical cuing position.[124] Others, using phoneme monitoring tasks ("listen for 'p' as in please") concluded that manipulations of driving rhythms (i.e., as in relative timing of stresses) had no significant effect on attending[125]

Eventually, the tide turned on the issue of timed attending. Subsequent phoneme-monitoring studies indicated a powerful role for contextual timing of stressed sounds.[126,127,128] Also, Zheng and Pierrehumbert[129] found that listeners are more accurate in detecting lengthening of stressed (vs. unstressed) syllables in running speech where contexts were based on iambic, trochaic, and dactyl rhythms.[130] Converging support for the influence of contextual driving rhythms (vs. lexical or semantic factors) continues to accumulate.[131,132,133,134]

Prosodic context is a critical variable. According to DAT, such contexts establish a speaker's opening articulation rate. This referent driving rhythm sets in motion related expectancies in listeners.[135] Speaking rate has long been a topic of interest for its normalizing function and long-lasting effects on perception.[136,137,138,139] Indeed, Gary Kidd and colleagues discovered that a speaker's articulation rate is one of several related rhythms that form listeners' expectancies.[140,141] Although the speaking rate of a talker may vary, it rarely shifts randomly. Instead, rate changes deliver systematic local modulations in timing and/or intensity that highlight meaningful groups. That is, speech rate variations reveal crafted tempo response curves with the potential for signaling the beginning and ends of prosodic groups, a process detailed later.

Grouping and the Iambic/Trochaic Law

Prosodic grouping cannot be discussed without acknowledging Woodrow's Iambic/Trochaic law, which provides one of psychology's most esteemed descriptions of determinants of grouping perceptions.[142,143] Although Woodrow

acknowledged inherent relative timing biases (e.g., in producing/perceiving groups of two or three tones), his law focuses on determinants of perceived beginnings and endings of tone groups (see Figure 12.5). He proposed that linguistic stress patterns: iambic (*weak–strong*) and trochaic (*strong–weak*) operate differently when considering continuously alternating stress patterns, as in *weak-strong-weak-strong* . . . . Specifically, if a recurring strong stress is defined *only* by increments in intensity (or frequency), it is perceived differently than a stressed sound defined only by a lengthened sound duration.[144]

The Iambic/Trochaic law stipulates that listeners presented with an unbroken recurring time pattern, as in . . . *long-short-long-short* . . . will hear *iambic* groups. That is, within this sequence, the perceived prosodic group is one that *ends* with the longer sound (i.e., not long-short). Figure 12.5 also illustrates this law with a continuously recurring (i.e., ambiguous) anapest pattern. Despite its ambiguity, this sequence is also uniformly reported to contain groups that end with a longer sound (i.e., short-short-long). By contrast, isochronous sequences outlined by markers alternating in intensity (or frequency), as in *H-Lo-H-Lo,* are universally heard as trochee groups. Specifically, the perceived group *begins* with an intense (or higher frequency) sound: H-Lo . . . and *ends* with the softer/lower sound.[145] Also, this figure shows that an ambiguous recycled dactyl pattern is always heard as beginning with a strong stress (intensity/frequency).

The Iambic/Trochaic law is fascinating. Arguably, it is universal. It holds in domains of speech and music, and it is found cross-culturally in infants and adults. Adult native speakers (English or French) hear both iambic and trochaic percepts based on systematic local variations of intensity and duration despite the fact that trochees are more prevalent in English and iambic end-lengthening is more common in French.[146,147] There is even evidence that these grouping biases extend to other species, such as the lowly rat.[148] (Note: Unlike intensity increments, which seem universal, some argue that lengthened durations may be learned as harbingers of endings.[149,150])

Finally, the Iambic/Trochaic law offers a widely respected description of people's inborn grouping tendencies. However, reasons for its success are vague. They leave unanswered an important question: "*Why* do people hear iambic (and anapest) rhythms as ending with a long time interval, but trochaic (and dactyl) rhythms as beginning with heightened intensity?" One answer springs from entrainment theory and the role of tempo response curves.

Perceiving Speech Groups: A Different View

This section tackles prosodic parsing by exploring the role of tempo response curves on people's grouping percepts. The general attending hypothesis implies that properties of force and temporal regularity are important aspects of any driving rhythm. With regard to speaking rate, these properties figure in the local fluctuations that a speaker creates when producing a referent driving rhythm. This should not be surprising. Speakers routinely, often unwittingly, shape their utterances by modulating these fluctuations via vocal tract constrictions that turn on and off articulatory gestures.[151] The resulting modulations affect a speaker's tempo response curve by introducing momentary changes in the intensity and timing of syllable time markers.[152]

A listener exposed to a speaker's production experiences temporal expectancies largely based on entrainment that originates in speaking rate of opening portions of a speaker's utterance (T_R). These expectancies are manifest as anticipatory expectancy pulses, $p' \sim p$, gauged to the unfolding context. Consequently, local fluctuations in T_R are experienced as expectancy violations, which automatically evoke corresponding reactive pulses. These momentary disparities between expected and reactive pulses (in intensity or timing) contribute to a listener's experience of perceptual contrasts. Ultimately perceptual contrasts determine how listeners perceive the beginnings and ends of prosodic groups.

To illustrate how this happens in more detail, let's consider a very simple phrase such as "Rap on the door." As with Port's phrase, this simplifies into two metric time scales, T_{RM}: T_R (n:m of 1:3), outlined respectively by stress and syllable onset markers. There is, of course, an overall temporal envelope that decomposes into component, fluctuating, waveforms. In addition, the string of monosyllables creates an approximately isochronous waveform as a syllabic context (i.e., markers of vowel onsets). Thus, this speaker's articulation rate, T_R, is roughly constant spelling out a fuzzy rhythm that hides a very simple attractor profile based on time spans of successive syllables (i.e., a series of n:m = 1:1 attractors). Next, imagine a listener who responds to this unfolding utterance with a contextually induced oscillator that generates a series of temporal expectancies manifest as a series of expectancy pulses. This is suggested in in Figure 12.6 where expectancy pulses appear in dark gray. Note that natural fluctuations of this fuzzy driving rhythm (solid line as tempo response curve), give rise to timed local expectancy violations. These reflect different timed phrasings of "Rap on the door" which varies in this fuzzy rhythm. For instance, prosodic groupings may superficially manifest as

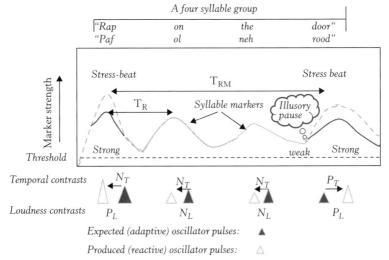

Prosodic grouping hypotheses
Entraining within a speech phrase

FIGURE 12.6 Four types of momentary perceptual contrasts have different grouping effects in entrainment. Loudness contrasts (positive, negative) affect stability. Timing contrasts (positive, negative) are linked to phase corrections. See text for discussion.

"Rapon" the "door" or even "Raponthedoor." In other words, speakers unwittingly vary both the local tempo and marker intensity of the referent (syllable) driving rhythm (ordinate) and timing (abscissa), thus influencing a listener's manifest responses. One version of such phrasing appears in this figure (i.e., simplified to convey the gist of only two external driving rhythms.[153,154])

Figure 12.6 suggests the nature of such impacts of on listeners. For instance listener's timed expectancies (dark gray pluse), yields quasi isochronously timed expectancy pulses that are fallible; thus, small expectancy violations arise from fluctuating articulation rate. Importantly, each violation triggers a momentary *perceptual contrast* between an expectancy (as an expectancy pulse) and the immediate stimulation (as a reactive pulse); this ushers in a phase correction.

Perceptual contrasts, albeit fleeing, are important. They come in two forms: loudness and timing contrasts. Both appear in Figure 12.6 and are detailed in Figure 12.7. Positive contrasts, **P**, are distinguished from negative contrasts, **N**. A positive loudness, P_L, contrast happens if a fluctuating sound (reactive pulse intensity) is unexpectedly loud relative to a contextually expected levels. Similarly, a positive timing contrast, P_T, happens

if an expectancy pulse arrives early (or the syllable onset is late). Also shown in Figure 12.7 are negative contrasts. These happen when an expected sound is either softer (N_L) or later (N_T) than contextually anticipated values.

In sum, Figure 12.6 shows how perceptual contrasts figure into tacit percepts of prosodic grouping in running speech. And Figure 12.7 summarizes theoretical predictions about perceived grouping that shed new light on the Iambic/Trochaic law.

Loudness Contrasts: An On–Off Rule

An unexpected loud sound has a more potent effect on a grouping percept than an unexpected soft one. This loudness contrast reflects the difference between two energy pulses: expectancy and reactive pulses. This contrast gauges the relative strength of a driving rhythm, hence it registers effective coupling strength.[77] Thus, a local increment in the intensity of an external driving rhythm (i.e., a louder sound) delivers a positive loudness contrast, P_L. This contrast predicts a momentary strengthening in coupling between driving and driven rhythms. In an entrainment account, this implies heightened stability. The reverse holds for a driving rhythm that locally weakens dyadic

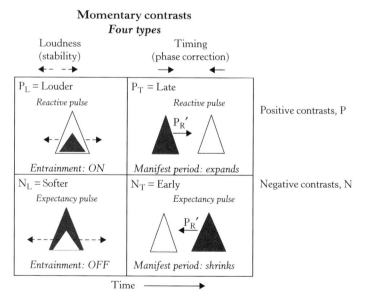

FIGURE 12.7 Four types of contrasts on a listener's grouping tendencies during entrainment to a four-syllable phrase, with a T_{RM}: T_R ~1:4; this covers individual transient mode-locking groups of n:m = 1:1 for syllables. Syllables are highlighted by temporal and loudness contrasts, shown by reactive versus expectancy pulses (lower diagram). Dark gray expectancy pulses reflect listener's internal timing of the referent (articulator) rate; empty pulses (triangles) are reactive pulses in the produced phrase. Note that expectancy pulses lag reactive ones for the first three syllable, but the expectancy pulse anticipates the fourth reactive pulse when preceding "door," thus creating an illusory pause which segments syllable from preceding ones.

coupling. It creates a negative loudness contrast that lowers stability, N_L.

In short, the *on–off rule* offers important stability predictions. Greater stability means stronger entrainment. In terms of prosodic grouping, it suggests that a listener senses a local increase in stability as a "turning on" of entrainment. In turn, this sense of "turning on" distinctly signals the beginning of prosodic group. Figure 12.7 (*left column*) indicates that heightened stability, with P_L values, occurs with the stressed syllables (such as *Rap* and *door* in the present example). Accordingly, listeners treat these points as beginnings of syllable groups (i.e., beginnings of words). Conversely, local drops in a speaker's vocal intensity at the end of "on" and "the" create negative loudness contrasts, N_L. Lower stability indexes weaken entrainment; conversely, this is sensed as a "turning off" of entrainment, namely, it directly cues a group ending. In this case, the N_L (for *on, the*) reflects weak coupling, leading to "attentional wandering." Thus, loose couplings bias listeners to hear "Rap onthe door."

Temporal Contrasts: An Expand–Shrink Rule

Other aspects of prosodic grouping percepts are linked to temporal contrasts arising from violations of temporal expectancies. Speakers rarely talk with precise isochrony. Typically, a talker will create fuzzy tempo response curves either unwittingly or intentionally for emphasis. Yet, even a momentary hesitation of a few milliseconds, or a sudden speeding up of a speaker's talking rate creates time changes that are automatically calibrated by a listener's ever-tunable brain. In turn, these subtle timing changes afford another way of influencing the listener's percepts of prosodic groups. When listeners exogenously entrain to (i.e., track) a speaker's syllable driving rhythm, even small timing variations (e.g., 5–30 ms) yield meaningful time contrasts, given contextually generated expectancies. Consequently, listeners automatically phase-correct in reacting to momentary time violations, whether these are unexpectedly early or late violations (Figure 12.7; *right column*). An automatic phase adaption delivers a manifest period, p_R', of the driven oscillation's intrinsic period ($p_R \sim T_R$). Recall that time percepts are based on the manifest oscillator period, not its latent period.

The *expand–shrink rule* offers important predictions about perceived groups that arise from *temporal illusions*. It maintains that a variable referent driving rhythm (i.e., a tempo response curve) induces in listeners hear groups

segregated by temporal illusions that derive from manifest periods: specifically, illusions of larger time intervals arise from fleeting corrections that adaptive expand the manifest period, p_R'. This results with positive contrasts (P_T). On the other hand, brief shrinking corrections yield negative (N_T) time contrasts as illusions of reduced time intervals, shown in Figure 12.7. Arrows in this figure indicate that positive time contrasts, from an unexpectedly late reactive pulse, spark an automatic percept of an *expansion* of the oscillator's manifest period, p_R', whereas negative temporal contrasts invite a corrective *shrink* p_R'.[155,156]

Time expansions create illusory pauses that happen in listeners' heads, not in an acoustic speech signal. For instance, in Figure 12.6, an illusory pause is predicted when the expectancy pulse to *door* precedes its reactive pulse, creating a positive time contrast, P_T. This leads to a corrective expansion of the manifest period, p_R'. Importantly, waveform acoustics register only reactive, not expectancy, pulses. Yet listeners persist in reporting these timing illusions.

Time shrinkages are also illusory. They are based upon a shortened manifest period, p_R'. As with time expansions, shrinkages, too, are missing in an acoustic signal. They arise from a listener's experience of negative temporal contrasts, N_T, and are most common with fast speaking rates.[157] Figure 12.6 suggests the effects of negative contrasts on a listener's percepts of "on" and "the" in this phrase. Here, the driven oscillator's manifest period shortens, leading to a perceptual pulling together of "on" and "the" in this phrase, and moving these words closer to "Rap." Together this illustrates proximal grouping. As such, it explains a common observation that the syllables within words seem to "stick" together. Echoing the role of timing in musical contour groupings (Chapter 11), here, time shrinkage exaggerates perceived proximities thereby enhancing the perception of "groupiness" among syllables in a word.[158]

Revisiting the Iambic/Trochaic Law: The On–Off Rule

The puzzling success of the Iambic/Trochaic law, described earlier, can now be viewed through the lens of entrainment as just outlined. For instance the on–off rule, which applies to percepts of group beginnings and endings, explains these percepts in terms of intensity modulations of a local driving rhythm (e.g., articulation rate). Therefore, intensity changes (as loudness) effectively "turn on" or "turn off" the coupling strength of dyads leading, respectively, to stronger or weaker connections. This explains iambic/trochaic descriptions of beginnings and ends of prosodic groups due to intensity variations.

The Iambic/Trochaic law is also famous for aptly describing percepts of group endings signaled by a lengthened time intervals. Following the on–off rule, a single lengthened sound is perceived as a group ending because it inevitably contains at least one silent expectancy pulse created by a persisting driven rhythm with a latent period, p_R. Figure 12.5 illustrates this. A silent pulse (ligher gray) inside the longer sound, L, creates a negative loudness contrast, N_L hence weakening coupling and signaling a group ending.[159]

Revisiting Speech Segmentation Issues: The Expand–Shrink Rule

Word segmentation is a topic central to speech perception. Theoretically, it is also a source of debate. It seems inexplicable that listeners report hearing segmenting silences in utterances when these silences are distinctly *absent* from the acoustic signal. Recall that certain lexical theories attribute this phenomenon to the consumed time of a lexical access process that occurs prior to a strongly stressed syllable.

The expand–shrink rule offers a different explanation of segmentation. In an entrainment framework, a driving–driven context induces certain expectancies that deliver positive time contrasts. A Positive time contrast occurs whenever a speaking context induces corresponding fast-paced expectancies of the driven oscillation that tracks the syllable level. Such expectancies deliver expectancy pulses that typically precede a future reactive pulse due to a local slowing of the driving rhythm. Positive contrasts (P_T) automatically emerge from phase corrections to an unexpectedly late reactive pulse. These phase corrections yield manifest lengthening of the period, p_R', of this entraining oscillation. Consequently, the listener will experience a localized illusory pause preceding (i.e., segmenting) a group of syllables (with an initial stressed word). Such an illusory pause precedes "door" in Figure 12.6.

Finally, not all segmenting pauses are illusory. Segmenting time gaps between phrases, for example, are true time gaps.[160] In these, the distinctive time intervals separating phrases usually contain one or more *silent pulses*. For instance, the phrase "Rap on this door" might be followed, after a true silence, by another phrase. However, typically this silence is calibrated by talking rate, meaning that the true pause will contain one or two silent expectancy pules.[161]

Summary of Prosodic Groups and the Tempo Response Curve

In sum, a dynamic attending approach offers new ways to conceive of prosodic grouping. It rests on basic entrainment assumptions as well as related rules that explain the percepts of prosodic speech groups responsible for segmenting speech attractor profiles. These rules lead to predictions that accommodate long-standing psychological descriptions of group perception stipulated by the Iambic/Trochaic law. This dynamic attending approach features the behavior of driven temporal expectancies operating in the context of fluctuating rhythmic time markers of a tempo response curve that is created by a speaker. In brief, in fluent speech, local modulations of a speaker's talking rate produce unexpected changes in stimulus intensity and/or timing, changes that automatically facilitate parsing of groups of syllables. A speaker's modulations of these referent rhythm properties shape a listener's expectancies and their responses to expectancy violations.

Finally, this showcases one avenue to explore when considering how linguistic knowledge affects perceived grouping. Here, intensity variations figure into percepts of beginnings and ends of groups. And timing fluctuations in a speaker's articulation rate contribute to listeners' percepts of prosodic groups due to segmentation by illusory pauses and percepts of meshed syllables due to time shrinkage. The resulting prosodic groups preserve or obscure hidden attractor relationships.

The major points of this section are:

- Contextually induced expectancies in listeners result in expectancy violations due largely to local driving rhythm fluctuations in intensity and timing.
- Two kinds of expectancy violations appear in running speech. Respectively, they deliver contrasts in loudness and in timing.
- An on–off entrainment rule addresses loudness violations. Consistent with the Iambic/Trochaic law, these either "turn on" entrainment signaling a group beginning or they "turn off" entrainment signaling an ending.
- An expand–shrink entrainment rule addresses temporal expectancy violations (i.e., of late or early time markers). Respectively, these violations create illusory expansions (pauses) or illusory shrinkages (connections).

CHAPTER SUMMARY

Against a historical background that toyed with, then abandoned isochrony, this chapter introduces a new way of thinking about speech timing. It proposes that production profiles of speakers hide multiple hierarchically related, quasi-isochronous driving rhythms. Together, these rhythms form compelling time relationships that invite synchronous attending. Specifically, a speech production profile affords both relative time relations (as attractors) and a tempo response curve (as a changing referent driving rhythm).

Major sections of this chapter expand an entrainment interpretation of speech timing in which speech affords multiple driving rhythms. Moreover, interdependencies among such rhythms express time ratios that approximate attractor time relations. At least two fuzzy driving rhythms in a speaker's production profile are highlighted in this chapter; these correspond to speaking rate, marked by syllable features, and a slower rhythm, marked by stressed beats. As such, these rhythms participate in inducing a parallel expectancy profile in listeners. This interaction is a theoretical core of speaker–listener dynamics.

In this chapter, rhythmic relations in speech that have puzzled scholars for decades are cast as attractors within an entrainment framework. And, of course, given the prevalence of fuzzy speech rhythms, these attractors are often hidden. Thus, teasing out evidence for such attractors depends on special techniques involving recycling groups or phrases, which have a potential for isolating metrical time relationships. However, more complicated speech productions cannot be captured by recycling paradigms. Thus, the time structure of speech falls along a continuum that ranges from meter-like configurations of simple attractors, which induce metric oscillator clusters, to rhythm-like configurations, which induce attractor profiles. The former derive from traditional mode-locking of listeners' attending, whereas the latter requires transient mode-locking of attending. Whereas some ordinary phrases and poetry lend themselves to traditional mode-locking, ordinary, running speech often engages transient mode-locking. Generally, in normal conversational discourse, listeners experience both internal metric oscillator clusters and attractor profiles.

A fundamental component of speech perception, whether involving traditional or transient mode-locking, concerns the role of a referent driving rhythm. In speech, this referent reflects a speaker-specific speaking rate, which can vary over time and lead to a fluctuating tempo response curve. As a driving rhythm, articulation rate is important for several reasons. One overlooked function of articulation rate is its role in stimulating context-driven expectancies while concurrently delivering local changes that violate these expectancies. The result is a new way of specifying percepts of beginnings and ends of attractor groups and group segmentation.

Finally, this chapter opened with a dialogue on the demise of isochrony theories due to apparent unruliness of surface timing in speech. Statistical analyses of interstress intervals, for example, led to the downfall of several early attempts to understand speech rhythms. It is worth noting that early fateful assumptions about the variability of speech timing fed into theories that assumed the time structure of speech is inherently stochastic. Such assumptions linger today, inspiring approaches to speech timing and prosody that rely on statistical coding models. This chapter disputes this view. It asserts that speech timing, in its various forms, is *really* rhythmical.

NOTES

1. David Abercrombie, *Elements of General Phonetics* (Edinburgh: Edinburgh University Press, 1967).

2. R. M. Dauer, "Stress-Timing and Syllable-Timing Reanalyzed," *Journal of Phonetics*, 11, no. 1 (January 1983): 51–62, http://psycnet.apa.org/psycinfo/1983-29886-001.

3. Amalia Arvaniti, "The Usefulness of Metrics in the Quantification of Speech Rhythm," *Journal of Phonetics* 40, no. 3 (May 2012): 351–73, doi:10.1016/j.wocn.2012.02.003.

4. Klaus J. Kohler, "Rhythm in Speech and Language," *Phonetica* 66, no. 1–2 (2009): 29–45, doi:10.1159/000208929.

5. Klaus J. Kohler, "Whither Speech Rhythm Research?" *Phonetica* 66, no. 1–2 (2009): 5–14.

6. E. Mendoza et al., "Temporal Variability in Speech Segments of Spanish: Context and Speaker Related Differences," *Speech Communication* 40, no. 4 (June 2003): 431–47, doi:10.1016/S0167-6393(02)00086-9.

7. Laurence White, Sven L. Mattys, and Lukas Wiget, "Segmentation Cues in Conversational Speech: Robust Semantics and Fragile Phonotactics," *Frontiers in Psychology* 3 (2012): 375.

8. Oded Ghitza, "The Theta-Syllable: A Unit of Speech Information Defined by Cortical Function," *Frontiers in Psychology* 4 (2013), https://doi.org/10.3389/fpsyg.2013.00138.

9. C refers to consonant and V to vowels.

10. Amalia Arvaniti, "Rhythm, Timing and the Timing of Rhythm," *Phonetica* 66, no. 1–2 (2009): 46–63, doi:10.1159/000208930.

11. Ilse Lehiste, "Isochrony Reconsidered," *Journal of Phonetics* 5, no. 3 (1977): 253–63.

12. Hugo Quené and Robert F. Port, "Effects of Timing Regularity and Metrical Expectancy on Spoken-Word Perception," *Phonetica* 62, no. 1 (2005): 1–13, doi:10.1159/000087222.

13. Kenneth L. Pike, *The Intonation of American English* (Ann Arbor: University of Michigan Press, 1945), http://eric.ed.gov.proxy.library.ucsb.edu:2048/?id=ED077259.

14. Stress is often disputed as the single marker of timing across cultures. Hence, English is described as a *stress-based* language, not a stress-timed language. Also, some interpret stress as the result of a speaker's effort, allowing a positive correlation of higher vocal intensity (stress) with higher vocal pitch (F0).

15. Beth M. Tingley and George D. Allen, "Development of Speech Timing Control in Children," *Child Development* 46, no. 1 (March 1975): 186, doi:10.2307/1128847.

16. George D. Allen, "The Location of Rhythmic Stress Beats in English: An Experimental Study I," *Language and Speech* 15, no. 1 (January 1, 1972): 72–100, doi:10.1177/002383097201500110.

17. Variability ranged from 4% to 11% of average tap rate in these studies.

18. Greg Kochanski and Christina Orphanidou, "What Marks the Beat of Speech?" *Journal of the Acoustical Society of America* 123, no. 5 (May 1, 2008): 2780–91, doi:10.1121/1.2890742.

19. Pascale Lidji et al., "Listeners Feel the Beat: Entrainment to English and French Speech Rhythms," *Psychonomic Bulletin & Review* 18, no. 6 (September 13, 2011): 1035–41, doi:10.3758/s13423-011-0163-0.

20. Peter Roach, "On the Distinction Between 'Stress-Timed' and 'Syllable-Timed' Languages," *Linguistic Controversies*, 1982, 73–9.

21. Dauer, "Stress-Timing and Syllable-Timing Reanalyzed."

22. Natasha Warner and Takayuki Arai, "The Role of the Mora in the Timing of Spontaneous Japanese Speech," *Journal of the Acoustical Society of America* 109, no. 3 (March 2001): 1144–56, doi:10.1121/1.1344156.

23. Franck Ramus, Marina Nespor, and Jacques Mehler, "Correlates of Linguistic Rhythm in the Speech Signal," *Cognition* 73, no. 3 (December 1999): 265–92, doi:10.1016/S0010-0277(99)00058-X.

24. Dauer, "Stress-Timing and Syllable-Timing Reanalyzed."

25. Mendoza et al., "Temporal Variability in Speech Segments of Spanish."

26. Thomas H. Crystal, "Segmental Durations in Connected-Speech Signals: Current Results," *Journal of the Acoustical Society of America* 83, no. 4 (1988): 1553, doi:10.1121/1.395911.

27. Thomas H. Crystal, "Segmental Durations in Connected Speech Signals: Preliminary Results," *Journal of the Acoustical Society of America* 72, no. 3 (1982): 705, doi:10.1121/1.388251.

28. Takayuki Arai and Steven Greenberg, "The Temporal Properties of Spoken Japanese Are Similar to Those of English," presented at EUROSPEECH, Rhodes, Greece,1997, http://ftp.icsi.berkeley.edu/ftp/pub/speech/papers/euro97-japeng.pdf.

29. Warner and Arai, "The Role of the Mora in the Timing of Spontaneous Japanese Speech."

30. Warner and Arai used a large sample of Japanese utterances where mora durations ranged from 72 ms to 141 ms comparable to English syllables (87 ms to 275 ms).

31. Alessandra Sansavini, Josiane Bertoncini, and Giuliana Giovanelli, "Newborns Discriminate the Rhythm of Multisyllabic Stressed Words," *Developmental Psychology* 33, no. 1 (1997): 3–11, doi:10.1037/0012-1649.33.1.3.

32. Thierry Nazzi, Josiane Bertoncini, and Jacques Mehler, "Language Discrimination by Newborns: Toward an Understanding of the Role of Rhythm.," *Journal of Experimental Psychology: Human Perception and Performance* 24, no. 3 (1998): 756–66, doi:10.1037/0096-1523.24.3.756.

33. F. Ramus, "Language Discrimination by Human Newborns and by Cotton-Top Tamarin Monkeys," *Science* 288, no. 5464 (April 14, 2000): 349–51, doi:10.1126/science.288.5464.349.

34. M. Pena et al., "Sounds and Silence: An Optical Topography Study of Language Recognition at Birth," *Proceedings of the National Academy of Sciences* 100, no. 20 (September 30, 2003): 11702–05, doi:10.1073/pnas.1934290100.

35. Laurent Demany, Beryl McKenzie, and Eliane Vurpillot, "Rhythm Perception in Early Infancy," *Nature* 266, no. 5604 (1977): 718–19, doi:10.1038/266718a0.

36. Lehiste, "Isochrony Reconsidered."

37. Ilse Lehiste, "Role of Duration in Disambiguating Syntactically Ambiguous Sentences," *Journal of the Acoustical Society of America* 60, no. 5 (1976): 1199, doi:10.1121/1.381180.

38. Stephen Handel, *Listening: An Introduction to the Perception of Auditory Events*, vol. xii (Cambridge, MA: MIT Press, 1993).

39. James G. Martin, "Rhythmic (Hierarchical) Versus Serial Structure in Speech and Other Behavior," *Psychological Review* 79, no. 6 (1972): 487–509, doi:10.1037/h0033467.

40. Mari R. Jones, "Time, Our Lost Dimension: Toward a New Theory of Perception,

Attention, and Memory," *Psychological Review* 83, no. 5 (1976): 323–55, doi:10.1037/0033-295X.83.5.323.

41. Mari R. Jones and Marilyn Boltz, "Dynamic Attending and Responses to Time," *Psychological Review* 96, no. 3 (1989): 459–91, doi:10.1037/0033-295X.96.3.459.

42. Sam Tilsen and Keith Johnson, "Low-Frequency Fourier Analysis of Speech Rhythm," *Journal of the Acoustical Society of America* 124, no. 2 (August 2008): EL34–39, doi:10.1121/1.2947626.

43. Rob Drullman, Joost M. Festen, and Reinier Plomp, "Effect of Temporal Envelope Smearing on Speech Reception," *Journal of the Acoustical Society of America* 95, no. 2 (1994): 1053, doi:10.1121/1.408467.

44. Rob Drullman, Joost M. Festen, and Reinier Plomp, "Effect of Reducing Slow Temporal Modulations on Speech Reception," *Journal of the Acoustical Society of America* 95, no. 5 (1994): 2670, doi:10.1121/1.409836.

45. Taffeta M. Elliott and Frédéric E. Theunissen, "The Modulation Transfer Function for Speech Intelligibility," *PLoS Computational Biology* 5, no. 3 (March 6, 2009): e1000302, doi:10.1371/journal.pcbi.1000302.

46. Nandini C. Singh and Frédéric E. Theunissen, "Modulation Spectra of Natural Sounds and Ethological Theories of Auditory Processing," *Journal of the Acoustical Society of America* 114, no. 6 (2003): 3394, doi:10.1121/1.1624067.

47. Ramus, Nespor, and Mehler, "Correlates of Linguistic Rhythm in the Speech Signal."

48. Nazzi, Bertoncini, and Mehler, "Language Discrimination by Newborns."

49. Thierry Nazzi and Franck Ramus, "Perception and Acquisition of Linguistic Rhythm by Infants," *Speech Communication* 41, no. 1 (August 2003): 233–43, doi:10.1016/S0167-6393(02)00106-1.

50. Ramus, Nespor, and Mehler, "Correlates of Linguistic Rhythm in the Speech Signal."

51. William J. Barry et al., "Do Rhythm Measures Tell Us Anything About Language Type," in *Proceedings of the 15th ICPhS* (Barcelona, 2003), 2693–2696, https://www.internationalphoneticassociation.org/icphs-proceedings/ICPhS2003/papers/p15_2693.pdf.

52. Kohler, "Rhythm in Speech and Language."

53. Arvaniti, "Rhythm, Timing and the Timing of Rhythm."

54. Arvaniti, "The Usefulness of Metrics in the Quantification of Speech Rhythm."

55. Esther Grabe and E. Ling Low, "Durational Variability in Speech and the Rhythm Class Hypothesis," *Papers in Laboratory Phonology* 7, no. 515–46 (2002), http://wwwhomes.uni-bielefeld.de/~gibbon/AK-Phon/Rhythmus/Grabe/Grabe_Low-reformatted.pdf.

56. David Poeppel, "The Neuroanatomic and Neurophysiological Infrastructure for Speech and Language," *Current Opinion in Neurobiology* 28 (October 2014): 142–49, doi:10.1016/j.conb.2014.07.005.

57. Nai Ding et al., "Cortical Tracking of Hierarchical Linguistic Structures in Connected Speech," *Nature Neuroscience* 19, no. 1 (December 7, 2015): 158–64, doi:10.1038/nn.4186.

58. Anne-Lise Giraud and David Poeppel, "Cortical Oscillations and Speech Processing: Emerging Computational Principles and Operations," *Nature Neuroscience* 15, no. 4 (March 18, 2012): 511–17, doi:10.1038/nn.3063.

59. Mark A. Pitt, Christine Szostak, and Laura C. Dilley, "Rate Dependent Speech Processing Can Be Speech Specific: Evidence from the Perceptual Disappearance of Words Under Changes in Context Speech Rate," *Attention, Perception, & Psychophysics* 78, no. 1 (January 2016): 334–45, doi:10.3758/s13414-015-0981-7.

60. Jonathan E. Peelle and Matthew H. Davis, "Neural Oscillations Carry Speech Rhythm Through to Comprehension," *Frontiers in Psychology* 3 (2012), doi:10.3389/fpsyg.2012.00320.

61. Ding et al., "Cortical Tracking of Hierarchical Linguistic Structures in Connected Speech."

62. Colin Humphries et al., "Hierarchical Organization of Speech Perception in Human Auditory Cortex," *Frontiers in Neuroscience* 8 (December 11, 2014), doi:10.3389/fnins.2014.00406.

63. Oded Ghitza, "The Theta-Syllable: A Unit of Speech Information Defined by Cortical Function," *Frontiers in Psychology* 4 (2013), https://doi.org/10.3389/fpsyg.2013.00138.

64. Crystal, "Segmental Durations in Connected-Speech Signals: Current Results."

65. Huan Luo and David Poeppel, "Phase Patterns of Neuronal Responses Reliably Discriminate Speech in Human Auditory Cortex," *Neuron* 54, no. 6 (June 21, 2007): 1001–10, doi:10.1016/j.neuron.2007.06.004.

66. Giraud and Poeppel, "Cortical Oscillations and Speech Processing."

67. Oded Ghitza and Steven Greenberg, "On the Possible Role of Brain Rhythms in Speech Perception: Intelligibility of Time-Compressed Speech with Periodic and Aperiodic Insertions of Silence," *Phonetica* 66, no. 1–2 (2009): 113–26, doi:10.1159/000208934.

68. John Morton, Steve Marcus, and Clive Frankish, "Perceptual Centers (P-Centers)," *Psychological Review* 83, no. 5 (1976): 405–08, doi:10.1037/0033-295X.83.5.405.

69. P-centers are located near onsets of nuclear vowels, but shift with surrounding consonants.

70. Stephen Michael Marcus, "Acoustic Determinants of Perceptual Center (P-Center) Location," *Perception & Psychophysics* 30, no. 3 (May 1981): 247–56, doi:10.3758/BF03214280.

71. Aniruddh D. Patel, Anders Löfqvist, and Walter Naito, "The Acoustics and Kinematics of Regularly Timed Speech: A Database and Method for the Study of the p-Center Problem," in *Proceedings of the 14th International Congress of Phonetic Sciences*, vol. 1, 1999, 405–408, http://web.haskins.yale.edu.proxy.library.ucsb.edu:2048/Reprints/HL1137.pdf.

72. Sophie K. Scott, "The Point of P-Centres," *Psychological Research Psychologische Forschung* 61, no. 1 (March 5, 1998): 4–11, doi:10.1007/PL00008162.

73. Sophie K. Scott, "P-Centres in Speech: An Acoustic Analysis," *Journal of the Acoustical Society of America* 92 no. 4 (1993).

74. Morton, Marcus, and Frankish, "Perceptual Centers (P-Centers)."

75. Marcus, "Acoustic Determinants of Perceptual Center (P-Center) Location."

76. Carol A. Fowler, "Perception of Syllable Timing by Prebabbling Infants," *Journal of the Acoustical Society of America* 79, no. 3 (1986): 814, doi:10.1121/1.393472.

77. Rudi C. Villing et al., "Measuring Perceptual Centers Using the Phase Correction Response," *Attention, Perception, & Psychophysics* 73, no. 5 (July 2011): 1614–29, doi:10.3758/s13414-011-0110-1.

78. Scott, "The Point of P-Centres."

79. Peter Howell, "Prediction of P-Center Location from the Distribution of Energy in the Amplitude Envelope: II," *Perception & Psychophysics* 43, no. 1 (January 1988): 99, doi:10.3758/BF03208980.

80. Fred Cummins, "Rhythm as Entrainment: The Case of Synchronous Speech," *Journal of Phonetics* 37, no. 1 (January 2009): 16–28, doi:10.1016/j.wocn.2008.08.003.

81. Keith B. Doelling et al., "Acoustic Landmarks Drive Delta–theta Oscillations to Enable Speech Comprehension by Facilitating Perceptual Parsing," *NeuroImage* 85, Part 2 (January 15, 2014): 761–68, doi:10.1016/j.neuroimage.2013.06.035.

82. Kochanski and Orphanidou, "What Marks the Beat of Speech?"

83. Specifically, prominence judgments of speech elements depend on intensity increments of syllables with stress beats and, to a lesser degree, duration.

84. Kochanski and Orphanidou, "What Marks the Beat of Speech?" p. 2780.

85. Using a coupled oscillator algorithm, they isolated local loudness contrasts as determinants of participants' stable phase alignments between produced words/syllables and metronome ticks.

86. Note that with syllables of less than 300 ms, loudness contrast depended on *both* intensity and sound duration.

87. Dilley and Pitt, "Altering Context Speech Rate Can Cause Words to Appear or Disappear."

88. Pitt, Szostak, and Dilley, "Rate Dependent Speech Processing Can Be Speech Specific."

89. Tuuli H. Morrill et al., "Distal Rhythm Influences Whether or Not Listeners Hear a Word in Continuous Speech: Support for a Perceptual Grouping Hypothesis," *Cognition* 131, no. 1 (April 2014): 69–74, doi:10.1016/j.cognition.2013.12.006.

90. E. Reinisch, A. Jesse, and J. M. McQueen, "Speaking Rate Affects the Perception of Duration as a Suprasegmental Lexical-Stress Cue," *Language and Speech* 54, no. 2 (June 1, 2011): 147–65, doi:10.1177/0023830910397489.

91. Pitt, Szostak, and Dilley, "Rate Dependent Speech Processing Can Be Speech Specific."

92. Howard Giles and Robert N. St. Clair, *Language and Social Psychology* (Oxford: Blackwell, 1979), http://www.ulb.tu-darmstadt.de/tocs/57332967.pdf.

93. Bruce L. Brown, Howard Giles, and Jitendra N. Thakerar, "Speaker Evaluations as a Function of Speech Rate, Accent and Context," *Language & Communication* 5, no. 3 (January 1985): 207–20, doi:10.1016/0271-5309(85)90011-4.

94. Xiaoju Zheng and Janet B. Pierrehumbert, "The Effects of Prosodic Prominence and Serial Position on Duration Perception," *Journal of the Acoustical Society of America* 128, no. 2 (2010): 851, doi:10.1121/1.3455796.

95. Personal communication from R. F. Port.

96. Robert F. Port, "Meter and Speech," *Journal of Phonetics* 31, no. 3–4 (July 2003): 599–611, doi:10.1016/j.wocn.2003.08.001.

97. Fred Cummins and Robert Port, "Rhythmic Constraints on Stress Timing in English," *Journal of Phonetics* 26, no. 2 (April 1998): 145–71, doi:10.1006/jpho.1998.0070.

98. J. A. Scott Kelso, *Dynamic Patterns: The Self-Organization of Brain and Behavior* (Cambridge, MA: MIT Press, 1997), https://books-google-com.proxy.library.ucsb.edu:9443/books?hl=en&lr=&id=zpjejjytkiIC&oi=fnd&pg=PR9&dq=Book++++Kelso,+J.+A.+S.+1995+dynamic+patterns&ots=-bjBWye6fw&sig=BBH9-1-whqxlxSuyd-VqQiZTTJY.

99. B. Tuller and J. A. S. Kelso, "Environmentally-Specified Patterns of Movement Coordination in Normal and Split-Brain Subjects," *Experimental Brain Research* 75, no. 2 (April 1989), doi:10.1007/BF00247936.

100. Tilsen and Johnson, "Low-Frequency Fourier Analysis of Speech Rhythm."

101. Tilsen and Johnson, "Low-Frequency Fourier Analysis of Speech Rhythm."

102. Sam Tilsen and Amalia Arvaniti, "Speech Rhythm Analysis with Decomposition of the Amplitude Envelope: Characterizing Rhythmic

Patterns Within and Across Languages," *Journal of the Acoustical Society of America* 134, no. 1 (July 1, 2013): 628–39, doi:10.1121/1.4807565.

103. Tilsen and Arvaniti, "Speech Rhythm Analysis with Decomposition of the Amplitude Envelope."

104. N. E. Huang et al., "The Empirical Mode Decomposition and the Hilbert Spectrum for Nonlinear and Non-Stationary Time Series Analysis," *Proceedings of the Royal Society A: Mathematical, Physical and Engineering Sciences* 454, no. 1971 (March 8, 1998): 903–95, doi:10.1098/rspa.1998.0193.

105. Stefan J. Kiebel, Jean Daunizeau, and Karl J. Friston, "A Hierarchy of Time-Scales and the Brain," ed. Olaf Sporns, *PLoS Computational Biology* 4, no. 11 (November 14, 2008): e1000209, doi:10.1371/journal.pcbi.1000209.

106. Port, "Meter and Speech." p. 610.

107. Mark Yoffe Liberman, "The Intonational System of English." (Thesis, Massachusetts Institute of Technology, 1975), http://dspace.mit.edu/handle/1721.1/27376.

108. Mark Liberman and Alan Prince, "On Stress and Linguistic Rhythm," *Linguistic Inquiry* 8, no. 2 (1977): 249–336.

109. J. Pierrehumbert and M. Beckman, "Japanese Tone Structure," *Linguistic Inquiry Monographs*, no. 15 (1988): 1–282.

110. Mary E. Beckman, "The Parsing of Prosody," *Language and Cognitive Processes* 11, no. 1–2 (April 1996): 17–68, doi:10.1080/016909696387213.

111. E. O. Selkirk, *Phonology and Syntax*, 1984.

112. E. O. Selkirk, *Phonology and Syntax: The Relationship Between Sound and Structure* (Cambridge, MA: MIT Press, 1986).

113. Lidji et al., "Listeners Feel the Beat."

114. George D. Allen, "The Location of Rhythmic Stress Beats in English: An Experimental Study II," *Language and Speech* 15, no. 2 (April 1, 1972): 179–95.

115. Speakers of French and English were either monolinguals or proficient bilinguals (French, English).

116. Ding et al., "Cortical Tracking of Hierarchical Linguistic Structures in Connected Speech."

117. Because conditions randomized the order of syllables, averaged responses prevented precise assessments of attractor profiles. In theory, transient mode-locking predicts evidence favoring a series of local attractors as, for instance, in 1:1-1:4-1:2 referenced to an articulation rate of 250 ms (4 Hz),

118. Anne Cutler and Dennis Norris, "The Role of Strong Syllables in Segmentation for Lexical Access," *Journal of Experimental Psychology: Human Perception and Performance* 14, no. 1 (1988): 113–21, doi:10.1037/0096-1523.14.1.113.

119. Anne Cutler and Sally Butterfield, "Rhythmic Cues to Speech Segmentation: Evidence from Juncture Misperception," *Journal of Memory and Language* 31, no. 2 (April 1992): 218–36, doi:10.1016/0749-596X(92)90012-M.

120. Strong syllables have full vowels; i.e., they are reduced—shorter or softer—than counterparts. Access means activating a word meaning in a mental lexicon.

121. James L. McClelland and Jeffrey L. Elman, "The TRACE Model of Speech Perception," *Cognitive Psychology* 18, no. 1 (January 1986): 1–86, doi:10.1016/0010-0285(86)90015-0.

122. Dennis Norris, "Shortlist: A Connectionist Model of Continuous Speech Recognition," *Cognition* 52, no. 3 (September 1994): 189–234, doi:10.1016/0010-0277(94)90043-4.

123. Paul A. Luce and Emily A. Lyons, "Processing Lexically Embedded Spoken Words," *Journal of Experimental Psychology: Human Perception and Performance* 25, no. 1 (1999): 174–83, doi:10.1037/0096-1523.25.1.174.

124. Sven L. Mattys, Laurence White, and James F. Melhorn, "Integration of Multiple Speech Segmentation Cues: A Hierarchical Framework.," *Journal of Experimental Psychology: General* 134, no. 4 (2005): 477–500, doi:10.1037/0096-3445.134.4.477.

125. Mark A. Pitt and Arthur G. Samuel, "The Use of Rhythm in Attending to Speech.," *Journal of Experimental Psychology: Human Perception and Performance* 16, no. 3 (1990): 564–73, doi:10.1037/0096-1523.16.3.564.

126. Anne Cutler and Donald J. Foss, "On the Role of Sentence Stress in Sentence Processing," *Language and Speech* 20, no. 1 (January 1, 1977): 1–10, doi:10.1177/002383097702000101.

127. Joyce L. Shields, Astrid McHugh, and James G. Martin, "Reaction Time to Phoneme Targets as a Function of Rhythmic Cues in Continuous Speech.," *Journal of Experimental Psychology* 102, no. 2 (1974): 250–55, doi:10.1037/h0035855.

128. Quené and Port, "Effects of Timing Regularity and Metrical Expectancy on Spoken-Word Perception."

129. Zheng and Pierrehumbert, "The Effects of Prosodic Prominence and Serial Position on Duration Perception."

130. For example, people were better at detecting lengthening in the stressed word *freezes* than in the unstressed word *cream* in a dactyl rhythmic sentence: *"Butter cream freezes well."* Here, stress corresponds to pitch accents.

131. Janet Pierrehumbert, "Tonal Elements and Their Alignment," in *Prosody: Theory and Experiment*, ed. Merle Horne, vol. 14 (Dordrecht: Springer Netherlands, 2000), 11–36, http://www.springerlink.com/index/10.1007/978-94-015-9413-4_2.

132. Laura C. Dilley and J. Devin McAuley, "Distal Prosodic Context Affects Word Segmentation and

Lexical Processing," *Journal of Memory and Language* 59, no. 3 (October 2008): 294–311, doi:10.1016/j.jml.2008.06.006.

133. Laura C. Dilley, Sven L. Mattys, and Louis Vinke, "Potent Prosody: Comparing the Effects of Distal Prosody, Proximal Prosody, and Semantic Context on Word Segmentation," *Journal of Memory and Language* 63, no. 3 (October 2010): 274–94, doi:10.1016/j.jml.2010.06.003.

134. C. Heffner et al., "When Cues Collide: How Distal Speech Rate and Proximal Acoustic Information Jointly Determine Word Perception," *Language and Cognitive Processes*, 2012, 1–28.

135. Joanne L. Miller and Emily R. Dexter, "Effects of Speaking Rate and Lexical Status on Phonetic Perception.," *Journal of Experimental Psychology: Human Perception and Performance* 14, no. 3 (1988): 369–78, doi:10.1037/0096-1523.14.3.369.

136. Thomas H. Crystal and Arthur S. House, "A Note on the Variability of Timing Control," *Journal of Speech Language and Hearing Research* 31, no. 3 (September 1, 1988): 497, doi:10.1044/jshr.3103.497.

137. David B. Pisoni, "Long-Term Memory in Speech Perception: Some New Findings on Talker Variability, Speaking Rate and Perceptual Learning," *Speech Communication* 13, no. 1–2 (October 1993): 109–25, doi:10.1016/0167-6393(93)90063-Q.

138. Joseph C. Toscano and Bob McMurray, "The Time-Course of Speaking Rate Compensation: Effects of Sentential Rate and Vowel Length on Voicing Judgments," *Language, Cognition and Neuroscience* 30, no. 5 (May 28, 2015): 529–43, doi:10.1080/23273798.2014.946427.

139. Stephen D. Goldinger, David B. Pisoni, and John S. Logan, "On the Nature of Talker Variability Effects on Recall of Spoken Word Lists," *Journal of Experimental Psychology: Learning, Memory, and Cognition* 17, no. 1 (1991): 152–62, doi:10.1037/0278-7393.17.1.152.

140. Gary R. Kidd, "Articulatory-Rate Context Effects in Phoneme Identification," *Journal of Experimental Psychology: Human Perception and Performance* 15, no. 4 (1989): 736–48, doi:10.1037/0096-1523.15.4.736.

141. Gary R. Kidd and Larry E. Humes, "Tempo-Based Segregation of Spoken Sentences," *Journal of the Acoustical Society of America* 136, no. 4 (October 2014): 2311, doi:10.1121/1.4900367.

142. Herbert Woodrow, "Time Perception," in *Handbook of Experimental Psychology* (Oxford: Wiley, 1951), 1224–36.

143. Jessica S. F. Hay and Randy L. Diehl, "Perception of Rhythmic Grouping: Testing the Iambic/Trochaic Law," *Perception & Psychophysics* 69, no. 1 (January 2007): 113–22, doi:10.3758/BF03194458.

144. Or, AM and FM modulations, respectively.

145. According to Woodrow, if the time interval following the H sound is lengthened, people should revert to reporting an iambic percept (Lo-H).

146. Hay and Diehl, "Perception of Rhythmic Grouping."

147. Michael D. Tyler and Anne Cutler, "Cross-Language Differences in Cue Use for Speech Segmentation," *Journal of the Acoustical Society of America* 126, no. 1 (2009): 367, doi:10.1121/1.3129127.

148. Daniela M. de la Mora, Marina Nespor, and Juan M. Toro, "Do Humans and Nonhuman Animals Share the Grouping Principles of the Iambic–trochaic Law?," *Attention, Perception, & Psychophysics* 75, no. 1 (January 2013): 92–100, doi:10.3758/s13414-012-0371-3.

149. John R. Iversen, Aniruddh D. Patel, and Kengo Ohgushi, "Perception of Rhythmic Grouping Depends on Auditory Experiences)," *Journal of the Acoustical Society of America* 124, no. 4 (October 1, 2008): 2263–71, doi:10.1121/1.2973189.

150. Katherine A. Yoshida et al., "The Development of Perceptual Grouping Biases in Infancy: A Japanese-English Cross-Linguistic Study," *Cognition* 115, no. 2 (May 2010): 356–61, doi:10.1016/j.cognition.2010.01.005.

151. D. Byrd and E. Saltzman. "The Elastic Phrase: Modeling the Dynamics of Boundary-Adjacent Lengthening," *Journal of Phonetics* 31, no. 2 (April 2003): 149–80, doi:10.1016/S0095-4470(02)00085-2.

152. This does not exclude contributions from local fluctuations in the overall envelope.

153. Tilsen and Arvaniti, "Speech Rhythm Analysis with Decomposition of the Amplitude Envelope."

154. Amplitudes also vary with sound intensity at different time scales (Table 12.1). And amplitudes defining one time scale may impact amplitude at another, as in co-modulation.

155. Peter Ulric Tse et al., "Attention and the Subjective Expansion of Time," *Perception & Psychophysics* 66, no. 7 (October 2004): 1171–89, doi:10.3758/BF03196844.

156.

157. Yoshitaka Nakajima et al., "Time-Shrinking: The Process of Unilateral Temporal Assimilation," *Perception* 33, no. 9 (September 1, 2004): 1061–79, doi:10.1068/p5061.

158. This explanation of proximity is similar to that involving Gestalt proximities in faster time scales of music in Chapter 11.

159. This also sets the stage for the subsequent heightening of a heightened positive loudness contrast, P_L, with the next sound.

160. L. Frazier, K. Carlson, and C. Clifton, "Prosodic Phrasing Is Central to Language

Comprehension," *Trends in Cognitive Sciences* 10, no. 6 (June 2006): 244–49, doi:10.1016/j.tics.2006.04.002.

161. M. G. Boltz, "Temporal Dimensions of Conversational Interaction: The Role of Response Latencies and Pauses in Social Impression Formation," *Journal of Language and Social Psychology* 24, no. 2 (June 1, 2005): 103–38, doi:10.1177/0261927X05275734.

162. Elliott, T. and Theunissen, F. "The Modulation Transfer Function for Speech Intelligibility," *PLoS Computational Biology*, 5, no. 3 (March 2009): 1–14.

163. N. Ding and J. Z. Simon, "Neural Representations of Complex Temporal Modulations in the Human Auditory Cortex," *Journal of Neurophysiology* 102, no. 5 (November 1, 2009): 2731–43, doi:10.1152/jn.00523.2009.

164. Drullman, Festen, and Plomp, "Effect of Reducing Slow Temporal Modulations on Speech Reception," *The Journal of Acoustical Society of America*, 95, no. 2670 (1994): 2670–80, doi:10.1121/1.409836.

165. Drullman, R. Festen, J. M. and Plomp, R. "Effect of Temporal Envelope Smearing on Speech Reception," *The Journal of Acoustical Society of America*, 95, no. 1053 (1994): 1053–64, doi.10.1121,408467.

13

Melodies of Speech

Melody brings to mind music. We might imagine a soaring stream of pitches in a rendition of "Somewhere over the rainbow . . ." with its frequencies shaped over time in an arc, rising then falling. Even if we simply speak a phrase, such as "over the rainbow," there remains a melodic aspect to our vocal intonations. In both cases, melody derives from the human voice, which conveys a continuously changing pitch pattern. These speech phrases have a kinship with musical melodies in that both exhibit a dynamic pitch contour as a fleeting series of changes in stimulus frequencies, perhaps shaped emotionally by the producer. For instance, a happy or excited voice has contours shaped by rising frequencies, whereas a melancholy voice tends to fall in pitch. Vocal modulations, whether produced involuntarily or voluntarily, are ubiquitous, assuming a variety of forms in normal speech. This raises fundamental questions about the role of extended vocal modulations in acoustic communications and the ability of listeners to follow the dynamics of the resulting pitch trajectories.

Of course, speech melodies differ from musical melodies. One obvious domain difference centers on the absence of musical scales in speech patterns. Instead, the resemblances between music and speech are largely found in similarities with pitch contour patterns (i.e., not scalar tonal patterns). Indeed, this chapter draws heavily on earlier discussions of musical contour to describe listeners' pitch tracking activities while attending to speech. In Chapter 11 musical pitch tracking to melodic contours was defined as continuous adaptive adjustments of oscillations entraining exogenously to a modulating, external, driving rhythm (typically an F0). In other words, pitch tracking is a form of frequency-following based on stimulus-driven i.e., exogenous, entrainment.

The present chapter continues to draw on pitch tracking to explore how people follow rapid and virtually continuous vocal changes in speech frequency. Essentially, this chapter concentrates on *intonation* in speech prosody. In contrast to the preceding chapter, which touched on prosodic features of intensity and timing that shape words and phrases, this chapter extends the focus of speech prosody to modulations of frequency-driving rhythms. Also, the stimulus frequencies of interest here exhibit more extensive modulations than those of intensity discussed for speech groupings in Chapter 12. In this case, speech intonations create true pitch contours that travel over several melodic contour groups in speech.

A foundation for discussing speech melodies was also laid in Chapter 6, where listeners' pitch perception was described as exogenous entrainment to a sound's fundamental frequency. In particular, a complex speech sound leads to a complex pitch percept that is strongly determined by its fundamental frequency, underscored by its repetition rate. Yet Chapter 6 did not consider percepts of sound patterns arising from systematic variations over time of this fundamental frequency. The present chapter tackles this topic. It explores ways in which dynamic changes in a speaker's vocal frequency, i.e., one's *intonation,* allow a listener to follow, in real time, systematic rising and falling shapes of this frequency. Although we draw on parallels with the musical contour described in Chapter 11, the intriguing intonation contours of speech deserve a separate chapter.

The main themes of this chapter, then, center on frequency modulations. Although local frequency modulations involve specific rises and falls that shape speech intonation curves, beyond such local ups and downs of frequency modulations lie the challenge of explaining percepts of grander excursions of intonation paths in speech. In fact, a full discussion of this topic is beyond the scope of this chapter, which addresses only a piece of this formidable puzzle. This piece concerns the potential roles of traditional versus transient mode-locking in describing entrainment to the slower rhythms of speech contours. Finally, to tackle speech melody, whether local or global, it is essential to begin with the micro-rhythms that define the fundamental frequency of speech.

CHAPTER GOALS

This chapter focuses on speech prosody as expressed by intonations. An overriding goal is to illustrate ways in which certain frequency modulations in speech instill in listeners percepts of speech melody (i.e., intonation patterns). This chapter has three main sections.

The first section extends the entrainment framework to embrace melodic shapes in speech. In this respect, it shares with other Part II chapters a goal of selectively illustrating applications of entrainment concepts of Part I. Here, we return to focus upon fast speech events. Specifically, this section addresses modulations of vocal micro-driving rhythms carried by a vocal fundamental frequency. It concentrates on a listener's capacity to engage in *pitch tracking* (i.e., frequency following) of changing vocal intonations. The aim is to illustrate how fast exogenous entrainments of a listener's driven micro-rhythm(s) are modified as a speaker's voice rapidly shifts rates of significant micro-driving rhythms. In short, we zoom into the tiny time zone of instantaneous velocities to explore those *pitch expectancies* which emerge in listeners as they automatically follow changing fine time scales through the local ups and downs of a speech melody.

This section also returns to the topic of *perceptual contrasts*, now as *pitch contrasts*. This application of entrainment principles resembles that for time and loudness contrasts developed in the preceding chapter. But formalizing pitch contrasts requires introduction of an important entrainment construct: the *detuning curve*. A by-product of this construct allows for identification of certain *pitch accents*. These accents are defined as time markers, which elicit pronounced perceptual (pitch) contrasts that figure locally in prosodic groups.

A second section addresses more global aspects of a melodic context associated with slower prosodic rhythms created by multiple intonation groups. In contrast to the fast external driving rhythms of pitch tracking, in this section, the relevant external rhythms are the slower macro-rhythms of a melodic contour that arise from time markers based on pitch accents.[1] These resulting macro-rhythms function as slower driving rhythms that initiate temporal expectancies at rates spelled out by the time structure of intonation groups.

The third and final section distinguishes Dynamic Attending Theory (DAT) intonation concepts from corresponding concepts found in prominent linguistic approaches. This dynamic view of speech prosody extends entrainment concepts developed in earlier chapters. Few new theoretical concepts appear in this chapter. Nevertheless, this application of dynamic attending concepts highlights aspects of prosody that do not figure in leading linguistic theories. That is, DAT hypothesizes that prosodic structure determines listeners' melodic expectancies based on entrainment activities, whereas contemporary linguistic theories concentrate largely on indexing the function of salient surface properties of intonation contours.

TRACKING MELODIC SHAPES OF SPEECH: PITCH EXPECTANCIES

Our capacity to attend to a speech pattern, in the moment, depends on our ability to rapidly synchronize attending. And, as previous chapters have shown, a pattern's time structure is critical to advancing certain modes of synchronized attending. This is true even at time scales of very fast events. Indeed, at the micro-time scales of pitch, we can argue that a listener's attending is driven by a speaker's vocal micro-rhythms that convey fast driving rhythms. As a speaker's vocalizations unfold over time, the most compelling frequency component, the fundamental frequency, F0, varies in nonrandom ways.

Consider, for instance, that vocal pitch excursions of average adult speakers range between 100 and 300 Hz, with such frequencies modulating into different prosodic shapes. These shapes result from continuous changes in pitch contour which resemble the musical contour patterns discussed earlier. That is, they involve glides and hat patterns that grow out of rapidly rising and falling vocal frequencies. This section unpacks a listener's percepts of such shapes in speech. As with musical contours, it assumes that percepts of pitch contours in speech depend on a listener's ongoing exogenous entrainment to rapidly changing frequencies in sounds, i.e., pitch tracking. Generally, it explores how speakers and listeners unknowingly "keep in touch" with each other through dynamic synchronies that link the listener's driven rhythm to the speaker's driving rhythm even with rhythms operating on microscopic time scales.

Paths of Pitch Expectancies in Speech

In any entrainment scenario, the driving and driven dyad is a central concept. Important dyads in conversational exchanges are those originating from the fast time scales of vocal pitch. At these micro-time scales, we begin by considering a series of instantaneously changing dyadic states where a fast driving stimulus rhythm is created by a speaker and an equally fast driven rhythm is elicited, via resonance, in the listener. The speaker's micro-driving rhythm is the fundamental vocal frequency, F0, of a complex speech sound. At these time scales, any instantaneous frequency (velocity) is denoted by its angular velocity, ω; also, as in prior chapters, the external driving rhythm is similarly denoted as ω_i, with its resonant neural counterpart: ω_{oi}. (This assumes that a driving rhythm may be the repetition rate of a complex sound [~F0].)

Past chapters have established that fast entrainment is robust. Thus, exogenous entrainment to very fast driving rhythms continues to reflect adaptive coupling of an entraining neural oscillation to its fast-paced driving rhythm. In this case, attending activity is based on coupling of these rhythms, thereby delivering a pitch percept. Unlike Chapter 6 (on pitch perception), this chapter aims to explain the impact of *continuous changes* in the fundamental frequency of a complex speech sound. For a listener to follow such a frequency, the entraining neural correlate of F0 undergoes corresponding continuous changes. This driven oscillation must momentarily adapt its phase and period to keep pace with the glide path of its partner. Moreover, given entrainment region limits of any entrainment activity, a driving rhythm exhibiting an extended glide path will also awaken successive (possibly overlapping) activities of near-neighbor gradient oscillations. This means that the ERO hypothesis, involving dynamic proximity, may also be involved, as described in Chapter 11.[2]

This adventure, then, involves an adaptive following of changing micro-rhythms which naturally results in *pitch tracking*. Recall that pitch tracking applies to fast events; it is based upon fast successive exogenous entrainments of one or several driven micro-rhythms.[3] This is an automatic activity that allows a listener to perceptually "ride" the hills and valleys of a melodic contour. Along this ride, a listener's pitch tracking continually updates ongoing driven rhythm expectancies about the sound's pitch. These internal responses are *pitch expectancies*.

To pursue pitch expectancies and their violations more thoroughly, this chapter focuses on activities of the neural correlate; i.e., of a pertinent driving rhythm (F0), namely, its intrinsic driven rhythm, ω_{oi}. This oscillator continuously adapts its manifest frequency, Ω, as it momentarily tracks the frequency of the external driving rhythms, ω_i.[4]

Melodic Contour and Pitch Tracking: An Example

To simplify matters, let us reduce the world of rapid F0 changes to the toy phrase "*We just dislike fog*" in Figure 13.1A. Because intonation contours vary, two different speaker contours are shown in this figure (black and gray curves). Each of the two versions of this utterance reflects rapid pitch changes based on correspondingly small time periods. Also, each curve for this phrase, over a stretch of time, qualifies as a distinct *intonation curve*, which begins with an F0 = 200 Hz. Notice, however, the black curve shows a micro-driving rhythm journey that deviates more widely from its opening frequency than does the gray curve. Yet each contour has a path based on minor F0 modulations of micro-driving rhythms that progress from a relatively low frequency to a higher one (accented), then fall to a lower information point. The minor speaker fluctuations of F0 along both paths justify a simplification which allows acknowledgment of the adaptivity of a single driven rhythm, not shown in the figure. (Note: H*, and etc. are linguistic codes for high and low pitch accents, discussed in a later section; see Box 13.1.)

In a tutorial spirit, let's briefly review the notation of angular velocity (Chapter 3). This expresses a frequency change as an angular velocity in radians per second (or ms): $\omega = 2\pi$ F0. As such, angular velocity nicely captures the brevity of frequency modulations that continuously undulate in time. Simply put, higher frequencies reflect faster spinning oscillations. That is, imagine velocities as describing toy spinning tops. Then tops should spin faster and faster as frequencies rise. Figure 13.1A shows rising, then falling, F0 values, denoted by ω (or ω). However, such a phrase can be shaped in various ways. Note that the intonation shape is more pronounced for ω than for ω. Thus, in Figure 13.1A, the initial F0 value of 200 Hz has a 5 ms cycle (or 1,256.6 radians per second). For simplicity, momentary frequency values are reported in the more familiar unit of Hertz.

Several important DAT constructs emerge from Figure 13.1 which shows a speaker-listener dyad. First, each modulating stimulus (i.e., a speaker's driving rhythm) initially induces a resonant neural correlate. For instance, the black curve, ω, of a speaker initially taps into a listener's latent oscillation, hence eliciting the

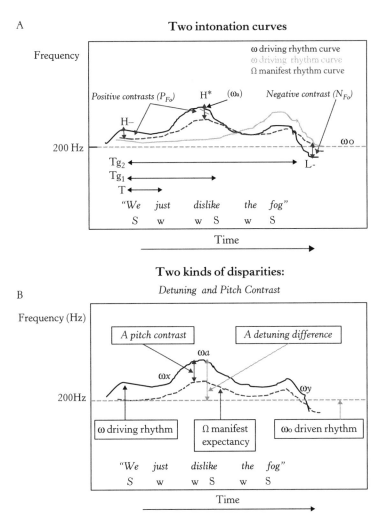

A   **Two intonation curves**

FIGURE 13.1 Two intonation curves to the same phrase. Panel **A** shows hypothetical intonation driving rhythms of a speaker's curves for two different frequency contours (black, gray) which vary in intonational emphasis, hence creating different accents. A listener's manifest driven rhythm (dashed dark gray curve, Ω) shows attempts to track the black driving rhythm of a speaker. Also shown is the latent frequency of the listener's driven rhythm, ωo, as a flat dashed gray line. Panel **B** distinguishes between differences of a speaker's driving rhythm (solid black line) relative to the listener's manifest driven rhythm (dashed curve) and its detuning differences, which is referenced to the listener's latent oscillation (flat dashed line).

intrinsic neural frequency, ω_o (dashed flat line), that is near the initial ω. Together, an exogenous driving–driven dyad ($\omega{:}\omega_o$) forms a coupled oscillator unit: a *micro-dyad*. In this coupling, ω_o remains invariant while the external driving rhythm, ω, modulates, forming melodic peaks and valleys. This interaction revives another familiar construct; namely, a listener's manifest frequency designated as Ω (dashed curve). Up to a point, a listener's latent oscillation tolerates frequency modulations in the driving rhythm; this is evident in Ω adjustments to local driving rhythm changes in ω. Pitch tracking of

an attender then refers to an oscillation's observable adaptive behavior to a changing external stimulus. Thus, responses to ω are gauged by changes in Ω. Therefore, we can say this listener's Ω realizes *pitch tracking* the changes in ω produced by a speaker. In short, here a listener tracks the vocalized shape of a speaker's utterance (ω) with the manifest frequency (Ω) automatically speeding up or slowing down, but adaptively growing closer to the driving rhythm over time. Importantly, these adaptive changes in a driven rhythm's period *do not affect its intrinsic period*: ω_o remains stationary.

BOX 13.1

DYNAMIC ATTENDING THEORY AND LINGUISTIC THEORIES

Five differences between dynamic attending and linguistic theories are listed.

1. *Driving–driven rhythms and expectancies*: A basic DAT unit, the dyad, derives from speaker–listener exchanges. A driving rhythm produced by a speaker entrains a listener's driven rhythm that carries expectancies. Violated expectancies create pitch contrasts. AM Theory (with ToBI) indexes surface speech properties not interpreted as driving rhythms.

2. *Linguistic oscillator cluster and attractor profile*: In DAT, an *oscillator cluster* comprises multiple, simultaneous neural oscillations endogenously entrained. An *attractor profile* emerges when a series of different, fleeting driving rhythms entrain to a common referent oscillation. AM/ToBI features neither construct.

3. *Definitions: Accents and contrast*: DAT defines accents as local physical changes in some dimension (e.g., intensity, F0, etc.). A *joint accent* is a co-occurrence of two (or more) such accents (e.g., F0 + intensity; F0 + intensity + duration). ToBI defines accents categorically, based on pragmatic function. Some categories (codes: H*, L*) depend on joint accents (e.g., pitch-plus-stress).

4. *Context: Multiple expectancies*: In DAT, a speech context is a temporal distribution of multiple time markers which outline various driving rhythms. Driving rhythms induce in listeners driven rhythms that express temporal expectancies. In AM/ToBI, temporal context is not a source of expectancies.

5. *Local frequency modulations: Intonation groups*: In DAT, beginnings and ends of intonation groups are associated, respectively, with local rising and falling vocal changes (ω). Respectively, they strengthen or weaken entrainments, signaling the beginning and ends of intonation groups (fast–slow rule). ToBI also distinguishes beginning (L+) from ending (L−) pitch accents, but the impact of such changes is not attributed to differences in entrainment strength.

Pitch Tracking and Pitch Expectancies

Pitch tracking is effortless. It enables listeners to involuntarily "keep pace" perceptually with stimulus changes in a speaker's fundamental frequency. Normally, an average adult male speaker has a fundamental frequency that averages between 140 Hz and 170 Hz. But, realistically, people do not speak in monotones. So, male speakers readily exhibit vocal variations of F0 that deviate from this average (by e.g., +/− 4 semitones). Nevertheless, the typical listener exposed to such vocal excursions readily copes with such variations by engaging manifest driven rhythms that continuously adapt to changing intonations in a speaker's driving rhythm. Also, as with melodic contours, pitch tracking of large vocal excursions may involve overlapping activities of near-neighbor oscillations, as described in the ERO (cf. Chapter 11).

Importantly, recall that pitch tracking rests on two different types of expectancies: the latent expectancy of the driven oscillation, ω_o, and the active manifest expectancy, Ω. Theoretically, listeners' overt expectancy responses reflect Ω. In turn, Ω depends on the adaptive proficiency of the driven, but latent, oscillation and certain driving rhythm properties. To review, the general attending hypothesis implies that phase-coupling depends on the force and regularity of a driving rhythm (ω). However, a qualifying tension on coupling during entrainment rests with the opposing strength of the driven oscillation (ω_o). This revives the push–pull scenario, wherein a strong oscillation is less responsive to perturbations within a driving rhythm than is a weak oscillation. For instance, in Figure 13.1, a stronger latent oscillation will tend to "pull" the dashed curved line of Ω closer to ω_o, whereas a stronger external driving rhythm, ω, "pushes" Ω closer to it. Finally, we need to keep in mind that these various factors are always in play

Let's focus on the manifest frequency, Ω. It is rarely identical to ω_o or to ω; it can waffle back and forth between these opposing forces. However, in an entrainment scenario, over time the manifest frequency tends to gravitate toward a persisting driving rhythm frequency: $\Omega \rightarrow \omega$, as suggested in Figure 13.1A. In other words, a listener's momentary pitch percept is based on aligning a manifest expectancy with a to-be-perceived stimulus.

Expectancy Violations and Pitch Contrasts

As with all expectancies, pitch expectancies are fallible. Even at micro-time scales, a preceding speaking context that establishes in a listener a manifest expectancy, Ω, can lead to a subsequent expectancy violation due to an unanticipated local change in a speaker's driving rhythm, ω. Figure 13.1A illustrates this idea. Note that the more expressive (solid black curve) driving rhythm creates certain frequency modulations that lead to momentary, but significant, ω-Ω disparities. (These disparities translate into local differences between expectancy and reactive pulses, thus resembling the loudness and timing contrasts outlined Chapter 12.) In Figure 13.1A, all ω-Ω disparities express *pitch contrasts* (see double arrows). In addition to loudness and temporal contrasts, we now have pitch contrasts.

Intuitively, these contrasts arise from expectancy violations which create larger pitch contrasts at high and low ω points in a speech melody. In fact, this is generally true.

Notice that the pitch tracking example in Figure 13.1A suggests that a pitch peak of the ω trajectory coincides with the word *dislike*. This is interesting because it creates a significant pitch contrast which, in turn, catches a listener's attending. This creates a *pitch accent*, ωa. Such accents vary in strength as a function of contrast i.e., due to a local (physical) change in ω.

Clearly, pitch contrasts are linked to manifest expectancies. However, Figure 13.1B also shows another disparity, one linked to the latent expectancy, ω_o. The momentary (i) difference between a driving and driven rhythm: $\omega_i - \omega_o$ is termed a *detuning difference*. This is an important distinction which is spelled out in an equally important plot, termed a *detuning curve*.

Detuning Curves

The detuning curve is fundamental to entrainment analysis. It is a basic technique that specifies the limits of manifest expectancies for a given entraining oscillation. It plots pitch contrasts

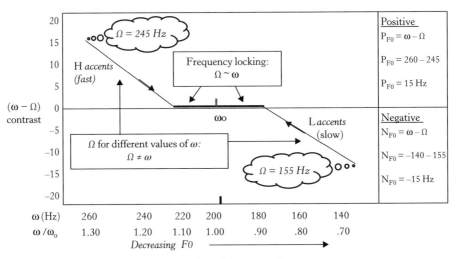

A detuning curve: F0 contrasts

ω: instantaneous F0 of speaker's modulated driving rhythm
ω_o: instantaneous listener's intrinsic (resting) driven rhythm
Ω: instantaneous manifest driven frequency (i.e., corresponding to $1/p'$)

FIGURE 13.2 A detuning curve based on frequency contrasts between the driving rhythm (ω) and the manifest driven rhythm tracking it (Ω) on the ordinate is plotted as a function of driving rhythm frequency for a latent oscillator ωo. As driving rhythms speed up in frequency (relative to ωo), positive contrasts (ω–Ω) increase in value; the reverse holds for relative slowing of the driving rhythm. Extreme contrasts are defined, respectively, as High (H) and Low (L) pitch accents.

as a function of the frequency of a prevailing driving rhythm and the limiting latent oscillation. Basically, this curve depends on a *detuning (frequency) difference*, Δf_D (for any time scale). For these fast frequencies, $\Delta f_D = \omega_1 - \omega_2$ where ω_2 is identical to the intrinsic frequency, ω_o.

An example detuning curve appears in Figure 13.2. This curve describes the impact of a latent oscillation on pitch contrasts experienced by listeners exposed, for instance, to a phrase such as "We just dislike fog" in Figure 13.1. Thus, assume a listener responds throughout this phrase by relying on a resonant latent oscillation with $\omega_o = 200$ Hz (flat dashed line). (Note that ω_o is activated by the initial ω of 200 Hz.) As a hypothetical listener encounters this micro-driving rhythm, ω, her ostensible adaptive responses, Ω, are limited by ω_o. This leads to a pitch contrasts, $\omega - \Omega$, for momentary ω values, according to the detuning curve in Figure 13.2. A pitch contrast depends on three factors: ω_o, ω, and Ω.

A detuning curve incorporates all three factors just identified. The curve illustrated in Figure 13.2. is one of several possible detuning curves. It exhibits values of ω ranging from 260 Hz to 140 Hz (abscissa). In this example, note that during pitch tracking both positive, **P**, and negative, **N**, pitch contrasts emerge, depending on whether the driving rhythm frequency, ω, is faster (a positive contrast) or slower (a negative contrast) than expected, Ω (i.e., for $\omega \neq \omega_o = 200$ Hz).

Adaptive limits always exist for entraining oscillations. In light of this, it is remarkable that the adaptivity of this oscillation allows the manifest rhythm, Ω, to change from complete adaptation to a stimulus driving rhythm ($\Omega = \omega$) between 180 Hz and 220 Hz (abscissa) to significant corrections for extreme driving rhythms. For instance, consider corrections with fast ω rhythms above 220 Hz ($\Omega \neq \omega$). If ω is 260 Hz, then the corrected manifest frequency shows a $\Omega \sim 245$ Hz. This creates a positive pitch contrast of 15 Hz ($\mathbf{P}_{F0}$, right ordinate).

Detuning plots are useful, in part, because they spell out the limits of pitch contrasts. Detuning curves also stipulate various adaptive responses open to listeners during pitch tracking. For instance, in Figure 13.2, a range of different corrected (manifest) pitch expectancies, Ω, are portrayed given a driving rhythm and its latent counterpart, ω_o. Complete corrections show a listener's expectancy precisely matching the driving rhythm, thus eliminating any pitch contrast; this indicates perfect pitch tracking where l$\omega - \Omega$l = zero. Furthermore, very small differences, where ω is close to ω_o, fall within a *frequency-locking region*. In this example,

the frequency-locking region, which varies with the force of ω, ranges from 220 Hz to 180 Hz. Essentially, this region is a comfort zone around the natural frequency, ω_o, with a center defined by a powerful attractor ratio: $\omega/\omega_o = 1.00$. In other words, this exogenous entrainment, known as pitch tracking, is governed by a simple attractor of $n{:}m = 1{:}1$.

At a general level, three aspects of detuning curves are worth highlighting. Respectively, they involve pitch tracking, detuning differences, and pitch accents.

Pitch Tracking

A detuning curve documents listeners' ostensible reliance on the manifest pitch expectancy, rather than on ω_o, as a source of pitch tracking. Generally, this tracking of intonation contours involves the activity of a single entraining oscillator, as implied in Figure 13.1. However, in some cases, it can involve overlapping activities of several, near-neighbor oscillations (as in Chapter 11). In any case, it is the manifest frequencies of a driven oscillation that realize listeners' *pitch tracking behaviors*.

Pitch Contrasts Versus Detuning Differences

Detuning curves reveal an important distinction involving tones that differ in frequencies. The frequency-locking region in Figure 13.2 specifies a detuning difference in which listeners cannot differentiate between sounds with two different frequencies: ω and ω_o. That is, if Ω ($= \omega_1$) functions as standard stimulus and ω_o is a comparison stimulus in a psychophysical task assessing discrimination limits, then the detuning region reflects threshold limits. Alternatively, in an entrainment task, a whole range of l$\omega - \Omega$l differences, including those outside the frequency-locking region, are relevant.

This distinction has interesting implications. It means that psychophysics measurements of discrimination thresholds, which often specify a 5% time discrimination threshold, do not tell the whole story about listeners' percepts of periodic differences associated with frequencies. Also important are the pitch contrasts plotted by detuning curves. This chapter broadens that discussion.

Pitch Contrasts and Pitch Accents

Listeners routinely encounter intonation modulations in utterances of others. Indeed, listeners are often unaware of their effortless tracking of these pitch changes. In part, this is because the motivating attending mechanism is involuntary at tiny time scales. The virtual continuity of frequency modulations in ordinary speech enables effective adaptations during pitch tracking to a broad range of frequency changes (e.g., as in Figure 13.2). Typically, many pitch contrasts are so small that they are ignored because involuntary corrections are performing as they should.

Nevertheless, certain driving rhythm excursions can create distinctive pitch contrasts. The brings up the topic of pitch accents. Figure 13.2 shows some extreme pitch contrasts, where pitch tracking, conveyed by variable values of Ω, undershoots high F0 values or overshoots low ones. In the context of spontaneous speech, three types of intonation contrasts distinguish certain pitch accents. One accent type is a pitch peak accent. This is illustrated in Figure 13.3 for the familiar

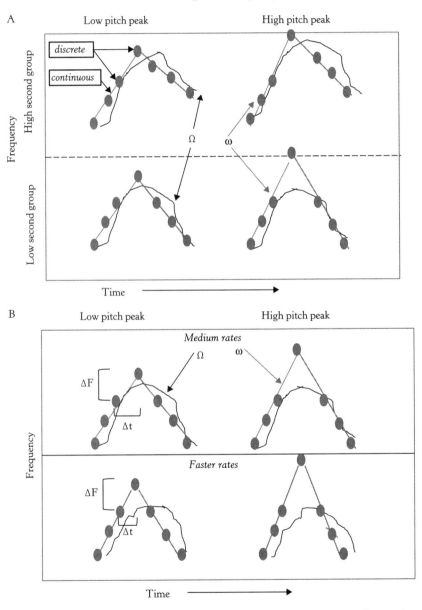

Pitch tracking of HAT groups

FIGURE 13.3 Examples of pitch tracking of hypothetical hat contours, continuous or discrete (separated tone) frequencies, with low and high central pitch peaks. (**A**) Seven tone sequences with declining tones either in a relatively high frequency range (top) or low range (bottom). (**B**) Symmetric groups as a function of rate differences (slow, fast). Exceptions occur when highest pitch is not included in group. Also adaptive pitch tracking tends to lag, as shown by Ω values during rising/falling tone groups.

hat patterns (at different rates). Pitch peak accents depend on relatively large pitch contrasts (positive and negative). The other accent types shown in this figure involve positive and negative contrasts that distinguish different boundary accents, respectively, from rising and falling driving rhythm frequencies.

Imagine that Figure 13.3 depicts pitch tracking (Ω, as variable lines) of a hypothetical listener presented with a speech pattern conforming to this melodic hat pattern. The listener's manifest frequency is shown to lag rising and falling glides that define this contour pattern. These are partially corrected Ω values. Returning to the spontaneous speech depicted in Figure 13.1. In this figure, a pitch peak accent, **ωa**, is shown as a local increase in the speaker's driving frequency of **ω**. Here, **ωa** accents the word *dislike* (H* is linguistic code). Boundary accents (H⁺, H⁻) are also shown. All these accents, by definition, capture a degree of attention.

This account also adds clarity to different versions of accent "salience." *Objective salience* of an accent refers to an actual physical change in local driving rhythm points as in, for example, **ωa** – **ω**$_i$. By contrast, *subjective salience* of an accent depends on the magnitude of a pitch contrast, **ωa** – **Ω**. Although correlated, both properties contribute to the strength of accents as time markers.

The Fast–Slow Intonation Rule: Perceiving Prosodic Groups

Pitch contour, whether in music or speech, can be described in terms of frequency modulations of one (or several) micro-driving rhythms. A fast–slow rule, based on these modulations in music, was introduced in Chapter 11. This prosodic contrast rule describes perceptual grouping as a function of local frequency changes. Chapter 12, added other prosodic rules for grouping. These rules focused on percepts of beginnings and endings of speech groups; namely, the on–off rule (loudness/intensity) and the expand–shrink rule (time).

Importantly, the fast–slow rule joins the panetheon of grouping rules. When it is applied to intonation contours, this rule describes adaptive oscillator responses to driving rhythm changes that affect a listener's sense of changing entrainment strength. Specifically, rising frequencies of driving rhythms, **ω**$_i$, as in glides, reflect a speeding up of angular velocity, yielding positive pitch contrasts (**P** in Figure 13.4A). Alternatively, falling **ω**$_i$ values slow angular velocities, yielding negative pitch contrasts (**N** in Figure 13.4A). The fast–slow rule goes further to stipulate that positive pitch contrasts signify a strengthening of entrainment due to its speeding up. To a listener's tunable brain, this announces the beginning of a group.

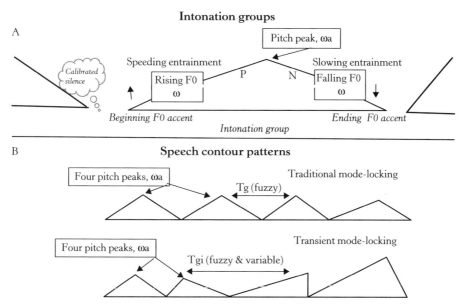

FIGURE 13.4 (A) Micro-driving rhythm paths for a hypothetical intonation group showing rising and falling contours. A pitch peak determines a pitch accent, denoted **ωa**. **(B)** Top row. Macro-driving rhythms of group time spans, Tg$_3$, outlined by pitch peak accents (**ωa**). Rising and falling pitch accents are boundaries for shorter (embedded) phrases of Tg$_2$. Regular group time spans invite Traditional mode locking. Bottom row of **(B)**. Time spans marked by irregularly timed pitch peak accents invites Transient mode-locking.

Alternatively, negative pitch contrasts due to a falling ω reflect entrainment weakening, which signals the end of prosodic group.

Figure 13.4A sketches the fast–slow rule for a hypothetical intonation group based on a hat pattern. This pattern opens with a speeding up of ω that conveys rapid strengthening of entrainment at a group's onset. Also shown are slowing ω values that accompany a falling glide, signaling a weakening of dyadic coupling. The latter is a harbinger of a group ending. Rising glides offer increasingly more phase-locking opportunities (cycles) per second than do falling ones. Entrainment naturally happens rapidly as a listener tracks a boundary accent at the onset of an intonation group where the driving rhythm actually is speeding up. Conversely, a falling frequency validly signals an ending because this micro-driving rhythm truly is slowing down. Consequently, a listener's experience is one of "tuning in" to a rising F0 and "tuning out" with falling F0 profiles.

Evidence consistent with this interpretation of rising and falling pitch contours in speech is overwhelming. Beginning and ending F0 changes are commonly coded linguistically as important group boundaries or edge features in prosody (Box 13.1). This widely acknowledged status of rising versus falling sound frequencies in intonation contours of speech strongly supports the idea that rising frequencies open a phrase while falling frequencies are boundary accents that end a phrase.

Fast–Slow Versus On–Off Rules

The fast–slow rule of frequency modulations shares with the on–off rule (from the prior chapter) a focus on features that increase or decrease *entrainment strength*. Both rules appeal to waxing versus waning of entrainment activity at group boundaries.[5,6,7] They lend credence to the employment of sharp changes in frequency as effective time-markers.[8] Although it is likely that driving rhythm changes involving intensity and frequency are correlated, this account implies that they can operate independently as well.[9]

Summary of Pitch Expectancies

Few of us speak in monotones. In fact, when we do, listeners become passive, annoyed, or simply fall asleep. It is the engaging, even fleeting, variations in the frequency of a speaker's voice that keeps people awake and listening. Vocal frequencies and their modulations actively awaken adaptive resonant oscillations in the tunable brains of listeners. Along with prosodic modulations of intensity and timing, frequency modulations are critical components of lively prosody.

This section offers a theoretical backdrop for understanding listeners' dynamic engagements with speech melodies. In speech, a speaker may unconsciously control a listener's involuntary attending. That is, listeners who experience a speaker's utterance unconsciously operate in parallel with that speaker's production by automatically tracking the peaks and valleys of its intonation contour. This dynamic speaker–listener unit, formalized as a dyad, depends on exogenous entrainments of listeners' neural oscillations that realize pitch tracking. Pitch tracking in speech operates much as it does in music (Chapter 11). That is, it involves fleeting expectancies along with momentary corrected violations (pitch contrasts); expectancies literally ride along all the ups and downs of a speaker's intonation contour. This section concentrates on listeners' grouping percepts based on changing intonation frequencies in speech.

Listeners' percepts of intonation groups are created by modulations in vocal pitch arising from local changes in a speaker's F0 (micro-driving rhythm). Exogenous entrainment enters into this picture with pitch tracking and correlated expectancies which, when violated, create pitch contrasts. During entrainment, relatively large pitch contrasts determine pitch accents. The fast–slow entrainment rule (of musical contour) also describes a listener's reactions to pitch contrasts, including those which specify beginnings and endings of intonation groups.

The major points of this section are:

- *Pitch tracking* reflects a listener's exogenous entrainment to modulations of vocal frequency in a speaker's utterances.
- *Pitch tracking* involves listeners' pitch expectancies about changing vocal micro-driving rhythms (ω) in a speech signal.
- An observable *pitch expectancy* carries corrected (manifest) frequencies (Ω) of the latent oscillation (ω_o).
- *Pitch contrasts* happen with expectancy violations (i.e., when a manifest pitch expectancy differs from a driving rhythm ($\omega - \Omega$)).
- *Detuning curves* depict pitch contrasts ($\omega - \Omega$) as a function of the micro-driving rhythm, ω, and ωo.
- A *fast–slow* hypothesis explains differential effects of local F0 changes in ω at beginnings versus ends of intonation groups.

SPEECH CONTOUR PATTERNS

Images of prosodic intonations in speech call up sweeping patterns of rising and falling pitches. Preceding sections describe a listener's responses to an individual contour group in the ongoing speech of a speaker. These responses involve pitch tracking at micro-time levels and the pitch expectancies that grow out of this entrainment activity. However, a single hat pattern or one glide does not describe the whole contour pattern of a sentence. Sentences and phrases typically comprise many, often different, intonation groups. This section focuses on speech contour patterns and the slower driving rhythms they bring.

A speech contour pattern involves a series of intonation groups within a spoken sentence. As we have seen, percepts of these groups depend on the ups and downs of pitch tracking of frequency modulations. Although local changes in frequency mark beginnings and ends of groups, it is also common to find intensity changes reinforcing one or another frequency accent (e.g., **SwSw**. . . of strong–weak stress patterns). Simply put, the local strength of a time marker (or accent) can depend on both a frequency modulating (FM) time marker and a coinciding amplitude modulating (AM) time marker, when present.

The Shape of Speech Melodies

A speech melody, as described, is shaped by the ups and downs created by successive frequency glides. As in music, speech contour is shaped by the nature of a whole series of such groups. Two abstract profiles of speech contour patterns appear in Figure 13.4B. These patterns combine several individual intonation groups (as in Figure 13.4A). Note that, in addition to the up and down glide features of micro-driving rhythms, these melodic shapes are outlined by pitch accents that figure in creating a slower (i.e., a macro) driving rhythm. That is, as salient time markers, pitch accents outline the slower speech-driving rhythms implicated by melodic contours.

This broad definition of speech contour patterns leaves room for variations among melodic speech patterns. That is, prosodic variations arise from different speakers, different linguistic cultures, and so on. Contour patterns may operate on different levels and change with speaker and culture, among other things. Addressing the wider variety of melodic speech patterns that humans have developed is not possible in this book. Instead, this chapter aims more narrowly to consider certain ways in which speech contour patterns provide distinctive speech-driving rhythms that govern the dynamic attending activities of listeners.

To begin, Figure 13.4A abstracts a single intonation group arising from micro-driving rhythms that induce exogenous entrainments, described previously as pitch tracking. Moreover, this contour group features the pitch accents just discussed. A *pitch peak* accent, **ωa**, corresponds to a local, but relatively high-frequency central point within a hat-like contour. *Boundary accents* occur at the beginning, ↑**ω**, and ending, ↓**ω**, of groups. All accents have subjective salience conferred locally by pitch contrasts.

From a DAT perspective, pitch accents serve several functions. First, their salience captures a listener's attending. That is, accents can deliver strong reactive pulses that may or may not coincide with expectancy pulses generated by a preceding context. Second, as a set, pitch accents outline slower driving rhythms that, in turn, promote listener entrainments to an unfolding contour pattern at relatively slower time scales. This is suggested by the two speech contour patterns in Figure 13.4B. A variety of such contour patterns affords slower driving rhythms that invite listeners' entrainment at time scales marked by accented groups (e.g., Tg).

One argument against the hypothesis that speech contours carry functional, accent-marked driving rhythms has a familiar ring: *in speech, there is just too much temporal variability of pitch accents (i.e., pitch peak, boundary accents) for them to outline recurring (i.e., functional) driving rhythms.* In short, critics will argue that the variability of pitch accents renders them unreliable markers of effective speech-driving rhythms.

Setting aside issues surrounding the vague criteria of "too much" temporal variability, such arguments have merit only if we are bound to the assumption that successive groups within an extended utterance must have the same group length; that is, that Tgi, the time span of melodic group i, must be identical to group time spans of all surrounding groups. Clearly, this does not happen. Spontaneous speech is "spontaneous" because of its variability. In ordinary speech, utterances are afloat with a speaker's hesitations and seemingly arbitrary pauses, with idiosyncratically placed emphases as in: "Well, . . . Ummh . . . I think I'll take the chocolate cookie . . . ah, NO, . . . Hmmm, well . . . the FRUIT-bar." Yet, despite the hesitations and vagaries of everyday speech, which admittedly appear to render implausible the regularity of any accents, there remains room for hidden, contextual, regularities in time in entrainment models.

The magic of entrainment lies in the hidden pattern of attractors. Recall how moderate irregularities in time markers are routinely handled in entrainment theory. Moderate irregularities define a fuzzy rhythm that, nonetheless, succeeds (within limits) in engaging adaptive oscillations. With many fuzzy rhythms, entrainment can describe synchronized attending in a listener who relies on the traditional mode-locking protocol. This is suggested in Figure 13.4. This figure shows a driving rhythm comprising contour groups (Tgi) at the slower time scale of pitch peaks; although variations are not shown in this figure, in theory, such group time spans vary modestly over time (as in Chapters 7 and 8). Yet, despite such fuzziness, these group time spans can elicit/entrain a resonant oscillation with a matching period (p ~ Tg). And, upon recurrence of this we find a quasi-isochronous stimulus rhythm that supports traditional mode-locking, as suggested in Figure 13.4B (*top row*).

But what about *real* variability of accented time spans? Sometimes a speaker delivers a significantly expressive utterance that is so irregular, it does not belong to the category of quasi-isochronous, Tgi, driving rhythms. Such a case is shown in Figure 13.4B. The bottom row shows a contour pattern exhibiting significant temporal variability of speech accents that define successive melodic groups. Nevertheless, transient mode-locking operates in this case (from Chapter 7). With the transient mode-locking protocol, a persisting neural referent oscillation, elicited, initially, for instance, by speaking rate, prevails throughout a succession of variable contour groups, Tgi. In both cases shown in Figure 13.4B, mode-locking takes place with the aid of an internal referent periodicity. This referent might correspond to an opening group time span, supplied by the initial rate of a tempo response curve, and/or the period of a preferred subdivision.

Articulation rate usually plays a referential role in both traditional and transient mode-locking. As Chapter 12 showed, many emerging neuroscience studies verify the persisting presence of strong cortical oscillations in listeners linked to speech talking rate. This is consistent with the present view. What may be new, given earlier discussions, is acknowledgment that the articulation rate in a speaker's production supplies a possibly variable *tempo response curve* (Chapter 8).

Finally, a general caveat regarding criteria for "too much" variability cautions that variance, as gauged by psychoacoustic threshold limits, does not apply to entrainment. If "too much" reflects, 5% deviations as with psychoacoustic thresholds, that is "too little." As detuning curves suggest, entrainment limits applied to natural events invite more liberal limits (deriving from entrainment regions and bifurcation limits in phase space). For instance, the adaptivity an entraining oscillation can survive variations in time marker deviations as large as 20% of the driven rhythm's intrinsic period. In other words, even with the traditional entrainment protocol, moderate irregularity involves greater variability than is typical given discrimination threshold criteria. And, with transient mode-locking, greater flexibility abides.

Linguistic Oscillator Clusters and Attractor Profiles

The preceding chapter tackled issues of temporal variability of successive speech time spans by arguing that normal speech is described in terms of a continuum of temporal relationships which ranges from globally metrical time relationships, similar to musical meter, to distinctly quite nonmetrical patterns of time relations involving successions of rhythmic groups, thus resembling musical rhythms. This continuum applies as well to descriptions of speech contour configurations where time spans are outlined by pitch accents.

Figure 13.4B illustrates two idealized speech patterns that represent, respectively, traditional and transient modes of synchrony. Sometimes pitch contours are highly regular in speech, almost metrical, as in the top row in panel B. Such patterns invite traditional mode-locking, even if this temporal regularity hides beneath modest variance in timing of pitch accents (i.e., with fuzzy rhythms). In other contexts, speech contour patterns are distinctly variable. They form coherent time patterns, as illustrated in the bottom row of panel B. Consequently, such patterns invite transient mode-locking even if there exists some fuzziness in these fleeting driving rhythms (Chapter 7). The claim is that entrainments involving pitch contour follow a continuum already suggested for speech rhythms in general.

Traditional Mode-Locking

The special case of traditional mode-locking happens within patches of speech exhibiting regular contour patterns. These are created by speakers who produce an almost regular up-and-down undulating speaking pattern, either due to habit or for emphasis in speaking, as indicated in the top row of Figure 13.4. Here pitch accents outline relatively regular, possibly fuzzy, time spans at two different time scales. Pitch peaks outline the shower of the two scales, where rising and falling glides embed shorter time spans. Listeners involuntarily fall in pace with such a pattern, thus tacitly employing the traditional mode-locking protocol. Especially important are opening time spans of groups, Tg, as they usually provide a melodic context that awakens a related, but possibly faster, referent neural correlate (e.g., p_R). At the same time, the activity of any contextually elicited oscillation has a potential to endogenously synchronize with other active oscillations possessing related periods. Finally, both couplings and bindings can occur to connect faster with slower activated oscillations. The result is a meter-like *linguistic oscillator cluster*.

More generally, Figure 13.5 illustrates a typical linguistic oscillator cluster. Let the referent oscillation be based on articulation rate, T_R. Thus, for instance, $p_R \sim T_R = 200$ ms (for $T_R \sim$ Tg/2). In a meter-like fashion, the p_R can endogenously entrain to various other oscillations, including those excited by slower, accented, time spans. Thus, these three different resonating oscillations can form endogenous couplings among several harmonically related oscillations. In other words, this oscillator cluster results from endogenous couplings of multiple harmonically related oscillations; a set of global attractors have n:m ratios of 1:2, 1:1, and 2:1. In general, traditional mode-locking leads to such clusters and to sets of global attractors. Although this example shows simple global attractors,

more complex attractors of different cultures and circumstances follow similar principles.

Evidence for Traditional Mode-Locking: Research of Laura Dilley

The preceding discussion leads to the hypothesis that listeners will be sensitive to the opening contexts of spoken phrases. In particular, if exposed to a somewhat regular intonation context that excites a linguistic oscillator cluster, via traditional mode-locking, they will generate expectancies about future contour groups based on dominant oscillations in this cluster. So, is there any evidence for such context effects on listeners' percepts of prosody?

Indeed there is. Laura Dilley and Devin McAuley created regular speech contexts by controlling pitch (and stress) accents in two-syllable words (e.g., *skirmish, princess*, etc.).[10] Two conditions contained words that differed, respectively, in contour groupings such that contours highlighted either monosyllable properties, using falling glides, or disyllable properties, using rising glides. As shown in Figure 13.6. word contours highlight either monosyllable properties, using falling pitch glides, or they highlighted disyllables using rising pitch glides. In both conditions, these sequences ended with the same ambiguous test word. The task required that listeners report their percept of a final test word. Results showed that listeners heard the test word as a monosyllable in the monosyllable context but as a disyllable in the disyllable context.

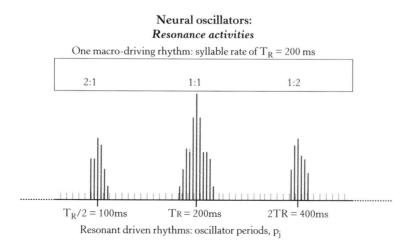

FIGURE 13.5 Resonance among different levels of a macro-rhythm. The referent-level oscillation (e.g., of syllables) is T_R. Periodic (pj) activity at this level resonates with oscillations of lower (faster) and higher (slower) periods.

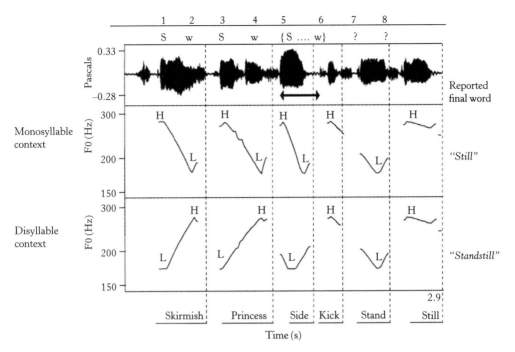

FIGURE 13.6 Context effects in syllable sequences. See text for details.

Adapted from figure 1 in Laura C. Dilley and J. Devin McAuley, "Distal Prosodic Context Affects Word Segmentation and Lexical Processing," *Journal of Memory and Language* 59, no. 3 (October 2008): 294–311, doi:10.1016/j.jml.2008.06.006.

Why does this happen? DAT offers a two-part explanation. One part focuses on the loci of fast micro-driving rhythms in individual contours, the other focuses upon the macro-driving rhythms of accent timings. Basically, the first part compares features of experimental conditions with falling glides to those with rising glides. Preceding DAT analyses of intonation contours implies that groups with falling contours elicit pitch tracking over the glide that weakens entrainment near the ending, signaling negative pitch contrasts, N. This means entrainment is strongest for the first syllable. For instance, in Figure 13.6, the high/low (HL) contour of *skirmish* accents, the syllable *skir* sparks a stronger entrainment than *mish* receives a weakening entrainment. Consequently, a listener's attending energy is greater for individual syllable time scales, in fact segregating the two syllables into percepts of monosyllables (cf. Figure 13.5 for a syllable of T_R). Conversely, in the condition with rising glides, pitch tracking gains strength over time span of glide, signaled by positive pitch contrasts, **P**, throughout (also see Figure 13.4A). This glues together the two syllables, leading to percepts of disyllables.

The second part of this DAT story is straightforward. It concerns the regularity of pitch peak accents (H) in both conditions. These macro-rhythms support traditional mode-locking of attending, as outlined in Figure 13.4B (*top row*). In turn, this protocol contributes to a listener's tendency to anticipate "when" test items will occur.[11] Underlying expectancies involve respectively different oscillations entraining at syllable (p_R) and dissyllable (np_R; n=2) macro-time levels for monosyllable and disyllable conditions, respectively. This underscores the importance of an opening context. It shows that we can "hear" the same word differently depending on the nature of a preceding context. Related studies of these context effects rule out semantic factors.[12,13] Together, such findings implicate a role for context-driven expectancies.[14]

Finally, in theory, traditional mode-locking delivers oscillator clusters, with oscillator members inter-related by global attractor ratios (here, duple meter ratios of Figure 13.5). However, listeners develop expectancies specific to individual periodicities. That is, focal attending can shifts among driving rhythms by selectively heightening the energy of one or another driven oscillation. Specifically, an expectancy typically rides on the dominant (most energetic) oscillation of a cluster. But dominance changes with an attender's goals.

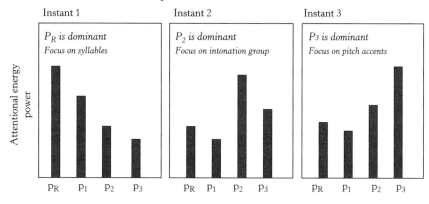

FIGURE 13.7 Attending in the moment, as shown by changing power spectra of the four oscillator components of speech oscillator cluster. The dominant oscillation (not to be confused with the referent; here with period, p_R) changes from moment to moment to focus on different time levels of a phrase.

At one moment, a dominant oscillation reflects a focus on syllables; hence, the dominant oscillation is the referent period (i.e., the talking rate period, p_R). Then, later, attending might shift with an energy boost to a slower, related oscillation (period, $pi \sim 2\ p_R$).[15,16] Figure 13.7 portrays selective attending dynamics within an oscillator cluster. Each bar in this figure reflects the hypothetical activity of an oscillation in a meter-like cluster. It indicates that the oscillation with most energy at a particular point in time (i.e., the dominant oscillation) determines a listener's momentary expectancy. The power spectrum reflects the momentary strength of cluster oscillations.

Transient Mode-Locking

Ordinary speech abounds in irregularities of accent timings. Often temporal variations of strong accents are too great to support traditional mode-locking. In these cases, speech exhibits distinctly irregular contour patterns; one example is seen in Figure 13.4B (*bottom*). As with the top pattern of Figure 13.4B the bottom pattern contains contour groups outlined by fast micro-driving rhythms in the form of rising and falling glides. However, the two example sequences in panel B differ with respect to the slower time pattern of contour groups marked out by pitch accents. The grouping pattern in the top row of this panel has regular accent

timing (both pitch peak accents and boundary accents). By contrast, the speech contour pattern in the bottom row has irregular accent timing and that creates variable driving rhythm time spans of groups, Tgi.

Transient mode-locking happens when successive driving rhythm time spans vary substantially. Here, transient mode-locking develops as successive macro-driving rhythms lock into a persisting referent oscillation. In this protocol, let's assume that the referent oscillation, awakened early in an unfolding context, is based on articulation rate. This entrainment protocol will then eventually yield an internalized attractor profile, a *linguistic attractor profile*.

Expectancies in Transient Mode-Locking

Traditional mode-locking promotes the growth of expectancies in linguistic metric clusters. An analogous story holds for expectancies resulting from transient mode-locking. Transient mode-locking builds on the concept of parallelism between attractor profiles in a speaker's produced contour patterns and corresponding attractor profiles induced in a listener's expectancy profile. In speech contour patterns, such as that in Figure 13.4B (*bottom row*), a listener's transient mode-locking leads to development of low level expectancies that accrue to the contextually induced, and persisting, referent period. This internal referent period initially entrains to a speaker's talking rate. However, higher level entrainments to successive intonation group time spans are inevitably weaker for irregular speech contours (e.g., Figure 13.4B, bottom) than for regular ones (e.g., Figure 13.4B, top). Nevertheless, parallelism of a speaker's production with a listener's expectancy applies to the example patterns in Figure 13.4B (*bottom row*) as well as to a wide variety of speech contour patterns with variable intonation groups as suggested in Chapter 8; Box 8.1). The main point of this exercise holds that irregularly timed accents in an utterance generally signal transient mode-locking. This delivers to listeners a culture-specific attractor profile.

In sum, context-generated expectancies, stimulated by speech contour patterns, guide a listener's attending to future intonation accents. Effectively, at different time scales, they guide heightened attending to future, expected accents. Finally, this account does not mandate that expectancies are infallible. Indeed, contextually driven expectancies often project future attending to incorrect targets. However, the resulting errors spark sometimes voluntary corrections elicited by an unexpected accent.

Expectancies, Speaking Rate, and Accent Timing in Speech

Life is boring if all things are regular. So, too, with highly regular speech contours. Indeed, it is the spontaneity of speech, with its manageable irregularities, that keeps us responsive. Irregularities may be small, as with fuzzy rhythms in many patches of ordinary conversations, thereby supporting traditional mode-locking (Figure 13.4B, *top row*). But irregularities are also often large, thus commanding transient attending (Figure 13B, *bottom row*).

Although natural irregularities are commonplace in speech, speakers (and listeners) are rarely aware of them. Speakers' tendencies to slow or speed their talking rates are casual or habitual involuntary acts. Common modulations in speaking rate are routine; they happen unwittingly in various situations, as when speakers unknowingly talk more slowly and regularly to older listeners ("elder speech"[17,18], or in directing speech to infants, where most speakers favor timed, regular, higher pitched intonation contours (infant-directed speech[19,20,21]). Tempo response curves, which shape speaking rate, are essential in speech as well as in music. This lends emphasis and/or expression, again often without the awareness of either speaker or listener.

Contributing to these natural variabilities in speech is the fact that speaking rates also vary across speakers. Some people are "fast talkers," while others just drawl at slower rates. Individuals also differ in their characteristic timing of pitch accents as they attempt to deliver a communicative message. With all this variability, it seems impossible that communications succeed. However, one normalizing constraint comes with articulation rate—*syllable rate*. In turn, this referent waveform calibrates speaker-specific inter-accent time spans. In spite of variations of a tempo response curve, speakers who create characteristically different rates as well as characteristic accent rhythms can nonetheless entrain listener's attending and stimulate (fallible) expectancies about forthcoming accents (cf. Chapter 8).

An Example Sentence

Transient mode-locking describes listeners' responses to variably timed accents in sentences studied by Frazier and colleagues.[22] Figure 13.8 shows intonation contours produced by two different speakers with different speaking rates. Both speakers produced the sentence "I met the daughter of the colonel who was on the balcony." The slow talker had a mean speaking rate[23] of $T_R \sim p_R = 186$ ms (panel A) while the fast talker produced a $T_R \sim p_R$ of 145 ms (panel B), where p_R is the hypothesized period of this listener's referent oscillation. Not surprisingly, these speakers also differ in timing of pitch peak accents (**ωa**, linguistically coded, H*).[24] Yet, in spite of this, both speakers plant strong pitch accents on the same three target words (i.e., *daughter, colonel, balcony*). Linguistically, such accented words are *focus points*.

To understand how synchronized attending may fit into this picture, a DAT explanation of listener's attending addresses the variability of slow, accented driving rhythms in the speech contour pattern created by this utterance (e.g., as in Figure 13.4, *bottom*). This sentence should provoke transient mode-locking in listeners' attending. Specifically, listeners hear such sentences by calibrating them with the speaker's speaking rate, T_R. From the opening phrase, a listener exogenously entrains to the speaker-specific talking rate of "I met the *daughter. . . .*" Syllable timing initially awakens a resonant referent oscillation, with period, p_R.[25] In turn, this internal periodicity persists to facilitate synchronized attending via transient mode-locking, with intonation contour groups defined by varied pitch-accented time spans, Tgi.[26]

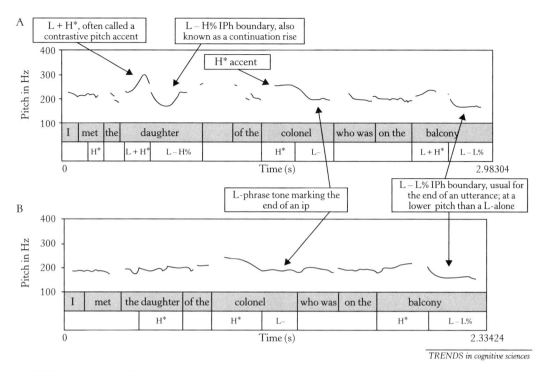

FIGURE 13.8 A brief illustration of ToBI analysis of prosody (top) with an example of a pitch track of intonation curves for two speakers. (**A**) Slow speaker and (**B**) fast speaker.

Reprinted from figure 1 in Lyn Frazier, Katy Carlson, and Charles Clifton Jr, "Prosodic Phrasing Is Central to Language Comprehension," *Trends in Cognitive Sciences* 10, no. 6 (June 2006): 244–49, doi:10.1016/j.tics.2006.04.002.

The referent period, then, supports coordination of attending over these different inter-accent time intervals.

Consider the slow speaker in panel A. This speaker delivers a series of three Tgi:T$_R$ relations.[27] To the ears of a listener relying on an activated referent, p$_R$, this speaker hides a linguistic attractor profile of 2:1-4:1-8:1.[28] Similarly, although the fast speaker (panel B) produces a different accent timing pattern, the intonation profile captures the same pitch-accented words. However, this talker has a different talking rate (i.e., hence a different p$_R$), thus leading to a different hidden linguistic attractor profile: 4:1-8:1.

A critical point in this exercise centers on delivery of an attractor profile. Both attractor profiles afford a listener comprehension. The particular profile is less important than simply arriving at a reliable profile that recognizes appropriately accented words. Despite different linguistic attractor profiles, both talkers lead listeners to the same targets of attending: *daughter, colonel, balcony*. This is because dynamic speech tracking requires that listeners use expectancies based on the relative timing of referent rate and interaccent time intervals that are specific to an individual speaker.[29]

Expectancies and "the Future"

One implication of a dynamic attending approach involves the readiness of a listener to attend to a speaker. In theory, readiness rides on the listener's predisposition to exploit initial time spans of a speaker's utterance to establish a referent period, hence a workable expectancy. Failure to establish a referent explains why listeners sometimes gasp "What?' to the opening utterance of a newly met speaker. Other common listening failures happen with misguided expectancies.

All expectancies, by definition, concern the future, especially future accents. Expectancies usually ride on entrainments involving the referent oscillation which subtly prepares a listener for a future happening. And, the future is unpacked by a speaker using a slower (higher level) external driving rhythms, one related to the referent. Such slower rhythms, with longer group time spans, are typically outlined by prominent accents. Assuming

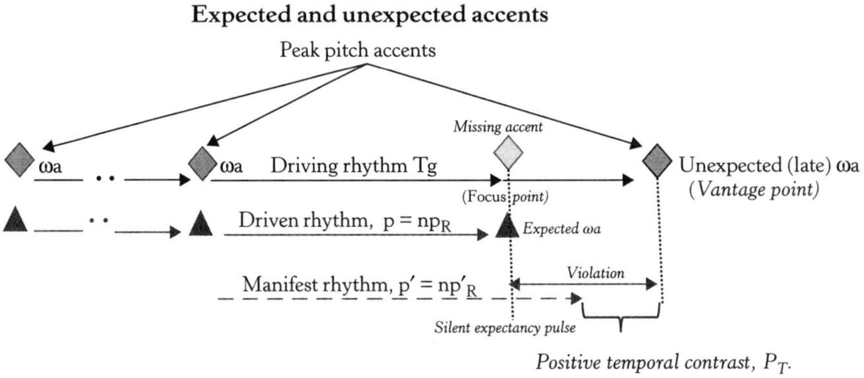

Expected and unexpected accents

Peak pitch accents

FIGURE 13.9 A driving rhythm opens with a group time span Tg_3 marked by strong pitch accents, ωa, (cf. Figure 13.4). This driving rhythm induces a driven rhythm (below) that carries a contextually generated expectancy pulse (dark triangles) for 'when' future pitch accents will occur. The expected accent fails to occur; it is unexpectedly late creating a silent pulse and manifest rhythm (dashed line) that attempts to match it. The result is an expectancy violation and positive temporal contrast, P_T (from Chapter 12). Focus and vantage points are corresponding linguistic terms described later in the text.

the listener's expectancies reflect a reliance on an entraining referent oscillation with a period, p_R, simple higher order expectancies involving slower driving rhythms then are generated by multiples of this referent. Thus, an expected slower oscillator period, pj, assuming $p_j \sim npR$. However, activating such a slower oscillation often leads to fallible expectancies about onsets of future accents.

Figure 13.9 illustrates a fallible expectancy at work. An induced driven rhythm delivers an expectancy based on its oscillatory period, p_j, where $p_j = npR$ (second solid line). A late peak pitch accent, ωa, occurs (see vantage point). However, despite this failure, the sustaining power of the induced expectancy continues through the missing (expected) accent, creating a *silent pulse* (dark gray triangle). This expectancy violation instills an adaptive lengthening of this oscillation's period, thus creating its manifest period, $p_j{}'$ (dashed line, bottom).

Surprisingly, speakers often strategically create phrases as in Figure 13. 9. They reflect a subtle tendency to defy listeners' expectancies in this manner. Future accents are planted in unexpectedly late timing locales where they violate a context-driven expectancy. Theoretically, this unconscious ploy of speakers serves an interesting communicative goal. The expectancy violation surprises a listener, who then boosts voluntary control over relevant phase corrections. Thus, a delayed ωa accent can heighten one's attention and

motivate corrective action (e.g., lengthening p'). Imagine the facile orator who pauses . . . just before . . . delivering an anticipated word, leaving the audience with heightened attending.

Persisting expectancies, while fallible, serve as preparatory crutches. They enable listeners to project attending to promising temporal regions where a key word *might* occur. In linguistic terminology, this provides *vantage points* for detecting unexpected time markers later in a sentence.

Overall, this discussion has portrayed a listener's perception of running speech as a dynamic affair involving a context-sensitive, flexible, attending mechanism. Clearly, attending to speech requires a flexible listener who instantly adapts to talking rates of different speakers and who automatically calibrates accent timings and fallible expectancies relative to a speaker's talking rate. Such a picture is in line with that portrayed for musical listeners who must also engage in momentary attending that is guided to spots in time where future pitch accents might happen.

Summary of Speech Contour Patterns
Speech melodies embed many different, related time scales. These include micro-time scales of pitch velocities which rise and fall to create the contours of speech intonation that afford pitch tracking. They also include macro-time scales created by intonation contours because they are shaped by pitch accents. Pitch accents outline various exogenous

driving rhythms in speech, whether these are regular or variable time spans of contour groups. Together, fast and slow speech rhythms generate in listeners tentative temporal expectancies that guide attending, rightly or wrongly, toward important focal points in a speaker's utterance. Although fallible, expectancies about forthcoming pitch accents guide attending to temporal regions wherein future accents "might" occur. As such, the dynamic context created by a speaker entrains a listener in different ways (e.g., pitch tracking, oscillator clusters, attractor profiles) that keep a listener engaged.

Major points of this section are:

- Speech contour patterns outline multiple slow driving rhythms, often marked by strong pitch accents.
- Speaking rate functions as a referent driving rhythm for calibrating slower rhythms of contour groups. It also supplies fallible expectancies about "when" future accents many occur in running speech.
- Speech prosody supports two entrainment protocols: traditional mode-locking, which leads to linguistic oscillator clusters, and transient mode-locking, which leads to linguistic attractor profiles.

LINGUISTIC APPROACHES TO INTONATION

The psychological perspective on prosody perception just presented emphasizes in-the-moment dynamics of listeners responding to pre-lexical speech contours. It shares some explanatory constructs with the DAT treatment of musical contours. Both entail pitch tracking based on exogenous entrainment to frequency modulations. And with longer, accented time spans, speech shares with music grounds for the operation of both traditional and transient entrainment protocols. Moreover, the commonality of a referent period in both musical and speech domains means that in speech perception listeners seek a speech form of the musical "tactus," i.e., the musical referent periodicity. However, in speech, this referent, as well as related tempo curves, may differ with speaker to a greater degree than in musical events. Each speaker carries his or her own "tempo" to which listeners readily adapt.

Analogies between speech and music can be questioned, however. One reason for questioning them points to extensive domain differences between speech and music, evident in the many

linguistic concepts applicable to speech but not music. Possibly, entrainment theory is more appropriate for explaining attending/perceiving musical events than for explaining attending to speech patterns because the latter uniquely require encoding by linguistically determined constructs. In this spirit, many influential approaches to speech prosody derive from linguistic, not psychological, theories.

Finally, however, it can be argued that the goals of linguistic approaches differ from those of psychological theories. Linguistic theories aim to find codes for spoken sound patterns that clarify certain pragmatic communicative functions of speech. By contrast, psychological approaches aim to understand how listeners attend to and perceive acoustic events provided by speech as well as musical patterns. Although goals in these domains differ, fortunately there is overlap in the two approaches. Agreement is found in central roles granted to fundamental frequency modulations and pitch accents in both approaches. For instance, both DAT and many linguistic theories assume that the continuous modulation of a speaker's vocal frequency in phrases is a primary vehicle for creating intonation contours and pitch accents.

This section has two parts. The first part outlines relevant concepts of prominent linguistic/psycholinguistics accounts of prosody. The second part highlights similarities and differences between linguistic and dynamic attending theories. Throughout this section, the practice observed in prior chapters applies. Accordingly, one or two prominent linguistic theories about prosody are described to compare with DAT.

Linguistic Theories of Intonation Theories and ToBI

Several linguistic theories of prosody have guided research on intonation.[30,31,32] Thus, Bolinger's theory laid the foundation for emphasizing pitch accents as critical to intonation forms. Also important is the analytic system of indexing speech accents developed by Pierrehumbert[33]; namely, the *Tone and Boundary Indices* (ToBI) system. This system catalogs the intonation patterns and accents of typical speakers. Fruits of the ToBI system led to the highly influential intonation theory, the Autosegmental-Metrical (AM) Theory of Pierrehumbert and Beckman.[34]

AM Theory and the ToBI system offer detailed descriptions of critical intonation features in utterances. This approach labels and categorizes surface features of F0 contours that serve important pragmatic functions. Thus, the AM Theory does not aim to explain the attending/perception of prosodic features. Rather, its success rests in reliable indexing of important aspects of speech prosody in acoustic speech signals.

ToBI Codes

Frequency modulations are the heart of AM Theory, which builds on ToBI codes. Melodic contours arise from interpolations between many discrete frequencies, termed "tones." Tones differ in pragmatic function; hence, they are categorized collectively by their accenting functions. A few ToBI features appear in Figures 13.1, 13.8 and 13.9. For instance, some tones are categorized as *pitch targets* if they exhibit a local F0 shift to a higher (H) or lower (L) pitch in a speaker's melodic contour. Other tones at ends of whole phrases belong to different accent categories, as boundary accents. For instance, initial and final tones of *short* phrases are categorized as high (H-) and low (L-) accented pitches; those of longer phrases have different codes (e.g., L%, H%). Hence, ToBI differentiates pitch accents.[35]

One important ToBI category involves strong pitch accents. These accents fall on tones that reflect an F0 change central to an intonation group that coincides with stress points. Two strong accent categories are labeled high (H*) or low *(L*)* pitch accents (see Figure 13.8). Here, * specifies strength due to a stress-plus-frequency aligned tone. Thus, accent categories of L* or H* and H-L* are strong accents. For instance, Figure 13.1A shows a strong pitch accent on a stressed "tone" for the syllable ("Like"); linguistically, it belongs to the H* pitch accent category.

Two other concepts stem from AM Theory. One recognizes the tendencies of speakers to place important pitch accents at relatively late time points in an utterance, where they serve a *focus point* function. This is illustrated in Figure 13.9. The other concept captures a speaker's tendency to violate the precise timing of a future target (its focus point) and situate this pitch accent at a still later time. Linguistically, this region is a *vantage point,* also illustrated in Figure 13.9.

In short, numerous ToBI constructs exemplify its descriptive approach to intonation profiles. This attention to detail paid off. ToBI is a successful, widely used method for analyzing vocal pitch paths of speech. AM Theory, associated with ToBI, places great weight on these measurable, discrete features of melodic contours. It conveys a growing validation that rising and falling pitch patterns indeed form the core of intonations. In fact, these descriptions converge with other accounts that specify the prominence of certain kernel melodic configurations (e.g., of LHL, HL, LH, HLH).[36,37,38] Interestingly, these root melodic forms, variants of the hat pattern, which are popular in various linguistic analyses also happen to resemble common pitch contours of musical melodies.

Linguistic Versus Dynamic Attending Approaches: A Comparison

Although the goals of linguistic and psychological approaches differ, they share certain assumptions. One shared assumption holds that modulation of a speaker's vocal frequency is a primary vehicle for creating intonational prosody. In addition, both approaches recognize different kinds of pitch accents. These two approaches also agree that boundary accents of phrases (rising vs. falling F0 segments) in speech differ from strong, centrally located pitch peak accents in successive phrases. And both recognize that adding stress accents to pitch accents creates stronger central (pitch peak) accents. Finally, other curious parallels also hold. In particular, one involves a comparison between vantage points and focus points of linguistic and corresponding concepts in DAT: a *focus point* corresponds to a listener's temporally expected time point in DAT, whereas a *vantage point* corresponds to the unexpected (but salient) time of a future, compelling accent, as in Figure 13.9.

The preceding commonalities are instructive. Also instructive are ways in which linguistic and attending approaches differ (detailed in Box 13.1). Three central differences are described here.

Theoretical Primitives

First, entrainment and linguistic approaches rest on different primitives. The basic explanatory unit of DAT is a driving–driven dyad. A speaker's F0 becomes a micro-driving rhythm (ω) that elicits in a listener a resonant driven rhythm. Moreover, the neural oscillation (ω_o) is joined by a manifest pitch expectancy (Ω) as both are entrainment primitives. While a modulating F0 appears in both theories, linguistic approaches do not describe F0 as a fast-driving rhythm that elicits pitch tracking neural correlates.

Expectancies and Their Violations

Second, DAT posits that listeners contextually entrain to driving rhythms, which leads to future expectancies. This holds even for the tiny time scales of micro-driving rhythms that activate neural activity, generating both intrinsic (ω_o) and manifest (Ω) expectancies. These attending constructs, as well as expectancy violations (hence, contrasts, ω-Ω), have no counterparts in linguistic theories.

Resonance/Entrainment Principles
Third and most important is that DAT mechanisms of resonance and entrainment, which lead respectively to the activation and coupling of internal (driven) oscillations to external (driving) rhythms, are not found in linguistic theories. In this regard, linguistic theories tell only half the story. They concentrate on external driving rhythm properties, whereas the other half of the story concerns perception/attending associated with driving rhythms.

Summary of Linguistic Approaches to Intonation
In sum, commonalities between linguistic theories and DAT largely involve similar identifications of accents and their roles in outlining intonation patterns in the surface of speech. Important differences surround the impact of these intonational properties on attending dynamics (see Box 13.1 for details).

CHAPTER SUMMARY
This chapter explores the role of intonation in prosody from a psychological perspective. It continues a theoretical focus on speech timing established in preceding chapters. Intonation is formalized as the patterned shaping of a speaker's vocal frequencies, expressed as modulating micro-driving rhythms. For listeners, these modulations drive the fast exogenous entrainments of pitch tracking. As an intonation pattern unfolds, a speech melody opens up with additional time levels of rhythms that are variously marked by accents.

The first major section describes the fast micro-rhythms (F0) that shape pitch contours in speech. At micro-time scales, listeners track fast external driving rhythms with adaptive driven oscillations that deliver fast-paced expectancies which characterize pitch tracking. Adaptive pitch tracking at these micro-time levels relies on exogenous entrainments that lead to pitch contrasts, including contrasts that function as pitch accents.

A second major section describes slower speech-driving rhythms, outlined by various, contour-generated pitch accents. Together, several slower speech rhythms in an utterance create in listeners a dynamic context that includes linguistic oscillator clusters or linguistic attractor profiles, analogous to dynamic constructs identified in musical contexts. These internalized constructs involve driven oscillations that support the slower, sometimes fallible, expectancies of listeners.

This dynamic approach to speech prosody rests on constructs also functional in listening to music. In its domain-general approach, DAT departs from prominent linguistic approaches to prosody, as discussed in a final (third) section of this chapter. That is, DAT interprets speech structure as a source of driving rhythms, whereas linguistic approaches do not. Also, the dynamic attending view rests on concepts of expectancies, oscillator clusters, and attractor profiles which have no parallels in linguistic theories.

NOTES
1. This does not deny a role for accents, strong time markers, based on other objectively salient changes.
2. See discussion of overlapping entrainment regions used to explain proximity percepts.
3. Micro-rhythmic periods here are measured in fractions of seconds.
4. As F0 reflects repetition rate of a complex sound, partials change as well.
5. Philip Lieberman, "Intonation, Perception, and Language," *MIT Research Monograph* 38 (1967): xiii, 210.
6. Johan Sundberg, "Maximum Speed of Pitch Changes in Singers and Untrained Subjects," *Journal of Phonetics* 7, no. 2 (1979): 71–9.
7. These frequency differences also reflect corresponding differences in speaking effort of speakers.
8. Keith B. Doelling et al., "Acoustic Landmarks Drive Delta–theta Oscillations to Enable Speech Comprehension by Facilitating Perceptual Parsing," *NeuroImage*, New Horizons for Neural Oscillations, 85 (January 15, 2014): 761–68, https://doi.org/10.1016/j.neuroimage.2013.06.035.
9. This reasoning is also compatible with breath group explanations of longer intonation contours.
10. Laura C. Dilley and J. Devin McAuley, "Distal Prosodic Context Affects Word Segmentation and Lexical Processing," *Journal of Memory and Language* 59, no. 3 (October 2008): 294–311, doi:10.1016/j.jml.2008.06.006.
11. Oliver Niebuhr, "The Effect of Global Rhythms on Local Accent Perceptions in German," in *Proceedings of the 4th Conference on Speech Prosody, Campinas* (Citeseer, 2008), 331–34, http://citeseerx.ist.psu.edu/viewdoc/download?doi=10.1.1.532.6028&rep=rep1&type=pdf.

12. Meredith Brown et al., "Expectations from Preceding Prosody Influence Segmentation in Online Sentence Processing," *Psychonomic Bulletin & Review* 18, no. 6 (October 4, 2011): 1189–96, doi:10.3758/s13423-011-0167-9.

13. Tuuli H. Morrill et al., "Distal Rhythm Influences Whether or Not Listeners Hear a Word in Continuous Speech: Support for a Perceptual Grouping Hypothesis," *Cognition* 131, no. 1 (April 2014): 69–74, doi:10.1016/j.cognition.2013.12.006.

14. This leads to attractor relations, n:m of 1:1 and 2:1, respectively, throughout monosyllable and dissyllable contexts.

15. This idea was prefigured in Mari R. Jones and Marilyn Boltz, "Dynamic Attending and Responses to Time," *Psychological Review* 96, no. 3 (1989): 459–91, doi:10.1037/0033-295X.96.3.459.

16. Jones and Boltz, "Dynamic Attending and Responses to Time."

17. Jessica A. Hehman and Daphne Blunt Bugental, "Responses to Patronizing Communication and Factors that Attenuate Those Responses," *Psychology and Aging* 30, no. 3 (2015): 552–60, doi:10.1037/pag0000041.

18. Jessica A. Hehman, Randy Corpuz, and Daphne Bugental, "Patronizing Speech to Older Adults," *Journal of Nonverbal Behavior* 36, no. 4 (December 2012): 249–61, doi:10.1007/s10919-012-0135-8.

19. Anne Fernald, "Four-Month-Old Infants Prefer to Listen to Motherese," *Infant Behavior and Development* 8, no. 2 (April 1985): 181–95, doi:10.1016/S0163-6383(85)80005-9.

20. Laurel J. Trainor and Renée N. Desjardins, "Pitch Characteristics of Infant-Directed Speech Affect Infants' Ability to Discriminate Vowels," *Psychonomic Bulletin & Review* 9, no. 2 (June 2002): 335–40, doi:10.3758/BF03196290.

21. T. R. Bergeson and S. E. Trehub, "Absolute Pitch and Tempo in Mothers' Songs to Infants," *Psychological Science* 13, no. 1 (January 1, 2002): 72–75, doi:10.1111/1467-9280.00413.

22. L. Frazier, K. Carlson, and C. Clifton, "Prosodic Phrasing Is Central to Language Comprehension," *Trends in Cognitive Sciences* 10, no. 6 (June 2006): 244–49, doi:10.1016/j.tics.2006.04.002.

23. Average speaking rate for this example was calculated by dividing the total utterance length by the number of syllables. For simplicity of illustration, T_R is assumed to be constant (i.e., the tempo response curve was flat).

24. Linguistic codes are based on the ToBi system which requires trained listeners to follow rules of segmentation of intonation patterns. More details on the ToBi systems appear in later sections and in Box 13.1.

25. Joanne L. Miller and Emily R. Dexter, "Effects of Speaking Rate and Lexical Status on Phonetic Perception," *Journal of Experimental Psychology: Human Perception and Performance* 14, no. 3 (1988): 369–78, doi:10.1037/0096-1523.14.3.369.

26. Tgi are estimated by the number of speaker-specific syllable durations between accents, based on average syllable durations.

27. To calculate these, estimates of p_R were rate means, under the assumption of constant articulation rate. Also, the Tgi were treated as fuzzy rhythms, with time lengths estimated from the figure.

28. The 8:1 ratio accommodates the first syllable of *balcony*.

29. The actual measurement of speaking rate is tricky as it is quite variable (cf. tempo response curve and speaker specificities, among other features). Here, plausible estimates based on averages are assumed to reflect a particular limit cycle oscillation for talking rate in a given context for a given listener.

30. Elisabeth Selkirk, "Phonology and Syntax: The Relation Between Sound and Structure," MIT Press, Cambridge, Massachusetts, 1986.

31. D. Robert Ladd, *Intonational Phonology* (New York: Cambridge University Press, 2008), https://books-google-com.proxy.library.ucsb.edu:9443/books?hl=en&lr=&id=T0aIk3GUJoQC&oi=fnd&pg=PR9&dq=+Ladd,+Phonology+book+and++Bolinger,++&ots=B6XwA9M7un&sig=UyAgVyuEwcodtlWjoA1NgOSahdw.i

32. Dwight L. Bolinger, "Intonation and its Uses: Melody in Grammar and Discourse," Stanford University Press, Stanford, Californiz, 1989.

33. Janet Breckenridge Pierrehumbert, "The Phonology and Phonetics of English Intonation" (Thesis, Massachusetts Institute of Technology, 1980), http://dspace.mit.edu/handle/1721.1/16065.

34. Janet Pierrehumbert, "Tonal Elements and Their Alignment," in *Prosody: Theory and Experiment*, ed. Merle Horne, vol. 14 (Dordrecht: Springer Netherlands, 2000), 11–36, http://www.springerlink.com/index/10.1007/978-94-015-9413-4_2.

35. ToBI also distinguishes tones temporally, coding end lengthening and/or silences between phrases.

36. Carlos Gussenhoven, "Focus, Mode and the Nucleus," *Journal of Linguistics* 19, no. 2 (September 1983): 377, doi:10.1017/S0022226700007799.

37. Carlos Gussenhoven, "Types of Focus in English," in *Topic and Focus*, ed. Chungmin Lee, Matthew Gordon, and Daniel Büring, vol. 82 (Dordrecht: Springer Netherlands, 2007), 83–100, http://link.springer.com/10.1007/978-1-4020-4796-1_5.

38. D. Robert Ladd, "Intonational Phrasing: The Case for Recursive Prosodic Structure," *Phonology* 3 (May 1986): 311, doi:10.1017/S0952675700000671.

14

Learning Speech

From Phonemes to Syllables to Words

This chapter explores how listeners, young and old, acquire skills that enable them to follow everyday speech. These skills include tracking, in real time, speakers' utterances involving elements such as phonemes, syllables, and words. Although such an endeavor sounds far-reaching, this chapter has limited goals. It is confined to explaining a few behavioral phenomena central to perceptual learning of the categories of such speech elements. Against a historical background, the aim is to suggest threads of a different way of viewing speech perception/learning. These threads relate to familiar dynamic concepts and to speculative applications of these concepts to a few central topics surrounding implicit speech learning.

An amazing aspect of speech learning is its speed. For instance, infants rapidly learn phoneme categories in the first year of life. Given that this learning comes with an infant's early exposure to a wide variety of ambient, novel speech sounds, the acquisition is not only mysteriously speedy but it also implicates a selective, or self-guided, quality. This chapter explores how this process might happen. For infants, this revives assumptions of age-specific sensitivities, discussed in Chapter 5, involving fast driving rhythms of speech phonemes. And, for listeners of any age, ideas entertained in this chapter concern how people automatically engage with, then tacitly learn, categories of novel speech sounds.

The underlying fundamentals featured in this chapter arise from two basic hypotheses: the general attending hypothesis and the aging hypothesis. Together, these hypotheses are responsible for the spinoff of various, by now familiar, constructs involving entrained attending, such as pitch (i.e., frequency) tracking, oscillator clusters, and attractor profiles. These three constructs come together in this chapter to lay a foundation for category learning. In particular, they figure into category learning of speech units such as phonemes, syllables, and words. Learning, by its very nature,

depends on exposure frequency. Consequently, this chapter considers issues associated not only with couplings involving entraining oscillations, but also with bindings among oscillations that grow stronger with repeated coupling opportunities during exposure to speech time patterns (from Chapter 10).

CHAPTER GOALS

Perceptual learning of speech begins so early in life that tempting themes of innate predispositions weave in and out of discussions of this learning. Generally, it is useful to conceptualize innate tendencies and their place in learning. Thus, Dynamic Attending Theory (DAT) posits that certain innate prosodic tendencies surrounding rate and rhythm "jump start" implicit speech learning.

To pursue these ideas, this chapter is divided into four parts. An opening section provides an essential historical background concerning themes of innate versus learned aspects of speech properties. These themes continue to color contemporary thinking about speech categories. The following three sections trace mastery of timing levels in speech, beginning with early learning of fast speech units such as phonemes and their categories. This section builds on entrainment concepts associated with the psychoacoustics of complex sounds where multiple micro-rhythms contribute to pitch perception (Chapter 6). Familiar concepts of exogenous entrainment (i.e., as a stimulus driven construct of frequency tracking) and endogenous entrainments (i.e., as oscillator clusters, attractor profiles) also return to describe infants' early learning of phonemes. The next section tackles syllable learning, which revives the topic of attractor profiles. A final section addresses research on the slower periodicities where both traditional and transient mode-locking figure in adults' learning of novel words.

Addressing learning generally invites exploring answers to two questions: "What is learned?" and

"How is it learned?" Several answers to these questions are reviewed in this chapter. Although most agree that the "how" of learning involves exposure frequency in some form, opinions differ regarding "what" is learned. However, in considering speech units such as phonemes, syllables, and words, it is generally conceded that "what" is learned is somehow related to properties of these speech categories.

An overarching aim of this chapter entails enlisting familiar entrainment concepts, applicable in the musical domain, to address these questions in the speech domain. Unquestionably, this is a daunting goal. Therefore, this chapter should be viewed as a tentative first step toward uniting concepts underlying perceptual learning in speech and music. Accordingly, each section in this chapter addresses a different aspect of speech learning with the goal of illustrating how a dynamic attending approach might address attending/learning of phonemes, syllable, and words.

In this spirit, the specific questions tackled in this chapter concern people's abilities to recognize individual instances of various speech categories (e.g., phonemes, syllables, words). For instance, one section asks how we recognize the word "bet" as that word (and not "bit") even when the syllable is spoken by different speakers in different contexts and with wildly differing acoustic features. Finally, this recognition skill depends on learning some abstract properties of phonemes and syllables that transcend superficial differences among individual instances (tokens) of a category.

This chapter builds on the broad hypothesis that entrained attending is a gateway to perceptual learning (Chapter 10). No new constructs appear in this culminating chapter. Instead, Chapter 14 brings together many familiar constructs from earlier chapters to suggest how they figure in new, and challenging, contexts. Basic entrainment mechanisms, such as exogenous entrainments, oscillator clusters, and attractor profiles, all applicable to musical events, are shown to also apply in speech sounds but in somewhat disguised forms. Finally, broad constraints on attending dynamics are ever-present, as described in the aging hypothesis (for driven rhythms) and in the general attending hypothesis (for driving rhythms).

BACKGROUND: ORIGINS OF LINGUISTIC SKILLS

A simple narrative on the origins of linguistic skills is impossible given the colorful history of this subject. Over decades, lively debates have bubbled up around topics such as innate endowments, maturation, evolutionary determinism, domain specificities, and more. These discussions provide a rich background for addressing issues surrounding speech acquisition. In a quest for clarity on this important subject, it is questionable to ignore a role for innateness, just as it is foolhardy to ignore the power and universality of learning. As preceding chapters imply, the theoretical position of DAT is that innate biases pave the way for learning. This interactional perspective features both innate and acquired factors. Both factors supply universal but complementary mechanisms. Yet, as this background section illustrates, even such a moderate position is debatable.

Innate Issues and "Speech as Special"

An age-old issue concerning innate determinants of speech/linguistic skills was reignited in modern times by the influential linguist, Noam Chomsky.[1,2] He argued that humans have an inborn, species-specific, general language faculty. Noting that infants in all cultures show early and rapid speech acquisition, he claimed that this confirms operations of an innate and universal grammar mechanism. This domain-specific theory of speech perception assumed operation of an inborn grammar, generally known as Universal Grammar. This grammar included broad syntactic principles, along with culture-specific parameters, which presumably determined infants' early percepts of speech units. Clearly, an answer to the question of "what" is learned is constrained by grand limits imposed by this innate grammar. Although some of Chomsky's contemporaries, such as Lenneberg,[3] appealed instead to innate biological predispositions and internal rhythms as grounds for developing speech skills, these ideas were out of step with the thinking of this era.

Also sounding a domain-specific theme in this era, psychologists approached innateness from a very different angle. Liberman and colleagues[4] proposed a "speech is special" motor theory of speech perception. Although instantly popular, this theory proved controversial due to its grounding of speech perception in motor production, specifically in motor gestures of the human vocal tract. Articulatory motor patterns (for consonants, vowels) were deemed to specify different categories of phonemes. Specifically, articulatory gestures determined percepts of different phoneme categories. For instance, although tokens of the phoneme, /d/, in /di/ and /du/ differ in certain observable formants, they nonetheless share a common motor gesture that denotes a whole category of /d/ instances (tokens). Accordingly, this theory joined a camp of theories proposing innate, species-specific determinants of perceived speech categories (e.g., of phonemes). In these views, "what" defined a phoneme category was a set of neural motor commands. Presumably, these determine listeners' sense of governing, but hidden, gestures underlying different tokens of the same phoneme category.[5] Arguably a more parsimonious, less restrictive motor theory was offered by Carol Fowler.[6,7,8] Her direct realism approach eschewed neural commands; rather, it proposed that listeners directly perceive cues to the hidden motor sources of speech units (i.e., unifying gestures). Thus, listeners respond to phonological properties of speech based on a directed sense of articulatory gestures of a speaker's vocal tract.[9]

Categorical Perception: A Critical Experimental Paradigm

Motor theories of speech perception shared with early linguistic theories a tendency to downplay learning in the perception of speech elements such as phoneme categories. Support for motor theory came with hallmark studies of categorical perception. This support rested on an indispensable experimental paradigm for studying phoneme categorization skills, a paradigm that remains useful today.

Classically, the categorization paradigm involves two tasks. One, an *identification task*, assesses a listener's sense of the defining category core, namely its prototypical features (e.g., of /d/). This task requires that listeners identify (label) a phoneme category when presented with a single token sound (e.g., the consonant sound in /ba/ or /pa/). The accompanying task assesses a listener's ability to *discriminate* category boundaries between two token phonemes. People must differentiate phonemes that may (or may not) straddle a category boundary. Thus, the motor theory of speech correctly predicts best discrimination for pairs of phonemes that straddle a gesture-defined category boundary. This paradigm garnered substantial support for this theory. As such, it promoted acceptance of the claim that phoneme categories are defined by hidden motor vocal gestures.

The "speech is special" approach became very influential. Not only did it establish an invaluable experimental paradigm for codifying categorical percepts, it also led to provocative predictions about categorical speech perception in humans. Theoretically, this approach spawned

a more sweeping proposal that confined categorization of certain sounds to the human speech domain. Philosophically, this view converged with the *modularity concept* proposed by Fodor.[10] Modularity theory codified domain specificity. Spatially segregated brain modules purportedly govern a listener's processing of different stimulus domains, thus distinguishing musical categories from speech categories, each operating within a special brain module. Issues of domain specificity remain alive and well today.

A General Approach to Auditory Perception

Despite the popularity of such domain-specific theories, challenges to these approaches to speech perception surfaced. At least with regard to motor theory approaches, enthusiasm for a "speech is special" perspective waned. Observing mounting contrary evidence, Diehl et al.[11] identified two major shortcomings of the motor theory of speech. One concerns species-specific claims that categorical perception of phonemes applies only to humans; the other relates to the idea that phoneme perception is domain-specific. In fact, Diehl et al. report support for neither assumption. Categorical phoneme perception appears in several nonhuman species (chinchillas, monkeys[12,13,14,15]). Categorical parallels also appear in other domains.[16,17] In addition, questionable aspects of the motor theories relate to their de-emphasis of contributions of speech contexts and learning in categorization.[18,19,20]

Diehl and colleagues argue persuasively for a general approach to auditory perception. They refer to the impact of various acoustic features, including prosodic ones, that motivate perceptual learning of speech and music based on general principles of perception and learning: "The results of comparing speech and non-speech perception and speech perception in humans and nonhumans strongly indicate that general auditory mechanisms (common to human adults and infants, other mammals, and even birds) contribute to the categorical perception of speech sounds."[21,22]

Specificity of Domains and Species: A Theoretical Update

The domain-general approach championed by Diehl and others has gained a foothold in recent years. As a result, contrary views found in classic linguistic approaches have been updated, with new hypotheses about roles of innateness, domain specificity, and species specificity in speech perception.

One current view updates Chomsky's original theory.[23,24] This new view assumes that humans evolved a *broad language faculty* (FLB) that encompasses phonological skills (e.g., sensory-motor activities) found in other species. Importantly, certain inborn human abilities distinguish a species-specific, *narrow language faculty* (FLN). This hypothesis holds that FLN has evolved only in humans for use in syntax. Furthermore, general psychological activities, such as attending and perceptual learning, play a minor role relative to that of innate grammar constraints of FLN. Moreover, a clear line distinguishes prosodic (phonology) from syntactic (grammar) features, and FLN applies *only* to syntactic grammars. In particular, FLN reflects grammars with recursive nesting of phrases, used uniquely in human languages. Accordingly, only humans can decipher/learn acoustic patterns that are true linguistic sequences, as defined by FLN recursion rules. Moreover, grammar learning takes shape independently of prosodic features.

Perceptual Learning as Rule Learning

This updated theory clearly disputes a domain-general approach (e.g., of Diehl et al.). Importantly, it also challenges any theory, including DAT, which rests on general psychological mechanisms. Instead, FLN/FLB theory revives the joint specter of domain-specificity for speech (vs. music) and species specificity for humans. Only humans can learn the FLN rules of recursive grammars. In other words, perceptual learning of speech amounts to *rule learning*: "What" is learned are syntactic rules that do not include prosody.

FLN Rule Learning: An Example

To illustrate FLN constraints, consider two grammar systems: a *context-free grammar* and a *finite state grammar*. Let the sequences of interest contain only two elements, **a, b** (e.g., two phonemes). A *context-free grammar* allows for recursive embedding, as in the formula; $a^n b^n$ (integer, $n \to \infty$). This rule generates strings such as **ab** ($n = 1$) **aabb** ($n = 2$), and **aaabbb** ($n = 3$) with n as a repeat rule. Thus, learning such a context-free FLN rule enables humans to acquire categories with token sequences sharing the same abstract recursive embeddings. By contrast, a *finite state grammar* (FSG), denies recursions. Instead, an FSG of (**ab**) n specifies *serial attachments*, such as **ab** ($n = 1$), **abab** ($n = 2$), **ababab** ($n = 3$). In principle, categorization depends on applications of the same rule system to different sets of tokens

(**a, b** vs. **c, d**). In other words, only context-free grammars facilitate categorization.

In sum, this linguistic approach describes "what" humans (vs. other species) can learn. Specifically, regardless of phonological features (e.g., pitch contour), humans learn linguistic categories based on two types of grammatical rules, whereas other species only learn FSG grammars.

This update of Chomsky's theory has stimulated lively debates. Some rightly note that FLN constraints rest on untenable domain-specific distinctions because phonological properties exhibit relevant embedding relationships in both music and speech.[25,26] Relatedly, both grammars lead to correlated prosodic features of sound sequences, such as runs or alternations of elements, which are notoriously salient, perceptually. For instance, people group (i.e., chunk) runs of identical items in ways that facilitate sequence learning.[27,28,29,30] Finally, species-specific predictions about grammar learning are dubious in light of discoveries by Gentner and colleagues.[31,32] They found that European starlings easily learn both finite state (FSG) and context-free (FLN) grammars (**a, b** units were bird "phonemes" of "rattle" and "warble"). These clever birds even showed *transfer of training* to novel sequences of the same grammar.

Summary of Origins of Linguistic Skills

So where does this leave us? Against this historical background, current thinking about "what" is learned in speech is at a crossroads. We can rule out motor gestures as a primary source of speech categorization, and it seems clear that perceptual categorization is not specific to human speech. It remains possible that "what" people learn involves to-be-determined abstract grammatical rules that cross domain and species boundaries. Alternatively, it is also possible that "what" is learned in these cases are prosodic features that happen to correlate with certain rules.

Sticky problems also remain about what exactly defines a category. For instance, most agree that phonemes can be categorized, but what are the critical categorizing features? What allows so many very different spoken versions (tokens) of one phoneme (e.g., /ɛ/) to be judged as belonging to the same category? Do speech categories have some abstract and/or defining feature(s)? If so, are these invariants innate, or must they be learned, or both? Furthermore, it remains unclear how learning enables mastery of categorization skills. That is, is the nature of learning so general that it is independent of "what" is learned? Is it possible, with enough repetitions, to learn *any set of arbitrary sounds* as a category, or must member sounds of a category share some unifying property? In other words, do learning hypotheses necessarily mean abandonment of hypotheses about innate factors?

The remainder of this chapter struggles with such questions. It draws on basic assumptions of dynamic attending to suggest ways that DAT might apply to the development of speech categories for phonemes, syllables, and even words. These reflect tentative forays into a challenging field of research. They explore the generality of synchrony and synchronous modes of entrained attending by extending these concepts to suggest new ways of defining speech categories and category learning.

Major points in this background section are:

- Historically, debates over speech skills juxtapose views embracing innate predispositions (motor gestures, inborn grammars) with more general approaches to perceptual learning.
- Issues of skill specificity involving different domains (music, speech) and species are challenged by evidence showing a generality of perceptual skills across domain and species.
- Questions remain concerning "what" is learned and "how" it is learned in speech categories.

LEARNING PHONEMES: THE FIRST YEAR OF LIFE

Learning starts even before birth. Any approach to learning must begin where learning begins, namely in infants' early experiences. Consistent with a general auditory learning orientation, the dynamic attending approach assumes that infants' early responses to speech depend on universal principles for guiding attending which then paves a route to learning. This section examines the "what" and "how" of learning by applying these ideas to infant learning of phoneme categories in the first year of life.

Background

As Chomsky observed, impressive learning feats happen in the first year of life. This is most evident in the elegant research of Patricia Kuhl and others.[33,34,35] Kuhl showed that by the end of the first year infants have acquired knowledge of phoneme categories and are on the threshold of word learning. Her *Native Language Magnet Theory*

identifies three developmental stages of infant learning, as infants "grow" an ability to categorize speech sounds in their first year of life.

This research rekindles issues about category learning. In addressing these issues, Arthur Samuel and Tanya Kralic[36] distinguish category learning theories, such as Kuhl's and Goldstone's,[37] from an earlier Gibsonian account.[38] The latter assumes that exposure to a variety of category tokens motivates learners to make increasingly finer distinctions among tokens, leading then to the discovery of a residual category defined by invariants common to all tokens. Alternatively, Kuhl and Goldstone both emphasize the import of a significant turning point in category learning, an "Ah-Ha" experience in perceptual restructuring which unveils a critical, defining, category invariant. This insight point presumably sparks a cognitive shift in the learner from relying on superficial physical features to using abstract categorical features. For Kuhl, this shift happens within the first year of life when infants' have accumulated sufficient exposures to a certain common token in a category; this token then functions as that category's prototype.

Finally, both Gibsonian differentiation and Kuhl's and Goldstone's restructuring proposals have merit. As Samuel and Kralic observe, both perspectives touch on an overriding characteristic of perceptual learning of categories: namely, that it is "aggressively adaptive."

Perceptual category learning in Infants

Perhaps the best way to begin to address category learning is to start when life starts. Even very young infants are exposed to speech sounds of their caretaker. And clearly, infants eventually succeed in learning basic elements of speech very early in life. In particular within the first year of life they master category learning of phonemes, seemingly by simply experiencing people talking. *So, how do infants do this?*

Two answers to this question that address the early category learning of speech elements displayed by infants are considered in this section. In particular, they consider category learning of phonemes. One answer, provided by Patricia Kuhl,[39] outlines the progression of learning through three behavioral stages in an infant's first year. This is shown in Table 14.1 (column 2). A second answer, provided by DAT, builds on Kuhl's descriptions of these stages, translating them into comparable stages of attending/entrainment that become platforms for implicit learning in the first year of life. DAT stages

TABLE 14.1 INFANT STAGES OF PHONEME LEARNING

Stages: Ages	Infant Behavior	Attending/Learning
Stage 1: (prenatal → on)	Detects frequency changes	*What*: Frequency contours*How*: Exogenous entrainments: Tracking
Stage 2: (2/3 months → on)	Reacts to universally tofrequency relationships	*What*: Token oscillator clusters*How*: Multiple endogenous entrainments.
Stage 3: (6 months → on)	Perceives phoneme categories	*What*: Attractors of oscillator clusters*How*: Include referent oscillator

too are briefly summarized in Table 14.1 (column 3). Both approaches are described in more detal in this section.

The Perceptual Magnet effect

Patricia Kuhl's brilliant research on perceptual magnets holds that older infants begin to categorize phonemes using a phoneme prototype acquired strictly by exposure frequency.[40] Once learned, this prototype then functions as a magnet that '*pulls*' a listener's token percept toward it, thus warping a perceptual vowel space. Warping predicts perceptual distortions of tokens near a prototype, such as mistaking a token close to the prototype as the prototype. Figure 14.1 shows two examples of vowel prototypes (for /i/ and /y/ categories) at respectively different loci in a two dimensional space of varying formant frequencies (F1, F2).[41,42,43]

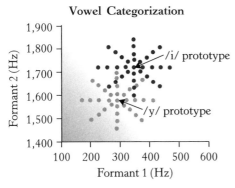

Vowel Categorization

FIGURE 14.1 In a two-dimensional plot of formant frequencies (F1 and F2), two prototypical phoneme categories are illustrated. Two stimuli that align with the defining prototype are shown as matching the central point according Kuhl.

Reprinted from figure 1a in P. Kuhl, "Early Language Acquisition: Cracking the Speech Code," *Nature Reviews Neuroscience* 5, no. 11 (November 2004): 831–43, doi:10.1038/nrn1533.

According to Kuhl, this sort of true categorical perception does not emerge in infants until around six months of age. At this point, it results from repeated exposures to a particular token that strengthens its role as a category prototype.[44] This explains perceptual distortions of phoneme tokens *near a prototype*. Moreover older infants differentiate among token phonemes that *straddle* two different category boundaries.[45] And data support the claim that the magnet effect is domain general, extending to musical stimuli, as well as to other species, appearing in chinchillas, monkeys and quails.[46,47]

So, how do older infants arrive at this asymptotic stage? Kuhl traced the evolution of phoneme categorization over the first year of life arriving at distinct behaviors for each of three developmental stages outlined in column 2 of Table 14.1.

Stage 1: In stage 1 very young infants, including newborns, exhibit a clear sensitivity to individual frequency components of phonemes that cuts across linguistic cultures.[48,49]

Stage 2: In the second stage (over 2–3 months of age) infants gain sensitivity to relative timing, i.e., inter-dependencies among micro-driving rhythms within a phoneme, thus accounting for their differentiation of rhythms among various languages (cf. Table 14.1).

Stage 3: Older infants (around six months) begin to exhibit phoneme categorizations. These infants show classic categorical phoneme perception. Around 7.5 months, they master both identity and discrimination categorization tasks. Kuhl explains this behavior in terms of a *perceptual magnet* that restructures previously acquired token knowledge.

A Dynamic Attending Approach to Category Learning of Phonemes

A different perspective on infants' acquisition of speech (phoneme) categories is developed in this section, one that is strongly influenced by Kuhl's research. This approach speaks to "what" is learned and "how" it is learned in each of the stages Kuhl has identified. In some respects, the DAT stages resemble those outlined by DAT for category learning in adults (Chapter 10). However, to fully understand applications of entrainment principles that promote early phoneme learning from a DAT, a detour is required to detail "what" infants attend to and learn about phonemes produced by adults.

A DAT Overview: Detailing "What" Is Learned

A basic premise of DAT holds that learning depends on binding, which happens during an entrainment episode. To flesh out relevant attending dynamics for category learning of phonemes, recall that the phonemes produced by adult caretakers reflect fast complex sounds that mix waveforms of harmonic and nonharmonic (formant) components (cf. Chapter 6). From a DAT perspective, these adult-generated waveforms function as sets of phoneme micro-driving rhythms in which the slowest waveform is associated with an adult's fundamental frequency, F0 (e.g., from Chapter 6). These sets may combine certain harmonics (nF0) with more distinctive, high-energy formants (Fi). Finally, given the aging hypothesis, infants should readily resonate/entrain (through coupling) to such fast micro-driving rhythms, thereby forming pitch-like clusters containing neural correlates of these driving rhythms. With maturation and exposure to more adult phonemes, infants also learn (through binding) relationships among these phoneme waveforms as well as the attractors implied by hidden harmonic relationships. In short, phonemes set the stage for cluster formations.

More details about micro-driving rhythms

To be more concrete, a DAT approach requires assessments of exactly 'what' infants confront when hearing an adult speaks. This, of course, also speaks to issues of attending, namely 'what' attracts a listener's attending? With respect to phonemes, Table 14.2 provides some example micro-driving rhythms provided by the English vowel frequencies of an adult female. Imagine that each phoneme of this caregiver delivers to a young listener a set of micro-driving rhythms with different rates. For a single vowel, then, an infant experiences several different micro-driving rhythms that form a cluster of driving–driven dyads ($\omega_i{:}\omega_{oi}$). Driving rhythms (ω_i) supplied by adults are found in vowels which feature high-energy micro-rhythms

of defining formants. Given the aging hypothesis, very young infants' tend to "tune in" to fast waveforms (in the adult's voice), activating via resonance, corresponding neural correlates. Moreover, stimulus-driven infants rely more on weaker driven oscillations than do adult listeners. In a push/pull configuration between a hidden harmonic's attractor 'pull' and a fluctuating stimulus formant, the latter will' push' young infants to adapt toward the 'deviant' formant. In general, infants are more reactive to the fuzziness of fuzzy rhythms than adults.

Very young infants involuntarily follow certain stepping stones to achieve category learning. According to DAT, this process begins with stimulus-driven entrainments to several signature micro-rhythms within a phoneme, and it winds up, 6 months later, with older infants' showing an internalized mastery of these complex vocal sounds characterizing true vowels. How does this happen?

The return of Tokens and Attractors

Table 14.2 allows a closer look at adult phonemes (i.e., vowels). Something about these sounds draws infants' attending. The idea is that this attending provides a platform for vowel learning. This table details relevant vowel frequencies/waveforms plus their attractor properties. From a DAT perspective, a phoneme category is defined by a set of global attractors that characterize a category prototype. In this prototype set, each attractor reflects an distinct internalized n:m ratio. By contrast, vowel tokens express only approximations to these attractors. Yet, recall that in dynamic attending terms, an attractor defines a category's core (i.e., its prototype), and bifurcations (category boundaries) limit the attractor's entrainment region i.e., the region of tokens.

Consider a detailed example. The vowel category of /ɛ/ in Table 14.2 (row 5) contains many tokens, all differing in various fuzzy micro-rhythms. A single token of such a vowel contains several different signature waveforms: for formants such as F1, F2, F3, plus a referent F0 (plus others). It is the timing relationships, i.e., period ratios, among these waveforms that turn out to *approximate* a given phoneme's defining (but hidden) attractor ratios. Thus, tokens within the /ɛ/ category share similar sets of formant frequencies (F1′, F2′, F3′); their ratios deliver fuzzy estimates of phoneme's defining attractor ratios. Nevertheless, in spite of fuzzy ratios, all /ɛ/ tokens occupy a particular entrainment region, meaning all "point to" the same defining attractor (i.e.,of the set of phoneme defining

TABLE 14.2 MICRO-DRIVING RHYTHMS IN VOWEL PHONEMES (FEMALES)

1	2		3		4		5	
	F1 (Hz) Nearest Harmonic (Hz)	F2	F1 (periods, ms) Attractor periods (for F1 only)	F2	F1/F0 (period ratios) From Tokens	F1/F2	F1/F0 (period ratios) Near attractors Ai Aj	F1/F2
i	325	2,900	3.077	.345	.615	.112	.625 (5:8)	.111(1:9)
	400	*2800*	*3.125*					
I**	450	2,300	2.222	.435	.444	.195	.444 (4:9)M	.200(1:5)*
	400	*2400*	*2.22*					
E	550	2,500	1.818	.400	.364	.220{378}!	.375(3:8) {.375{3:8}!}	.222(2:9)
	600	*2,400*	*1.82*					
ε**	600	2,200	1.667	.454	.333	.272	.333 (1:3) M* or .250 (3:12)	.273 (3:11) M
	600	*2,200*	*1.665*					
Æ	1,000	1,950	1.000	.513	.200	.513	.200 (1:5) M*	.500 (1:2)*
	1,000	*2,000*	*1.000*					
A	875	1,175	1.143	.851	.229	.745{.249}!	.200 (1:5) M*	.500 (1:2)*
	800	*1,200*	*1.135*					
Λ	700	1,400	1.429	.714	.286	.500	.286 (2:7) M	.500(1:2)M*
	600/800	*1,400*	*1.430*					
O	500	800	2.000	1.25	.400	.625	.400 (2:5) M*	.625 (5:8)M
	400/600	*800*	*2.000*					
ʊ	500	1350	2.000	.741	.400	.371	.400 (2:5) M*	.375 (3:8)
	400/600	*1,400*	*2.000*					
U	250	850	4.000	1.176	.800	.294	.800 (4:5) M*	.286 (2:7)
	200	*800*	*4.000*					

Not bold/italic entries: These are recorded data are in columns 1–4 for F1, F2, and F0 values from Kewley-Port and Watson (1994), given a constant F0 of 200 Hz. Column 3 shows periods (ms) for column 2 (in Hz). Vowels were synthesized directly from spectrographic measures of female talkers. Brackets indicate normative periods and ratios (columns 2, 4) from other data for different F1 values (Bakan, 1996). Note that nearest attractors change (column 5).

Bold/italized entries: These entries denote hypothesized internal frequencies as harmonics nearest to F1 or F2 (column 2). Column 3 shows attractor periods of F1 (relative observed in bold italics) predicted by a mode-locking attractor of F1/F0 for hypothetical token (*ωo*) values (column 5). Column 5 presents calculated mode-locking attractors nearest to observed F1/F0 and F2/F1 formant relationships. The asterisk (*) in this column reflects simpler attractors (higher stability); M superscripts connote good matches of attractor with period ratios. Not shown are other hidden attractors such as F2/F0 (or generally Fk/Fj), also functional in determining attractor sets. See Figure 14.5 for a depiction of mode-locking at micro-time scales of phoneme /ɛ/.

** Designates example phonemes discussed in the text and in Figures 14.5 and 14.6

attractors). Prototypical tokens correspond to attractors. Moreover, each protype is surrounded by a wide entrainment region populated by token ratios that implicate the attractors. All tokens of a given phoneme category then hide the same set of global attractors (notation for a set of global attractors is {Aj = A1, A2, A3 . . . }). Only the category prototype, which shares the same global attractor set, is not hidden.

Table 14.2 illustrates these ideas for tokens of several English vowels (column 1). These are adult female formant vocalizations with an F0 of 200 Hz (from Kewley-Port and Watson).[50] Although each vowel contains many formant waveforms, for tutorial reasons, these examples reflect only the two most important formants (i.e., F1, F2 in column 2). Here, formants and their nearest harmonics (below in Hz) are labeled "frequency," but it is important to recognize that formants are fluctuating micro-driving rhythms.[51] Period ratios of formant waveforms and nearby attractors appear in columns 4 and 5, respectively, for F1/F0 and F1/F2. In this presentation, formant relationships are critical to identifying category tokens, whereas attractor relationships are pertinent for defining category prototypes. (For other dynamic system approaches, see Huange, Gentili, and Reggia[52] and Tokuda et al.[53]).

To be specific, let's dig inside a few token vowels. Two phoneme examples involving the vowels /I/ and /ɛ/ in rows 3 and 5 are instructive for they distinguish "bit" from "bet." These vowels have different attractors. Compare the observable (i.e., token) formant ratios of column 4 with unobservable (near attractors) in column 5 and note that in each case the token formant ratio provides a plausible estimate of its hidden attractor ratio. And the attractors differ for these two vowels. In fact, within an entrainment region of each ($n{:}m$) attractor ratio, category tokens approximate their *nearest harmonic ratio*.

Some token ratios are closer to nearby attractors than others. For instance, in this table the /I/ vowel (see**) has token ratios of .444 and .195 (column 4), which are good approximations of two respective attractors for this vowel: .444 and .200 (column 5). Different token ratios for /ɛ/ (.333, .273 in column 5) are also close to their attractors, Ai. Here the set of hidden attractors (A1, A2) defines the vowel category, /I/ where A1 is .444 ($n{:}m$ of 4:9) and A2 is .200 ($n{:}m$ of 1:5), whereas the attractor set of category /ɛ/ is A1 is .333 ($n{:}m$ of 1:3) and A2 is .273 ($n{:}m$ of 3:11).

These two examples happen to illustrate tokens with close approximations to their attractors. Keep in mind that many tokens vary significantly from

their attractor within the attracor's entrainment region. Indeed, other vowels in Table 14.2 exhibit poorer estimates of nearest attractors, but these still remain functional tokens within the confines of an entrainment region. This means they still "point to" their hidden categorical *attractor* ratios. Also, for simplicity, Table 14.2 provides examples with a small set of the most important attractors (with three frequency components: F0, F1, F2). Finally, not only does a token's sound draw attending toward an implied prototype (attractor), it simultaneously establishes an entrainment region that plays a major role in explaining listeners' ability to categorize a range of different phoneme tokens.

In sum, this detailed glimpse inside phonemes highlights a relatively simple and recurring theme of this book: namely, that special synchronous relationships (attractors) identify a category, but they are usually hidden by a variety of different fuzzy (and here fast) driving rhythms. This holds for young infants and fast sounds, where a stable, hidden, attractor ratio is contrasted with variable, manifest token ratios. Token ratios can be quite fuzzy, with distinctly smeared time ratios due to articulatory and contextual factors. Yet, in theory, the defining (hidden) attractors do not change.[54,55] Attractors guide how we sense the same phoneme because it appears in different guises (tokens) across a range of different contexts and speakers. Typically, token formant ratios, which populate an attractor's entrainment region, are quite changeable. In this way, entrained attending paves a path to learning.

Perceptual Learning of phonemes in Infants

The preceding discussion outlines the '*what*' of phoneme properties that infants must master in their first year. However, along the way, it lays the groundwork for understanding how infants begin to learn phoneme categories as Patricia Kuhl[56] has neatly outlined for the first year Table 14.1 (column 2).

Table 14.1 also summarizes a DAT approach to these stages of phoneme learning (column 3). This adds attending dynamics as a platform for implicit learning. It suggests that three entrainment mechanisms are operative in determining attending behaviors, i.e., couplings, over the stages Kuhl has observed. In turn, entrained attending in each stage leads to learning, through binding, as summarized in Table 14.1 (column 3). A fuller description of these stages from a DAT perspective is considered next.

Stage 1: Very Young Infants: Attending to and Learning Simple Micro-Rhythms

Stage 1, entails behaviors of very young infants, including newborns. These infants show an early sensitivity to individual waveform components of phonemes that cuts across linguistic cultu res.[57,58,59,60]

Attending in Stage 1

According to DAT, attending early in life is stimulus-driven. "What" is learned involves individual waveform components. Early in life, attending is controlled by the fast exogenous entrainments of driven rhythms. It awakens weak cortical oscillations that are largely reactive to external stimuli (cf., phase response curves [PRCs] as described in Chapter 4).[61,62] And, resulting driving-driven dyads rely on simple attractors (e.g., $n{:}m$ = 1:1) that determine exogenous tracking of individual waveforms. That is, frequency (or pitch) tracking characterizes this early stage. Given the aging hypothesis, these micro-driving rhythms involve the faster, high-frequency formants within an adult's token phoneme. Hence young infants can *independently* track (exogenously entrain) one (or several) of micro-driving rhythms. Moreover, even small deviations in these stimulus rhythms create noticeable perceptual (pitch) contrasts for these infants (cf. detuning curves, Figure 13.2).

Learning in Stage 1

Early learning depends on the exogenous entrainment of attending with a given formant waveform (a guiding attractor is $n{:}m$ = 1:1). Resulting dyad synchronies during entrainment yield implicit learning based on reinforced bindings between a token's micro-driving rhythm and its correlated driven oscillation.[63] In turn, more entrainment episodes promote learning from strengthened bindings of driving with driven rhythms, thus familiarizing infants with individual frequencies.

Figure 14.2 outlines aspects of Stage 1. It distinguishes between *attending* (arrows of coupling) and *learning* of formants (lines of period bindings). These infants are aggressively adaptive in responding to perceptual *contrasts*, echoing a refrain from the Gibsonian position on category learning.

Evidence for Stage 1 Attending/Learning

Newborns appear to spontaneously track fast phoneme waveforms in speech.[64,65,66] Newborns' cries reveal implicit, indeed prenatal, learning. Mampe and colleagues[67] found that the cries of French

Stages of Category leaning

Phoneme micro-rhythms

Stage 1: Young Infants learn simple micro-rhythms

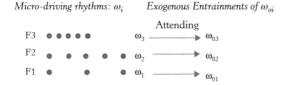 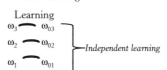

Stage 2: Older infants Learning complex micro-rhythms

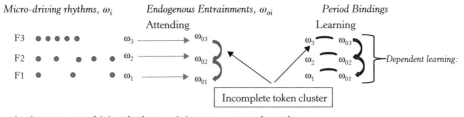

ω_i is a instantaneous driving rhythm; ω_{oi} is its resonant neural correlate.
gray ovals, connotes period-coupled dyads; Black connotes period-bindings of learning.

FIGURE 14.2 Two of the three stages of phoneme category learning, according to Dynamic Attending Theory (DAT). Stage 1 (*top*) involves independent frequency (e.g., pitch) tracking (attending) to individual micro-driving rhythms that enable learning (period binding). Stage 2 (*bottom*), shows endogenous coupling (attending) among oscillations from Stage 1; this enables binding (learning) among oscillations in an incomplete token oscillator cluster.

newborns revealed acquisition of culture-specific rising frequency contours, whereas the cries of German newborns followed acquired (culture-specific) falling contours. In short, these infants prenatally learned frequency contours, suggesting their mastery of pitch tracking. Other research confirms that stage 1 stimulus-driven infants can differentiate frequency changes in phonemes, supporting the validity of these contrasts.[68,69,70]

In sum, in stage 1 infants acquire familiarity with individual spectral components of a phoneme. They *independently track, then learn, different fast waveforms (of formants, harmonics) in caretakers' vocalizations*. Moreover, these infants *are not sensitive to relationships* among component waveforms. Loosely speaking, the newborn's tunable brain is "tuned to" track the frequency contours of independent melodic lines.

Stage 2: Attending and Learning with Complex Micro-Rhythms of Phonemes

Stage 2 describes older infants (more than 2–3 months of age) gaining sensitivity to relative timing (i.e., inter-dependencies) among micro-driving rhythms within a phoneme, thus accounting for their differentiation of rhythms among various languages (cf. Table 14.1).

Attending in Stage 2

Following DAT, stage 2 attending dynamics continue, but they now involve exogenous entrainments among multiple frequency components. Moreover, now endogenous relationships are found in couplings among the driven rhythms of these formant waveforms (see Table 14.1). Consequently, oscillators (ω_{oi}) form an *incomplete token oscillator cluster*, as depicted in Figure 14.2

In this stage, incomplete clusters reflect an important and telling aging constraint: *incomplete token oscillator clusters do not include* oscillations capable of reso1ating to the very slow frequency components, in particular to the F0 of adult speech. Micro-driving rhythms of an F0 are slow, falling outside these infants' temporal niche. Note that oscillations that mirror F0 oscillations are missing from these clusters.

Learning in Stage 2

"What" is learned during endogenous entrainments of oscillations of a cluster depends on bindings among oscillations with repeated exposures. Nevertheless, this learning is instance-(token-) specific. Stage 2 infants remain unaware of commonalities among different tokens of the same phoneme. Thus, if the same phoneme, for example, /ɛ/, is spoken by a male, its similarity to /ɛ /spoken by a female (with a higher F0) is missed by these infants. Although stage 2 infants have learned different tokens of the same vowel, they have not discovered the critical invariant relationships that unite the range of different tokens belonging to the same vowel category. In other words, stage 2 infants cannot pass the classic identify/discrimination tests for phoneme categories.

Stage 3: Phoneme Categories

A final stage happens around 6 months of age. Stage 3 (according to Kuhl), emerges near the end of an infant's first year. In this stage, infants show classic categorical phoneme perception, evident in Figure 14.2. Around 7.5 months, these infants master both identity and discrimination categorization tasks. Kuhl has explained this behavior in terms of a *perceptual magnet* that restructures previously acquired token knowledge.

The Perceptual Magnet Effect

Patricia Kuhl's brilliant research on perceptual magnets holds that older infants begin to categorize phonemes using a phoneme prototype acquired by exposure frequency.[71] Once learned, this prototype then functions as a magnet that "pulls" a listener's token percept toward it, warping a perceptual vowel space. Warping predicts perceptual distortions of tokens near a prototype, such as mistaking a token close to the prototype as the prototype. Figure 14.1 shows two examples of vowel prototypes (for /i/ and /y/ categories) at respectively different loci in a two-dimensional space of varying formant frequencies (F1, F2).[72,73,74]

By way of contrast, Kuhl has proposed that true categorical perception in stage 3 results from repeated exposures to a particular token, which then assumes the role of category prototype.[75] This explains perceptual distortions of phoneme tokens *near a prototype*. Conversely, stage 3 listeners also differentiate token phonemes that *straddle* category boundaries.[76] Also, other data support the claim that the magnet effect is domain-general, extending to musical stimuli, as well as to other species, appearing in chinchillas, monkeys, and quails.[77,78]

Categories and Phoneme Oscillator Clusters in DAT

A different, domain-general explanation of stage 3 behavior is offered by DAT. In important respects, Kuhl's concept of a perceptual magnet resembles DAT's explanation of attractor effects in stage 3.

Key to the DAT approach is the idea that infants in this stage restructure attractors. True phoneme attractors emerge which unite different token phonemes of a given phoneme category. "What" is learned in this stage is a complete oscillator cluster which incorporates true phoneme attractors. A complete cluster is depicted in Figure 14.3 to illustrate a DAT interpretation of stage 3. Theoretically, 'Ah Ha' learning happens because in this stage a common referent oscillation (from F0) is 'discovered' and incorporated into the incomplete token oscillator clusters of stage 2 as the infant discovers the complete cluster.

An example of a *complete oscillator cluster* is shown in Figure 14.4A. This figure depicts one of several /ɛ/ attractors with its entrainment region. This attractor is n:m of 1:3 (from Table 14.2; row 5, column 5) sets the stage for restructuring. It determines the vertical line which specifies the prototype.[79] Tokens, by definition, exhibit ratios that more or less approximate this attractor. For instance, one token for F1/F0 in the adult phoneme /ɛ/ (Table 14.2) is .334; this is quite close to that of the nearby hidden attractor of .333. This token is shown as a lighter gray dot in Figure 14.4A. Also, nearby is a prototype token (open circle) that expresses the attractor ratio, while other tokens are more remote (darker dots).

Tokens spoken by this or other speakers at different times naturally vary, exhibiting a great variety of frequency deviations from a common attractor, as suggested in this figure. Tokens may also vary in effective coupling strength (shown on the ordinate of this figure). All of these variations are accommodated within boundary limits. As Figure 14.4A shows, token disparities do not deny a listener the sense of the "what" of a phoneme (see "pointing to" arrows).

A wide range of tokens with measurably deviant ratios typically surround attractors. Thus, we should not expect to find fixed attractor ratios in produced tokens. Even tokens with quite remote ratios may fall inside an entrainment region, experiencing some "attractor pull." However, an attractor pull is likely to be stronger in older infants (than in younger ones) due to learning, which strengthens an underlying oscillation. Hence, for older infants, bifurcation boundaries (white lines) narrow an entrainment region (relative to young infants; dark gray lines).

Figure 14.4A depicts stage 3 tokens in the context of a discovered attractor. It arises with a restructuring of oscillator clusters in maturing infants. With age, an infant's temporal niche enables "tuning in" to the slower phoneme waveforms which include the F0. The oscillator

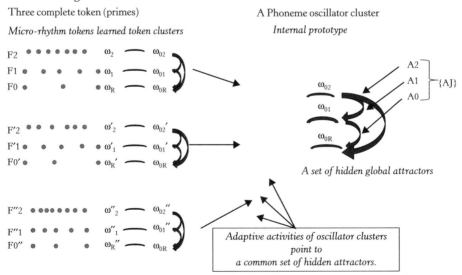

FIGURE 14.3 The third stage of phoneme category learning. With discovery of F0, senior infants complete token oscillator clusters of stage 2. Left side shows driving and driven rhytms for three (of many) different token clusters with an added oscillator (F0) component. All three point (arrows) to the abstract phoneme oscillator cluster expressed by a set of attractors (right side).

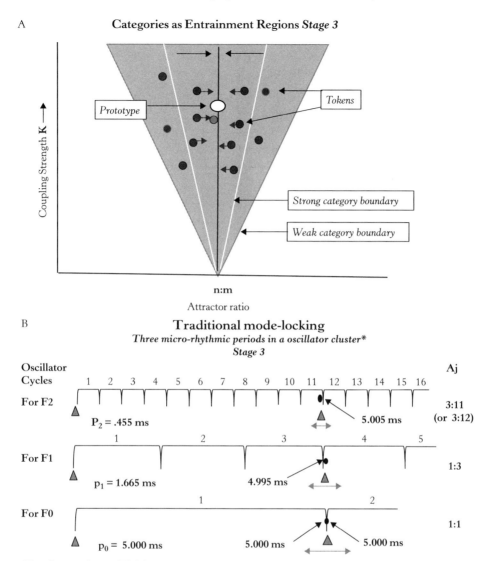

A **Categories as Entrainment Regions** *Stage 3*

B **Traditional mode-locking**
Three micro-rhythmic periods in a oscillator cluster*
Stage 3

*For the vowel /ɛ/ of Table 14.2: Three oscillations (cycles as three ωo periods) activated by respective spectral driving rhythms (not shown F0, F1, F2). Gray triangles as reactive pulses reflect persisting oscillation of the F0 as an internalized referent driving rhythm. Period ratios to the F0 and other oscillations serve as estimates of implied attractors, Aj, that belong to the larger set of all attractors defining a given phoneme.

FIGURE 14.4 (A) Expression of categories as tokens and prototype within an entrainment region. A prototype corresponds to a stimulus phoneme consistent with a token ratio identical to the attractor ratio; a token is any stimulus within an entrainment region that does not fall on the vertical attractor line. In this example, n:m might be 1:3, as in panel **B**. Ratios reflect micro-time levels among nested time layers in a phoneme F1/F0; the lighter gray token reflects a time ratio very close to the .333 attractor ratio i.e., given pi/p_0. (**B**) This panel shows three micro-driven phonemes (oscillations) entraining, respectively, to different micro-driving rhythms for the vowel /ɛ/ (Table 14.1). Stimulus periods are only shown for F0 oscillator (light gray pulses). Black brackets outline the periods of each of three external micro-driving rhythms (F0, F1, F2); triangle pulses outline internal oscillator periods. Note that mode-locked synchronies of oscillations of F1 and F2 with F0 validate hidden attractors Aj on the right.

cluster of Figure 14.4A depicts results of restructuring. The F0 becomes a critical invariant. F0 is an ever-present reference periodicity in all adult tokens of the same phoneme. In Gibsonian terms, access to F0 permits discovery of invariant time ratios that complete the category. As such, an infant's acquisition of the capacity to entrain to this slower rhythm introduces a heretofore missing internal referent period that completes a phoneme oscillator cluster.

The oscillator cluster operating in stage 3 involves endogenous entrainments among multiple oscillations. Together, these waveforms participate in traditional mode-locking, featuring a role for the F0 oscillation as a referent periodicity in this token cluster. Portions of this cluster are outlined in Figure 14.4B, where F0 contributes a waveform with a 5 ms period for the vowel /ɛ/ (from Table 14.2). This slow periodicity was effectively missing for infants in stage 2.

Finally, in stage 3 all token clusters of a phoneme now "point to" a signature set of hidden attractors {**Aj**}. Figure 14.4B shows three different attractor ratios (right side). (Note the ratio for F2 and F1 periods imply attractors of either 3:11 or 3:12; although both are possible, most likely the more stable, 3:12 attractor, prevails). Together, these and other attractors (not shown) form a full attractor set, denoted by {**Aj**}. In theory, all attractors contribute to defining a phoneme category. Thus, for older infants, a sensitivity to the fundamental frequency means that multiple oscillations in a token cluster are suddenly restructured to include the same, slow internal counterpart of this external referent, ω_{oR}. Adding the F0 referent oscillation to an incomplete token cluster changes everything; it sparks an *Ah-Ha moment*. This normalizing force ushers in perceptual restructuring, wherein all tokens of a given phoneme implicate the same set of attractors. Finally, incomplete token oscillator clusters become true *phoneme oscillator clusters*.

Practically speaking, restructuring means that a 6-month-old infant perceives that a /ɛ/, spoken by his mother with a high vocal frequency is perceived as the same vowel (/ɛ/) spoken by his father with a lower F0. Such restructuring of relative time relations acknowledges the normalizing function of the fundamental frequency.

Learning in stage 3 depends on strengthening new bindings among oscillator periods through repetition. These bindings now include ω_{oR}. Following restructuring, bindings swiftly grow stronger with exposures to relevant token phonemes as all implicate the same set of hidden attractors {**Aj**}. In short, tacit learning of guiding attractors involves both an initial discovery state plus relevant reinforced bindings. Binding is also strengthened with exposures to a range of different tokens with similar attractor relations.[80,81,82,83,84] Ultimately, "what" is learned is *a category prototype* defined by a *set of hidden attractors*.

Recapitulation

Category learning of phonemes happens early in life, beginning with stimulus-driven attending and ending with multiple endogenous links that reflect defining abstract (i.e., hidden) synchronous states, termed *attractors*. At each stage, learning depends on a strengthening of links between micro-rhythms that engage infants' attending. Although learning may be Hebbian in nature, its bindings depend on synchronies among micro-rhythms established by three basic entrainment mechanisms: exogenous (tracking) entrainments, oscillator clusters, and attractors. In this way, attending paves the way for implicit learning by binding as it delivers relevant synchronizing oscillators during entrainment.

A Plausibility Test

This, necessarily detailed portrait of phoneme learning has the merit of explaining the developmental findings of Kuhl and others. Moreover, it achieves this without modifying theoretical DAT constructs developed in earlier chapters. But does it really pass the plausibility test? As Micheyl and Oxenham note in their review,[85] vowel perception is a knotty problem, and, admittedly, the preceding discussion glided rather lightly over several psychoacoustic issues. Furthermore, DAT requires that we cease viewing formants as fixed frequencies and consider instead the (less familiar) concept that formants are rhythms; they are dominant, speaker-specific, micro-driving rhythms that can activate an adaptable neural correlates in a perceiver.

In addition, others may more pointedly question the proposal that listeners rely on a speaker's fundamental frequency to normalize percepts of other, concurrent, frequency components (e.g., formants) because their respective micro-rhythms arise from different sources (glottal vs. vocal tract filtering). However, the source-based interpretation has been disputed.[86] But, more to the point, this use of fundamental frequency garners some plausibility from an important line of research that validates these proposed relationships in vowel perception. For instance, similar vowels are easier to perceptually differentiate when their fundamental frequencies differ.[87] Generally, F0 differences induce separate groupings of phonemes.[88,89] Perhaps the clearest evidence for this relationship is provided by Summers et al.[90] and also Maurer.[91] The former found perceived grouping of F1-F2-F3 only when it was accompanied by a common F0. Mauer used synthesized vowels containing formant patterns (F1 to F5), with several different F0s (e.g., 200–600 Hz) and discovered that, in rating vowel quality, expert listeners indicated significant vowel differences as a function of F0. Although direct evidence favoring entrainment to individual high-frequency components is sparse, perhaps due to narrow cortical localizations of high-frequency oscillations, selective high-frequency cortical oscillations in the range of formants have certainly been recorded.[92,93,94] Finally, a few studies confirm the importance of joint neural activities related to F0, F1, and F3 in vowels (in superior temporal gyrus, or the primary auditory cortex)[95,96]

The singular focus on micro-timing relationships in this DAT account of phoneme categorization can also be questioned. However, this DAT account does not exclude a concomitant role for learning of various phonemic features. In fact, a recent review of models on learning phoneme categories emphasizes the importance of a number of other features in defining phoneme categories. The models considered phoneme categorization as a statistical inference problem, using, for instance, mean and variance of known phoneme properties in a Bayesian framework.[97] By contrast, the present approach highlights a greater role for relative timing than implied in this Bayesian framework. Indeed, one might argue that early mastery of micro-time structure facilitates phoneme feature learning by automatically allowing for heightened attending energy at the "right" times (e.g., from attending energy profiles [AEPs]).

Finally, the plausibility of this focus on implied attractor timing relationships, as shown in Table 14.2, is strengthened by the fact that these attractors parallel those found operative in pitch perception (Table 6.1; Figure 6.4) as well as attractors used in music perception (Table 11.1). All three tables show striking similarities of the attractor ratios involved in pitch perception, musical scales, and vowel sounds. In fact, at time scales of phonemes, these attractors have a curious resemblance to certain complex melodic tones of music. This domain generality of special synchronous states not only adds to the plausibility of this account of phoneme categories, but it also underscores an important theme of this book: namely, attending to speech and music relies on similar underlying attending mechanisms.

Finally, this story of infant phoneme categorizations, Table 14.1 summarizes infants'

growing mastery over special micro-time patterns in a world rich with intriguing micro-rhythms. And "what" infants learn (frequency contours, token oscillator cluster, categorical attractors) depends on age as well as exposure frequency. Each overlapping stage reflects general principles of entrainment and learning. In this sense, speech signals present *learnable problems* for infants inclined to tune in to micro-driving rhythms of their temporal niche. These young children eventually discover general states of synchrony. According to Gerken and colleagues, infants attend *more* to learnable than to unlearnable problems, where "[a] learnable problem is one that allows the learner to find deeper level patterns or generalizations in the stimuli themselves."[98]

Summary of Infants' Speedy Learning

The rapidity of infants' progress through learning stages remains remarkable. Speedy learning of solvable problems invites explanations based on automatic and universal mechanisms. This chapter opened with Chomsky's observations that an infant's speedy learning is so unusual it must arise from innate grammars that govern early language learning. In his famous retort to Skinner's response learning approach, Chomsky aptly cited infants' rapid language learning across all cultures as compelling evidence for an innate and universal grammar.[99] This recurring theme of innate versus learned origins of speech skills continues today.

On reflection, Chomsky is correct in two respects. First, some mechanisms underlying early speech learning are innate. Second, it is true that these mechanisms are universal. But, in updating his approach, Chomsky and colleagues are incorrect in inferring that the critical universal language mechanism is an innate grammar (e.g., an FLN).[100] Instead, the answer is much simpler; it involves an infant's natural gravitation to various forms of synchrony. Early speech learning relies on infants' inherent attending proclivities for synchronies, and these tendencies follow principles more fundamental and universal than grammar rules. They are principles of resonance and entrainment that are applicable to other domains (e.g., music) and other species (e.g., birds, whales). In human speech, these principles suggest that infants are selectively tuned to fast driving rhythms, posited by the aging hypothesis, and they also have innate orienting biases, based on modes of synchrony.

Early, speedy learning springs readily from dynamic attending. Entrainment and learning happen rapidly because both are *time-scaled to periodicities of micro-rhythms in speech*. Assuming infants quickly and involuntarily marshal requisite fast neural periodicities, then phoneme learning rapidly achieves asymptotic stability (cf. Chapter 6). For instance, often asymptotic phase-locking performance levels happen in less than eight cycles of a driving rhythm (for 1:1 dyadic mode-locking).[101] For very fast micro-rhythms, this really is speed learning. Consequently, exogenous dyads with fast micro-driving rhythms inevitably promote quick entrainment. Amazingly, asymptotically stable attending to a novel phoneme token can happen within 50 ms!

Given a fast entrainment platform, learning through binding then is also very rapid. Finally, speedy infant learning also has a self-guided aspect for playful 6-month-old babies. For these infants, phoneme learning is strengthened by their own repetitions in babbling, which they joyfully pursue. Although infants are novices, in self-guided learning they are "busy bees" progressing rapidly through different stages of learning phoneme categories.

Major points of this section are:

- Infants progress through three stages of learning phoneme categories in their first year, as described by Kuhl.
- DAT hypothesizes three stage-specific entrainment mechanisms that propose "what" infants learn in Kuhl's stages.
- Stage 1 relies on infants' primitive (i.e., exogenous) entrainments (stimulus-driven) and binding of driven with driving components of complex sounds.
- Stage 2 of older infants develop incomplete token oscillator clusters. Infants endogenously entrain, then bind, oscillations activated by frequency components of token phonemes.
- Stage 3 of still older infants relies on discovery of a normalizing referent oscillation (from F0) that effectively complete (normalize) token oscillator clusters. Learning through binding incorporates all token oscillator clusters that "point to" the same phoneme category defined by hidden attractors.

PHONEME CATEGORIZATION SKILLS OF ADULTS

Let us leap ahead to adults. From any perspective, adults are facile in deciphering rapid and complex sound patterns within familiar speech. Amazingly,

this happens even when phoneme tokens whip by at rates exceeding 30 phonemes per second. Some explain this skill in terms of internalized grammars or prototypes, whereas others assume that adults' category recognition skills rely strictly on learning common statistical properties of a phoneme's frequency spectrum.

This section explores a different path that includes a role for attending dynamics during adults' acquisition of phoneme skills. It addresses the well-honed habits of adults that govern their ability to track a spoken context containing rapidly changing phonemes. By adulthood, people are proficient in the three basic stage 3 entrainment mechanisms evident in childhood learning of phoneme categories: namely, exogenous rhythm tracking, oscillator cluster formation, and category (attractor) identification (Table 14.1). In adults, all these skills are enlisted simultaneously to tackle novel speech utterances, where they foster short-term learning.

This section has two parts. The first part expands on DAT mechanisms underlying adult phoneme categorizations. The second part offers examples of adult's use of these entrainment mechanisms in short-term category learning with speech contexts.

Categories and Boundaries: Underlying Entrainment Mechanisms

How do adults effortlessly identify vowels, as in "bit" versus "bet," in natural speaking contexts? The ability to tease out phoneme categories in fast-breaking speech contexts seems daunting. Indeed, it justifies a retreat to a simplified laboratory paradigm. The defining paradigms have required that people engage in a *category identification task* and/or perform a *pair-wise phoneme discrimination task*. Not surprisingly, in both tasks, adults are at least as proficient as stage 3 infants in categorizing various token vowels (as in "bit" versus "bet"). So how do adults do this? This section addresses this question using the same dynamic attending mechanisms outlined for infant stage 3 in Table 14.1.

Identifying Phoneme Categories

An adult's knowledge of phonemes stems from internalized phoneme oscillator categories (i.e., stage 3). Any task requiring an adult listener to identify the category of a particular phoneme token draws on the listener's sense of proximity between this phoneme's token cluster and the relevant attractors of this category. Theoretically, this proximity is reflected in the distance between a given token and its attractor within the attractor's entrainment region, as suggested in Figure 14.4A.

Phoneme Identification: An example

Let us assume that a listener recognizes the isolated syllable "bit" by sensing the nearest hidden attractors to the vowel token of /I/. From Table 14.2, this vowel consists of fuzzy frequency ratios that approximate two hidden attractor ratios of .444, .200 (i.e., F1/F0, F2/F1, column 5). A token stimulus with exactly these attractor ratios functions as an internalized prototype. Of course, this doesn't happen often; instead, as Figure 14.4A suggests, most tokens do not match these ratios. Rather, tokens exhibit variable proximity relative to the pertinent (hidden) attractor. The example token of /I/ in Table 14.2 (column 4) happens to be one with significant proximity to the above attractors with formant ratios of .444 and .195. As such, the proximity of this token vowel is likely to awaken ("point to") nearby attractors. Nevertheless, this analysis applies to any token, close or far from its attractors.

A different graphic portrayal of this token–prototype relationship appears in Figure 14.5. This figure depicts two quite different attractor-defined entrainment regions, each with a single attractor. In this framework, attractors are assumed to govern identification of categories, whereas entrainment region's boundaries influence discrimination performance. Here, tokens and attractors are situated in the respective entrainment regions of attractors from two different vowels (i.e., for /I/ and /ɛ/). Each region places boundaries (weak or strong) on perceptual limits of the category defined by its attractor ratio.

Consider now the standard category identification task mentioned earlier. Let this task involve the presentation of a single (isolated) token of the vowel /I/ with an attractor of .200 (as in "bit") to a listener who must name its category. With the centered attractor line in Figure 14.5 specifying this category, one token (star) is proximal to this attractor. Specifically, this vowel expresses a fuzzy formant ratio of .195, which is quite close to the attractor ratio of the /I/ prototype. Of course, this happens in an entrainment region, so the attractor exerts "pulls" (arrows) on such token oscillator clusters, thereby enhancing proximity percepts in listeners. Pull strength is inversely related to token–attractor proximity and positively related to attractor simplicity. Thus, in this example, a simple, nearby attractor exerts a strong "pull" on the token. In turn, this

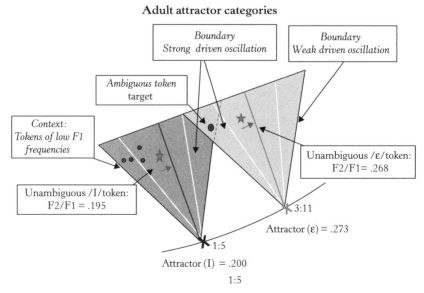

FIGURE 14.5 Schematic of two attractor categories postulated for listeners encountering adult produced vowels /I/ or /ɛ/. In Dynamic Attending Theory (DAT), a phoneme category is expressed by an attractor and its surrounding entrainment region (with bifurcation boundaries). Narrow regions (white lines) occur in adult listeners' strong driven oscillations. Attractors (vertical lines) define a category; tokens (light gray dots, stars) are either close or far from attractors. In identification tasks, adults hearing low-frequency contexts tokens (light gray dots) experience them in a remote (left) part of the entrainment region. The dark blue dot inside an overlapping entrainment regions reflects an ambiguous token.

leads to a prediction that listeners will readily identify this token as belonging to the /I/ category. Hence, the syllable is heard as "bit", not "bet." This account also implies that listeners are likely to mistake some very proximal tokens for their prototypes, which is a common finding in these identification tasks.

Context and Phoneme Categorization

Rarely do phoneme tokens occur in isolation. Even "bit" comes in a consonant envelope. A more realistic setting introduces a longer preceding speech context. In light of discussions about speech context in Chapter 13, it should not be surprising to learn that context also has an impact on the nature of listeners' percepts of individual phonemes. One way to explain these particular context effects, however, focuses on the biasing role of short-term learning, during a context, on listeners' responses to a future target token. Views differ on this topic. So let's first consider what we know about such context effects.

Context and Phoneme Categorization: Short-Term Learning

A classic study of Ladefoged and Broadbent[102] first revealed short-term context effects on phoneme perception. Listeners heard the phrase, "Please say what this word is . . ." prior to presentation of a target word, which was either *bit* or *bet*. Two different speech contexts were created in which F1 formants of relevant context phonemes were consistently low (under 450 Hz) or consistently high (above 600 Hz). And, although typically /ɛ/ has a higher F1 than does /I/ (Table 14.2), the target syllable listeners were asked to identify contained an ambiguous F1 vowel (synthesized between 450 and 600 Hz) in "bit" and "bet." Ladefoged and Broadbent discovered that this ambiguous target was heard as "bet" after a low F1 context, but as "bit" after high F1 contexts. In other words, target phonemes are judged *relative to* an established speech context.

One way to think about this effect rests on the DAT assumption that a spoken context induces entrainment, thereby promoting short-term learning. This then biases listeners toward one attractor over another. An illustration of this idea appears in Figure 14.5, which shows context tokens (lighter/smaller gray dots) preceding a presented (target) sound (star) within an entraining region. As with Ladefoged and Broadbent, these context tokens have relatively low F1 frequencies. Nevertheless, they fall inside wide category boundaries of the /I/ vowel attractor with an F2–F1 attractor relationship

of 1.5. Context tokens containing low F1 frequencies nonetheless will consistently "point to" the nearest F1–F2 attractor, given a fixed F2 frequency. In this case, the Attractor (I) = .200 is the nearest attractor for these context tokens. Also shown is the Attractor (ɛ) =.273 (or more likely .250).

Finally, ascertaining if a particular target token belongs to a particular attractor's category depends on the proximity of this token to a contextually active attractor.[103] This schematic shows three different target sounds. One target contains an unambiguous low F1 frequency (star) in the region of attractor (I); another unambiguous target (star), has a higher F1 frequency in the entrainment region of (ɛ). However, of most interest is the ambiguous target (dark gray oval) with an intermediate F1 frequency that could belong to either attractor category. But, if a prior context effectively installs the attractor for /I/, then the ambiguous target will be identified as belonging to the /I/ category (i.e., in "bit"). Alternatively, if very high F1 frequency context tokens (not shown in this figure) repeatedly precede the same ambiguous token, this should activate the /ɛ/ attractor and listeners will be increasingly biased to judge this target as "not /I /." This DAT prediction is consistent with findings about phoneme categorization reported by Ladefoged and Broadbent.

Finally, DAT assumes that adult listeners respond, in real time, to ongoing contexts. An adult listener's experience with a context depends on the same entrainment and learning mechanisms operative in infants (Table 14.1). However, in adults, these mechanisms are refined and they operate simultaneously to entrain to unfolding phonemes in speech. With repeated entrainment episodes, all three domain general entrainment mechanisms outlined in Table 14.1 are in play: *endogenous entrainments, token oscillator clusters,* and *context-implicated attractors.* Thus, adults concurrently track multiple frequency components, form token oscillator clusters, and recognize attractor relationships as they entrain to an unfolding speech pattern. Moreover, these context-generated entrainment activities support short-term learning based on repeated opportunities for bindings among active oscillations, including the referent oscillation, that strengthen knowledge of certain phonemes.

This explanation of short-term learning differs from one developed by Lori Holt and colleagues. They also propose that listeners acquire perceptual biases from a speech context, but in this approach these biases reflect a listener's extraction of the average of component frequencies in a preceding speech context. This *long-term average spectrum* (LTAS) model successfully explains phoneme context effects.[104] In this case, short-term learning yields a spectral average which functions as an internal referent from which to judge an ambiguous target. For instance, listeners learn that contexts with mostly high F1 frequencies define the category /ɛ/ (as in "bet"); then statistical deviants from this average are judged as "not bet."

Domain Specificity?

Recently, Holt and colleagues ruled out the domain specificity of context effects, using a context-oriented category identification task. They presented listeners with targets (XXX) of two consonant categories using syllables ranging from /ga/ to /da/. Using the context "Please say what this word is XXX," now F3 consonant frequencies were varied (denoted ω_3). Specifically, F3 was varied relative to a fixed F1, creating F3:F1 ratios designed to bias listeners to hear a token phoneme as /da/ or /ga/ (i.e., with lower or higher F3, respectively).[105] To assess domain specificity, two different contexts were speech, **S**, and nonspeech, **N**, shown in Figure 14.6. The **N** contexts had random musical notes for F3 values that matched formants in **S** contexts.[106]

Clear context effects emerged, replicating findings of Lagefoged and Broadbent. Also important were findings that these short-term learning effects appeared in *both* speech and nonspeech

contexts, favoring a domain-general approach. In fact, surprisingly, listeners' responses revealed greater sensitivity to modulations of the nonspeech context. Although this supports predictions of LTAS, it is also consistent with preceding interpretations of DAT.

Finally, the LTAS approach and the DAT approach both appeal to a domain-general internalization of context properties. However, they differ in two respects: (1) DAT reflects adaptive in-the-moment entrainments, whereas LTAS rests on the retrieval of a complete sequence; and (2) DAT relies on internal defining factors of attractors and entrainment regions, whereas LTAS rests on statistical properties of means and variances.

From Phonemes to Syllables: Syllable Attractor Profiles

Phonemes of the preceding sections feature micro-time structures that live inside syllables. For instance, syllables such as *bet* and *bit* provide a local context of consonants that surround the center vowel. Some accounts lump such phonemes together to conceive of syllables as *perceptual primitives*. This might, for instance, apply to infants' first struggles in speech learning, where consonants and vowels emerge together in infants' recurrent babbling of rudimentary syllables such as "ga" and "da."

Yet, the status of syllables as "the" perceptual primitive speech unit remains a matter of debate. Perhaps it is more appropriate to view syllables as

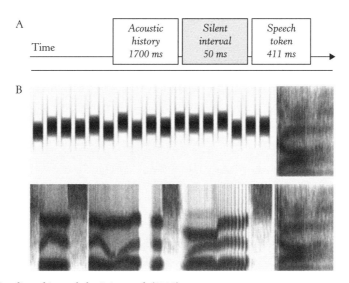

FIGURE 14.6 Stimuli used in study by Laing et al. (2012).

Reprinted from figure 1 in Erika J. C. Laing et al., "Tuned with a Tune: Talker Normalization via General Auditory Processes," *Auditory Cognitive Neuroscience* 3 (2012): 203, doi:10.3389/fpsyg.2012.00203.

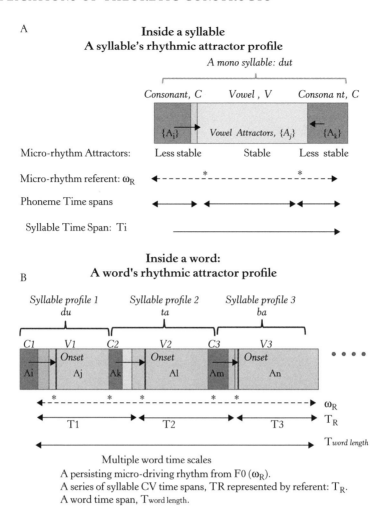

FIGURE 14.7 (A) Inside a hypothetical CVC syllable are determinants of a syllable attractor profile. This syllable elicits in a listener three oscillator sets (clusters) carrying phoneme attractors. Mode-locking holds this together (for attending, then learning) with two persisting speaker-specific internal references. At micro-time levels, a fluctuating internalized referent of vocal frequency, ω_R (i.e., F0) persists to hold phonemes within a syllable together in a syllable attractor profiles. Asterisks (*) show group-inducing ω_R points that outline phoneme time spans. **(B)** Inside a word are determinants of a word attractor profile. A nonsense word, *dutaba*, continues the persisting referents at micro-time levels (e.g., rhythm, ω_R). In addition, at macro-time levels, syllable durations, Ti, fluctuate relative to a persisting external articulation rate, T_R. Both traditional (meter-like) and transient (rhythm-like) mode-locking are possible for individual words depending on Ti variations.

bridges between phonemes and words. Certainly their apparent role in serving as referent driving rhythm with a tempo response curve is consistent with such a position. Nevertheless, a single syllable also lends itself to an interpretation as a serial pattern of phonemes in which successive phoneme attractors fit within certain time spans to form a brief syllabic time pattern. Figure 14.7A shows this for the syllable "dut." To be sure, during a speech utterance a speaker's normal articulatory constraints create carryover effects from one phoneme to the

next that shape successive consonants and vowels. Factors such as contextual smearing, formant transitions, and articulatory modulations not only modulate phoneme durations, but they also reinforce the notion of fuzziness of the micro-driving rhythms that comprise phoneme time spans. In spite of this, hidden attractors that define phoneme clusters, remain operative as core perceptual forces within syllables.

Moreover, certain unifying forces shape the stream of phonemes that tumbles out in speakers' utterances. For instance, both a speaker's fundamental frequency and her talking rate may serve as unifying/even normalizing forces for phonemes within and between syllables of this speaker. Given an entrainment framework, these two stimulus properties feature external, talker-specific referent levels. More specifically, during production, such referent driving rhythms realize tempo response curves with fluctuations that elicit momentary perceptual contrasts in listeners (recall perceived groupings from tempo response curves of Chapter 8; and Chapters 12 and 13).

Figure 14.7A highlights the role of a speaker's fundamental frequency in uniting phoneme attractors of phoneme clusters within a single, idealized, CVC syllable. For a given speaker, all phoneme attractors in the syllable incorporate the same referent waveform, ω_R (from a fluctuating F0).[107] Phoneme clusters resemble complex tones. Two or three phoneme clusters endogenously entrain, successively, to the persisting neural correlation of ω_R, namely ω_{oR}. Hence, they conform to a transient mode-locking protocol. This normalizing role of ω_{oR} is often overlooked, but imagine how unsettling it would be if each phoneme cluster in CVC syllables was synthesized using the F0s of different speakers.

Figure 14.7 recognizes natural fluctuations in the ω_R (suggested by *).[108] Such fluctuations highlight beginnings and endings of phoneme clusters, hence they encapsulate their respective attractors, {Aj}. Against the inherent fuzziness within a syllable, sets of phoneme attractors trace out a short serial pattern of attractor sets within each syllable. Given transient mode-locking, this forms a phoneme attractor profile that defines a syllable. Thus, a single syllable affords a brief profile of phoneme categories (attractor sets). For instance, the syllable *dut* of Figure 14.7A embeds a profile of three phoneme attractor states, {Aj}, in which each of three phoneme clusters contains several global attractors.[109] These are rich attractor sets containing attractors with different stabilities.[110,111]

As units, syllables become familiar because they are repeated in a wide range of entrainable contexts, leading to development of strong bindings among activated oscillations. In English, a typical syllable contains between one and four phonemes, with each phoneme eliciting a phoneme cluster and its global attractors.[112] As such, each syllable implicates a brief i.e., mini-melody conveyed by several constituent phoneme attractor profiles. And, a string of several syllables yields a longer speech 'melody' found in words. In this respect, syllables resemble short, speaker-specific, melodies.

A rhythmic pattern can also be identified, given subtle time markers in a melodic string of syllables. Indeed, a series of phoneme clusters across several syllables not only delivers a longer melody-like progression of abstract phoneme attractors, it also exhibits multiple time spans of the successive phonemes inside a syllable At one time level, phonemes are carved out by markers of phonemes (i.e., * in Figure 14.7A). And when these time spans vary significantly within a syllable, word or phrase, DAT predicts transient mode-locking of a listener's attending comes into play to form a sy*llable's rhythmic attractor profile.* As discussed in preceding chapters, this protocol assumes a normalizing referent period based upon a speaker's articulation rate.

Ultimately, still longer time spans are provided when considering multisyllabic words. In short, this leads to the emergence of a dynamic time hierarchy in speech in which the fastest time spans make-up waveforms embedded inside phoneme clusters; and, slower time times emerge with phoneme durations (about 12–60 ms), and still slower time spans, Ti, emerge to cover whole syllables such as *dut* (about 60–250 ms), and words (250–1,000 ms).[113,114,115]

Finally, mounting evidence supports the claim that many different speech time spans serve as driving rhythms in entrainment scenarios at different time scales. In other words, a variety of speaker-specific temporal configurations emerge from spoken phrases. Each projects a set of embedded external driving rhythms at a respectively different time scale. Furthermore a burst of recent research supports the idea that such driving rhythms elicit corresponding driven rhythms in the cortex.[116,117,118,119,120,121,122] Such temporal embeddings hark back to metric configurations which invite a traditional mode-locking attending protocol in listeners. Here multiple time scales range from very brief periodicities of micro-rhythms (e.g., of formants) within phonemes, to durations of phoneme clusters and syllables, and ultimately to the slower time scales of rhythms that fit onto words, phrases, and even sentences.

Summary of Adults' Phoneme Categorization Skills

Clearly, adults have mastered phoneme categories. However, short-term learning is essential for people to identify such categories in different speech contexts. Explanations vary regarding whether contextual biasing of phoneme identification depends on an acquired statistical summary of prior speech context properties or on listeners' sensitivity to contextually induced attractors.

Finally, we can assume that "what" adults learn about a syllable springs from entrainments involving both its melodic-like and its rhythmic content. The melodic content refers to a series of phoneme attractor sets; its rhythmic content refers to patterns of time spans at multiple time scales. With phoneme attractors, short-term learning contributes to strengthening (via binding) of token oscillator clusters that happens when a listener attends to phonemes within syllables; this invites the traditional mode-locking protocol. These are token clusters of defined sets of phoneme attractors, {Aj}. In syllables, listeners internalize these melodic-like sequences as a series of oscillator clusters where corresponding phoneme attractor sets lead to attractor profiles. Syllables also convey other attractors, specifically rhythmic attractors (from traditional or transient mode-lock protocols). Overall, this portrait of syllable strings in speech has intriguing parallels with the variety of attractor profiles found in music.

Major points in this section are:

- *Phoneme categories* arise from traditional mode-locking, which creates token oscillator clusters that "point to" hidden attractors defining a phoneme category.
- *Identification of phoneme categories* depends on category-specific sets of hidden global attractors. .
- Category identification and discrimination of phonemes are captured, respectively, in the entrainment concepts of attractor(s) and the boundaries surrounding attractors (prototype) that house tokens.
- Category identification of a phoneme is influenced by the speech context in which it occurs.
- *Syllables* comprise strings of phoneme attractors, forming melody-like sequences. They also carry time structure in the form of time patterns of phoneme durations. A *syllable's rhythmic attractor profile* refers to the rhythm formed by a series of different syllable time spans.

PRE-LEXICAL WORD CATEGORIES: WORD LEARNING

The narrative on speech learning developed in this chapter ends with word learning. Apart from semantic meaning, words belong to distinct, pre-lexical prosodic categories. For example, if a speaker simply utters the multisyllable word "yesterday" conversationally, as in: "Yesterday, I went to the store," this acoustic pattern differs drastically from its phonological form in the Beatles' song *Yesterday*. Vowel durations stretch in the musical rendition, together with increased variations in pitch and intensity modulations, among other phonological changes. Yet we easily recognize the same word in both contexts. There is "something" in these different versions of a word sound that transcends superficial acoustical differences in word tokens. Various word tokens all belong to the same, abstractly identified word category.

An obvious candidate for determining word categories immediately springs to mind: semantics. We learn to access the same "meaning node" in the brain's word lexicon. However, unanswered questions remain concerning how we get to the right node. This section entertains the possibility that learning prosodic aspects of a word jump-starts learning the word's meaning. The prosody of words leads to formation of word categories. However (yes, of course, a qualifier), a critical limitation is this: as with syllable categories, prosodic word categories themselves embody abstract time relationships that are shaped by a surrounding context.

This section has two parts. The first part considers ways in which attending dynamics constrain, pre-lexically, the learning of novel words in various contexts. The second part considers research on pre-lexical word learning.

Dynamic Attending: Word Categories

Words are strings of syllables. And syllables are strings of phonemes. Pre-lexically, word categories resemble syllable categories because both embody attractor profiles of phonemes. Both deal with serial changes in micro-driving rhythms as these are referenced to stable speaker-specific periodicities.[123] For syllables, the serial pattern of phoneme oscillator clusters is referenced to an internalized fundamental frequency, thus yielding phoneme attractor profiles that determine a syllable's melodic content. However, as a context expands with addition of more syllables, longer words are formed. This also means that the rhythmic attractor profiles of syllables grow into longer rhythmic attractor profiles. Words comprise longer strings of phoneme attractor profiles (i.e., as syllables). An idealized *rhythmic word attractor profile* of phonemes appears in Figure 14.7B.

Word Categories and Entrainment

Let's begin with the assumption that a prosodic word category includes a representation of the word's phoneme attractor profile. The simplest such category, of course, will be the phoneme attractor profile of a monosyllable, based on its F0 referent. By contrast, the prosodic frames of multisyllable words require adding in rhythmic constraints, including a second, slower referent period that captures speaking rate.

Figure 14.7B illustrates a three-syllable nonsense word, *dutaba,* containing both the fast referent waveform, ω_R (of F0). However, it also relies upon a slower temporal referent, namely the speaking rate, T_R. Note that both referents are speaker-specific; the former reflecting a melodic vocal property of a speaker and the latter reflecting a characteristic speaking rate, analogous to a speaker-specific tactus.

This entrainment analysis is clearly focused upon two different slices of time scales in the time hierarchy of speech. It presumes that entrainments essential to implicit learning happen concurrently with fast and slow stimulus speech driving rhythms arising respectively from micro-rhythms within phonemes (with periods of 12–20 ms) and macro-rhythms of syllables and words (e.g., periods ranging up to 2,000 ms and beyond; cf. Table 12.1). Current bursts of brain research support claims of entraining oscillations across this range of time scales. And, widespread, bilateral cortical synchronizations have been recorded in listeners entraining to the ordinary speech of a speaker at multiple time levels.[124,125]

In light of this, entrainments that engage phonemes within syllable and word attractor profiles happen simultaneously with entrainments of the slower macro-rhythms involving time spans of syllables and words in Figure 14.7B. As this figure illustrates, the fast time scales of phonemes are nested within the slower macro-rhythms of syllables and words. Let's now consider the macro-time spans of syllables, Ti. These stimulus time spans vary within and between words. As suggested in Figure 14.7B, changing Ti's are referenced to the period of speaking rate, T_R (see below). Specifically, exogenous entrainments happen with a listener's induction of a speaker-specific neural correlate of T_R (i.e., $p_R \sim T_R$). If all syllables in a word or phrase have roughly the same time span (i.e., a quasi-isochronous rhythm), then the traditional mode-locking protocol readily guides a listener's attending (all Ti = T_R). In this case, exogenous entrainment is likely, governed by a simple global attractor (e.g., *n:m* = 1:1).

What about rhythmic groups? If several groups of syllables (e.g., words) all have the same number of syllables/group (e.g., all are disyllables), then traditional mode-locking still applies, but it implicates a different global attractor (e.g., *n:m* = 2.1). Alternatively, with variable Ti values differ distinctly, as with words carrying different groups of syllables (monosyllables versus disyllables), then Ti ≠ T_R. In this case, listeners should automatically fall into using a transient mode-locking protocol to guide exogenous entrainment of attending. Respectively, these familiar entrainment protocols lead to meter-like (with global attractors) and rhythm-like (with attractor profiles) configurations of a word's syllable time structure.

The example in Figure 14.7B shows a word configuration that invites traditional mode-locking of attending. It assumes that, just as a speaker's vocalized F0 varies, a quasi-isochronous rhythm of the speaker's talking rate (i.e., the tempo response curve) will also vary depending upon a speaker's intentions (voluntary or involuntary, cf. Chapter 8). The result is subtle fluctuations of speaking rate, T_R. For instance, one speaker might slightly lengthen the beginning (*du*) and ending (*ba*) syllables in <u>*dutaba*</u>, creating a slow-fast-slow tempo response curve, whereas another speaker might produce a fast, medium, slow tempo response curve (cf. Chapter 8). Given limit cycle-driven oscillations, such fluctuations in speaking rate provoke only brief manifest (expressive) changes in a listener's percepts.[126] As illustrated in Chapter 8, modest modulation within a tempo response curve will nonetheless preserve an underlying attractor profile. Accordingly, listeners readily accommodate to the natural speaking habits of speakers, therein detecting the correct temporal grouping of a string of phoneme attractors.

Next lets examine the slower macro-rhythms of words. Spoken words also support a listener's entrainment, paving the route to implicit word learning. Also shown in Figure 14.7B is a word length variable, Twordlength, which registers the time spans of words. In research that holds word length constant, e.g., uses only syllables, or only disyllables, the driving-to-driven n:m ratio involving an unfolding driving rhythm, Twordlength, is calibrated by a driven speaking rate oscillation with period, p_R, elicited by the roughly stable contextually determined speaking rate (T_R). This T_R: Twordlength, relationship determines the mode-locking order. For instance, if this ratio is constant over a series of words, then again we find a metrical time structure based upon a traditional mode-locking protocol. This results in a single global attractor of $n{:}m = 1{:}1$, $1{:}2$, $1{:}3$, or $1{:}4$ and so on. Furthermore, any fixed meter-like frame should enhance temporal parsing of successive individual words; this has implications for word learning.

Implications for Word Learning

Learning through binding follows entrainment. Bindings strengthen with repetitions of syllables and words. At the time scales of syllables, bindings grow with repetitions of syllables. Typically, this learning is implicit; it happens automatically during entrainment. Moreover, bindings among entrainment-activated oscillations happen concurrently over multiple time scales. That is, during entrainments/bindings involving the brief time scales of phoneme clusters and syllable attractor profiles, described earlier, we also find that entrainments and bindings among oscillations of the longer time scales of syllables and words are automatically happening.

Typically, word learning in adults is studied using continuous sequences of novel (i.e., nonsense) words (notably, syllables and phonemes are not novel). From a DAT perspective, this methodology focuses on gaining mastery in segmenting strings of known syllable groups. The repetition of certain groups of phoneme attractors will foster entrainment, hence binding, of syllable attractor profiles. For instance, simply repeating a nonsense word attractor profile (e.g., for *dutaba*) enhances bindings.

Finally, research on word learning often overlooks the role of certain learning paradigm features that reside in the slower time structure of syllables and words. That is, typically, word length, Twordlength, is held constant throughout a learning session. This is pertinent because it insures recurring time spans of disyllables or trisyllables.[127] Specifically, this leads to a constant ratio of T_R:Twordlength and this determines fixed global attractors for disyllables (1:2) or trisyllables (1:3). These are familiar metric constraints. These constraints should not only advance learning via bindings for time relationships, they should also facilitate listeners' expectancies about "when" forthcoming words will occur. In short, these paradigms enhance learning of syllables within segmented words as well expectancies about word length.

Research on Word Learning

In a review of speech learning, Gervain and Mehler[128] distinguished nativistic approaches,[129,130] involving the innate grammars of Chomsky, from other approaches emphasizing syntactic biases proposed in perceptual learning theories. Prominent among the latter are contemporary approaches that focus on the facilitating effects of prosodic features and/or of statistical properties of word distributions. Clearly, these two broad approaches offer respectively different views on domain specificity.

Prosodic Bootstrapping: Domain-Specific

Approaches that emphasize the bootstrapping potential of various prosodic features were described in earlier chapters. They are of interest here because this line of thinking leads to a domain-specific orientation to word learning. For instance, specific prosodic properties, including phonemes, are viewed as statistically valid cues for word segmentation, which putatively bootstraps early learning.[131,132] Indeed, even newborns appear to rely on bootstrapping correlations between domain specific prosodic features and structural and grammatical regularities.[133,134,135]

Statistical Learning: Domain-General

Research in recent decades has challenged a domain-specific approach. To a large degree, this research centers on the generality of statistical properties in word learning. One example of statistical learning, based on feature averaging, was discussed with phoneme learning (i.e., the LTAS model). However, at time scales of words, statistical learning typically refers to the impact of conditional probabilities among successive syllables on implicit word learning.

This approach to word learning has been championed by Jennifer Saffran.[136,137] Saffran's domain-general approach applies to both word and melody learning. The basic idea is elegantly simple. It asserts that people acquire connections between successive syllables (or tones) due to relative probabilities of their joint occurrences. Syllables are deemed perceptual primitives that meld into words based on conditional probabilities, namely high transition probabilities (TPs) between successive syllables. Thus, high TPs between two syllables inside a longer, three-syllable, nonsense word speeds learning of this word. In this view, even infants are deemed "statistical learners."[138] Finally, to learn a word is to acquire a serial pattern of statistical contingencies.

Research Favoring Statistical Learning Theory

A gift of statistical learning theory is its simplicity. This contributes to its wide appeal. Following Hayes and Clark, Saffran and colleagues manipulated TP distributions in lengthy, temporally continuous sequences of monosyllables.[139,140,141] Trisyllable nonsense words contain two adjacent syllables connected by high TP values (TPs between 0.31 and 1.00), followed by a statistical boundary after a third syllable, namely a low TP (between .10 and 0.20). Higher TPs (e.g., 1.00) predict stronger connections. Hence, this TP pattern putatively signals novel 'word-like' groups of three syllables stripped of prominent prosodic features. All nonsense words in a session of trials typically have the same TP pattern, as in a continuous stream, such as: *babupu*dutaba*patubi* . . . etc. (* are low TP locations).

Amazingly, Saffran and colleagues discovered that even brief exposures to these nonsense words promoted learning in adults and also in 8-month-old infants. Both groups recognized "statistical words" (e.g., *babupu*), but not foil words (i.e., those crossing a low TP boundary; e.g., *puduta*; underlined).

These widely replicated findings generalize to musical sequences and to listeners of all ages.[142,143,144,145] Furthermore, infants transferred learning of nonsense words to learning real words.[146,147] This and other evidence suggests that word learning may depend primarily on statistical contingencies among syllables and not on phonemic/prosodic cues, as implied by a prosody bootstrapping hypothesis.

Limits of a Statistical Learning Hypothesis

Despite the success of the statistical learning hypothesis, some limits to this idea are instructive. One involves its restricted role for attending. With few exceptions, this research features statistical, TP patterns as the major factor in word learning.[148,149,150,151,152] The PARSER model offers an exception. It assumes that high TPs among adjacent syllables shift listeners' focal attending to chunks, thereby facilitating the learning of disyllables and trisyllables.[153,154] Another limit questions this domain general approach. It concerns the role of TP patterns themselves, given that cortical tracking of monosyllabic words does not exhibit sensitivity to statistical, i.e.,TP, patterns.[155] The focus of statistical learning on syllable primacy has also been questioned for its omission of a role for phonemes.

Not only do the discoveries of Kuhl on early phoneme learning (Table 14.1) seem to qualify the dominance of TP patterns, other research underscores the importance of phonemes in word learning.[156,157,158,159,160]

Finally, a most telling limitation involving the macro-rhythms of words has also surfaced. Statistical learning is most successful in paradigms that present to-be-learned nonsense words (disyllables or trisyllables) which *share the same syllable length and the same word length.*

Such findings implicate a role for word timing variables (e.g., Ti, T_R, Twordlength). Although the standard practice for controlling a "nuisance" variable is to hold it constant, ironically, treating timing as a nuisance variable does not work. To the contrary, a series of syllables or words in which all durations are held constant same creates isochronous rhythms! Not surprisingly, these rhythms may actually *increase* the impact of time, a phenomenon confirmed by Johnson and Tyler.[161] They found that infants (5.5–8 months) learned an artificial language when all nonsense words were of equal lengths, but not when word lengths varied. Notice, for instance, if word length, Tword length, and speaking rate, T_R, are both constant (i.e., Tword length = 600 ms; T_R = 200 ms), then the implicated time structure has attractors of n:m for trisyllables of 1:3 (triple meter) and 1:2 for dissyllables (duple meter). Over a session, such metrical attractors inevitably facilitate word learning. It should even motivate anticipations of beginnings and ends of future words. Confirming this, some speculate that "infants may have internalized a two or three part rhythm, which interacted with their perception of transition statistics."[162][p.244]

Beneficial effects of meter-like speech contexts on word learning cross ages and domains. Barbara Tillmann and colleagues[163] studied adults' learning of nonsense "word" groups in FSG-generated sequences as disyllables or trisyllables. These sequences contained meter-like groups with duple (1:2) or triple (1:3) metric relations (i.e., T_R:Tword length). Relatedly, Selchenkova and colleagues found that metrical timing boosts learning of an artificial grammar.[164,165] Such studies suggest that word learning benefits from meter-like timing properties. Generally, metrical contexts orient listeners' attending to beginnings of anticipated words. Indeed, Terry et al.[166] recently showed that random variations the time intervals between syllable groups weakened such anticipations. Consequently, relative to a meter-like time structure, such timing irregularities weakened the implicit learning of words. These and other studies suggest that learning is also influenced by rhythmic variations in patterns of external driving rhythm.[167,168,169,170,171,172,173,174,175]

Summary of Word Learning

From phonemes to syllables to words, a case can be made that attending dynamics play a role in word learning. Speech contains a variety of fuzzy driving rhythms that support entrainment activities at time scales of micro-rhythms (phonemes) and of macro-rhythms (syllables, words). In this regard, at the micro-time levels of phonemes and within syllable attractor profiles, it is hypothesized that entrainment and binding lead to learning of mini-melodies of phonemes. At the macro-time levels of words and groups of words, current research on word learning raises interesting new questions about the susceptibility of listeners' tunable brains to the macro-driving rhythms of a speaker's speaking rate and the rhythms of words themselves. At these slower speech time scales, the mini-melodies of syllable attractor profiles become encapsulated in different metrical or rhythmic capsules. These slower time scales bring to surface theoretically important periodicities in speech that involve a speaker's talking rate and word lengths. Furthermore, at these slower rates, learning continues to depend on entrainment protocols, namely traditional mode-locking (with metric clusters) or transient mode-locking (with attractor profiles).

Finally, word learning as a function of exposure frequency remains unchallenged. From a DAT perspective, this exposure comes with repeated entrainment episodes that lead to stronger reinforcement of bindings among activated oscillations. However, in this story, "what" is learned is not fully expressed as a statistical property. Instead, learning has stages, probably condensed in adults. Implicit learning begins automatically with stimulus-driven attending in exogenous entrainments and related bindings. And learning ends with activities of endogenous entrainments among many oscillations that implicate abstract synchronicities (i.e., innate attractors). All these ideas remain to be explored in the future.

Major points in this section are:

- Research on word learning suggests a major role for domain-general mechanisms.
- A DAT approach maintains that *word attractor profiles* consist of expanded syllable attractor profiles, thus implying that a string

of phoneme attractors represents a word's "mini-melody."
- Word learning research also indicates that macro-rhythms of a learning context affect learning of individual words.
- Meter-like timing in a context of words of similar durations facilitates individual word learning.
- Concepts pertaining to both melody and rhythm in speech offer parallels to those used to describe melody and rhythm in music.

CHAPTER SUMMARY

Major themes pertinent to language learning have traditionally centered on the respective roles of innate versus acquired factors. Certain long-standing innate factors, such as primitive grammar rules or inborn motor gestures, are questioned in this chapter as current thinking swings toward blank-slate assumptions in which perceptual learning depends largely on exposure frequency of speech units. The latter presents an appealing, domain-general, theoretical stance.

Yet ideas developed in this book, culminating in this chapter, question both strictly innate theories that feature domain-specific learning and blank-state learning approaches that imply domain generality. The former cannot handle commonalities in learning across different domains and species, whereas blank-slate approaches ignore certain innate biases that constrain learning

Following ideas developed in Part I of this book, innate tendencies are steeped in something so elementary that we simply take it for granted: *synchronicity*. We are naturally drawn to states of synchrony. Although an innate tendency, synchrony cannot happen unless at least two co-occurring activities share some, probably fuzzy, periodicity. Fuzzy rhythms across domains populate all time scales, fast and slow, and people of all ages simply cope with them. Humans, along with other species, adapt. Underlying this idea of adaptivity are various forms of synchrony, often hidden as attractors. Attractors are special states of relative timing that capture synchrony, regardless of time scale or domain. They govern various communicative interactions between conspecifics, via driving–driven dyads. In one way or another, dyadic interactions build on the inherent nature of synchronies between a speaker's sound-making and a listener's tunable brain.

In human speech, as in music, we find attractors hiding in the fuzzy micro-time scales of phonemes as well as in the fuzzy macro-time scales of syllables and words. In their innateness, attractors defy a blank-slate orientation. And in their formulation as abstract agents of relative timing, attractors also defy other innate proposals based on inborn grammars, motor gestures, and the like.

This chapter suggests how attractors may define prosodic categories of phonemes, syllables, and words, where the categories themselves embed a prototype, instantiated by some set of attractors, which is surrounded by related categorical tokens. Reigning attractor sets are implicated by ensembles of category tokens that populate hypothesized entrainment regions. Within the category boundaries of an entrainment region, each token "points to" common attractor sets. Attractor "pull" figures into adaptive entrainments (exogenous and endogenous). Attractors govern the operations of basic entrainment mechanisms; namely, exogenous pitch (frequency) tracking, endogenous oscillator clusters and innate attractor profiles. Moreover, as agents of relative timing, we find attractors at all time scales, from phonemes to word distributions.

Learning also enters this picture. Albeit eschewing blank-slate assumptions, learning builds on inherent synchronies that govern attending. Thus, DAT falls into the category of interactionist theories of skill acquisition. That is, innate attending predispositions pave the way for strengthening of connections (i.e., bindings) among active oscillations brought into play during entrainment episodes. Of course, exposure frequency remains a critical force in explaining the mastery of speech skills in infants and adults. It refines and strengthens bindings among active oscillations. Nevertheless, learning is triggered—and guided—by the pulls of synchronicity.

Finally, to conclude, let us return to the fundamental ideas underling constructs developed in this penultimate chapter. The universality of activities involved in attending (hence perceiving) and learning weaves throughout this chapter. Both attending and learning are seen as activities dependent on synchrony. Attending rides on various modes of synchrony between driving and driven rhythms, and learning follows suit because binding happens during adaptive entrainments when asymptotic synchrony elicits reinforcements. Universality is conveyed in principles of resonance and entrainment, both of which apply in some fashion to animate creatures of all ages, including humans. These principles ensure that attractor relationships serve as innate guardians of synchrony. This innate factor does not reflect specific grammar rules nor does it address special motor gestures or commands. Instead, attractors capture something much more basic: the power of synchrony.

NOTES

1. Noam Chomsky, *Syntactic Structures* (The Hague, Mouton and Co., 1965); *Aspects of the Theory of Syntax* (Cambridge, MA: MIT Press, 1957).

2. Noam Chomsky, *Syntactic Structures* (The Hague: Mouton and Co., 1965); *Aspects of the Theory of Syntax* (Cambridge, MA: MIT Press, 1966); *Cartesian Linguistics: A Chapter in the History of Rationalist Thought* (1957).

3. Eric H. Lenneberg, Noam Chomsky, and Otto Marx, *Biological Foundations of Language*, vol. 68 (New York: Wiley, 1967), http://tocs.ulb.tu-darmstadt.de/123135893.pdf.

4. A. M. Liberman et al., "Perception of the Speech Code," *Psychological Review* 74, no. 6 (1967): 431–61, doi:10.1037/h0020279.

5. Alvin M. Liberman and Ignatius G. Mattingly, "The Motor Theory of Speech Perception Revised," *Cognition* 21, no. 1 (October 1985): 1–36, doi:10.1016/0010-0277(85)90021-6.

6. Carol A. Fowler, "An Event Approach to the Study of Speech Perception from a Direct-Realist Perspective," *Journal of Phonetics* 14, no. 1 (1986): 3–28.

7. Carol A. Fowler, "Invariants, Specifiers, Cues: An Investigation of Locus Equations as Information for Place of Articulation," *Perception & Psychophysics* 55, no. 6 (November 1994): 597–610, doi:10.3758/BF03211675.

8. Carol A. Fowler and Dawn J. Dekle, "Listening with Eye and Hand: Cross-Modal Contributions to Speech Perception," *Journal of Experimental Psychology: Human Perception and Performance* 17, no. 3 (1991): 816–28, doi:10.1037/0096-1523.17.3.816.

9. Carol A. Fowler, "The Reality of Phonological Forms: A Reply to Port," *Language Sciences* 32, no. 1 (January 2010): 56–9, doi:10.1016/j.langsci.2009.10.015.

10. Jerry A. Fodor, *The Modularity of Mind: An Essay on Faculty Psychology* (Cambridge, MA: MIT Press, 1983), https://books-google-com.proxy.library.ucsb.edu:9443/books?hl=en&lr=&id=e7nrSeibJZYC&oi=fnd&pg=PP9&dq=Modularity+of+the+mind.+&ots=ooWNZyRA9T&sig=NC4iQXTrNgRG-4wAyKIlFZYX5QU.

11. Randy L. Diehl, Andrew J. Lotto, and Lori L. Holt, "Speech Perception," *Annual Review of Psychology* 55, no. 1 (2004): 149–79, doi:10.1146/annurev.psych.55.090902.142028.

12. Patricia K. Kuhl and Denise M. Padden, "Enhanced Discriminability at the Phonetic Boundaries for the Voicing Feature in Macaques," *Perception & Psychophysics* 32, no. 6 (November 1982): 542–50, doi:10.3758/BF03204208.

13. Patricia K. Kuhl, "Discrimination of Speech by Nonhuman Animals: Basic Auditory Sensitivities Conducive to the Perception of Speech-Sound Categories," *Journal of the Acoustical Society of America* 70, no. 2 (1981): 340, doi:10.1121/1.386782.

14. Charles K. Burdick, "Speech Perception by the Chinchilla: Discrimination of Sustained ||a|| and ||i||," *Journal of the Acoustical Society of America* 58, no. 2 (1975): 415, doi:10.1121/1.380686.

15. Mitchell Steinschneider, Kirill V. Nourski, and Yonatan I. Fishman, "Representation of Speech in Human Auditory Cortex: Is It Special?," *Hearing Research* 305 (November 2013): 57–73, https://doi.org/10.1016/j.heares.2013.05.013.

16. David B. Pisoni, "Identification and Discrimination of the Relative Onset Time of Two Component Tones: Implications for Voicing Perception in Stops," *Journal of the Acoustical Society of America* 61, no. 5 (1977): 1352, doi:10.1121/1.381409.

17. James D. Miller, "Discrimination and Labeling of Noise–buzz Sequences with Varying Noise-Lead Times: An Example of Categorical Perception," *Journal of the Acoustical Society of America* 60, no. 2 (1976): 410, doi:10.1121/1.381097.

18. Randy L. Diehl, "An Auditory Basis for the Stimulus-Length Effect in the Perception of Stops and Glides," *Journal of the Acoustical Society of America* 85, no. 5 (1989): 2154, doi:10.1121/1.397864.

19. David B. Pisoni, "Long-Term Memory in Speech Perception: Some New Findings on Talker Variability, Speaking Rate and Perceptual Learning," *Speech Communication* 13, no. 1–2 (October 1993): 109–25, doi:10.1016/0167-6393(93)90063-Q.

20. Gary R. Kidd, "Articulatory-Rate Context Effects in Phoneme Identification.," *Journal of Experimental Psychology: Human Perception and Performance* 15, no. 4 (1989): 736–48, doi:10.1037/0096-1523.15.4.736.

21. Diehl, Lotto, and Holt, "Speech Perception," p. 159.

22. I am indebted to these authors for their presentation of this topic.

23. Marc D. Hauser, Noam Chomsky, and W. Tecumseh Fitch, "The Faculty of Language: What Is It, Who Has It, and How Did It Evolve?" *Science* 298, no. 5598 (November 22, 2002): 1569–79, doi:10.1126/science.298.5598.1569.

24. W. Tecumseh Fitch, Marc D. Hauser, and Noam Chomsky, "The Evolution of the Language Faculty: Clarifications and Implications," *Cognition* 97, no. 2 (September 2005): 179–210, doi:10.1016/j.cognition.2005.02.005.

25. Ray Jackendoff and Steven Pinker, "The Nature of the Language Faculty and Its Implications for Evolution of Language (Reply to Fitch, Hauser, and Chomsky)," *Cognition* 97, no. 2 (September 2005): 211–25, doi:10.1016/j.cognition.2005.04.006.

26. Steven Pinker and Ray Jackendoff, "The Faculty of Language: What's Special about It?" *Cognition* 95, no. 2 (March 2005): 201–36, doi:10.1016/j.cognition.2004.08.004.

27. Blase Gambino and Jerome L. Myers, "Role of Event Runs in Probability Learning," *Psychological Review* 74, no. 5 (1967): 410.

28. Mari R. Jones and James R. Erickson, "Patterns of Event Runs in Probability Learning," *Psychonomic Science* 13, no. 6 (June 1968): 317–8, doi:10.3758/BF03342604.

29. Mari R. Jones, "From Probability Learning to Sequential Processing: A Critical Review," *Psychological Bulletin* 76, no. 3 (1971): 153–85, doi:10.1037/h0031338.

30. Pierre Perruchet and Barbara Tillmann, "Exploiting Multiple Sources of Information in Learning an Artificial Language: Human Data and Modeling," *Cognitive Science* 34, no. 2 (March 2010): 255–85, doi:10.1111/j.1551-6709.2009.01074.x.

31. Tiffany C. Bloomfield, Timothy Q. Gentner, and Daniel Margoliash, "What Birds Have to Say About Language," *Nature Neuroscience* 14, no. 8 (July 26, 2011): 947–8, doi:10.1038/nn.2884.

32. Timothy Q. Gentner et al., "Recursive Syntactic Pattern Learning by Songbirds," *Nature* 440, no. 7088 (April 27, 2006): 1204–7, doi:10.1038/nature04675.

33. P. K. Kuhl, "A New View of Language Acquisition," *Proceedings of the National Academy of Sciences* 97, no. 22 (October 24, 2000): 11850–7, doi:10.1073/pnas.97.22.11850.

34. Dennis Norris, James M. McQueen, and Anne Cutler, "Perceptual Learning in Speech," *Cognitive Psychology* 47, no. 2 (September 2003): 204–38, doi:10.1016/S0010-0285(03)00006-9.

35. James M. McQueen, Anne Cutler, and Dennis Norris, "Flow of Information in the Spoken Word Recognition System," *Speech Communication* 41, no. 1 (August 2003): 257–70, doi:10.1016/S0167-6393(02)00108-5.

36. Arthur G. Samuel and Tanya Kraljic, "Perceptual Learning for Speech," *Attention, Perception, & Psychophysics* 71, no. 6 (August 2009): 1207–18, doi:10.3758/APP.71.6.1207.

37. Robert L. Goldstone, "Perceptual Learning," *Annual Review of Psychology* 49, no. 1 (February 1998): 585–612, doi:10.1146/annurev.psych.49.1.585.

38. James J. Gibson and Eleanor J. Gibson, "Perceptual Learning: Differentiation or Enrichment?" *Psychological Review* 62, no. 1 (1955): 32–41, doi:10.1037/h0048826.

39. Patricia K. Kuhl, "Early Language Acquisition: Cracking the Speech Code," *Nature Reviews Neuroscience* 5, no. 11 (November 2004): 831–43, https://doi.org/10.1038/nrn1533.

40. Michael I. Posner and Steven W. Keele, "ON THE GENESIS OF ABSTRACT IDEAS.," *Journal of*

Experimental Psychology 77, no. 3, Pt.1 (1968): 353–63, https://doi.org/10.1037/h0025953.

41. Bert Schouten, Ellen Gerrits, and Arjan van Hessen, "The End of Categorical Perception as We Know It," *Speech Communication* 41, no. 1 (August 2003): 71–80, https://doi.org/10.1016/S0167-6393(02)00094-8.

42. Elaina M. Frieda et al., "Adults' Perception of Native and Nonnative Vowels: Implications for the Perceptual Magnet Effect," *Perception & Psychophysics* 61, no. 3 (April 1999): 561–77, https://doi.org/10.3758/BF03211973.

43. Andrew J. Lotto, Keith R. Kluender, and Lori L. Holt, "Depolarizing the Perceptual Magnet Effect," *The Journal of the Acoustical Society of America* 103, no. 6 (June 1998): 3648–55, https://doi.org/10.1121/1.423087.

44. P. K Kuhl et al., "Phonetic Learning as a Pathway to Language: New Data and Native Language Magnet Theory Expanded (NLM-E)," *Philosophical Transactions of the Royal Society B: Biological Sciences* 363, no. 1493 (March 12, 2008): 979–1000, https://doi.org/10.1098/rstb.2007.2154.

45. Paul Iverson and Patricia K. Kuhl, "Perceptual Magnet and Phoneme Boundary Effects in Speech Perception: Do They Arise from a Common Mechanism?," *Perception & Psychophysics* 62, no. 4 (January 2000): 874–86, https://doi.org/10.3758/BF03206929.

46. Patricia K. Kuhl, "Human Adults and Human Infants Show a 'Perceptual Magnet Effect' for the Prototypes of Speech Categories, Monkeys Do Not," *Perception & Psychophysics* 50, no. 2 (March 1991): 93–107, https://doi.org/10.3758/BF03212211.

47. K. Kluender, R. Diehl, and P. Killeen, "Japanese Quail Can Learn Phonetic Categories," *Science* 237, no. 4819 (September 4, 1987): 1195–97, https://doi.org/10.1126/science.3629235.

48. B. S. Kisilevsky et al., "Fetal Sensitivity to Properties of Maternal Speech and Language," *Infant Behavior and Development* 32, no. 1 (January 2009): 59–71, https://doi.org/10.1016/j.infbeh.2008.10.002.

49. Christine Moon, Hugo Lagercrantz, and Patricia K Kuhl, "Language Experienced *in Utero* Affects Vowel Perception after Birth: A Two-Country Study," *Acta Paediatrica* 102, no. 2 (February 2013): 156–60, https://doi.org/10.1111/apa.12098.

50. Diane Kewley-Port and Charles S. Watson, "Formant-Frequency Discrimination for Isolated English Vowels," *Journal of the Acoustical Society of America* 95, no. 1 (January 1, 1994): 485–96, doi:10.1121/1.410024.

51. Frequencies typically average over various fluctuations of formant waveforms, which are highly variable over time.

52. Di-Wei Huang, Rodolphe J. Gentili, and James A. Reggia, "Self-Organizing Maps Based on Limit Cycle Attractors," *Neural Networks* 63 (March 2015): 208–22, doi:10.1016/j.neunet.2014.12.003.

53. Isao Tokuda, Takaya Miyano, and Kazuyuki Aihara, "Surrogate Analysis for Detecting Nonlinear Dynamics in Normal Vowels," *Journal of the Acoustical Society of America* 110, no. 6 (2001): 3207, doi:10.1121/1.1413749.

54. E. Fireda, "Pitch, Harmonicity, and Concurrent Sound Segregation: Psychoacoustical and Neurophysiological Findings," *Hearing Research* 266, no. 1–2 (July 2010): 36–51, doi:10.1016/j.heares.2009.09.012.

55. Micheyl and Oxenham report that harmonic mistunings of 3–8% are detectable. Christophe Micheyl and Andrew J. Oxenham, "Pitch, Harmonicity and Concurrent Sound Segregation: Psychoacoustical and Neurophysiological Findings," *Hearing Research*, Special Issue: Annual Reviews 2010, 266, no. 1 (July 1, 2010): 36–51, https://doi.org/10.1016/j.heares.2009.09.012.

56. Patricia K. Kuhl, "Early Language Acquisition: Cracking the Speech Code," *Nature Reviews Neuroscience* 5, no. 11 (November 2004): 831–43, doi:10.1038/nrn1533.

57. B. S. Kisilevsky et al., "Fetal Sensitivity to Properties of Maternal Speech and Language," *Infant Behavior and Development* 32, no. 1 (January 2009): 59–71, doi:10.1016/j.infbeh.2008.10.002.

58. Jacques Mehler et al., "Infant Recognition of Mother's Voice," *Perception* 7, no. 5 (1978): 491–97, https://doi.org/10.1068/p070491.

59. A. DeCasper and W. Fifer, "Of Human Bonding: Newborns Prefer Their Mothers' Voices," *Science* 208, no. 4448 (June 6, 1980): 1174–76, https://doi.org/10.1126/science.7375928.

60. Christine Moon, Hugo Lagercrantz, and Patricia K. Kuhl, "Language Experienced *in Utero* Affects Vowel Perception After Birth: A Two-Country Study," *Acta Paediatrica* 102, no. 2 (February 2013): 156–60, doi:10.1111/apa.12098.

61. It is possible that reactive pulses are spikes discussed by Giraud and Poeppel in, Anne-Lise Giraud and David Poepple, "Cortical Oscillations and Speech Processing: Emerging Computational Principles and Operations," *Nature Neuroscience* 15, no. 4 (April 2012): 511–17, doi:10.1038/nn.3063.

62. Giraud and Poepple, "Cortical Oscillations and Speech Processing,"

63. More precisely, bindings grow between rhythms outlined by reactive pulses and resonant oscillations carrying expectancy pulses.

64. Barbara S. Kisilevsky et al., "Effects of Experience on Fetal Voice Recognition," *Psychological Science* 14, no. 3 (May 1, 2003): 220–24, doi:10.1111/1467-9280.02435.

65. Jacques Mehler et al., "Infant Recognition of Mother's Voice," *Perception* 7, no. 5 (1978): 491–97, doi:10.1068/p070491.

66. A. DeCasper and W. Fifer, "Of Human Bonding: Newborns Prefer Their Mothers' Voices," *Science* 208, no. 4448 (June 6, 1980): 1174–76, doi:10.1126/science.7375928.

67. Birgit Mampe et al., "Newborns' Cry Melody Is Shaped by Their Native Language," *Current Biology* 19, no. 23 (December 15, 2009): 1994–97, doi:10.1016/j.cub.2009.09.064.

68. Judit Gervain, Iris Berent, and Janet F. Werker, "Binding at Birth: The Newborn Brain Detects Identity Relations and Sequential Position in Speech," *Journal of Cognitive Neuroscience* 24, no. 3 (March 2012): 564–74, doi:10.1162/jocn_a_00157.

69. Judit Gervain et al., "The Neonate Brain Detects Speech Structure," *Proceedings of the National Academy of Sciences* 105, no. 37 (2008): 14222–27.

70. E. Partanen et al., "Learning-Induced Neural Plasticity of Speech Processing Before Birth," *Proceedings of the National Academy of Sciences* 110, no. 37 (September 10, 2013): 15145–50, doi:10.1073/pnas.1302159110.

71. Michael I. Posner and Steven W. Keele, "On the Genesis of Abstract Ideas," *Journal of Experimental Psychology* 77, no. 3, Pt.1 (1968): 353–63, doi:10.1037/h0025953.

72. Bert Schouten, Ellen Gerrits, and Arjan van Hessen, "The End of Categorical Perception as We Know It," *Speech Communication* 41, no. 1 (August 2003): 71–80, doi:10.1016/S0167-6393(02)00094-8.

73. Elaina M. Frieda et al., "Adults' Perception of Native and Nonnative Vowels: Implications for the Perceptual Magnet Effect," *Perception & Psychophysics* 61, no. 3 (April 1999): 561–77, doi:10.3758/BF03211973.

74. Andrew J. Lotto, Keith R. Kluender, and Lori L. Holt, "Depolarizing the Perceptual Magnet Effect," *Journal of the Acoustical Society of America* 103, no. 6 (June 1998): 3648–55, doi:10.1121/1.423087.

75. P. K. Kuhl et al., "Phonetic Learning as a Pathway to Language: New Data and Native Language Magnet Theory Expanded (NLM-E)," *Philosophical Transactions of the Royal Society B: Biological Sciences* 363, no. 1493 (March 12, 2008): 979–1000, doi:10.1098/rstb.2007.2154.

76. Paul Iverson and Patricia K. Kuhl, "Perceptual Magnet and Phoneme Boundary Effects in Speech Perception: Do They Arise from a Common Mechanism?" *Perception & Psychophysics* 62, no. 4 (January 2000): 874–86, doi:10.3758/BF03206929.

77. Patricia K. Kuhl, "Human Adults and Human Infants Show a 'Perceptual Magnet Effect' for the Prototypes of Speech Categories, Monkeys Do Not," *Perception & Psychophysics* 50, no. 2 (March 1991): 93–107, doi:10.3758/BF03212211.

78. K. Kluender, R. Diehl, and P. Killeen, "Japanese Quail Can Learn Phonetic Categories," *Science* 237, no. 4819 (September 4, 1987): 1195–7, doi:10.1126/science.3629235.

79. Technically, the prototype defends on several prominent n:m attractors involving other formants.

80. K. Nishi and D. Kewley-Port, "Nonnative Speech Perception Training Using Vowel Subsets: Effects of Vowels in Sets and Order of Training," *Journal of Speech, Language, and Hearing Research* 51, no. 6 (December 1, 2008): 1480–93, doi:10.1044/1092-4388(2008/07-0109).

81. Peter Ladefoged, *Three Areas of Experimental Phonetics: Stress and Respiration Activity, the Nature of Vowel Quality, Units in the Perception and Production of Speech* (New York: Oxford University Press, 1967).

82. Lynne C. Nygaard, Mitchell S. Sommers, and David B. Pisoni, "Speech Perception as a Talker-Contingent Process," *Psychological Science* 5, no. 1 (January 1994): 42–46, doi:10.1111/j.1467-9280.1994.tb00612.x.

83. Peter Ladefoged, "Information Conveyed by Vowels," *Journal of the Acoustical Society of America* 29, no. 1 (1957): 98, doi:10.1121/1.1908694.

84. Sarah C. Creel and Micah R. Bregman, "How Talker Identity Relates to Language Processing: Talkers and Language Processing," *Language and Linguistics Compass* 5, no. 5 (May 2011): 190–204, doi:10.1111/j.1749-818X.2011.00276.x.

85. Christophe Micheyl and Andrew J. Oxenham, "Pitch, Harmonicity and Concurrent Sound Segregation: Psychoacoustical and Neurophysiological Findings," *Hearing Research* 266, no. 1 (July 1, 2010): 36–51, doi:10.1016/j.heares.2009.09.012.

86. Lynn Maxfield, Anil Palaparthi, and Ingo Titze, "New Evidence that Nonlinear Source-Filter Coupling Affects Harmonic Intensity and Fo Stability During Instances of Harmonics Crossing Formants," *Journal of Voice* 31, no. 2 (March 2017): 149–56, doi:10.1016/j.jvoice.2016.04.010.

87. John F. Culling and C. J. Darwin, "Perceptual Separation of Simultaneous Vowels: Within and Across-Formant Grouping by F_0," *Journal of the Acoustical Society of America* 93, no. 6 (June 1993): 3454–67, doi:10.1121/1.405675.

88. C. J. Darwin, "Perceptual Grouping of Speech Components Differing in Fundamental Frequency and Onset-Time," *Quarterly Journal of Experimental Psychology Section A* 33, no. 2 (May 1981): 185–207, doi:10.1080/14640748108400785.

89. Robert J. Summers, Peter J. Bailey, and Brian Roberts, "Effects of Differences in Fundamental Frequency on Across-Formant Grouping in Speech Perception," *Journal of the Acoustical Society of America* 128, no. 6 (December 2010): 3667–77, doi:10.1121/1.3505119.

90. Summers, Bailey, and Roberts, "Effects of Differences in Fundamental Frequency on Across-Formant Grouping in Speech Perception."

91. Dieter Maurer et al., "Formant Pattern Ambiguity of Vowel Sounds Revisited in Synthesis: Changing Perceptual Vowel Quality by Only Changing Fundamental Frequency," *Journal of the Acoustical Society of America* 141, no. 5 (May 1, 2017): 3469–70, doi:10.1121/1.4987214.

92. B. Zoefel and R. VanRullen, "Selective Perceptual Phase Entrainment to Speech Rhythm in

the Absence of Spectral Energy Fluctuations," *Journal of Neuroscience* 35, no. 5 (February 4, 2015): 1954–64, doi:10.1523/JNEUROSCI.3484-14.2015.

93. Fernando Lopes da Silva, "EEG and MEG: Relevance to Neuroscience," *Neuron* 80, no. 5 (December 2013): 1112–28, doi:10.1016/j.neuron.2013.10.017.

94. György Buzsáki, Nikos Logothetis, and Wolf Singer, "Scaling Brain Size, Keeping Timing: Evolutionary Preservation of Brain Rhythms," *Neuron* 80, no. 3 (October 2013): 751–64, doi:10.1016/j.neuron.2013.10.002.

95. Nima Mesgarani et al., "Phoneme Representation and Classification in Primary Auditory Cortex," *Journal of the Acoustical Society of America* 123, no. 2 (February 2008): 899–909, doi:10.1121/1.2816572.

96. N. Mesgarani et al., "Phonetic Feature Encoding in Human Superior Temporal Gyrus," *Science* 343, no. 6174 (February 28, 2014): 1006–10, doi:10.1126/science.1245994.

97. Yakov Kronrod, Emily Coppess, and Naomi H. Feldman, "A Unified Account of Categorical Effects in Phonetic Perception," *Psychonomic Bulletin & Review* 23, no. 6 (December 2016): 1681–712, doi:10.3758/s13423-016-1049-y.

98. LouAnn Gerken, Frances K. Balcomb, and Juliet L. Minton, "Infants Avoid 'Labouring in Vain' by Attending More to Learnable than Unlearnable Linguistic Patterns: Infants Attend More to Learnable Patterns," *Developmental Science* 14, no. 5 (September 2011): 972–9, doi:10.1111/j.1467-7687.2011.01046.x. (page 973).

99. Noam Chomsky, "A Review of B. F. Skinner's Verbal Behavior," *Language* (1959), 35, no. 1(1959), 26–58. http://cogprints.org/1148/.

100. Hauser, Chomsky, and Fitch, "The Faculty of Language: What is it, Who has it, and How did it evolve?" Science, 22 Nov. 22, 298, no. 5598, 1569–79.

101. Adrián E. Granada and Hanspeter Herzel, "How to Achieve Fast Entrainment? The Timescale to Synchronization," *PLoS ONE* 4, no. 9 (September 23, 2009): e7057, doi:10.1371/journal.pone.0007057.

102. Ladefoged, "Information Conveyed by Vowels."

103. Alternatively, in a discrimination task, listeners rely on token information regarding category boundaries (i.e., entrainment region bifurcations).

104. Jingyuan Huang and Lori L. Holt, "General Perceptual Contributions to Lexical Tone Normalization," *Journal of the Acoustical Society of America* 125, no. 6 (June 1, 2009): 3983–94, doi:10.1121/1.3125342.

105. Erika J. C. Laing et al., "Tuned with a Tune: Talker Normalization via General Auditory Processes," *Frontiers in Psychology* 3 (2012): 1–9, doi:10.3389/fpsyg.2012.00203.

106. Jingyuan Huang and Lori L. Holt, "Listening for the Norm: Adaptive Coding in Speech Categorization," *Frontiers in Psychology* 3, no. 10 (2012): 1–6.

107. Variations of F0 in this capacity are a special case of tempo response curve modulations. For instance, perceptual contrasts caused by slight F0 changes contribute to grouping of successive phonemes (see Chapters 11 and 12).

108. Fluctuations of F0 at this time scale correspond to changes in a tempo response curve at a slower speech level.

109. Tokuda, Miyano, and Aihara, "Surrogate Analysis for Detecting Nonlinear Dynamics in Normal Vowels."

110. Shrikanth S. Narayanan and Abeer A. Alwan, "A Nonlinear Dynamical Systems Analysis of Fricative Consonants," *Journal of the Acoustical Society of America* 97, no. 4 (April 1, 1995): 2511–24, doi:10.1121/1.411971.

111. Tokuda, Miyano, and Aihara, "Surrogate Analysis for Detecting Nonlinear Dynamics in Normal Vowels."

112. See preceding chapter for grouping rules.

113. Recorded phoneme durations range from 12 to 60 ms, with vowels longer than consonants (see Table 12.1).

114. Elana M. Zion Golumbic et al., "Mechanisms Underlying Selective Neuronal Tracking of Attended Speech at a 'Cocktail Party,'" *Neuron* 77, no. 5 (March 2013): 980–91, doi:10.1016/j.neuron.2012.12.037.

115. Maria Chait et al., "Multi-Time Resolution Analysis of Speech: Evidence from Psychophysics," *Frontiers in Neuroscience* 9 (June 16, 2015), doi:10.3389/fnins.2015.00214.

116. Nai Ding et al., "Cortical Tracking of Hierarchical Linguistic Structures in Connected Speech," *Nature Neuroscience* 19, no. 1 (December 7, 2015): 158–64, doi:10.1038/nn.4186.

117. Jonathan E. Peelle and Matthew H. Davis, "Neural Oscillations Carry Speech Rhythm Through to Comprehension," *Frontiers in Psychology* 3 (2012), doi:10.3389/fpsyg.2012.00320.

118. David Poeppel, "The Neuroanatomic and Neurophysiological Infrastructure for Speech and Language," *Current Opinion in Neurobiology* 28 (October 2014): 142–9, doi:10.1016/j.conb.2014.07.005.

119. Catia M. Sameiro-Barbosa and Eveline Geiser, "Sensory Entrainment Mechanisms in Auditory Perception: Neural Synchronization Cortico-Striatal Activation," *Frontiers in Neuroscience* 10 (August 10, 2016), doi:10.3389/fnins.2016.00361.

120. Hong Zhou et al., "Interpretations of Frequency Domain Analyses of Neural Entrainment: Periodicity, Fundamental Frequency, and Harmonics," *Frontiers in Human Neuroscience* 10 (June 6, 2016), doi:10.3389/fnhum.2016.00274.

121. Giraud and Poeppel, "Cortical Oscillations and Speech Processing."

122. P. Lakatos, "An Oscillatory Hierarchy Controlling Neuronal Excitability and Stimulus Processing in the Auditory Cortex," *Journal of Neurophysiology* 94, no. 3 (September 1, 2005): 1904–11, doi:10.1152/jn.00263.2005.

123. This means that both rely on transient mode-locking, which leads to attractor profiles.

124. S. Dikker et al., "On the Same Wavelength: Predictable Language Enhances Speaker-Listener Brain-to-Brain Synchrony in Posterior Superior Temporal Gyrus," *Journal of Neuroscience* 34, no. 18 (April 30, 2014): 6267–72, doi:10.1523/JNEUROSCI.3796-13.2014.

125. Lauren J. Silbert et al., "Coupled Neural Systems Underlie the Production and Comprehension of Naturalistic Narrative Speech," *Proceedings of the National Academy of Sciences* 111, no. 43 (October 28, 2014): E4687–96, doi:10.1073/pnas.1323812111.

126. Debates over syllable onsets involve P-center locations (red vertical lines).

127. Grouping issues regarding word time lengths are discussed in Chapter 12.

128. Judit Gervain and Jacques Mehler, "Speech Perception and Language Acquisition in the First Year of Life," *Annual Review of Psychology* 61, no. 1 (January 2010): 191–218, doi:10.1146/annurev.psych.093008.100408.

129. Noam Chomsky, "On Certain Formal Properties of Grammars," *Information and Control* 2, no. 2 (June 1959): 137–67, doi:10.1016/S0019-9958(59)90362-6.

130. Fitch, Hauser, and Chomsky, "The Evolution of the Language Faculty."

131. Alessandra Sansavini, Josiane Bertoncini, and Giuliana Giovanelli, "Newborns Discriminate the Rhythm of Multisyllabic Stressed Words," *Developmental Psychology* 33, no. 1 (1997): 3–11, doi:10.1037/0012-1649.33.1.3.

132. Luca L. Bonatti et al., "Linguistic Constraints on Statistical Computations: The Role of Consonants and Vowels in Continuous Speech Processing," *Psychological Science* 16, no. 6 (June 1, 2005): 451–9, doi:10.1111/j.0956-7976.2005.01556.x.

133. Franck Ramus, Marina Nespor, and Jacques Mehler, "Correlates of Linguistic Rhythm in the Speech Signal," *Cognition* 73, no. 3 (December 1999): 265–92, doi:10.1016/S0010-0277(99)00058-X.

134. Bonatti et al., "Linguistic Constraints on Statistical Computations."

135. Ansgar D. Endress and Jacques Mehler, "Primitive Computations in Speech Processing," *Quarterly Journal of Experimental Psychology* 62, no. 11 (November 2009): 2187–209, doi:10.1080/17470210902783646.

136. Jenny R. Saffran, "Statistical Language Learning: Mechanisms and Constraints," *Current Directions in Psychological Science* 12, no. 4 (August 2003): 110–4, doi:10.1111/1467-8721.01243.

137. Alexa R. Romberg and Jenny R. Saffran, "Statistical Learning and Language Acquisition," *Wiley Interdisciplinary Reviews: Cognitive Science* 1, no. 6 (November 1, 2010): 906–14, doi:10.1002/wcs.78.

138. Casey Lew-Williams and Jenny R. Saffran, "All Words Are Not Created Equal: Expectations About Word Length Guide Infant Statistical Learning," *Cognition* 122, no. 2 (February 2012): 241–6, doi:10.1016/j.cognition.2011.10.007.

139. John R. Hayes and Herbert H. Clark, "Experiments in the Segmentation of an Artificial Speech Analog," *Cognition and the Development of Language*, 1970, 221–34.

140. Jenny R. Saffran, Elissa L. Newport, and Richard N. Aslin, "Word Segmentation: The Role of Distributional Cues," *Journal of Memory and Language* 35, no. 4 (August 1996): 606–21, doi:10.1006/jmla.1996.0032.

141. Richard N. Aslin, Jenny R. Saffran, and Elissa L. Newport, "Computation of Conditional Probability Statistics by 8-Month-Old Infants," *Psychological Science* 9, no. 4 (July 1, 1998): 321–4, doi:10.1111/1467-9280.00063.

142. Sarah C. Creel, Michael K. Tanenhaus, and Richard N. Aslin, "Consequences of Lexical Stress on Learning an Artificial Lexicon," *Journal of Experimental Psychology: Learning, Memory, and Cognition* 32, no. 1 (2006): 15–32, doi:10.1037/0278-7393.32.1.15.

143. Barbara Tillmann and Stephen McAdams, "Implicit Learning of Musical Timbre Sequences: Statistical Regularities Confronted With Acoustical (Dis)Similarities," *Journal of Experimental Psychology: Learning, Memory, and Cognition* 30, no. 5 (2004): 1131–42, doi:10.1037/0278-7393.30.5.1131.

144. Dilshat Abla, Kentaro Katahira, and Kazuo Okanoya, "On-Line Assessment of Statistical Learning by Event-Related Potentials," *Journal of Cognitive Neuroscience* 20, no. 6 (June 2008): 952–64, doi:10.1162/jocn.2008.20058.

145. Julia L. Evans, Jenny R. Saffran, and Kathryn Robe-Torres, "Statistical Learning in Children With Specific Language Impairment," *Journal of Speech Language and Hearing Research* 52, no. 2 (April 1, 2009): 321, doi:10.1044/1092-4388(2009/07-0189).

146. Bruna Pelucchi, Jessica F. Hay, and Jenny R. Saffran, "Statistical Learning in a Natural Language by 8-Month-Old Infants: Statistical Learning in a Natural Language," *Child Development* 80, no. 3 (May 2009): 674–85, doi:10.1111/j.1467-8624.2009.01290.x.

147. Bruna Pelucchi, Jessica F. Hay, and Jenny R. Saffran, "Learning in Reverse: Eight-Month-Old Infants Track Backward Transitional Probabilities," *Cognition* 113, no. 2 (November 2009): 244–47, doi:10.1016/j.cognition.2009.07.011.

148. Axel Cleeremans, *Mechanisms of Implicit Learning: Connectionist Models of Sequence Processing* (Cambridge, MA: MIT Press, 1993), https://books-google-com.proxy.library.ucsb.edu:9443/books?hl=en&lr=&id=aKPwAIIgdxgC&oi=fnd&pg=PR9&dq=Cleeremans,+1993&ots=jf1flMRnmH&sig=tRViO2SPLrFLX4-fpGSjj0yskLg.

149. Arthur S. Reber, "Implicit Learning of Synthetic Language," *Journal of Experimental Psychology: Human Learning & Memory* 2 (1976): 88–94.

150. Arthur S. Reber, "Implicit Learning and Tacit Knowledge," *Journal of Experimental*

Psychology: General 118, no. 3 (1989): 219–35, doi:10.1037/0096-3445.118.3.219.

151. Pierre Perruchet and Sebastien Pacton, "Implicit Learning and Statistical Learning: One Phenomenon, Two Approaches," *Trends in Cognitive Sciences* 10, no. 5 (May 2006): 233–38, doi:10.1016/j.tics.2006.03.006.

152. Pierre Perruchet, "Implicit Learning," *Cognitive Psychology of Memory* 2 (2008): 597–621.

153. Pierre Perruchet and Annie Vinter, "PARSER: A Model for Word Segmentation," *Journal of Memory and Language* 39, no. 2 (August 1998): 246–63, doi:10.1006/jmla.1998.2576.

154. Perruchet and Tillmann, "Exploiting Multiple Sources of Information in Learning an Artificial Language."

155. Ding et al., "Cortical Tracking of Hierarchical Linguistic Structures in Connected Speech."

156. Marcela Peña et al., "Signal-Driven Computations in Speech Processing," *Science* 298, no. 5593 (October 18, 2002): 604–7, doi:10.1126/science.1072901.

157. Bonatti et al., "Linguistic Constraints on Statistical Computations."

158. Juan M. Toro et al., "Finding Words and Rules in a Speech Stream: Functional Differences Between Vowels and Consonants," *Psychological Science* 19, no. 2 (February 2008): 137–44, doi:10.1111/j.1467-9280.2008.02059.x.

159. Elissa L. Newport and Richard N. Aslin, "Learning at a Distance I. Statistical Learning of Non-Adjacent Dependencies," *Cognitive Psychology* 48, no. 2 (March 2004): 127–62, doi:10.1016/S0010-0285(03)00128-2.

160. Sarah C. Creel, Elissa L. Newport, and Richard N. Aslin, "Distant Melodies: Statistical Learning of Nonadjacent Dependencies in Tone Sequences," *Journal of Experimental Psychology: Learning, Memory, and Cognition* 30, no. 5 (2004): 1119–30, doi:10.1037/0278-7393.30.5.1119.

161. Elizabeth K. Johnson and Michael D. Tyler, "Testing the Limits of Statistical Learning for Word Segmentation," *Developmental Science* 13, no. 2 (March 2010): 339–45, doi:10.1111/j.1467-7687.2009.00886.x.

162. Casey Lew-Williams, Bruna Pelucchi, and Jenny R. Saffran, "Isolated Words Enhance Statistical Language Learning in Infancy: Isolated Words," *Developmental Science* 14, no. 6 (November 2011): 1323–9, doi:10.1111/j.1467-7687.2011.01079.x.

163. L. Hoch, M. D. Tyler, and B. Tillmann, "Regularity of Unit Length Boosts Statistical Learning in Verbal and Nonverbal Artificial Languages," *Psychonomic Bulletin & Review* 20, no. 1 (February 2013): 142–7, doi:10.3758/s13423-012-0309-8.

164. Tatiana Selchenkova et al., "Metrical Presentation Boosts Implicit Learning of Artificial Grammar," *PLoS ONE* 9, no. 11 (November 5, 2014): e112233, doi:10.1371/journal.pone.0112233.

165. Tatiana Selchenkova, Mari Riess Jones, and Barbara Tillmann, "The Influence of Temporal Regularities on the Implicit Learning of Pitch Structures," *Quarterly Journal of Experimental Psychology* 67, no. 12 (December 2, 2014): 2360–80, doi:10.1080/17470218.2014.929155.

166. J. Terry et al., "Implicit Learning of Between-Group Intervals in Auditory Temporal Structures," *Attention, Perception, & Psychophysics* 78, no. 6 (August 2016): 1728–43, https://doi.org/10.3758/s13414-016-1148-x.

167. Creel, Tanenhaus, and Aslin, "Consequences of Lexical Stress on Learning an Artificial Lexicon."

168. Sarah C. Creel and Delphine Dahan, "The Effect of the Temporal Structure of Spoken Words on Paired-Associate Learning," *Journal of Experimental Psychology: Learning, Memory, and Cognition* 36, no. 1 (2010): 110–22, doi:10.1037/a0017527.

169. Benjamin G. Schultz et al., "The Implicit Learning of Metrical and Nonmetrical Temporal Patterns," *Quarterly Journal of Experimental Psychology* 66, no. 2 (February 2013): 360–80, doi:10.1080/17470218.2012.712146.

170. Nia Cason and Daniele Schön, "Rhythmic Priming Enhances the Phonological Processing of Speech," *Neuropsychologia* 50, no. 11 (September 2012): 2652–8, doi:10.1016/j.neuropsychologia.2012.07.018.

171. Nia Cason, Corine Astésano, and Daniele Schön, "Bridging Music and Speech Rhythm: Rhythmic Priming and Audio–Motor Training Affect Speech Perception," *Acta Psychologica* 155 (February 2015): 43–50, doi:10.1016/j.actpsy.2014.12.002.

172. Ahren B. Fitzroy and Lisa D. Sanders, "Musical Meter Modulates the Allocation of Attention across Time," *Journal of Cognitive Neuroscience* 27, no. 12 (December 2015): 2339–51, doi:10.1162/jocn_a_00862.

173. Daniele Schön and Barbara Tillmann, "Short- and Long-Term Rhythmic Interventions: Perspectives for Language Rehabilitation," *Annals of the New York Academy of Sciences* 1337, no. 1 (2015): 32–9.

174. Sonja A. Kotz and Maren Schmidt-Kassow, "Basal Ganglia Contribution to Rule Expectancy and Temporal Predictability in Speech," *Cortex* 68 (July 2015): 48–60, doi:10.1016/j.cortex.2015.02.021.

175. M. M. Baese-Berk et al., "Long-Term Temporal Tracking of Speech Rate Affects Spoken-Word Recognition," *Psychological Science* 25, no. 8 (August 1, 2014): 1546–53, doi:10.1177/0956797614533705.

15

Concluding Speculations

This chapter departs from preceding chapters because it entertains several implications of the dynamic attending perspective that go beyond ideas proposed in Parts I and II. Preceding chapters applied certain theoretical concepts to specific psychological phenomena with the aim of illustrating the explanatory potential of a dynamic approach to attending. In those chapters, my intentions were confined to presenting a few testable proposals that might illuminate a previously untold story about human listeners' timed tendencies to orient to and track sound events packaged within psychological laboratories.

Core ideas in this book have been uniformly grounded in synchronizations among driving rhythms of events and the driven rhythms of an attender with the basic theoretical unit cast as a driving–driven dyad. Driving rhythms were interpreted as productions of a human speaker/musician, and correlated driven rhythms were taken as internalized oscillations in the tunable brain of a human listener. Importantly, the overarching governing principles of resonance and entrainment are held as universals, thus justifying the development of a domain-general theory of dynamic attending to speech and well as music.

CHAPTER GOALS

In this closing chapter, this universality is shown to prompt other important implications. One goal then explores implications that that resonance and entrainment govern communications within all species, including humans, who flourish in natural environments where their community habitats are filled with a variety of interesting, naturally produced driving rhythms by conspecifics and other animals; hence, such events can involve chirps, hoots, trumpets, and other carriers of delightful time markers. With the aim of justifying universality, a sampling of such natural environments is discussed in the first portion of this chapter.

A related goal concerns considering another implication that can be drawn from the universality of these principles which is more alarming.

This envisions changes to or disruptions in natural communicative habitats that arise from the introduction of artifactual driving rhythms. Largely due to human advancement, evolving habitats for humans (and other species) are endangered by changes to our communicative environments. The second half of this chapter discusses implications of various artifactual environments on communications. These two topics form the major sections of this last chapter.

NATURAL ENVIRONMENTS OF NONHUMAN COMMUNICATIONS

In human communications, the major factors defining the driving rhythms are produced by other humans. This is also true for communicative exchanges among conspecifics in nonhuman species. Moreover, the driving rhythms created in communications of particular species are typically distinguished by a special range of rates as well as by certain species-specific timing relations (e.g., attractors). In this section, I speculate that the theoretical concepts based on resonance and entrainment applied in preceding chapters to explain dyadic relationships in humans also apply to other species. The driving rhythms of conspecifics and related species (e.g., predators versus prey) form a functional temporal niche for a given species.

This section offers a few examples of communicative dyads in animal species that are pertinent to this speculation. When considered together, crickets, birds, elephants, whales, and other species all illustrate species that flourish within respectively distinct species-specific temporal niches. All live in dynamic acoustic environments that are, to a large extent, shaped by the sounds of other natural inhabitants of their own locality. Although the specificities of these niches vary, there is an overriding commonality across species in that, regardless of species, temporal niches outline constraints on driving rhythms and rates and their relative time properties. These are properties at the core of entrainment.

To thoroughly address questions regarding universality of entrainment requires a rather exhaustive litany of members of all species. Instead, this section offers a few selective pieces of evidence consistent with dynamic attending principles by describing synchronicities in a sampling of nonhuman species. One aim is to deflect claims that only privileged species (e.g., humans) benefit from entrainment. Natural constraints on sound-making of various species will affect time markers, motor productions, and the neural capacities of "speakers," and, in turn, these impact "listeners" in any niche. Although the particular vehicles of entrainment may vary with species, entrainment as such does not.

Dyads: A Refresher

To probe entrainment in other species, it is useful to review the distinctions of dyads in entrainment theory. As already described, dyads assume two general forms. One form concerns attending oriented outward to external events; this involves *exogenous dyads* in which the driving rhythm is an external periodicity and the driven rhythm is an internal one. The other dyadic form is found in *endogenous entrainments*; in this, both driving and driven rhythms are internal periodicities. Experimental pursuit of endogenous entrainments in most species (including humans) is more challenging, requiring converging neuroscience measures of the stability of independent and correlated activities of neural oscillations. Consequently, the following discussions dwell mainly on evidence from exogenous entrainment as studies of endogenous entrainment are sparse.

In examining exogenous entrainment abilities across species, it is critical to identify the time markers of relevant driving rhythms in an animal's produced communications (i.e., its "songs"). Sometimes, these time markers are general and familiar, as with intensity and/or frequency changes, but, in other cases, time markers are actually species-specific. Nevertheless, one aim is to document species-specific rates of prominent driving rhythms in animal songs. Another aim is to probe species-specific time structures of animal songs (e.g., species attractors). One obvious possibility is that species differ in the nature of their defining attractors, with some communicating with more complex, even chaotic attractors while others communicate with simpler, even harmonic attractors. These ideas dovetail with the provocative writings of Tecumseth Fitch and colleagues on analogies among animal vocalizations.[1,2]

In exogenous entrainment, dyads are driving–driven pairs in which only the driven rhythm is an—often unobservable—internal oscillation. The only evidence of the driven rhythm emerges in a manifest (adaptive) form as a measureable overt tracking response, usually a motor response such as tapping or synchronized noise-making. For instance, in studies of birdsong, a dyad consists of a passive listening bird presented with a song (real or synthesized) produced by a singing bird. Thus, if the listener is a female bird and the singer a male, then attending of the former is confirmed by her subsequent mating choice, clearly an indirect index of possible exogenous entrainment. At the other extreme are paradigms and/or species that permit rather direct observations of driven rhythms during entraining episodes. For example, in various species, duets of two individuals reveal an observable synchrony of motor responses in both animals which emerges in simultaneously vocalized sounds and/or engagement of alternating (turn-taking) vocalizations.

Songs of Crickets

Let's begin with the humble cricket. Field crickets live in relatively fast-paced acoustic communities inhabited by companion crickets and other insects. In cricket communities, individual crickets are basically drummers. They drum out apparently unlearned species-specific time patterns with specific rates based on timed energy pulses created by wing motions. Produced pulses are brief, complex sounds (i.e., tones) comprising high-frequency components (e.g., 4 kHz–8 kHz); these are grouped tones defined as syllables. Together, the component frequencies plus a dominant frequency in cricket songs create the voice of an individual's cricket. Just as a human's vocal F0 pitch, plus timbre, differentiate one human speaker from another, crickets, too, have their individual identities. This is evident, for instance, in the selectivity of female crickets that is based on responding to a particular male's pulsed rate.

Furthermore, it is well known that crickets, along with katydids, frogs, and tropical birds, duet.[3] Converging evidence for this synchrony-guided behavior is found in the most famous duetting cricket species, the snowy tree cricket (*Oecanthus fultoni*). These cricket dyads systematically adjust inter-syllable time periods to achieve a precise phase synchrony of zero.[4,5] Although duetting (and chorusing) reflects synchronizations of overt motor gestures, other research confirms that precise neural synchronization occurs in the central neurons of crickets who listened to synthesized sounds of another cricket.[6]

In sum, both the rate and relative time structure of syllables contribute to defining a cricket's temporal niche. Generally, these time spans are marked by intensity, not frequency, changes. Crickets are basically drummers with a talent for entrainment.

Bird Songs

Song birds (Oscines) occupy quite different temporal niches than crickets. Relative to crickets, birds produce songs at tone rates significantly slower than the rates of cricket songs. Also, they feature sounds that are more complex than crickets, although they, too, create complex sounds (tones) with multiple frequency components in which one frequency dominates a bird's voice. And differentially marked tones lead to syllables and phrases. However, birds typically go beyond the drumming portfolio of crickets to include melodic time markers, sometimes captivating ones. For instance, the melodies of starlings (*Sturnus vulgaris*) famously inspired composers no less than Mozart. Also, other well-loved passages in the melodies of Beethoven and Chopin are hardly distinguishable from the songs of certain species of sparrows or wrens.[7] Furthermore, notations of the songs of adult birds reveal surprising melodic structure in pitch and in pitch transpositions.[8,9,10] Few crickets can claim such success with their drumming.

Producing Bird Songs

As with crickets, the time structure of bird songs is critical to establishing effective communications between members of the same species. A thorough assessment of birdsong time structure is beyond the scope of this chapter as it requires understanding the mechanics of song production, specifically of motor gestures governed by neural centers in bird's brain. Box 15.1 provides a brief summary of the elegant research on this topic.

The most critical aspects of birdsongs, when considering universal entrainment, concern

---

BOX 15.1
SONG PRODUCTION IN BIRDS

Elegant theories and research offer explanations of song productions in birds. Two premotor forebrain centers in the bird are the high vocal center (HVC), putatively responsible for syllable (and serial order) arrangements, and the nucleus archistriatalis, (RA), responsible for the timing of syllables. The HVC presumably sends signals to superfast muscles in a bird's syrinx (i.e., its voice box). The syrinx is divided by two medial membranes at the junction of two bronchi. These membranes (labial folds) are assumed to control airflow from the lungs. A working hypothesis holds that HVC neurons stimulate the RA to produce clock-timed neural pulses about every 50 ms during a bird's phrase production. Neural control projects to syrinx muscles, initiating oscillations that figure in sound productions (see Gardner et al. 2001; Suthers and Margoliash, 2002; Goller and Suthers 1996; Nowicki and Marler 1988 for a historical review[20-23]).

Also relevant are dynamic models that pinpoint neural and motor activities as the basis for driving rhythm productions in birdsongs. These models distinguish a labial fold resting state in which no vocalizations are produced from various oscillating states in which vocalizations emerge (i.e., a Hopf bifurcation). State changes are motivated by the actions of superfast syringeal muscles controlled (presumably) by the RA. As labial folds begin to oscillate, syringeal muscles control respiration, thus regulating air pressure. Produced sounds in birds usually accompany expiration of a breath, as birds take mini-breaths between syllables. Expiration of mini-breath air pressure from lungs builds; hence as it is forced through the labia, birds have less voluntary control over its course. Instead, its course is determined by a dynamic model's parameters (for air pressure, muscle tension) that initiate a motor gesture. Higher air pressure "drives" labial folds to greater oscillations, thus producing louder sounds. At the level of a sound pattern, song bird models hypothesize that these factors figure into the intensity and frequency of driving rhythms in breath-timed syllables.

the time structure created by produced driving rhythms. A core question is this: Are driving rhythms in a one bird's song capable of inciting entrainment (i.e., adaptive coupling) with neural oscillations of different, listening bird? It is clear that birdsongs contain elements such as tones and syllables, similar to ones in cricket sounds. And, as with cricket songs, bird songs exhibit nested time scales in which brief tones are embedded in syllables; in turn, syllables nest within longer phrases.[11] But, unlike crickets, bird vocalizations lead to productions of vocalized sequences that modulate both component frequencies and intensity over time. This adds a melodic component absent in cricket sounds. Given the basic entrainment protocols discussed in earlier chapters, we might speculate that birds are skilled in using *both* traditional and transient mode-locking protocols to communicate within their temporal niches, whereas crickets are confined to traditional mode-locking protocols.

There is also variability in the time structure across bird species. This is reminiscent of the variety of timing structures in linguistic categories or dialects in human languages. In birdsongs, timing variability is diagnostic of species-specific anatomical differences as well as geographical and communal influences.[12,13] The present discussion presents only a small slice of the vast knowledge accumulating on birdsongs. It focuses on the most studied songs of birds, including sparrows (e.g., song [*Melospiza melodia*], swamp [*M. georgiana*], and field [*Spizella pusilla*]), finches (e.g., zebra [*Taeniopygia guttata*], Bengalese [*Lonchura striata*]), canaries (*Serinus* sp.), starlings (European), and a few more exotic duetting birds (e.g., the Hornero [*Furnarius* sp.]).

Marler's classic work on sparrow songs first pinpointed species differences.[14,15] Swamp and song sparrows produce songs with a similar range of individual tone frequencies but with different time structures. Generally, song sparrow songs are slower (due to long frequency sweeps) than swamp sparrow songs, leading to a slower tone rate (~14 tones per second vs. 22 tones per second). Furthermore, the time structure of a song sparrow's song is more complex, with four different time layers (vs. two in the song of a swamp sparrow). Presumably, each layer of singer's production functions as a driving rhythm of particular rate that engages a driven rhythm in the tunable brain of a conspecific listening bird.

In sum, different bird species produce songs that differ not only in melodic structure (micro-timing profiles), but also in the rhythm of macro-timing properties involving tone rate and syllable rates and their timing relations. Members of a species are united in commonalities among these properties. And, finally, because micro-timing of melodies and macro-timing of rhythms can both be reduced to sound patterns based on relative timing, we may speculate that internal factors governing the production of micro-rhythms of melody and the macro-rhythms of rhythmic patterns in song birds include distinctive sets of species-specific attractors.

Perceiving Bird Songs

It is reasonable to assume that birds who produce certain sound patterns are capable of perceiving similar patterns created by their conspecifics. This parallelism holds for all creatures within a given communicative culture. A bird's voice is reflected in the spectral structure of the tones within his song; avian vocalizations have dominant frequencies of micro-driving rhythms centered in the narrow range of 2–3 KHz, with lower and upper perceptual limits around 1 kHz and 6 kHz frequencies, respectively. Note that birds' best frequencies are lower than those of crickets, but they are generally higher than prominent vocal frequencies in human speech (200 Hz to 2 kHz).

Marler's landmark research on sensitive developmental periods in song learning suggests that birds begin to tune in to fast-driving song rhythms early in life.[16] Thus, it is not surprising to find that adult birds are more sensitive to small time differences between sounds than are humans. For instance, zebra finches (budgerigars) who create complex songs have the ability to detect time changes as small as 1.225 ms, which are imperceptible to humans.[17,18]

If adult birds perceive the rate and the relative timing of syllables as well as the melodic arrangements of tones of conspecific songs, then we can infer that their internal neural mechanisms of attending parallel those of song production, as some research suggests[19] (e.g., for neural cells of the high vocal center [HVC] and/or nucleus archistriatalis [RA]; Box 15.1). This research contributes to the larger picture indicating parallelism between birds' perception/attending and song production[20,21,22]; also see Nowicki and Marler 1988.[23]

Duets

This brings us to duetting birds. As with some cricket species, birds, too, have champion duet singers. These are found particularly in tropical climates. Duets involve the synchronized motor acts of different individuals (i.e., both individuals interchange roles of perceiver and actor). This behavior provides dramatic evidence that both members of a dyad are keenly tracking the other's song in real time.

The artful synchrony of vocalizations in adult bird duets has been the object of both admiration and scientific inquiry. Indeed, the precision timing of duets originally led Thorpe[24] to distinguish expectancy-based response times based on a bird's sensitivity to an unfolding context from their reaction times, which reflect fast, context-independent actions. The telling feature of duets is that a bird's response times are temporally targeted in advance, apparently guided by expectancies, to synchronize with the overall rate and rhythm of an unfolding, jointly created, song in which birds' track the onset times of their cohorts. Amazingly, this resembles speech accommodation in humans.

Several reviews highlight the remarkable temporal synchrony of duets. Consistent with the temporal niche concept, they note its possible survival value (e.g., mate protection, territory etc.).[25,26,27] Manifest motor synchrony is found in either simultaneous sounds (of tones, syllables) delivered overtly by both feathered participants or in their antiphonal synchrony of precision-timed turn-taking (i.e., interleavings of vocalized sounds).

Perhaps the most dramatic example of turn-taking appears in songs of the South American duetting bird, the honero, studied by Mindlin and colleagues.[28,29] In this species, an antiphonal duet is created with the male bird producing lower frequency notes while the female creates a different melody of interleaved higher tones. The male opens a duet with a periodic sequence that speeds up over the course of his song (e.g., from periods of 166 ms to ones of 56 ms). The female jumps into this song after a few initial periods, with initial bids that outline a slower periodicity, half the rate of the male (i.e., her initial period is 332 ms, a 1:2 ratio). Interestingly, as the male speeds up, the female accommodates by shortening her period and also shifting the momentary time ratio between male and female productions. Thus, with a faster male period of 100 ms, the female shifts to a period of around 300 ms (now creating a 1:3 attractor ratio). In fact, as the male's tempo increases, the female's shifts to shorter periods to traverse a series of $n{:}m$ ratios of 1:2 . . . 1:2 . . . 1:3 . . . 1:3 . . . 1:4. This sequence of $n{:}m$ ratios is theoretically significant. It realizes an observable *attractor profile*. In fact, the authors claim that it resembles what is known as the *devil's staircase*, a special pattern of time ratios, varying in attractor complexity, that is

diagnostic of a dynamical system. In fact, Mindlin and colleagues outlined a dynamical model to explain these phenomena (Box 15.1).

Snowball. Although the duets discussed thus far involve conspecifics, this does not eliminate the possibility that one species can perceive the songs of another species—this is obvious to human bird watchers, many of whom both perceive and produce bird-like songs. But it becomes more interesting from the bird's perspective. To what degree can birds follow human sound productions? This is addressed in the behavior of the now-famous sulphur-crested cockatoo (*Cacatua galerita*) of YouTube fame, *Snowball*, who delightfully synchronized his motor behavior (and some vocalizations) to sound patterns of *Everybody* by the Backstreet Boys. Patel and his colleagues cleverly documented Snowball's affinity for this music.[30] They discovered that, as Snowball listened to this tune, synchronous head nodding appeared in bouts, with regular nodding evident at points consistent with a musical beat. In Western music, strong beats typically involve time periods that range from 430 ms (very fast) to 1,200 ms (very slow). Accordingly, Patel and his colleagues presented Snowball with different rates, ranging from fast (460 ms) to slow (644 ms) (550 ms was the original recorded period). Just as honeros' tracked rate changes, Snowball adjusted his motor responses to beat periods to accommodate tempo shifts (mainly for a synchronous mode of $n{:}m = 1{:}1$). Significantly, Snowball showed better synchronization as the tempo accelerated, suggesting that although functional rates overlap for cockatoos and humans, cockatoos prefer faster rates than humans. This suggests that species-specific rates may be one constraint on cross-species communications.

Current discussions of bird song productions describe cross-species synchronies in terms of the operations of a unique auditory-motor neural circuit common to a range of species, which presumably support entrainment activities.[31,32,33,34] Thus, to some extent, humans and birds share a common neural circuit underlying vocalizations. From an entrainment perspective, it is important to probe commonalities in rate, relative timing, and governing attractors across species.

Songs of Whales and Elephants

Finally, larger animals operate in correspondingly slower temporal niches. Body size does not solely determine the preferred or dominant time periods of a species, but these properties are correlated with the size of body structures that produce sounds. Relative to crickets, birds, and humans, elephants and whales rely on communications involving longer time spans at both micro-time levels (in tone frequencies) and macro-time levels (slower tone and syllable rates).

Elephants and whales share interesting characteristics. Both are social animals. Unlike birds, who tend to form family groups centered on a male–female dyad, elephants and whales form expanded family units, typically comprising many females and their immature offsprings; solitary adult males visit occasionally to mate. In these social communities, elephants and whales rely on low-frequency messages with several infrasonic frequency components.

Elephants

Both Asian elephants (*Elephas maximus*) and African elephants (*Loxodonta* sp.) rely on call vocabularies involving different vocalizations (e.g., trumpets, roars, barks, rumbles).[35,36,37] Although some elephant calls contain high-frequency components of 6 kHz (roars), it is the low-frequency rumbles (<250 Hz) that figure in communicative exchange. Again, certain component frequencies carry distinctive vocal information in formants and fundamental frequencies that individualize an elephant's "speaking" voice.[38] It is fair to speculate that elephants rely heavily on variations in rate and the relative rate of these sounds as driving rhythms in communications.

Finally, within female families, there is evidence for elephant conversations suggesting suggest synchronized exchanges. For example, well-timed antiphonal vocalizations of rumbles have been reported among affiliated females (i.e., "long-time friends"). Abstractly, there is a resemblance between such dyads and the duetting interactions of some bird species.

Whales

The largest mammals on the planet are whales. The two broad whale categories, toothed whales (Odontoceti) and Baleen whales (Mysticeti), differ in the time structures of their communicative vocalizations.

Toothed whales specialize in relatively high-frequency sounds as clicks/pulses (above 2 kHz), especially for echolocations. Overall, the relative timing of the whistles and clicks of these whales is fairly simple (an exception is the beluga whale's [*Delphinapterus leucas*] song). Sperm whales (*Physeter macrocephalus*), who are social creatures, exhibit click patterns suggesting slow rhythmic patterns, with several nested time scales.[39] In fact, fascinating findings revealed a group coherence in sperm whales where the click patterns of three different singers together formed a joint rhythm, with each whale contributing a different but synchronized click rate. Relative to the period of the dominant whale, the two nondominant singers produced cycle periods approximating time ratios of 2:1 and 3:2 that created a long-short-short rhythm. Not unlike the duetting honero birds, these whales learned to "keep time" in a manner resembling African polyrhythms!

On the other hand, baleen whales communicate primarily with low-frequency vocalizations (<100 Hz) that travel great distances in water. The largest whale, not surprisingly, produces the lowest of sound frequencies (12–200 Hz, due to a long vocal tract). Nevertheless, these whale songs share with very slow cricket songs relatively simple time patterns.

Finally, the famed songs of the humpback whale (*Megaptera novaeangliae*) are the most structured and intriguing of whale songs. Songs of these whales can last for hours, revealing themes based on multiple embedded time scales within a comfort zone of relatively slow rates.[40] Their themes, which embed marked phrases of around 15 seconds, come and go; phrases embed syllables, which in turn carry individual tones (of frequencies of 100 Hz–4 kHz). Recent analysis, provided by Stephan Handel and colleagues, confirms the song's time hierarchies and rhythmic patterns.[41] In short, the humpback whale song is distinguished by complex changes in melody and rhythm (time patterns).

Summary of Nonhuman Communications

Across a range of species, we find proof of the existence of synchronous modes of song production suggesting that driving–driven dyads abide in communicative exchanges of conspecifics. Vocalizations of crickets, birds, and whales contain complex sounds (tones) that carry micro-driving rhythms; these pulses or clicks (etc.) mark out slower (macro-) driving rhythms, revealing syllables and even phrases that, together, define species-specific habitats. This leads to speculations that, together, multiple rhythms of different rates function as species-specific driving rhythms in entrainment activities across species. Species occupy different temporal niches with respect to rates of driving rhythms, but also they differ in how various driving rhythms relate to one another as natural vehicles of communication. In these spotlight examples, clear evidence emerges for the universality of entrainment. I speculate that the prevalence of synchrony implies that related attractors distinguish species communications.

NATURAL AND ARTIFACTUAL ENVIRONMENTS OF NONHUMAN COMMUNICATIONS

Earlier chapters have concentrated on human communicative exchanges in natural environments in which driving rhythms, created by a human speaker, activate the resonant driven rhythms of a listener's tunable brain, which then entrains to these driving rhythms. In the larger panorama of species communications just provided, human "songs" falls somewhere between those of crickets and whales. For humans, the aging hypothesis has been enlisted to spell out age-related shifts in listeners' sensitivities to rates of external driving rhythms, leading to resonance predictions of age-related slowing; a corollary of this hypothesis holds that, over a life span, natural human communications depend on species-specific innate attractors that govern entrainment. Together with the general attending hypothesis, Dynamic Attending Theory (DAT) embraces the universality of resonance and entrainment that operate broadly, in different ways, in the lives of animate creatures. For instance, concepts outlined for humans, such as exogenous tracking of external events (e.g., as in pitch tracking) are not confined to humans. Nor are various forms of endogenous entrainments specific to the human species. This universality opens the door to speculations about the role of oscillator clusters and attractor profiles in species other than human listeners.

All of this assumes that the presence of certain communicative driving rhythms produced by conspecifics carves out a human habitat. Humans have evolved to thrive in natural environments created by other human communications. The critical driving rhythms are signals of natural, not artifactual, events. However, our environment is also peppered with events that deviate from the natural course of things, things that are too fast or too slow, or simply too erratic or artifactual. Yet, as intrinsically adaptable human beings, we are wired to attempt to react even to artifactual events and situations. In this final section, I speculate on two situations in which artifice may have unwelcome consequences for our species. The aim is to spark rethinking about environmental timing and its impact on humans and other organisms.

The Artifice of Methodology

Let's first consider the constrained environment of psychology laboratories. Throughout this book, I have tried to assess the impact of timing

constraints on listeners' abilities to perform assigned tasks in laboratory settings, particularly tasks where people must judge, perceive, or learn some sequential event. I have used data from these laboratory studies because the underlying science is committed to careful control of independent variables aimed at gaining decisive observable outcomes in dependent variables.

But, from another perspective, this is a tricky business for reasons not discussed in preceding chapters. Careful psychological experimenters are rightly trained to avoid confounding variables, and the best ways to accomplish this involves either randomizing a variable or holding it constant, ideally applying to all stimulus properties except the experimental variable of interest. A troubling aspect of the practice of holding constant a "nuisance" variable (to which we all adhere) is that, in real time, its constancy contributes to an experimental context.

The simplest example of this control is found in laboratory environments that traditionally constrain the timing of trials within an experimental session. These constraints can have unrecognized positive or negative influences on a participant's performance. For example, often we hold constant inter-trial time intervals in an experimental session in order to study a listener's perception of isolated stimuli (speech syllables, upright vs. inverted faces, etc.) presented in and/or over multiple trials. The isochronous rhythm of trials in a session is bound to have an effect on listener's attending—and hence performance—if we assume that such timing facilitates anticipations of successive stimuli. Although rarely acknowledged in reported results or anticipated in the theoretical hypotheses under examination, such subtle effects of rhythmic trial schedules are ever-present. Under scrutiny, the artifacts of laboratory time structures introduce a hidden, unrecognized contribution to the way people perform the tasks that we have so conscientiously designed. Yet it is telling that rarely do experimenters present trials in a session randomly in time. Perhaps this is because we intuitively "know" this can complicate the results. In this, we are tacitly granting the underlying importance of timing and synchrony in attending. In short, in "experimenter-speak," time is the ultimate confounding variable in experimental environments.

The Artifice of Machines in Our Everyday Environment

Next, step out of the laboratory to encounter another environmental setting: the big wide world. Today, there is rightly great concern about the environment, with fears largely centered on climate changes due to man-made activities. In some places, things are getting hotter! What has received much less focus, however, are other man-made environmental changes introduced in the nineteenth century. One very notable change has to do with the natural rate and rhythm of "things" in our natural environment. Things are also getting faster. "Things" here refer to all kinds of sound-making devices (and their time markers) to which people are exposed in their everyday environment.

This idea was introduced in past century by the music theorist R. Murray Schafer.[42] Schafer argued that with a shift from an agrarian society to an industrial society, the sound environment where people lived and worked shifted from natural noises of the wind and fields with various inhabiting creatures to the mechanical noises of machines in shuttered factories. In particular, he claimed that the soundscapes of people's everyday environments began to introduce intruding and harsh noises; these were sounds that offered things, i.e., time markers, of unusually high intensities which occurred with greater temporal density, repetitiveness, and/or droning continuity (i.e., flatline sounds). Schafer took us into the artifactual driving rhythms of the Industrial Age. Box 15.2 is Schafer's list of invading machines.

The Information Age
Schafer's insights ring true. So much so, that it is not difficult to extend his analysis to include another soundscape shift when, in the twentieth century, society entered the Information Age.

With this change, the environments in which people live and work are shifting from heavy machine noises to the softer noises (and images) of fast computers and iPhones. These soundscapes are characterized not so much by time markers of high-intensity machine sounds and as they are by soft, high-frequency sounds that occur densely in time (fast rates), often with deceptive temporal irregularities (arrhythmic) that persist over long time periods. Importantly, in this Information Age, where people sleep next to their mobile devices, humans now are inadvertently enmeshed in a fast-paced, dynamic environment on a 24-hour cycle. Mobile devices introduce a sustained, but rapidly changing, dynamic environment. I suggest this creates *sporadic human habitats*.

One can speculate about the introduction of sporadic habitats in contemporary society. For instance, it seems obvious that, over time, the inputs/outputs supplied by a mobile phone or a video game will not only entrain but, via binding, create an attending habit based on relatively fast rates of time markers. People's attending habits then become subtly and sporadically speeded up. Furthermore, with strong bindings, the tendency to anticipate a future 'message' will generalize to other times and situations. "Sporadic", then, implies the presence of artifactual time markers occurring at the irregular times of machine-driven messages. Arbitrarily timed messages typically disrupt ongoing natural contexts, such as ordinary conversations with a friend. Simply put, such inputs/outputs create not only fast, but also irregularly timed driving

---

BOX 15.2
THE INDUSTRIAL AGE

Dates	Machine
1711	Sewing machine
1714	Typewriter
1761	Air cylinders
1767	Cast iron rails
1781	Steam engine
1788	Thresher machine
1791	Gas engine
1796	Hydraulic press
To the present . . .	

(From Shafer)

rhythms. This presumes that the higher rates of stimulation imposed on a listener who relies on a mobile phone is due to greater transmission speeds and wider call access (e.g., Twitter, etc.). In general, sporadic habitats should lead to a listener's tunable brain being generally predisposed to orient to relatively fast events.

At least as problematic as the average rate established in sporadic habitats is the perturbing rhythmic effect of incoming signals. Rarely are the successive time markers (rings) of portable machines anticipated. This means that a listener's neural attending activity is under continual assault, captured recurrently by unexpected incoming signals of tweets, text messages, and the like. Reactive attending dominates, laying down uninvited and/or arbitrary time markers. The worst-case scenario is one in which dyadic bindings are strengthened (reinforced during entrainment) among sporadic, but automatically elicited, sets of fast neural rhythms that together manifest in the receiving listener unrelenting habitual orientations (i.e., anticipations) for fast-paced events. Diagnostic of this, for example, are illusions of iPhone vibrations that are not present (following DAT, these are simply silent expectancy pulses discussed in earlier chapters). Younger listeners whose temporal niche naturally orients them to faster events are at most risk for this type of co-opting of ordinary attending habits. When the speedy learning of youth (following binding principles) is taken into account, this scenario leads to young attenders acquiring unusually strong habits to tune in to fast events (an addiction). Conversely, as younger attenders become increasingly tethered to this sporatic or robotic world, older attenders are more likely to increasingly tune out. Neither is a promising outcome. More generally, it is worth thinking about the implications of unwanted entrainments associated with sporadic habitats. Despite all the real advantages the Information Age has bequeathed us, as a society, we have been promiscuous about introducing into our environment some machines that have unexamined impacts on our cognitive functions.

CHAPTER SUMMARY

The environment we inhabit and share with other species is a dynamically changing one. Humans, of course, contribute to these changes. As humans become more efficient in creating machines and vehicles that speed up our environment. And, this brings unheeded costs not only for the human species, but also for other creatures that share this accelerated environment. For instance, assume that a given species is distinguished by special sets of attractors and by a specific set of driving rhythm rates, as in a temporal niche. Events that "fit" into this niche allow this species to flourish, whereas filling this environment with artifactual rhythmic events that do not "fit" (i.e., they are too fast or slow) will be detrimental to that species. People are adaptable, to be sure. But humans and other animals have biological limits on their flexibility to adapt to changes in driving rhythms. Let's aim for a world that encourages successful synchrony among all its inhabitants.

NOTES

1. Roderick A. Suthers et al., *Vertebrate Sound Production and Acoustic Communication* (Springer, 2016), http://link.springer.com.proxy.library.ucsb.edu:2048/content/pdf/10.1007/978-3-319-27721-9.pdf.

2. W. Tecumseh Fitch, Jürgen Neubauer, and Hanspeter Herzel, "Calls out of Chaos: The Adaptive Significance of Nonlinear Phenomena in Mammalian Vocal Production," *Animal Behaviour* 63, no. 3 (March 2002): 407–18, doi:10.1006/anbe.2001.1912.

3. Megan A. Murphy, Nathan L. Thompson, and Johannes Schul, "Keeping up with the Neighbor: A Novel Mechanism of Call Synchrony in Neoconocephalus Ensiger Katydids," *Journal of Comparative Physiology A* 202, no. 3 (March 2016): 225–34, doi:10.1007/s00359-016-1068-1.

4. Thomas J. Walker, "Acoustic Synchrony: Two Mechanisms in the Snowy Tree Cricket," *Science* 166, no. 3907 (1969): 891–4.

5. Michael D. Greenfield, "Synchronous and Alternating Choruses in Insects and Anurans: Common Mechanisms and Diverse Functions," *American Zoologist* 34, no. 6 (December 1994): 605–15, doi:10.1093/icb/34.6.605.

6. H. Carl Gerhardt and Franz Huber, *Acoustic Communication in Insects and Anurans: Common Problems and Diverse Solutions* (University of Chicago Press, 2002), https://books-google-com.proxy.library.ucsb.edu:9443/books?hl=en&lr=&id=0ySUuQTNMpkC&oi=fnd&pg=PR9&dq=+%22Acoustic+Communication+in+Insects+and+Anurans%22&ots=uVvUt3hxlk&sig=Lnb_wwhOGnm8svA0raiD-jd9G24.

7. Luis Felipe Baptista and Robin A. Keister, "Why Birdsong Is Sometimes Like Music," *Perspectives in Biology and Medicine* 48, no. 3 (2005): 426–43, doi:10.1353/pbm.2005.0066.

8. Edward Allworthy Armstrong, *A Study of Bird Song*, vol. 335 (Oxford University Press London, 1963), http://library.wur.nl/WebQuery/clc/257601.

9. Charles Hartshorne, *Born to Sing: An Interpretation and World Survey of Bird Song* (Bloomington: Indiana University Press, 1992).

10. P. M. Gray, "BIOLOGY AND MUSIC: Enhanced: The Music of Nature and the Nature of Music," *Science* 291, no. 5501 (January 5, 2001): 52–4, doi:10.1126/science.10.1126/SCIENCE.1056960.

11. Todd W. Troyer, "Neuroscience: The Units of a Song," *Nature* 495, no. 7439 (February 27, 2013): 56–7, doi:10.1038/nature11957.

12. Peter R. Marler and Hans Slabbekoorn, *Nature's Music: The Science of Birdsong* (Academic Press, 2004), https://books-google-com.proxy.library.ucsb.edu:9443/books?hl=en&lr=&id=2iFmsVSyV4gC&oi=fnd&pg=PP1&dq=++++++++Marler,+2004+Birdsong+&ots=5r7Tg17Hpg&sig=2NPxRo2NYHQVdcWooCOvn5dmK2Y.

13. D. E. Kroodsma, "The Diversity and Plasticity of Birdsong," *Nature's Music: The Science of Bird Song*, 2004, 108e130.

14. Susan S. Peters, William A. Searcy, and Peter Marler, "Species Song Discrimination in Choice Experiments with Territorial Male Swamp and Song Sparrows," *Animal Behaviour* 28, no. 2 (May 1980): 393–404, doi:10.1016/S0003-3472(80)80048-0.

15. Peter Marler and Roberta Pickert, "Species-Universal Microstructure in the Learned Song of the Swamp Sparrow (Melospiza Georgiana)," *Animal Behaviour* 32, no. 3 (August 1984): 673–89, doi:10.1016/S0003-3472(84)80143-8.

16. Peter Marler, "Sensitive Periods and the Roles of Specific and General Sensory Stimulation in Birdsong Learning," *Imprinting and Cortical Plasticity*, 1987, 99–135.

17. Bernard Lohr, Robert J. Dooling, and Suzanne Bartone, "The Discrimination of Temporal Fine Structure in Call-like Harmonic Sounds by Birds.," *Journal of Comparative Psychology* 120, no. 3 (2006): 239–51, doi:10.1037/0735-7036.120.3.239.

18. Robert Dooling, "Auditory Temporal Resolving Power in Birds," *The Journal of the Acoustical Society of America* 138, no. 3 (September 2015): 1879, doi:10.1121/1.4933894.

19. Michele M. Solis and David J. Perkel, "Rhythmic Activity in a Forebrain Vocal Control Nucleus in Vitro," *The Journal of Neuroscience* 25, no. 11 (2005): 2811–22.

20. Tim Gardner, "Simple Motor Gestures for Birdsongs," *Physical Review Letters* 87, no. 20 (2001), doi:10.1103/PhysRevLett.87.208101.

21. Roderick A Suthers and Daniel Margoliash, "Motor Control of Birdsong," *Current Opinion in Neurobiology* 12, no. 6 (December 2002): 684–90, doi:10.1016/S0959-4388(02)00386-0.

22. R. Suthers, F. Goller, and C. Pytte, "The Neuromuscular Control of Birdsong," *Philosophical Transactions of the Royal Society B: Biological Sciences* 354, no. 1385 (May 29, 1999): 927–39, doi:10.1098/rstb.1999.0444.

23. Stephen Nowicki and Peter Marler, "How Do Birds Sing?," *Music Perception: An Interdisciplinary Journal* 5, no. 4 (July 1988): 391–426, doi:10.2307/40285408.

24. W. H. Thorpe, "Antiphonal Singing in Birds as Evidence for Avian Auditory Reaction Time," *Nature* 197 (1963): 774–6.

25. Susan M. Farabaugh, "The Ecological and Social Significance of Duetting," *Acoustic Communication in Birds* 2 (1982): 85–124.

26. Michelle L. Hall, "A Review of Hypotheses for the Functions of Avian Duetting," *Behavioral Ecology and Sociobiology* 55, no. 5 (March 1, 2004): 415–30, doi:10.1007/s00265-003-0741-x.

27. Cornelia Voigt, Manfred Gahr, and Stefan Leitner, "Repertoire and Structure of Duet and Solo Songs in Cooperatively Breeding White-Browed Sparrow Weavers," *Behaviour* 143, no. 2 (February 1, 2006): 159–82, doi:10.1163/156853906775900739.

28. Rodrigo Laje and Gabriel B. Mindlin, "Highly Structured Duets in the Song of the South American Hornero," *Physical Review Letters* 91, no. 25 (December 19, 2003): 258104, doi:10.1103/PhysRevLett.91.258104.

29. Ana Amador, M. A. Trevisan, and G. B. Mindlin, "Simple Neural Substrate Predicts Complex Rhythmic Structure in Duetting Birds," *Physical Review E* 72, no. 3 (September 13, 2005), doi:10.1103/PhysRevE.72.031905.

30. Aniruddh D. Patel et al., "Studying Synchronization to a Musical Beat in Nonhuman Animals," *Annals of the New York Academy of Sciences* 1169, no. 1 (July 1, 2009): 459–69, doi:10.1111/j.1749-6632.2009.04581.x.

31. W. Tecumseh Fitch, "Biology of Music: Another One Bites the Dust," *Current Biology* 19, no. 10 (May 26, 2009): R403–4, doi:10.1016/j.cub.2009.04.004.

32. Adena Schachner, "Auditory-Motor Entrainment in Vocal Mimicking Species: Additional Ontogenetic and Phylogenetic Factors," *Communicative & Integrative Biology* 3, no. 3 (May 2010): 290–93, doi:10.4161/cib.3.3.11708.

33. Adena Schachner et al., "Spontaneous Motor Entrainment to Music in Multiple Vocal Mimicking Species," *Current Biology* 19, no. 10 (May 26, 2009): 831–36, doi:10.1016/j.cub.2009.03.061.

34. Aniruddh D. Patel et al., "Experimental Evidence for Synchronization to a Musical Beat in a Nonhuman Animal," *Current Biology* 19, no. 10 (May 2009): 827–30, doi:10.1016/j.cub.2009.03.038.

35. Smita Nair et al., "Vocalizations of Wild Asian Elephants (Elephas Maximus): Structural Classification and Social Context," *The Journal of the Acoustical Society of America* 126, no. 5 (2009): 2768, doi:10.1121/1.3224717.

36. Joseph Soltis, Kirsten Leong, and Anne Savage, "African Elephant Vocal Communication II: Rumble Variation Reflects the Individual Identity and Emotional State of Callers," *Animal Behaviour* 70, no. 3 (September 2005): 589–99, doi:10.1016/j.anbehav.2004.11.016.

37. Ibid.

38. Joseph Soltis, Kirsten Leong, and Anne Savage, "African Elephant Vocal Communication II: Rumble Variation Reflects the Individual Identity and Emotional State of Callers," *Animal Behaviour* 70, no. 3 (September 2005): 589–99, doi:10.1016/j.anbehav.2004.11.016.

39. Peter L. Tyack and Christopher W. Clark, "Communication and Acoustic Behavior of Dolphins and Whales," in *Hearing by Whales and Dolphins*, ed. Whitlow W. L. Au, Richard R. Fay, and Arthur N. Popper, vol. 12 (New York, NY: Springer New York, 2000), 156–224, http://link.springer.com/10.1007/978-1-4612-1150-1_4.

40. R. S. Payne and S. McVay, "Songs of Humpback Whales," *Science* 173, no. 3997 (August 13, 1971): 585–97, doi:10.1126/science.173.3997.585.

41. Stephen Handel, Sean K. Todd, and Ann M. Zoidis, "Hierarchical and Rhythmic Organization in the Songs of Humpback Whales (*Megaptera Novaeangliae*)," *Bioacoustics* 21, no. 2 (June 2012): 141–56, doi:10.1080/09524622.2012.668324.

42. R. Murray Schafer, *The Tuning of the World* (Alfred A. Knopf, 1977).

INDEX